The Principles and Practice of Yoga in Cardiovascular Medicine

Indranill Basu-Ray
Editor-in-Chief

Darshan Mehta
Editor

The Principles and Practice of Yoga in Cardiovascular Medicine

Springer

Editor-in-chief
Indranill Basu-Ray
Cardiologist & Cardiac Electrophysiologist, Director of Cardiovascular Research
Memphis VA Medical Center
Memphis, TN, USA

Adjunct Professor of Public Health: The University of Memphis
Memphis, TN, USA

Adjunct Professor of Cardiology & Head of Integrative Cardiology
All India Institute of Medical Sciences
Rishikesh, UK, India

Editor
Darshan Mehta
Medical Director, Benson-Henry Institute for Mind Body Medicine & Director, Office for Well-Being, Center for Faculty Development
Massachusetts General Hospital
Boston, MA, USA

Education Director, Osher Center for Integrative Medicine
Harvard Medical School and Brigham and Women's Hospital
Boston, MA, USA

Assistant Professor of Medicine
Harvard Medical School
Boston, MA, USA

ISBN 978-981-16-6912-5 ISBN 978-981-16-6913-2 (eBook)
https://doi.org/10.1007/978-981-16-6913-2

This Springer imprint is published by the registered company Springer Nature Singapore Pte Ltd.
The registered company address is: 152 Beach Road, #21-01/04 Gateway East, Singapore 189721, Singapore

To my wife, Julie who made it all possible.
—Dr. Indranill Basu-Ray

This book is dedicated to my daughter, Asha, whose love and laughter continues to light my life with hope and joy.
—Dr. Darshan Mehta

Notice

Medicine is an ever-changing science. As new research and clinical experience broaden our knowledge, changes in treatment and drug therapy are required. The authors and the publisher of this work have checked with sources believed to be reliable in their efforts to provide information that is complete and generally in accord with the standards accepted at the time of publication. However, in view of the possibility of human error or changes in medical sciences, neither the authors nor the publisher nor any other party who has been involved in the preparation or publication of this work warrants that the information contained herein is in every respect accurate or complete, and they disclaim all responsibility for any errors or omissions or for the results obtained from use of the information contained in this work. Readers are encouraged to confirm the information contained herein with other sources. For example and in particular, readers are advised to check the product information sheet included in the package of each medication they plan to administer to be certain that the information contained in this work is accurate and that changes have not been made in the recommended dose or in the contraindications for administration. This recommendation is of particular importance in connection with new or infrequently used medications. Yoga procedures suggested are to be attempted only after medical advice and after ensuring that a trained and certified yoga teacher is present to teach and monitor the techniques. The editors, authors, and the publishers are not liable to any damage physical or mental on following one or any recommendations given in this work.

Foreword

Spending over six decades in learning, teaching, and mentoring studies in Indian philosophy, I was always intrigued by the almost magical powers that yoga is believed to confer. It has long been noted that yoga slows the aging process making it possible for a 90-year-old gentleman to look and function as if he were decades younger. It changes the brain to make it more powerful memory-wise. People with extended meditation practice are rarely known to be hypertensive. Such claims have been made from time to time down through the ages, often by people with little or no training in modern biology or medicine. Thus, it is impossible to know how many of these are real facts or just hyperbole by enamored practitioners of yoga worldwide.

Dr. Indranill Basu-Ray has spent most of his professional career as a cardiologist with research in yoga and heart disease. He is the author of the first guidelines on the role of Meditation in Cardiovascular disease written on behalf of the American Heart Association. One of the modern evils of civilization has been the epidemic spread of dangerous non-communicable diseases such as heart disease which is rampant as one out of every four people in this world is inflicted. Millions are suffering and maimed with it from all over the world, and it continues to kill twice the number of people than cancer which is the second largest killer of mankind. Modern research in the frontiers of medicine has revealed that the cause of heart disease can be traced to inflammation in our blood vessels due to the stress of day-to-day living. Blood vessels are the source of nutrition to the vital organs, including the heart, the brain, and the kidneys. Inflammation in these blood vessels and the resulting damages to these organs induces tremendous mortality and morbidity.

Dr. Basu Ray has been in the frontline of research into the role of yoga and heart disease. He had developed an interest in meditation since childhood. Formally trained in Kriya Yoga at a young age, along with following the strict yogic lifestyle, created an urge to understand the science behind such processes. Encouraged by his mentor Swami Hariharananda Giri, a self-realized yoga master, Dr. Basu-Ray decided to study cardiology. His guru's wish was to understand, unravel, and bring the biology behind yoga and meditation to the common man. Self-practice of meditation for hours deepened his understanding of the physical processes involved in yoga and meditation while studying the latest research in the field further helped cement an understanding of the process. He has passed on this knowledge to physicians, scientists, researchers, and yoga enthusiasts while trying to infuse a desire to understand

and practice yoga scientifically rather than being a blind believer. The book is part of that effort to present scientific research on yoga's role in the prevention and treatment of cardiovascular diseases.

This book talks about disease prevention and healing using yoga. Yoga has been a subject of extensive research in the last decade, which has proven its usefulness. Moreover, it is universal as both the poor and the rich can be benefitted. One does not need costly equipment or a loaded purse. Patience and determination to have daily practice are the only requirements. This book essentially outlines the updated research in every aspect of cardiovascular disease for the practitioner to use his art and science of healing. It also provides leads to researchers on lines that would need further investigation. Around seventy-five of the world's top physicians, scientists, and researchers have contributed to making this book the first complete encyclopedia of yoga for cardiovascular diseases, indeed a remarkable achievement.

Over the last few decades, scientific evidence of yoga and its effect has been found through genetic, epigenetic, molecular, and cellular studies. It is apparent how aberrant pathology created by stress results in heart disease and how yoga can reverse it to normal physiology restoring a harmonious balance. Despite its popularity the world over, yoga is entangled in the quagmire of unscientific deliberations, metaphysical debates, and unwanted wrangling by people with an inadequate scientific background. This situation is perpetuated by practitioners who claim knowledge about yoga by becoming "posture experts" but are wholly divorced from yoga's scientific rationale.

While yoga as a series of postures has become popular throughout the world, and indeed now we have a World Yoga Day, it is important to remember that though all these postures are useful, yoga is something deeper than only a physical exercise. It affects the body, the emotions, and the mind, all three of which need to be functioning harmoniously. This book helps us understand the science behind the use of yoga as a preventive and therapeutic modality and is a valuable addition to the growing volume of literature on various aspects of yoga. I commend Dr. Basu Ray for his pioneering work in bringing together so many expert views on this fascinating subject.

2nd January 2022

Dr. Karan Singh
Former Minister of Health and Family Planning,
Govertment of India
Former Chancellor, Jawaharlal Nehru University &
Benares Hindu University
New Delhi, India

Padma Vibhusan

Foreword

One of the present problems in today's society, which is also unfortunately reflected in scientific inquiry in medicine, is materialism. This philosophy automatically assumes that most events on this planet can be analyzed and expressed within the restricted lens of materialism. Materialism holds that there must be a physical explanation for every phenomenon. However, Indian sages from millennia taught that most phenomena have an extra materialistic basis that cannot always be explained by scientific determinism or mundane day-to-day materialistic thought. Though not patent with everyday science, this idea has enabled many scientific thinkers and philosophers to think "out of the box." They were able to conjure theories that were initially revolted as outlandish as they were totally against established concepts but accepted subsequently. A case in point is that many such "outrageous conclusions" such as "quantum entanglement" that have been accepted today in quantum physics, continues to defy established materialistic view.

Materialism left out the mind-body connection. Yoga which includes meditation is one such entity. The "mind" is not material. Yet yoga claims that mind and body are a single element with two entangled parts—the brain and the body. Moreover, there is a constant connect between them that ensures mind dictating every aspect of the body including its physiological constitution and genetic configuration. Ostensibly such a phantasmal claim made in a prehistoric treatise by Maharishi Patanjali was not precisely digestible for consumption to modern science and their torch bearers. Thus, relegated to just another physical exercise, yoga languished in this century and became restricted to yoga studios. Not particularly academically bright, but suave entrepreneurs made millions gaining from its popularity. Yoga, unfortunately, was thus hidden from the discerning eyes of scientists who would have subjected it to dissection using a standard scientific protocol to determine its true nature and effects on human physiology. Meanwhile, the already soaring popularity got skyrocketed when at the behest of India's prime minister, Mr. Narendra Modi, the United Nations accepted June 21 as the International Day of Yoga. The time-honored road to enlightenment devised by Hindu sages meanwhile soared to an $80 billion physical fitness business worldwide with over 50 million practitioners in the US alone and six times that number in the rest of the world.

This explosion in yoga's popularity as a fitness regime generated interest in the academic community to study yoga's effects on health and disease. In India, we have been doing clinical trials for over four decades on yoga's role in various diseases. The first scientific paper was published way back in

Circulation in the December of 1961. In 1986 in BMJ. The mentality to scientifically interrogate yoga started relatively late in the West but was a welcome change. Many researchers working at various universities started studying yoga's clinical effects in the last few decades. Numerous institutions like MD Anderson started implementing yoga protocols in their treatment strategies. Cardiovascular disease remains the largest killer on this planet. There is some evidence that multiple cardiac risk factors, including hypertension, diabetes mellitus, and hyperlipidemia, benefit from yoga, including meditation. Stress is now considered the predominant underlying cause for many non-communicable diseases responsible for 70% of mortality on earth. Accumulated evidence in the last decade point to the genetic and endocrinal changes that perpetuate inflammation in blood vessels leading to heart attack, stroke, or peripheral arterial disease. The origins of these have been deciphered to be induced by a pathophysiological reaction to stress. Though not any particular type of stress but all kinds, including the so-called mundane ones that we have to navigate in our daily existence. Yoga has been evidenced to reverse this aberrant pathophysiology. This book attempts to present the physiological changes including clinical evidence of yoga's role in cardiovascular diseases. It is written by over 75 eminent authors from multiple disciplines. This, to my knowledge, is one of the first attempts to provide a detailed but updated account of the clinical validity of using yoga, both as preventive and therapeutic modalities for cardiovascular diseases. Cardiologists, psychiatrists, neurologists, and integrative medicine experts have contributed, putting in their years of expertise in this book.

Dr. Indranill Basu-Ray, whose brainchild is this project, has been known to me for many years. Besides being an eminent cardiologist with research in yoga, Dr. Basu Ray is one of those few people with experiential knowledge of the system. He has been practicing yoga which includes deep meditation, since the age of six. Trained by various Himalayan masters, he has been a practitioner of Kriya Yoga. He was initiated into kriya yoga by Swami Hariharananda Giri, a disciple of Sri Yukteshwar Giri and the brother disciple of Paramhansa Yogananda of fame through his book "Autobiography of a Yogi." I mention this not for a historical reason, but this has scientific ramifications in studying and interpreting yoga's overall effect. It is imperative to understand that yoga is not a theoretical construct. Nor is it a practical protocol to develop physical fitness alone. Postural yoga inundated with an emphasis on physical prowess called Hatha yoga also is meant for one's evolution through mastery over the modifications of the mind. Sage Patanjali, in his yoga sutras, talks about how to use these physical practices also to achieve "enlightenment" referred to as merging of individual consciousness with the cosmic consciousness. It is a discipline couched in metaphysical constructs that is mostly inaccessible to anybody other than a practitioner guided by an experienced master. It is an experience-based science that highlights personal development through both mental and physical discipline. The meditation part of the construct, it may be remembered, is that it yields the major beneficial effects of rewiring the constructs in the psyche and the brain. Meditative practices induce changes that have the potential to reverse the stress-related inflammation that is known to be responsible for heart diseases. Surprisingly, this deeper understanding is lacking in today's popular way of practicing yoga postures. Although these physical postures performed like exercises are clearly beneficial for health, fitness, and a sense of well-being, the programs taught today under the name of physical yoga typically bear little resemblance to the tradition whose name they use. Thus, testing yoga protocols devoid of its valid construct though helpful, will never reveal the true extent of yoga's prowess to decrease aging, prevent heart diseases, or root out anxiety and depression. Since childhood, Dr. Basu Ray, being trained in the yogic system and philosophy, is best suited to understand real yoga's nuances outlined by Patanjali in his Yoga Sutra and many other authorities. In principle, this entails a silent and internalized journey that proceeds, independent of external input, through defined and progressive phases of relaxation, interiorization, and expansion. It begins with a withdrawal of the senses from their gross level of functioning termed pratyahara and proceeds through a stage of mindfulness called Dharana followed by deep meditation or dhyana, which results in successive levels of settled mental absorption termed samadhi.

I commend the editors and the authors for taking this arduous task of bringing to light the yoga's benefits, as evidenced by clinical studies. This endeavor, I am confident, will entice many clinicians and researchers to take-up yoga research. Moreover, it will entail millions who practice yoga to be assured that their health is protected by one of the best inventions in this universe ever discovered by mankind.

1st January 2022
Bengaluru, India

H. R Nagendra
Chancellor,
Swami Vivekananda Yoga
Anusandhana Samsthana (a Deemed University),
Prashanti Kutiram Vivekananda Road,
Kalluballu Post, Jigani, Anekal, Bengaluru

Padma Shri

Contents

About the Editors

Indranill Basu-Ray, MBBS,MD(Med),DNB(Card),FACP,FACC is a Cardiac Electrophysiologist and a Professor of Cardiology and Public Health, based in Memphis, TN, USA. He is the Founder Chairman of The American Academy of Yoga and Meditation. Dr. Basu-Ray went to medical school at the Nil Ratan Sircar Medical College in Kolkata, West Bengal, India. He has further trained in Cardiology and Interventional Cardiac Electrophysiology from Tulane University in New Orleans, LA, and Texas Heart Institute at the Baylor College of Medicine, Houston, TX. In addition, he trained in Cardiac Electrophysiology Research at the Massachusetts General Hospital, Harvard Medical School in Boston, MA. Dr. Basu Ray is an active researcher in cardiac electrophysiology and yoga and has numerous peer-reviewed research articles. In addition, he has contributed book chapters to multiple books in Cardiology and Medicine. He is the editor of *Clinical Cardiology*, a book for the medical curriculum for subspecialty training in cardiology with over forty authors contributing from worldwide. Dr. Basu-Ray has been a practicing yogi and started meditating at the age of six. He was initiated by Swami Hariharananda Giri, the brother disciple of Paramhansa Yogananda of the "Autobiography of a Yogi" fame. He has been practicing, teaching, and researching yoga and meditation for over three decades now. His research centers on the use of meditation and yoga in cardiovascular diseases. He wrote the American Heart Association's scientific statement on using meditation to treat cardiovascular diseases. He is the founder chairman of the American Academy for Yoga and Meditation (AAYM). AAYM is an organization of physicians, scientists, and researchers who work on scientific validation of Yoga and Meditation and hold regular international conferences worldwide where the latest research is presented. He was the program director of the "World's first conference on the role of Meditation in Cardiovascular Diseases" held at All India Institute of Medical Sciences, Rishikesh, UK, India. He also led the virtual conference—Yoga Conference USA 2021 held virtually with over a hundred speakers and fifty sessions. Dr. Basu-Ray played a pioneering role in developing multiple tools for atrial fibrillation and Ventricular Tachycardia ablation in humans today. He was involved in the initial proof of concept for cryotherapy and the laser balloon used for atrial fibrillation ablation. He contributed to the initial research of a new iteration of 3D mapping systems using multimodality imaging used for intracardiac mapping today. Dr. Basu-Ray performs complex ablations for Atrial Fibrillation and Ventricular Tachycardia. He also treats Heart failure with ICD's, Cardiac

Resynchronization Devices, and S-ICD's. He also implants Pacemaker and leadless Pacemakers for bradyarrhythmia therapy. Dr. Basu Ray lives with his wife Julie and son Ishan in Memphis, TN, USA.

Darshan Mehta, MD, MPH is a Medical Director and a Director of Medical Education for the Benson-Henry Institute for Mind Body Medicine at Massachusetts General Hospital (BHI-MGH) and a Director of Education at the Osher Center for Integrative Medicine, Harvard Medical School and Brigham and Women's Hospital (OCIM). In addition, he is the MGH site director for the Practice of Medicine curriculum required of all first-year Harvard Medical School students, and leads their well-being curriculum. Dr. Mehta received his BA in Biology from Illinois Wesleyan University and an MD from the University of Texas-Southwestern Medical School. He completed his residency in internal medicine at the University of Illinois-Chicago Hospital. In 2008, he completed a clinical research fellowship in complementary and integrative medicine at the Harvard Medical School Osher Research Center, during which he received a Master of Public Health degree from the Harvard School of Public Health. His educational and research interests include curricular development in complementary and integrative medical therapies, mind/body educational interventions in health professions training, and promotion of professionalism in medical trainees. He directs medical student and resident rotational electives at BHI-MGH and the Osher Center. Dr. Mehta sees patients at both locations in a consultative role for use of complementary and integrative medical therapies, as well as mind/body interventions for stress management and stress reduction. Dr. Mehta is active in the Massachusetts Medical Society and is a member of the American College of Physicians. Dr. Mehta is board-certified through the American Board of Integrative Medicine and has completed professional training in mindfulness-based stress reduction at the University of Massachusetts Medical School. He serves on the leadership for the Academic Consortium for Integrative Medicine and Health and is on the Editorial Board for the Journal of Alternative and Complementary Medicine.

Part I

Introduction

1 Cardiology: A Primer for the Uninitiated

Indranill Basu-Ray and Dibbendhu Khanra

1.1 Basic Anatomy

Human heart has four chambers—two atria and two ventricles. Atria work as a reservoir and ventricles have pumping capacities. Left atria (LA) is connected to pulmonary veins posteriorly and can produce pulmonary venous hypertension due to stretching when LA is dilated. LA appendage (LAA) is an important structure as it is the most common source of embolus in non-valvular atrial fibrillation causing stroke (Fig. 1.1) [1]. Complex anatomy of LAA is an independent predictor of stroke even in patients without AF (Fig. 1.2) [2]. Inferior vena cava is often guarded by Eustachian valve and is often too elongated to direct deoxygenated blood to patent foramen ovale (PFO) and to LA causing platypnea orthopnea syndrome. PFO is often associated with paradoxical embolism [3]. Crista terminalis is a structure inside the right atrium (RA), which is the commonest foci of atrial tachycardia [4]. Sinoatrial node (SA node) and atrioventricular node (AVN) both are right atrial structures and are mostly supplied by right coronary artery. Coronary sinus is an important venous structure, which is drained in RA. Important coronary sinus interventions include LV lead placement in cardiac resyncronization therapy (CRT). A device used in heart failure patients to improve cardiac function and indirect mitral annuloplasty for Mitral regurgitation [5]. Persistent left superior vena cava often drains into coronary sinus and unroofed coronary sinus can cause cyanosis. Fossa ovalis is a structure present on right side of interatrial septum and is an important site for transseptal puncture (TSP). Left ventricle (LV) is the smooth ventricle and non-compaction of left ventricle is genetic cardiomyopathy (Fig. 1.3). Chordo-papillary complexes are part of the left ventricular myocardium and are supplied by coronary arteries and ischemia can produce papillary muscle dys-

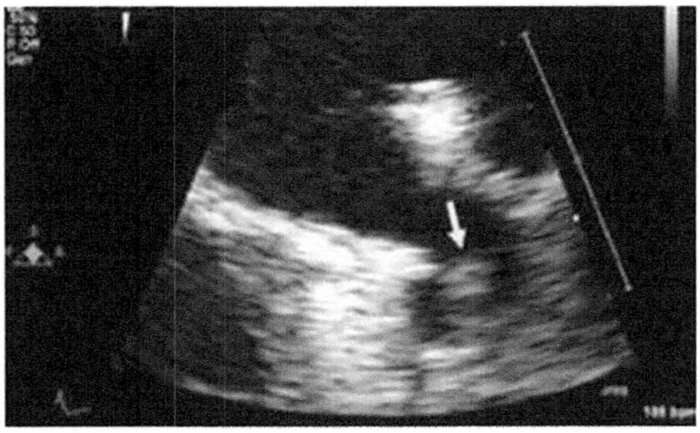

Fig. 1.1 Left atrial appendage (LAA) clot (Kawakami, T., Kobayakawa, H., Ohno, H. et al. Thrombosis J (2013) 11 26. doi: 10.11861477-9560-11-26)

I. Busu-Ray (✉)
Memphis VA Medical Center, Memphis, TN, USA

All India Institute of Medical Sciences, Rishikesh, Uttarakhand, India

School of Public Health, University of Memphis, Memphis, TN, USA
e-mail: ibr@ibasuray.com

D. Khanra
All India Institute of Medical Sciences, Rishikesh, Uttarakhand, India

Liverpool Heart and Chest Hospital, Liverpool, UK

I. Basu-Ray, D. Mehta (eds.), *The Principles and Practice of Yoga in Cardiovascular Medicine*,
https://doi.org/10.1007/978-981-16-6913-2_1

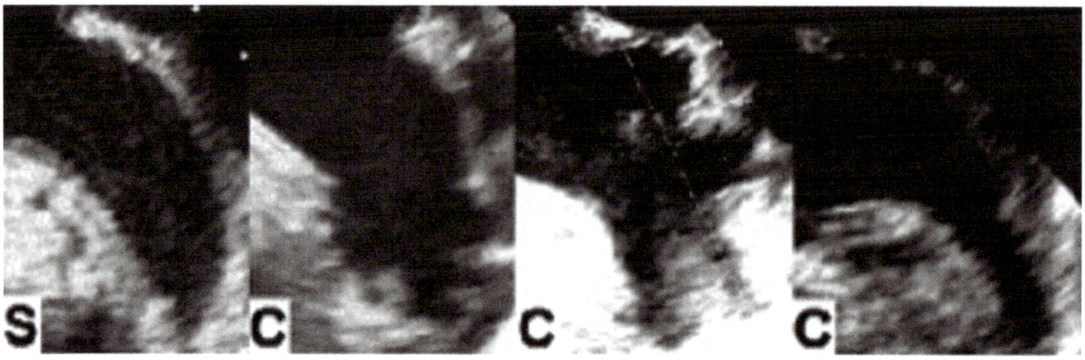

Fig. 1.2 Left atrial appendage (LAA) morphology. Left to right S, simple LAA or SLA2M (chicken wing based on prior classifications); C, Complex LAA or CLA2M (ref [2])

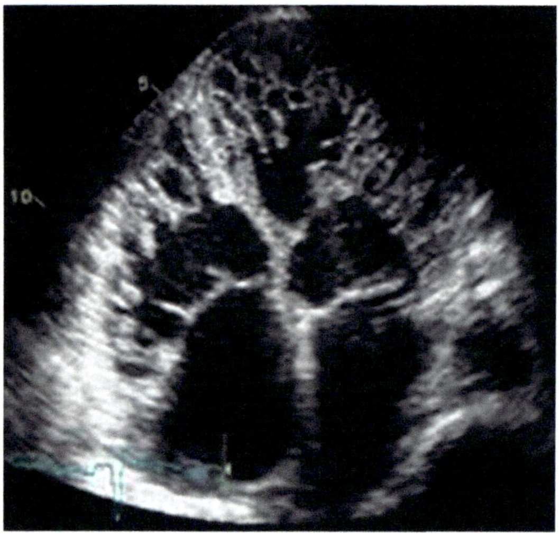

Fig. 1.3 Non-compaction cardiomyopathy (copyright springer)

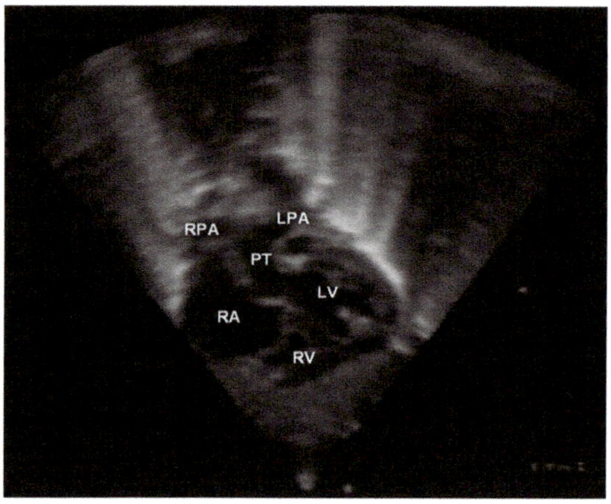

Fig. 1.4 Transposition of great arteries (TGA)

function. Right ventricle is an elongated retort-shaped structure composed of an inflow, body, and outflow tract. Moderator band is a right ventricular (RV) structure and is hypertrophied in endomyocardial fibrosis (EMF) described below [6]. LV and RV are connected to the aorta and pulmonary artery, respectively. Pulmonary artery is located anterior and left to aorta and this relation is reversed in the transposition of great arteries (TGA) (Fig. 1.4). Aortic valve is a tricuspid structure. Bicuspid aortic valve causes premature aortic stenosis, associated aortic regurgitation and dilated aortic root and often associated with coarctation of aorta (Fig. 1.5). Aortic arch is usually left sided and right sided aortic arch is often associated with ventricular septal defect (Fig. 1.6). Ascending aorta has three important branches include brachiocephalic artery, carotid artery, and subclavian artery (Fig. 1.8). Left main Coronary artery (LMCA) and right coronary artery (RCA) emerge from sinus of valsalva. LMCA is bifurcated into left anterior descending (LAD) artery and left circumflex (LCX) artery. In the right dominant coronary circulation, posterior descending artery (PDA) is a branch from RCA and in left dominant circulation PDA is a branch from LCX (Fig. 1.7).

1.2 Basic Physiology

Cardiac cycle consists of a shorter systole and a longer diastole of ventricles. Pressure inside ventricles (dp/dt) rises in isovolumetric contraction period where atrioventricular and semilunar

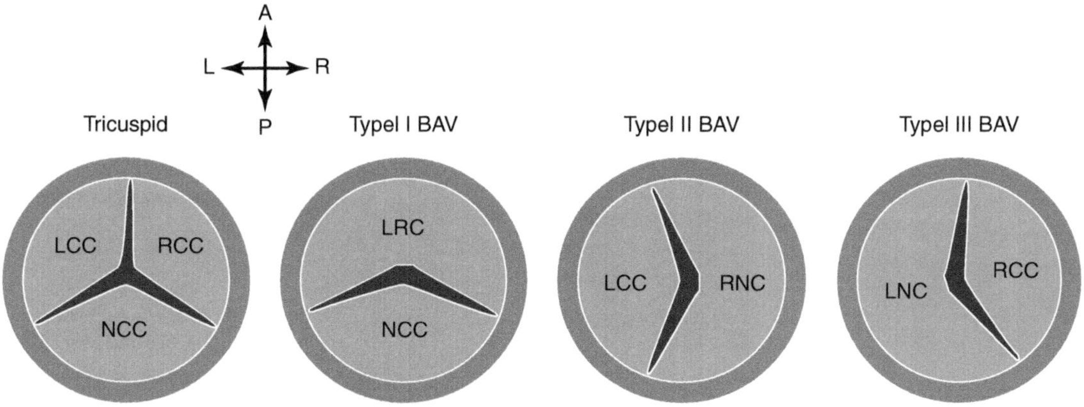

Fig. 1.5 Bicuspid aortic valve and its subtypes

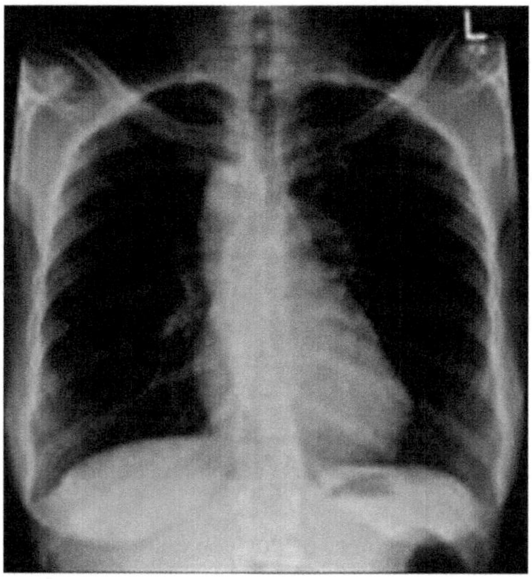

Fig. 1.6 Right-sided aortic arch

valves are closed. When ventricular pressure overcomes pressure in the great vessels, semilunar valves open and forward flow happens until pressure inside the ventricles falls below the pressure in the great vessels which takes place little longer than S2 and corresponds to the hang out interval and end of T of in electrocardiogram. Hang out interval in aorta is more than pulmonary artery and thus A2 occurs earlier than P2. Pressure inside the ventricle starts rising with inflow of blood from the atria during diastole and reaches maximum at end-diastole and when the ventricular pressure overcomes atrial pressure atrioventricular valve closes which corresponds to S1 and q waves in the electrocardiogram. Atrial contraction contributes significantly (25%) during the late diastolic filling of ventricles and this contribution rises in pressure overloaded conditions like outflow tract obstructions and that generates S4 which corresponds to P wave in electrocardiogram (Fig. 1.9).

Frank Sterling law states that more the diastolic filling of the ventricle more is the ventricular contraction due to increasing the calcium sensitivity of the myofibrils causing a greater number of actin–myosin cross-bridges (Fig. 1.10). But the Frank Sterling pressure curve plateaus in the face of maximal volume load. So, in failing heart increasing preload will not increase further contraction. Laplace law states that afterload or wall stress (T) is equal to pressure (P) multiplied by radius (r) divided by twice of thickness (d) [$T = P X r/2d$]. In the setting of increased LV pressure (e.g., systemic hypertension and LVOT obstruction), concentric hypertrophy is a protective mechanism to reduce afterload (Fig. 1.11).

1.3 Hypertension

Hypertension is a worldwide epidemic and one of the major harbinger of cardiovascular disease. According to recent ACC/AHA guideline, hypertension is defined as SBP and/or DBP >130/80 (Fig. 1.12) [7]. Initial treatment options for hypertension include ACEI/ARB, CCB and long-acting diuretic (Chlorthalidone, Indapamide). Optimal drug therapy with at least three different antihypertensive drugs (including a long acting diuretic),

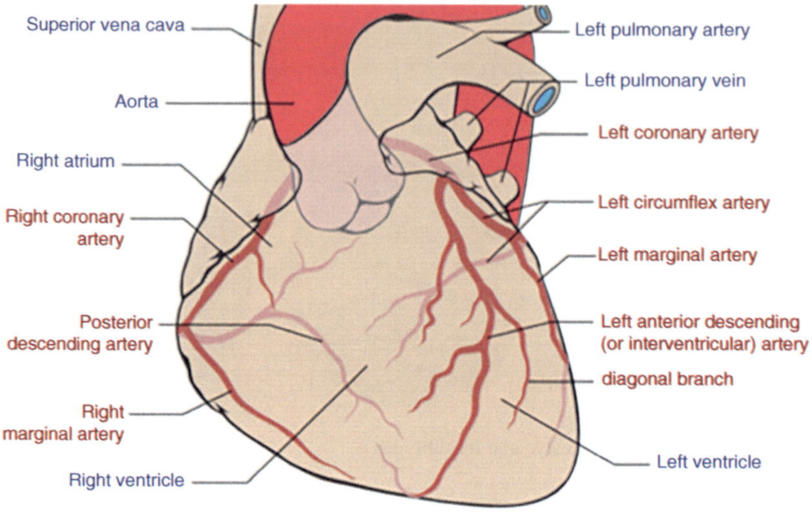

Fig. 1.7 Coronary artery branches

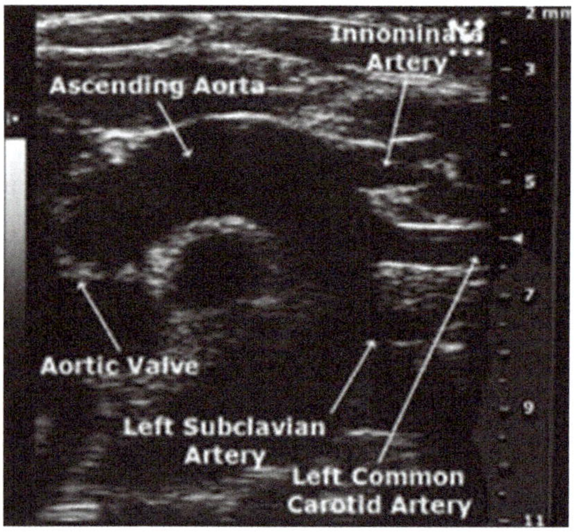

Fig. 1.8 Branches of ascending aorta in suprasternal view

proper measurement of blood pressure and adequate compliance of medicines are to be ensured before diagnosing resistant hypertension [8]. Ambulatory blood pressure monitoring (ABPM) is indicated in such rule out white coat hypertension and masked hypertension from truly resistant hypertension. In such patients, a serum potassium (k) level is important and in k > 5.5 mEq/L, additional blood diuretic can be given and in k < 3.5 mEq/L, spiranolactone is indicated (Fig. 1.13) [8]. If blood pressure is not controlled with five antihypertensives including a long acting thiazide-like diuretic and spironolactone, it is known as refractory hypertension is said to be a different phenotype than resistant hypertension. In refractory hypertension group, beta-blockers and centrally acting antihypertensives (like methyldopa and clonidine) is indicated [8]. Renal artery denervation is re-emerging as a viable treatment option in hypertension along with baroreceptor activating technique and central arterio-venous shunt procedure [9–11]. Chapter 23 discusses the role of yoga in hypertension.

1.4 Coronary Artery Disease

Predominant cause of coronary artery disease is atherosclerosis and atherosclerotic coronary vascular disease (ASCVD) can present as stable ischemic heart disease (SIHD) or acute coronary syndromes (ACS), which include ST elevated myocardial infarction (STEMI) or non-ST elevated ACS (NSTE-ACS). Based on the biomarker evidence of myocardial injury (e.g., Troponin), NSTEASC can be of Non-ST elevated myocardial infarction (NSTEMI) or Unstable angina (USA). Highly sensitive troponins have been found to detect myocardial injury within 3 h and are available to rule in/out heart attack. As per fourth international definition of myocardial infarction, high sensitivity troponin I (HsTnI)-it is a blood marker positivity or increase by >20% in subsequent testing suggests myocardial injury and any ongoing angina, ECG changes or imaging evidence of ischemia or angiographic evi-

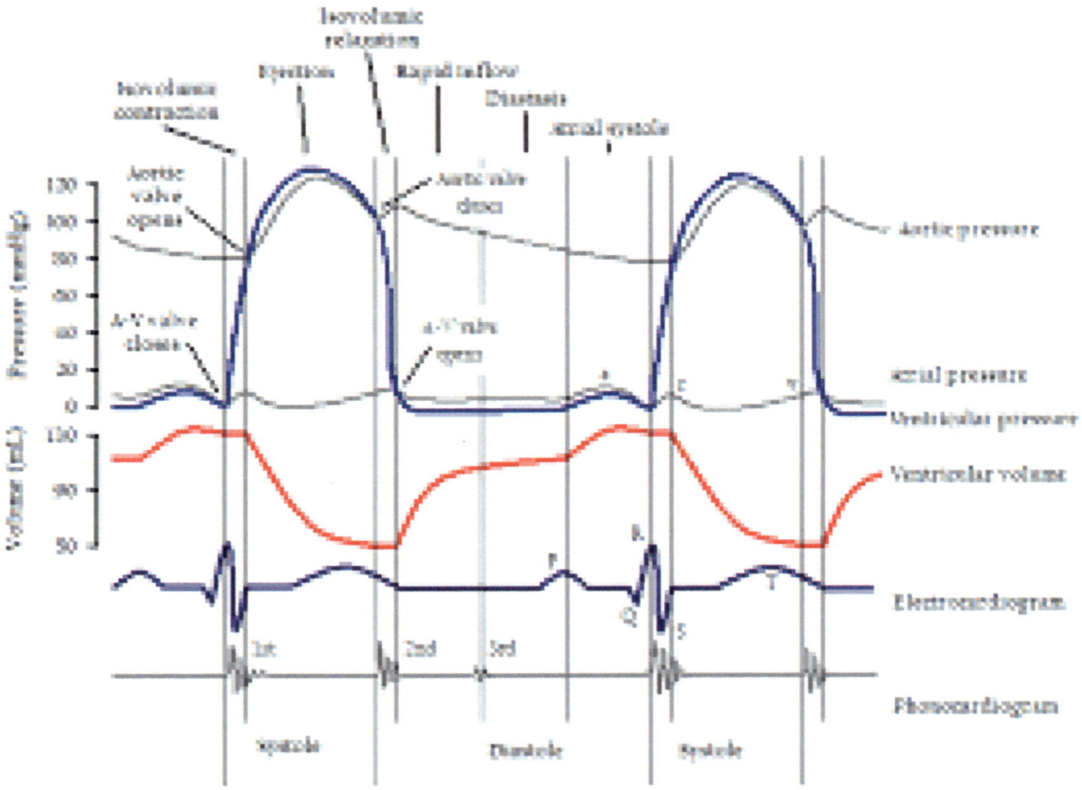

Fig. 1.9 Wiggers cycle

dence of thrombus will clinch the diagnosis of myocardial infarction (Fig. 1.14) [12].

Patients presenting with SIHD should be assessed for pre-test probability of having significant coronary artery disease (CAD) based on risk factors (old age, male sex, smoking, hypertension, diabetes mellitus, hyperlipidemia including elevated level of lipoprotein (a), family history of premature heart disease), baseline electrocardiographic changes suggestive of ischemia and regional wall motion abnormality found in baseline echocardiography. In patients with low pre-test probability no further testing is required. In patients with high pre-test probability, coronary angiogram is recommended without further testing. In patients with intermediate pre-test probability, stress tests like treadmill test or nuclear scan are reasonable to assess reversible ischemia. CT coronary angiogram is becoming a popular screening tool in the intermediate as well as high pre-test probability SIHD patients, as anatomical lesions are easily identified (in absence of severe calcification) and often plaque morphology is also understood in 320 slice CT scanner (even with heart rate > 60 bpm) [13]. Studies have also demonstrated good correlations between CT FFR and angiographic FFR to assess physiological significance of intermediate lesions [14]. CT coronary angiogram can also give idea about the length of lesion, severity of lesion and calcification precisely and thus planning for angioplasty can be done well. Thus CT angiogram is becoming a popular one-stop-shop for SIHD patients and NICE has also incorporated this tool as an important screening tool (Fig. 1.15) [15].

In significant stenosis involving left main alone or proximal LAD artery, angioplasty with drug eluting stent followed by dual antiplatelets for 6 months at-least is a class I recommendation to treat angina and reduce mortality due to heart attack [16]. In LMCA disease, using IVUS during PCI is a class I indication. In significant stenosis involving other coronary arteries, intervention is recommended only to reduce

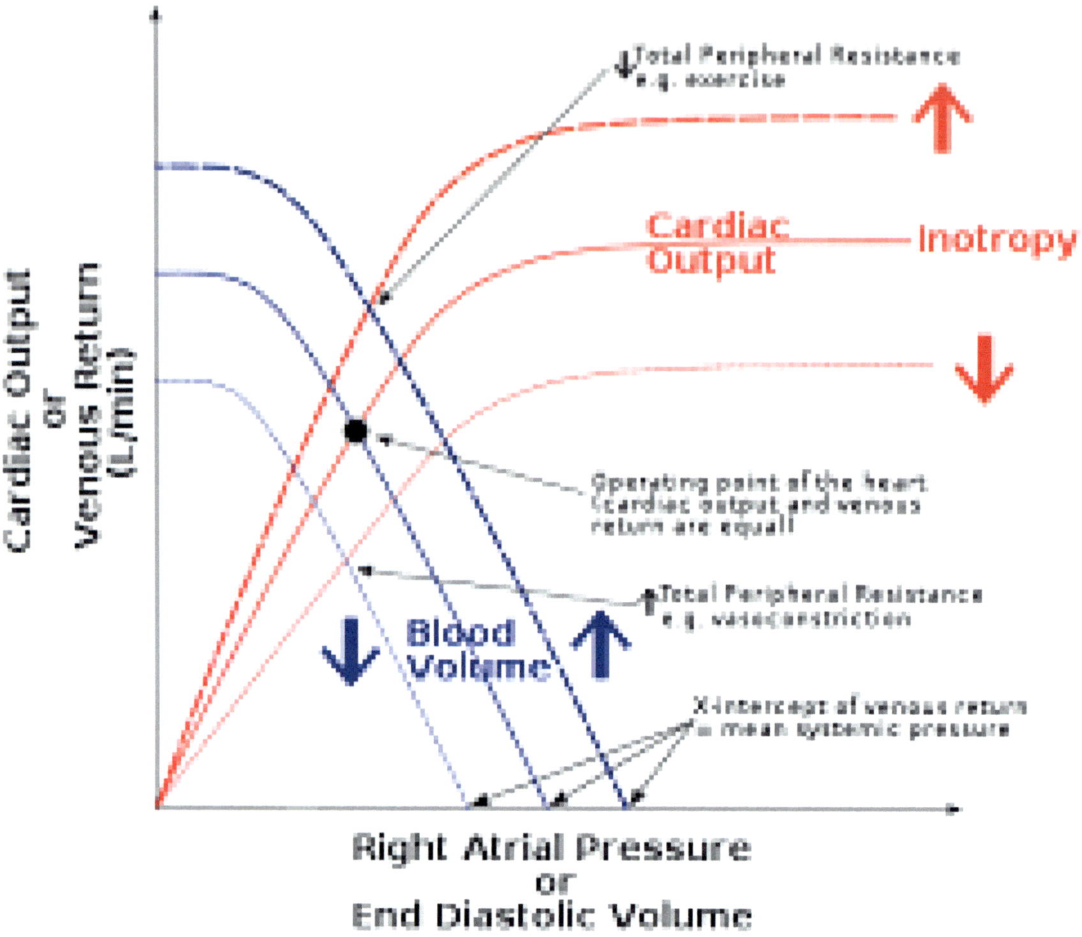

Fig. 1.10 Frank sterling law

angina when optimal medical (beta blockers, nitrates, and ivabradine) therapy is not adequately taking care of angina but no difference in mortality could be demonstrated in long term observational studies [16]. Newer anti-anginals like trimetazidine, nicorandil, and ranolazine can be tried. In patients with left main disease and triple vessel disease SYNTAX score calculation is important and in low or intermediate SYNTAX, percutaneous coronary intervention (PCI) is recommended and in high SYNTAX score patients, coronary artery by-pass graft (CABG) is recommended. In patients with low ejection fraction or diabetes, CABG performed better than PCI in large observational studies [16]. In SIHD patients with intermediate lesion (50–70%), FFR is a class I indication to asses functional significance of the lesion and stenting is only recommended if FFR < 0.7 [16]. IFR is also coming up as a new strategy, where adenosine is not required. Hybrid strategies with IFR/FFR with utilizing FFR only if IFR is between 0.86–0.93 has been found to be cost-effective strategy in literature [17].

All patients of ACS are to be loaded with aspirin 325 mg AND P2Y12 inhibitors (Clopidegreol 300 mg Pasugrel 60 mg and Ticagrelor 180 mg). Pasugrel is to used cautiously in patients with previous history of stroke, elderly patients and low body weight. Administrating oxygen has been found only beneficial when sPo2 < 92% [18]. In patients of STEMI, if the patient presents within 3 h of chest pain, thrombolysis and primary PCI (PPCI) performs similarly [16]. Thrombolysis can be done using streptokinase or

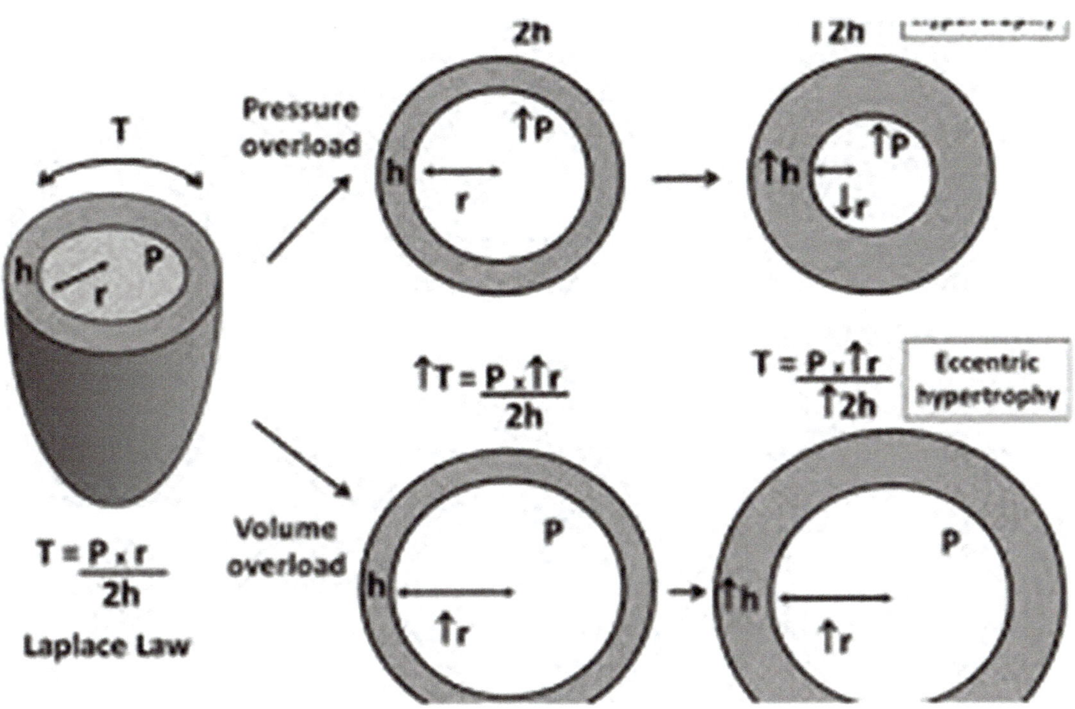

Fig. 1.11 Laplace law

Blood Pressure Categories

American Heart Association | American Stroke Association

BLOOD PRESSURE CATEGORY	SYSTOLIC mm Hg (upper number)		DIASTOLIC mm Hg (lower number)
NORMAL	LESS THAN 120	and	LESS THAN 80
ELEVATED	120 – 129	and	LESS THAN 80
HIGH BLOOD PRESSURE (HYPERTENSION) STAGE 1	130 – 139	or	80 – 89
HIGH BLOOD PRESSURE (HYPERTENSION) STAGE 2	140 OR HIGHER	or	90 OR HIGHER
HYPERTENSIVE CRISIS (consult your doctor immediately)	HIGHER THAN 180	and/or	HIGHER THAN 120

Fig. 1.12 Stages of hypertension as per 2017 ACC guideline

tenecteplase (single dose) or Reteplase (two doses). In elderly patients, streptokinase has the least chance of causing intracranial bleeding [19]. In STEMI patients, if the patient presenting within 3–6 h, PPCI is better than thrombolysis (Fig. 1.16) [20]. However, if PPCI is not available, phramcoinvasive strategy (i.e., thrombolysis followed by routine angiography) can be undertaken, which in many recent studies found to be equivalent to primary PCI. In patients of STEMI who are presenting after 6 h, primary PCI is the recommendation [20]. However, if ongoing

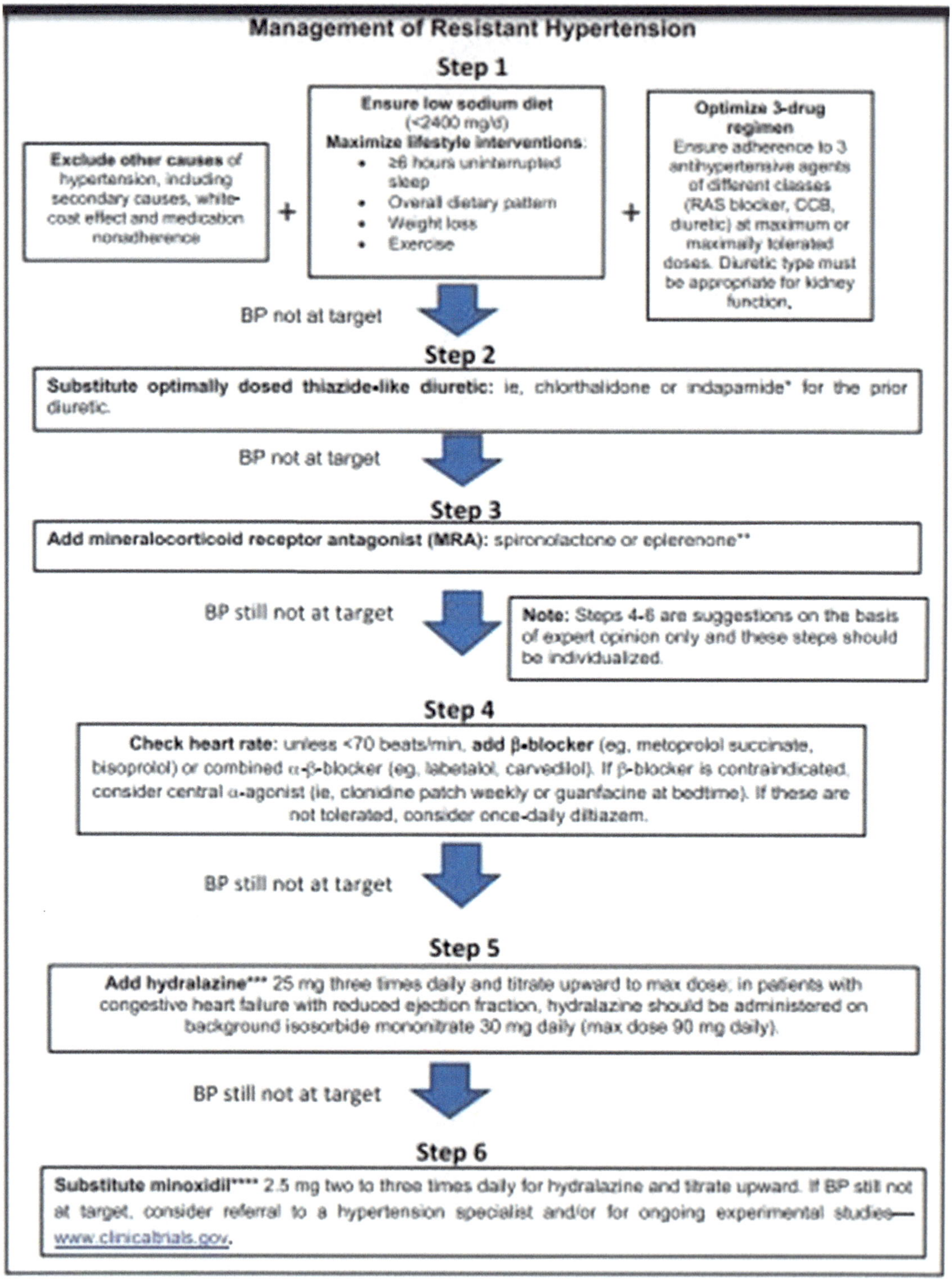

Fig. 1.13 Management of resistant hypertension (Source: 2017 ACC Hypertension guideline)

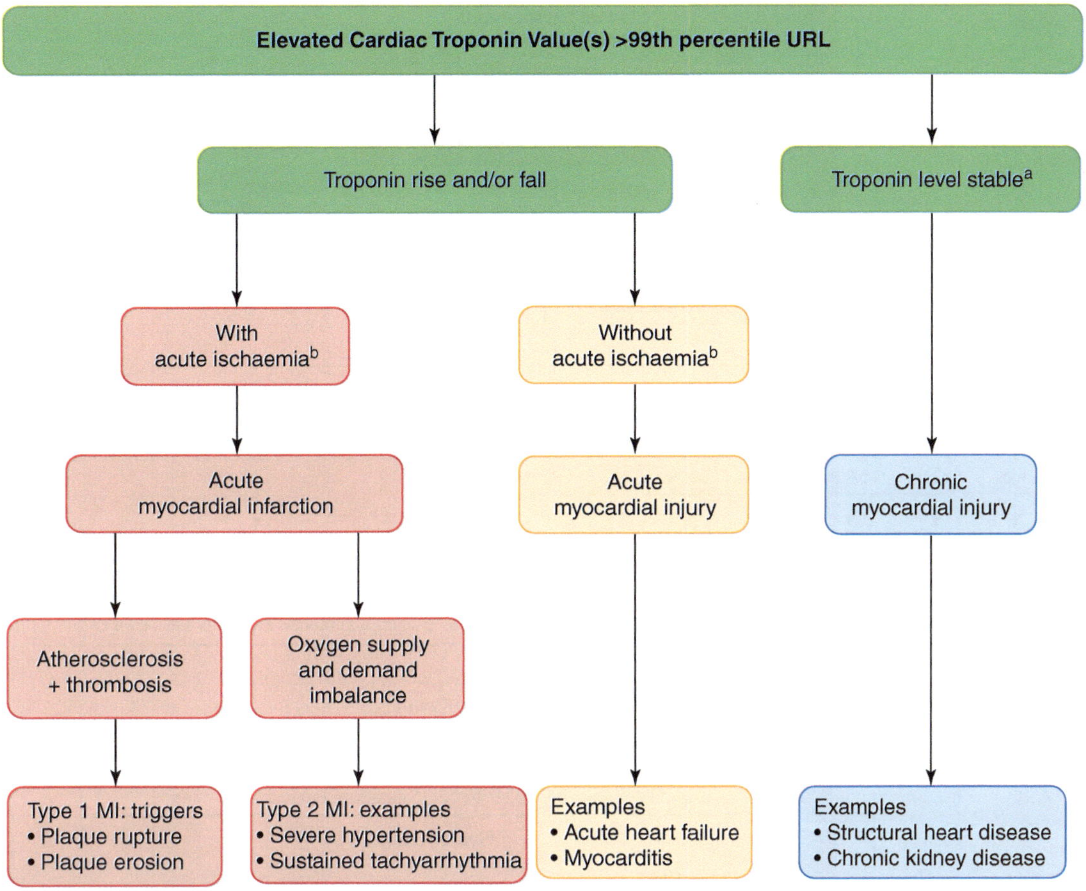

Fig. 1.14 Myocardial injury and infarction

angina is present, along with persistent ST elevation, pharmaco-invasive strategy is reasonable [20]. Time is muscle in saving myocardial damage, and thus primary PCI is a class I indication for STEMI till 24 h and class IIa indication till 48 h [21]. STEMI Patients presenting beyond 48 h are taken for PPCI only if ongoing angina or dynamic ECG changes or imaging evidence of viable myocardium are present [21]. STEMI Patients presenting beyond 48 h with complete occlusion of coronary artery should be intervened only if there is evidence of viable myocardium present [20, 21].

During primary PCI, routing manual thrombus aspiration is not recommended and non-culprit artery stenosis are to be stented only if not a complex lesion and significant (FFR < 0.7) and patient is not in shock [21]. In patient with heart failure and shock, use of IABP is falling out of grace after recent studies [22]. However, role of unloading first (with Impell, ECMO or Tandem-Heart) and then revascularization is becoming a popular strategy not only to prevent cath-lab mortality but also to prevent microvascular damage and revascularization injury [23]. Drug eluting stent followed by DAPT for at least 12 months is a class I recommendation after PCI for ACS (Fig. 1.17). Shorter or longer course of DAPT can be advised according to PRECISE DAPT or DAPT score, respectively (Fig. 1.18) [24]. Clopidogrel is going out of fashion in many centers, even in India due to its prevalent resistance profile and thus ticagrelor is becoming the default choice. Only problems with ticagrelor are dyspnea in some patients and cost factors. Pasugrel is a reasonable choice is stent thrombosis and diabetic patients. In patients who are not affordable or not tolerating ticagrelor or pasugrel

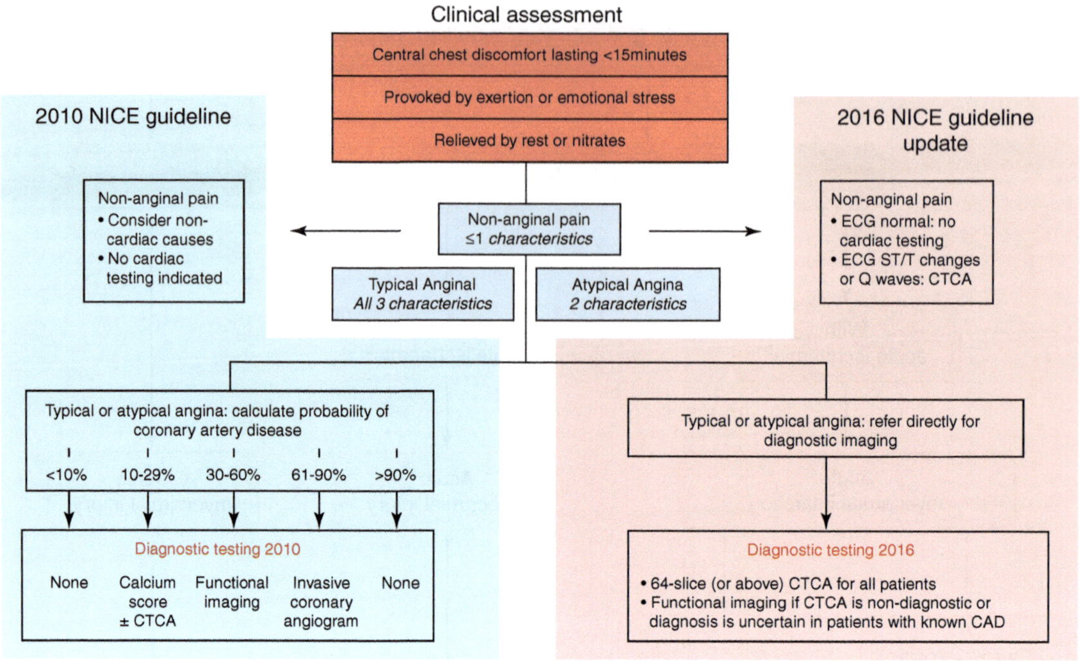

Fig. 1.15 Cardiac CT in decision-making of patients with acute chest pain

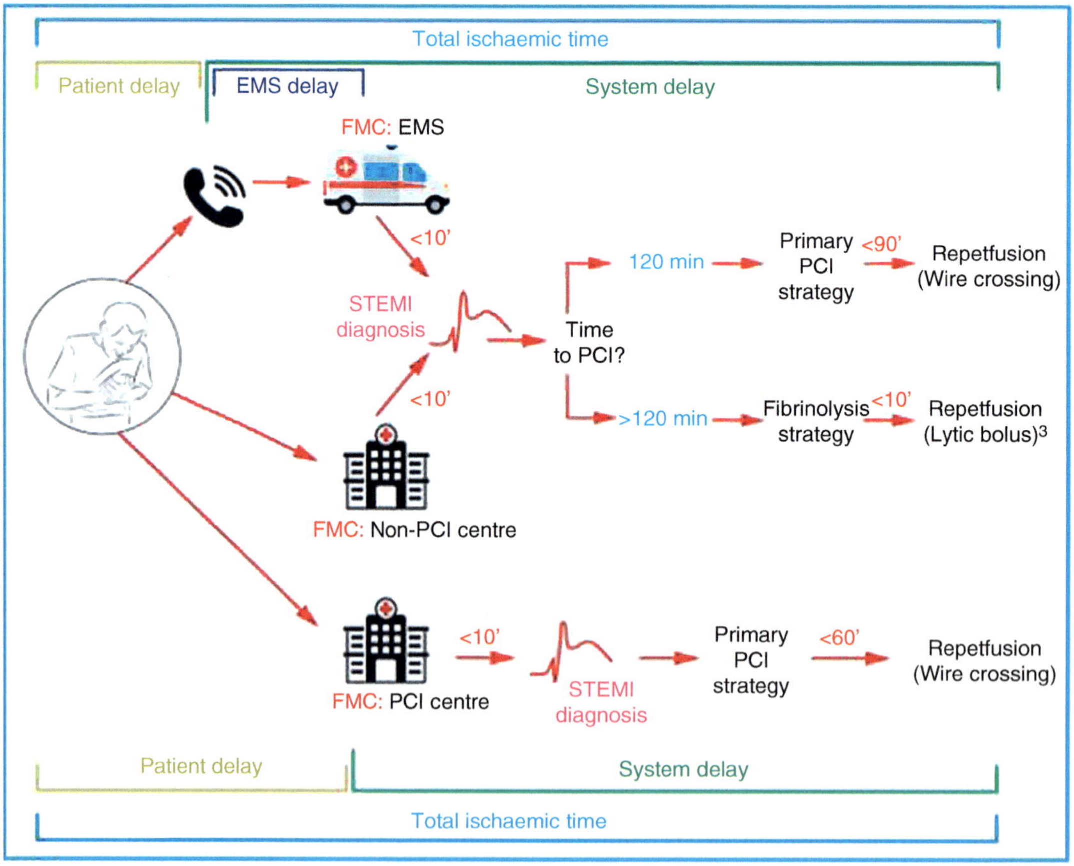

Fig. 1.16 STEMI management pathway (Source: ESC 2018)

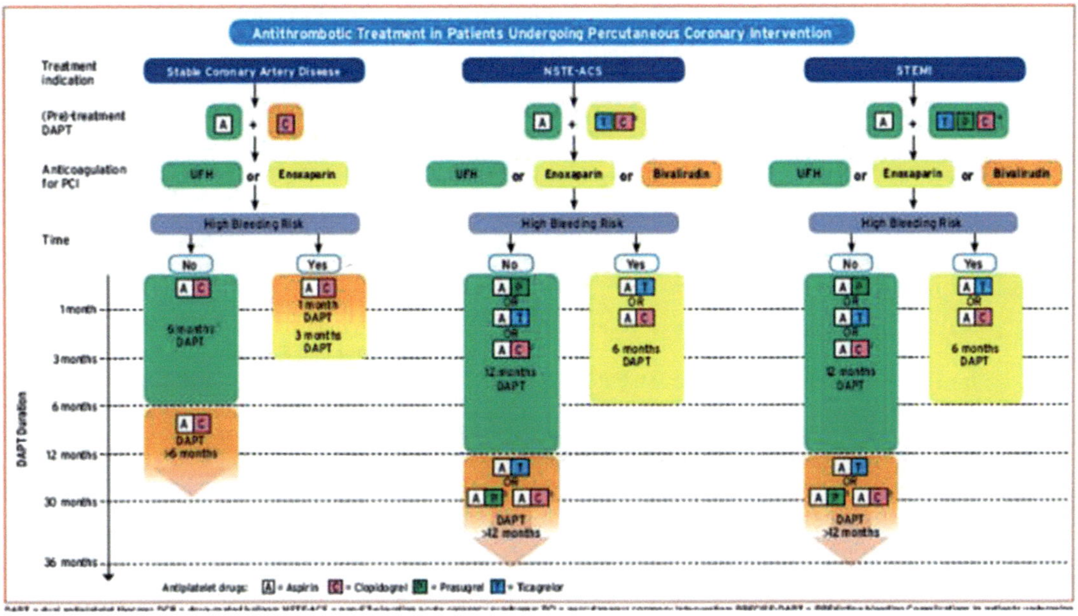

Fig. 1.17 Duration of antiplatelets in patients undergoing angioplasty (source: ESC 2018)

	PRECISE-DAPT score[15]	DAPT score[15]	
Time of use	At the time of coronary stenting	After 12 months of uneventful DAPT	
DAPT duration starategies assessed	Short DAPT (3–6 months) vs. Standard/long DAPT (12–24 months)	Standard DAPT (12 months) vs. Long DAPT (30 months)	
Score calculation[a]	HB ≥12 11-5 11 10-5 10-5 WBC 5 8 10 12 14 15 18 ≥20 Age 50 60 70 80 ≥90 CRCl ≥100 80 60 40 20 0 Prior Bleeding No Yes Score Points 0 2 4 6 8 10 12 14 16 18 20 22 24 26 28 30	Age ≥75 65 to <75 <65 Cigarecte smoking Diabetes mellitus MI at presentation Prior PCI or prior MI Paclitaxel-eluting stent Stent diameter <3 mm CHF or LVEF <30% Vein graft stent	 –2 pt –1 pt 0 pt +1 pt +1 pt +1 pt +1 pt +1 pt +1 pt +2 pt +2 pt
Score range	0 to 100 points	–2 to 10 points	
Decision making out-off suggested	Score ≥25 Short DAPT Score <25 Standard/long DAPT	Score ≥2 Long DAPT Score <2 Standard DAPT	
Calculator	www.precisedaptscore.com	www.daptstudy.org	

©ESC 2017

Fig. 1.18 Clinical scores for dual-antiplatelet therapy DAPT duration decision-making (Source: 2017 ESC Focused update on DAPT)

can be switched to clopidogrel after 3 months (Fig. 1.19) [24]. High intensity statin is also recommended after ACS with a target LDL below 70 mg/dL (Fig. 1.20) [25]. Beta-blockers are to be continued indefinitely unless patient is not tolerating heart rate < 60 bpm and ACEI for at least 1 year especially in large AWMI and EF < 40%. Spironolactone or Eplerenone is recommended in ACS patients with EF < 40% [24]. Chapter 19 profiles the use of yoga in the prevention and treatment of coronary artery disease.

1.5 Valvular Heart Disease

In developing countries like India, rheumatic heart disease still continue to be the leading cause of valvular heart disease and mitral valve

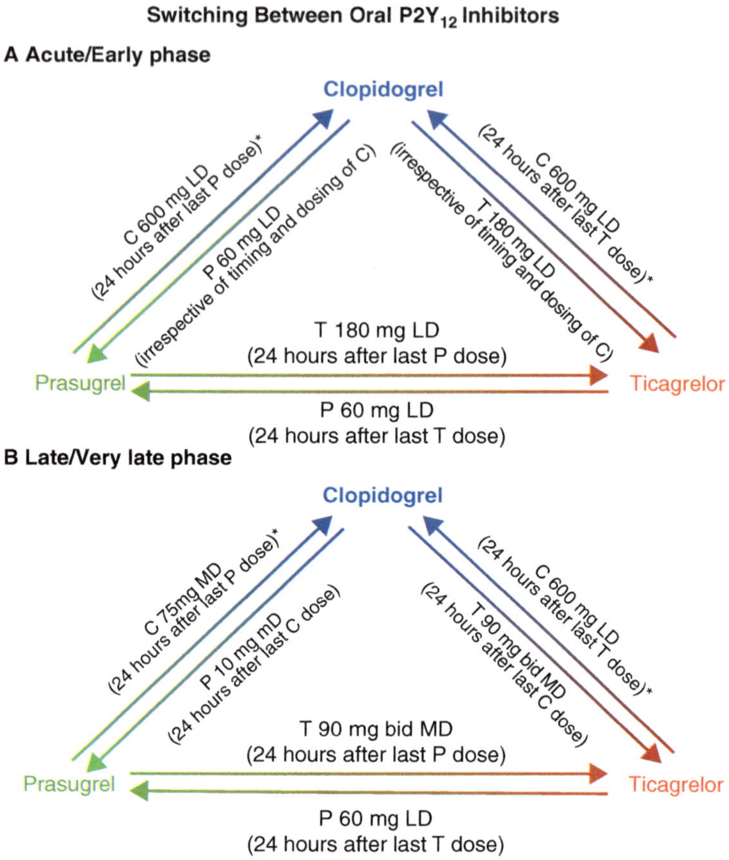

Fig. 1.19 Switching between P2Y12 inhibitor. (**A**) Acute/early phase. (**B**) Late/very late phase

involvement is the commonest in the form of mitral stenosis (MS) and mitral regurgitation (MR). In the developed world, degenerative mitral valve disease, also known as Fibroelastic Deficiency (FED), in its various shades is the commonest cause of MR [26]. Functional mitral regurgitation (FMR) is found in cardiomyopathies (ischemic as well as non-ischemic). Aortic valve disease is the second most common valve to be diseased in the form of aortic stenosis (AS) with or without regurgitation. In the developed world, AS due to degenerative conditions is the most common valvular disease found. Congenital valvular disease like bicuspid aortic valve (BAV) leading to aortic stenosis could be found in relatively younger age, often associated with coarctation of aorta (CoA). Isolated aortic valve disease due to rheumatic etiology is uncommon. Aortic regurgitation (AR) may be found in non-rheumatic causes which include aortopathies, bicuspid aortic valve or Marfan's syndrome, ankylosing spondylosis, connective tissue disorders, and rarely in syphilis. Tricuspid valve disease is found in nearly 10% of valvular heart disease [27]. The commonest cause of tricuspid regurgitation (TR) is left heart disease leading to severe pulmonary artery hypertension (PAH). Tricuspid stenosis (TS) is found in carcinoid, endomyocardial fibrosis, and uncommonly in rheumatic heart disease (almost always along with mitral stenosis). Pulmonary valve diseases are mostly congenital pulmonary stenosis (PS). Other causes of pulmonary stenosis include carcinoid diseases and rarely in rheumatic heart diseases. Pulmonary regurgitation is often functional due to severe PAH.

MS, the commonest valvular disease in the rheumatic background, presents as dyspnea on exertion, often associated with orthopnea and paroxysmal nocturnal dyspnea (PND). Often, patients with MS deteriorate in pregnancy due to volume overload and tachycardia. Significant palpitation denotes associated regurgitating lesions like MR or AR. Loud S1, opening snap, and rumbling mid-diastolic murmur are the telltale features of MS. Apical pansystolic murmur (PSM) with displaced apical impulse is classical of

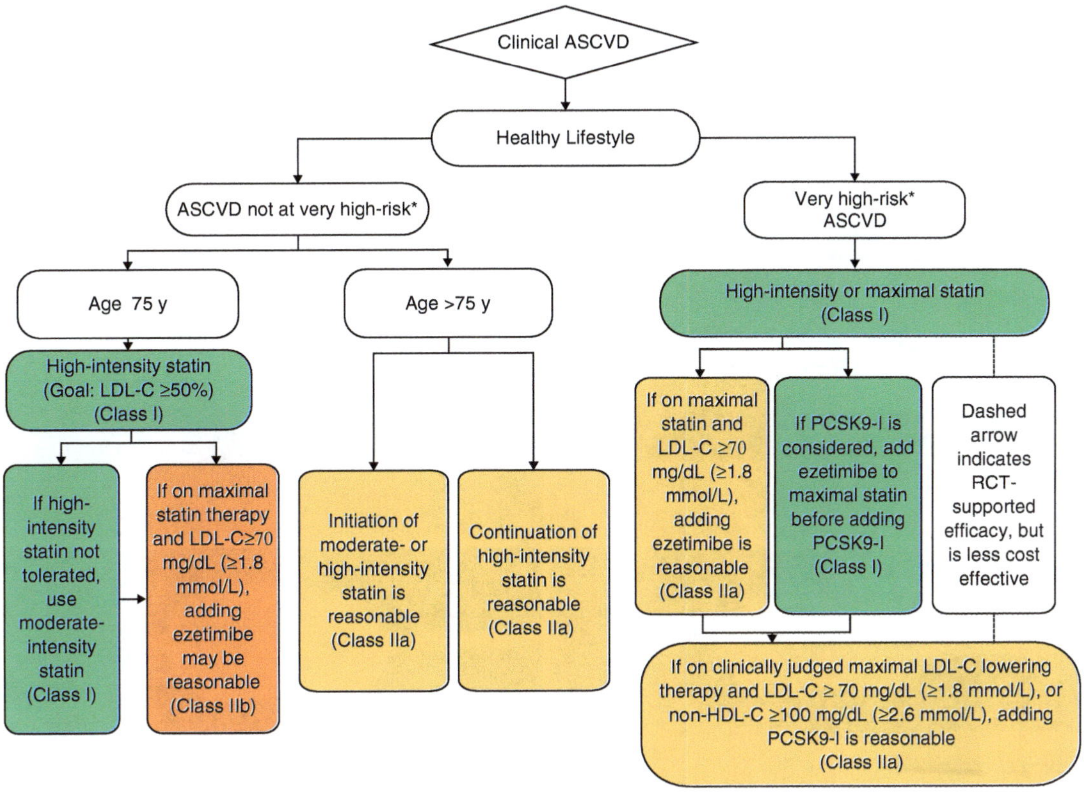

Fig. 1.20 Statin pathway for secondary prevention

MR. However, peripheral signs of aortic run-off like water hammer pulse in radial artery and pistol shots sound over femoral artery are often classical. Consequences like hemoptysis, PAH, and atrial fibrillation (AF) are common. AS presents with the classical triad of angina, syncope, and dyspnea, mostly on exertion. Aortic ejection systolic murmur (ESM) with radiation to bilateral carotid arteries are pathognomonic of AS. AR is rather well tolerated but identifying early diastolic murmur (EDM) of AR is often challenging clinically Severe TR often leads to right ventricular dysfunction and pedal swelling. Parasternal PSM which gets louder with inspiration and elevation of legs is classical of TR. Patients with PS are younger and are characterized by ESM in the pulmonary area with soft P2 and wide split. Basal EDM may be heard due to hypertensive PR (Graham Steel murmur) and often needs dynamic auscultation to differentiate with AR.

Medical therapies for MS include rate controllers like beta-blockers (BB) or calcium channel blockers (CCB), digoxin in patients with atrial fibrillation, and diuretics. Vasodilators, BB/CCB, and diuretics are to be used cautiously in patients with AS. Prophylactic antibiotics like penicillin or erythromycin are to be given in patients with rheumatic heart disease for lifelong. However, evidence of secondary prophylaxis in patients more than 40 years of age are less.

Intervention for mitral stenosis is percutaneous balloon mitral valvotomy (PBMV) using Inoue (Fig. 1.21) or Accura balloon and it is indicated in symptomatic severe MS (mitral valve area < 1.5 cm^2) in pliable mitral valve (Wilkins score < 7/16) without clot in left atrial body, more than moderate MR and bilateral commissural calcifications [28, 29]. Mitral valve separation index is a useful echocardiographic marker to assess the severity of MS [30]. With the advent of three-dimensional echocardiography (3DE) and intracardiac echocardiography (ICE), trans-septal puncture (TSP) became more guided. With the new software like MVQ in 3DE, reconstructing mitral valve annulus is possible which is informative for the surgeons contemplating surgical

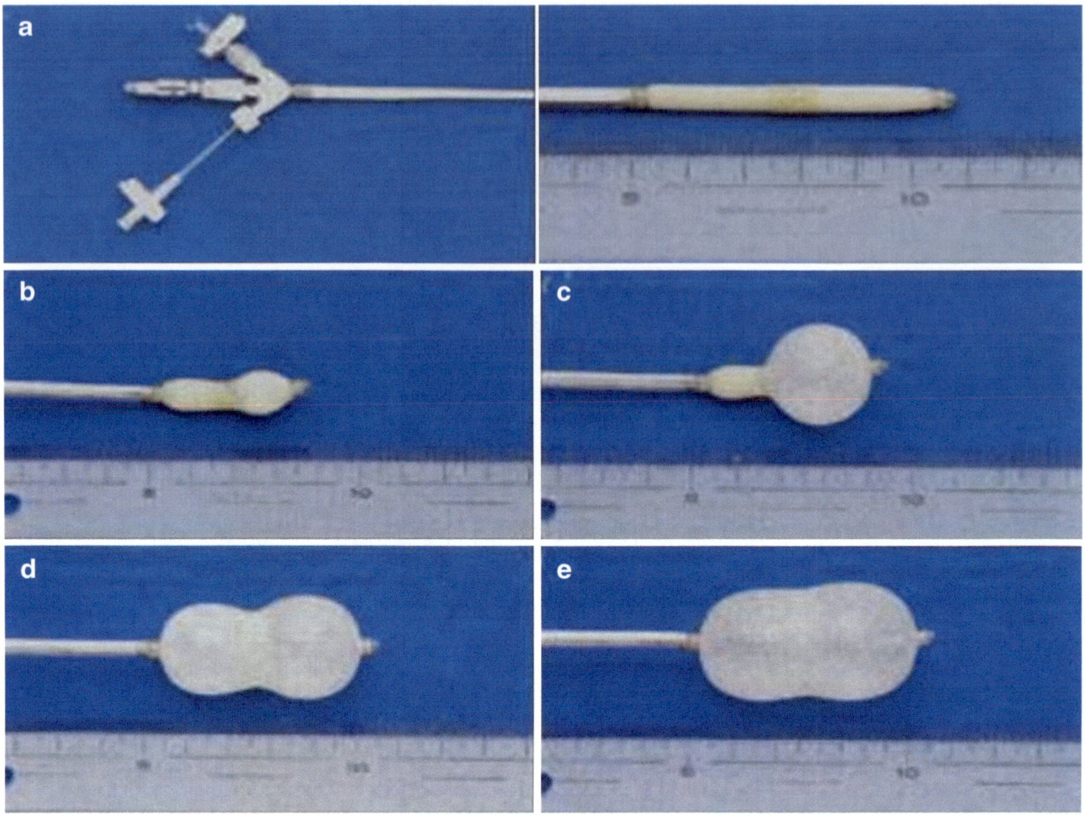

Fig. 1.21 Inoue-Balloon used for balloon mitral valvotomy (BMV). The figure shows the Inoue balloon catheter. (**a**) The top panel shows the length of the catheter. On the far left, at the hub, the stretching metal tube has been fully advanced, resulting in stretching and elongation of the balloon catheter, seen on the right side of the figure. This results in a minimized profile to facilitate passage through a femoral venous sheath or directly through the skin. Panels (**b**) through (**e**) show the stepwise inflation characteristics of the balloon. (**b**) the balloon is uninflated. (**c**) the distal portion has been inflated. This portion of the balloon can be "floated" or manipulated across the mitral valve from the left atrium to the left ventricle in a manner analogous to crossing the tricuspid valve with a right heart balloon floatation catheter. (**d**) the balloon in further inflated to create a "dog bone" configuration. This allows the balloon to self-position within the mitral valve. (**e**) Upon final inflation, as seen in panel 6, the waist of the balloon is fully expanded, ultimately resulting in commissural splitting

mitral valve repair (MVRe) using annuloplasty ring [31]. Percutaneous MVRe, is also becoming available in the form of edge-to-edge repair with Mitraclip, indirect mitral annuloplasty (Monarc, Carillon), and direct mitral annuloplasty (Mitrallign) (Fig. 1.22) [32]. For unrepairable MR and calcified MS, surgical mitral valve replacement (MVR) is the choice of treatment. Percutaneous MVR is also available with balloon (Edward sapiens) and self-expandable percutaneous mitral valve prosthetics (Tiara, Navigate, CardiAQ, etc.) (Fig. 1.23) [33].

Treatment for severe AS is surgical aortic valve replacement (AVR). In patients with prohibitive, high, and even intermediate surgical risk patients transcutaneous AVR (TAVR) is becoming the treatment of choice. There are two types of valve systems available for TAVR, including balloon expandable (Edward Sapiens) and self-expandable (Medtronic core valve). TAVR can be done by trans-apical or trans-caval route too in case of a severely calcified aorto-iliac artery. TAVR is also available Lotus is also a newer self-expandable valve available for TAVR which has promising results in newer studies. Made-in-India MyVal is a balloon-expandable valve for TAVR, which is being studied in India. Jena valve is the only percutaneous aortic valve, which is available for severe AR (Fig. 1.24).

Tricuspid valve is often called the forgotten valve but assessing the need for repair of tricuspid valve surgery of left heart valves has been

Target of therapy	Device name (manufacturer)	Mechanism of action
Leaflet repair	MitraClip (Abbott)	Clip-based edge-toedge repair
	Percu-Pro (Cardiosolutions)	Regurgitant orifice space occupying
	Mobius (Edwards)	Suture-based edge-to-edge repair
Chordal implant	NeoChord (Neochord)	Synthetic chordae tendineae
Indirect annuloplasty	Carillon (Cardiac Dimensions)	Coronary sinus reshaping
	Monarc (Edwards)	Coronary sinus reshaping
	PTMA Device (Viacor)	Coronary sinus reshaping
	Mitral Cerclage (NIH)	Coronary sinus-right atrial encircling
	PS3 System (MVRx)	Transatrial coronary sinus-atrial septal shortening
Direct annuloplasty	Mitralign (Mitralign)	2 2 plicating anchors through posterior annulus
	AccuCinch (Guided Delivery) Systems)	Plicating anchors in ventricular side of mitral annulus
	Cardioband (Valtech)	Plicating anchors on atrial side of mitral annulus
	QuantumCor (QuantumCor)	Radiofrequency energy shrinking annular collagen
	Millipede (Millipede)	Semirigid circumferential annular ring
Left ventricular reshaping	iCoapsys (Edwards)	Transventricular reshaping
	BACE (Mardil)	External basal myocardial reshaping

Fig. 1.22 Options available for percutaneous mitral valve repair

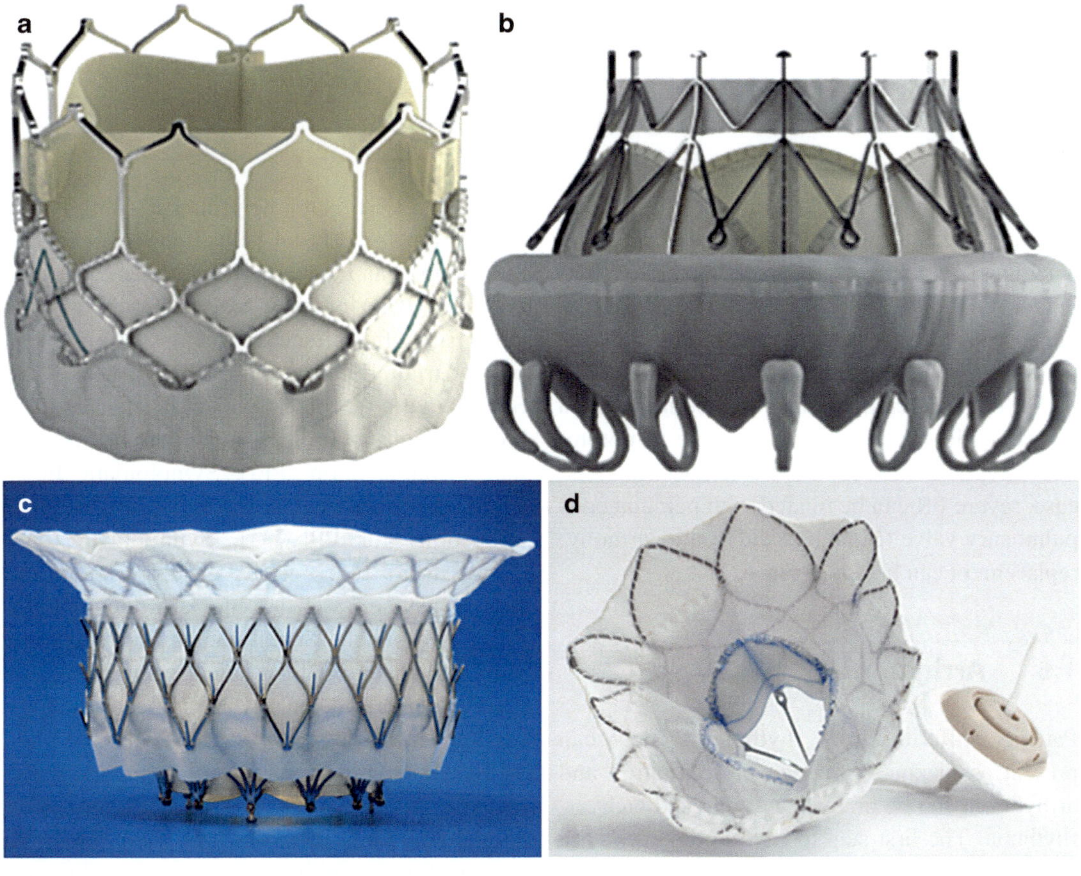

Fig. 1.23 Options available for percutaneous mitral valve replacement SAPIEN 3™ valve (**a**). CardiAQ-Edwards™ Transcatheter Mitral Valve (**b**). Medtronic Intrepid™ transcatheter heart valve (**c**). Tendyne™ Mitral Valve System (**d**)

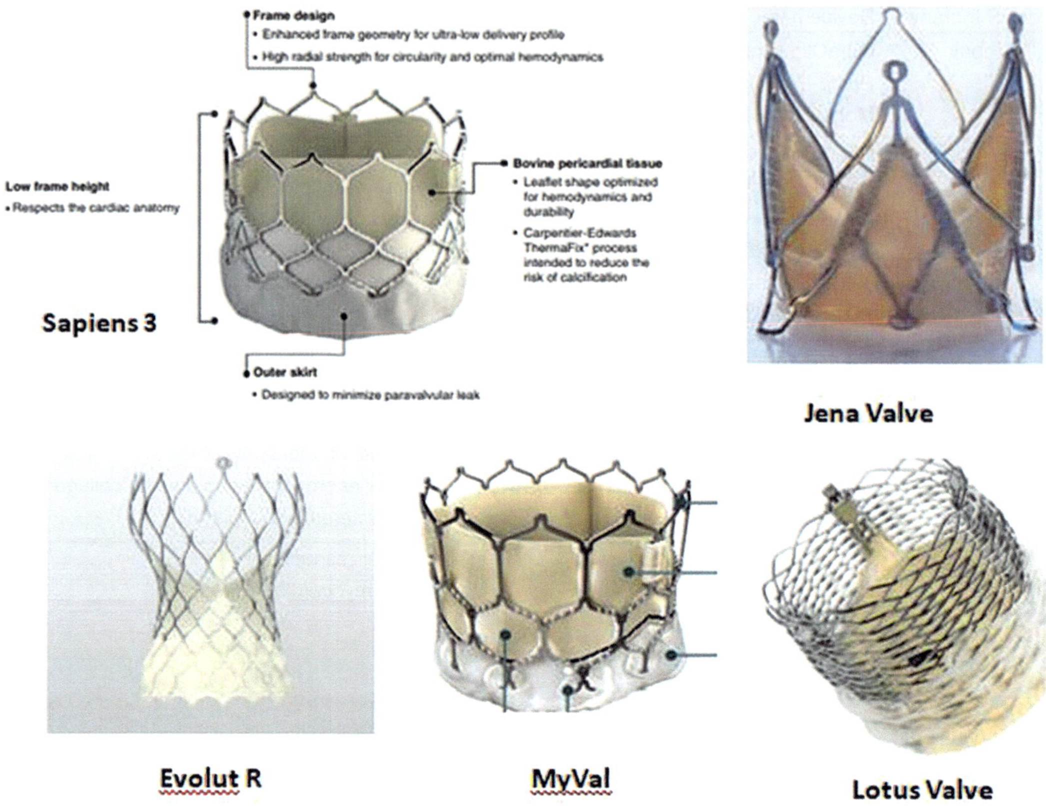

Fig. 1.24 Valves available for transcatheter aortic valve replacement (TAVR)

emphasized in current literature (Fig. 1.25). Percutaneous tricuspid valve repair using Trialign, Tricinch, Forma devices are being studied for functional TR (FTR). Percutaneous tricuspid valve replacement using Tric-valve is also in the experimental phase (Fig. 1.26).

For PS, balloon pulmonary valvotomy using a Tyshak balloon can be done in severe symptomatic valvular PS. In repaired cyanotic heart disease, severe PR can be treated with percutaneous pulmonary valve (Melody, Lotus, and Harmony) replacement can be done (Fig. 1.27).

1.6 Arrhythmias

Patients suffering from rhythm disorders can present as dizziness/syncope or palpitation and arrhythmia can be bradyarrhythmia and tachyarrhythmia. The first step to rhythm disorder is to take a proper history of syncope and interpretation of ECG during the episode (when available). If baseline ECG is not helpful, a 24–48 h Holter monitoring could be of help. Long-term rhythm monitoring can be achieved by implantable loop recorder (ILR) or even external loop recorder (ELR) and often clinch the diagnosis of paroxysmal Atrial Fibrillation (AF) (Fig. 1.28). Symptomatic second- and third-degree heart block is a class I indication for permanent pacemaker implantation (PPI). Symptomatic bifascicular or trifascicular block are also class I indications for PPI [34]. Symptomatic first-degree heart block needs electrophysiological study and if infra-Hisian block is demonstrated PPI is reasonable. Septal pacing is found to be more physiological than apical pacing [35] and dual-chamber pacemakers are more physiological than single chamber pacemakers [36].

Tachyarrhythmias can be of supraventricular tachycardias like AVNRT (Fig. 1.29) and AVRT (Fig. 1.30). Drug therapies have been the front-runner of treatment but never without failure and adverse reactions. Thus, in symptomatic patients

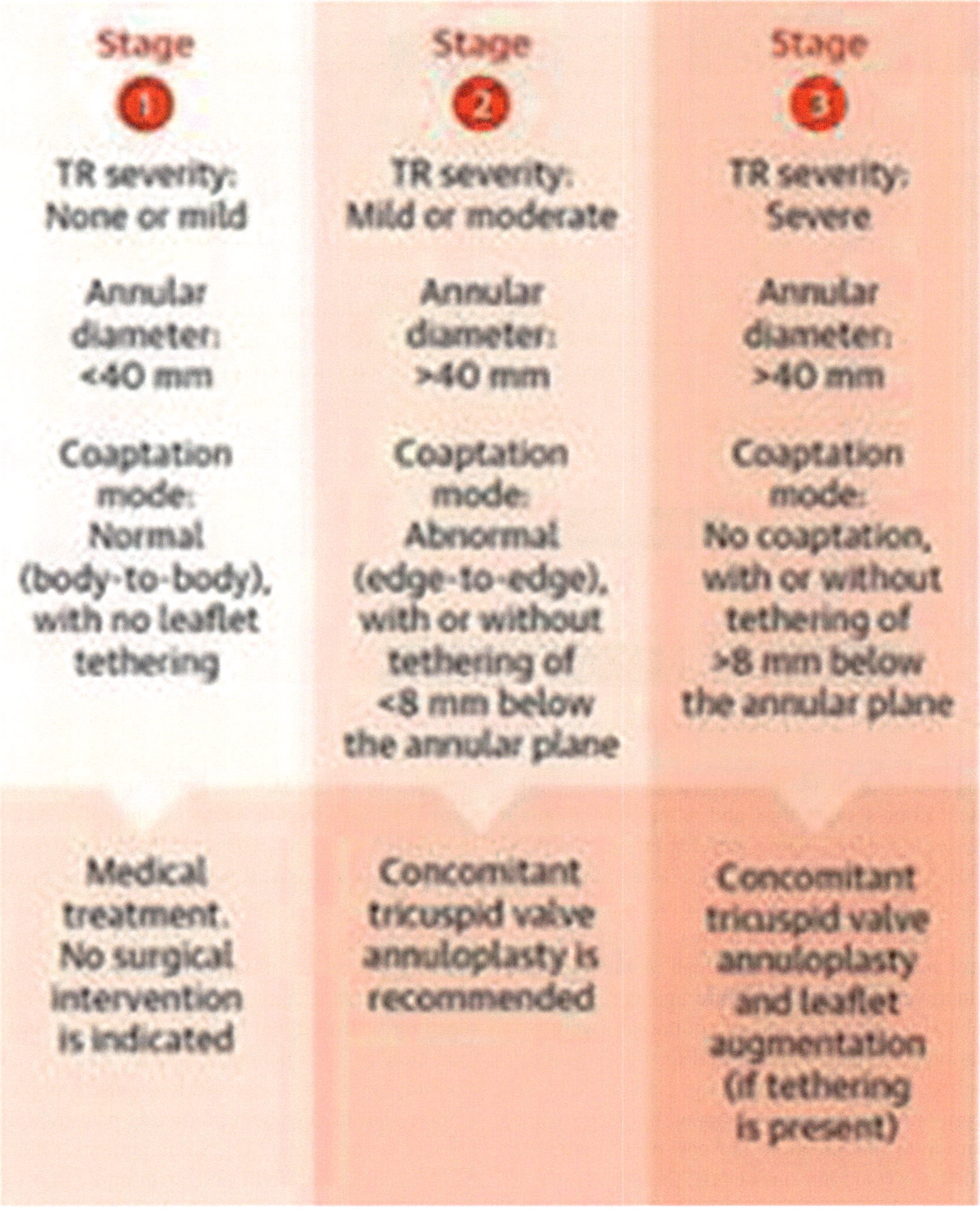

Fig. 1.25 Grades and recommended treatment functional tricuspid regurgitation (FTR)

with highly inducible PSVT in electrophysiological study (EPS), ablation of a slow pathway or accessory pathway (AP) can be achieved with high success rate in AVNRT or AVRT, respectively. In patients with Wolff-Parkinson-White (WPW) syndrome (Fig. 1.31) with anterograde conduction, Accessory pathway (AP) can be identified by Arruda's algorithm and can be confirmed in EPS and can be ablated with a high success rate [37]. Atrial Flutter (AFL) (Fig. 1.32) can be mapped by a 3D system and CTI-dependent AFL can be ablated whereas for left atrial AFL TSP is required and AFL can be ablated using anterograde technique. Origin of

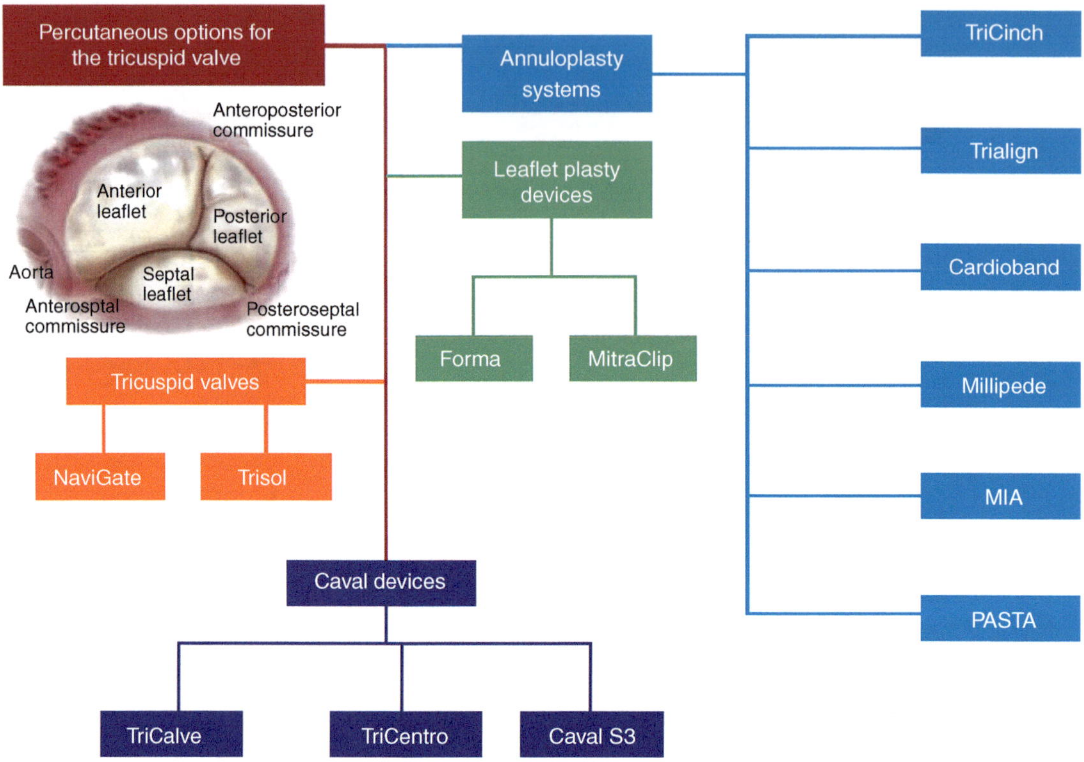

Fig. 1.26 Percutaneous interventions for tricuspid regurgitation

AT can be made out from surface ECG by modified Zhou's algorithm and after 3D mapping system, can be ablated with lesser success (65–70%) [38]. Atrial fibrillation (AF) in non-valvular etiology leading to heart failure patients have been studied for Afib ablation and in rhythm control was found to be better than rate control and improvement of heart failure and EF [39]. Afib ablation techniques include pulmonary vein isolation, roofline, and mitral line block with or without CTI ablation. VT (Fig. 1.33) in ischemic cardiomyopathy can be mapped by pace map or substrate modification and can be ablated with 3D CARTO (Johnson) or NAV X (Abott). VT in a normal structural heart can also be ablated using 3D guided endocardial technique but often epicardial ablation is required in this subset. Epicardial ablation of RVOT is coming up as a treatment of Brugada syndrome (Fig. 1.34) [40].

In atrial fibrillation, lenient rate control is the current consensus of therapy and anticoagulation is recommended calculating the risk of stroke and bleeding. NOACs are better than VKAs in terms of less bleeding chances and no need to monitor PT-INR. In CKD patients, Dabigatran is to be used cautiously. Rivaroxaban has the highest evidence in patients of AF also having ACS. Apixaban has the least gastrointestinal bleeding complication. Idarucizumab has emerged as a treatment for NOACs induced bleeding where urgent reversal of Dabigatran is mandated [41]. In patients of AF, complex LAA anatomy, low LA strain, and low-pulse Doppler velocity are independent predictors of thrombus formation and stroke [42]. So, in patients, where NOACs are contraindicated or complicated by serious adverse effects, LAA closure by watchman device or, ACP or Amulet can be contemplated (Fig. 1.35) [43]. In patients with atrial fibrillation who are undergoing stenting need triple therapy including dual antiplatelets and anticoagulants for at least 3 months (Fig. 1.36) [20]. Chapter 14 provides a current update on the role of yoga in arrythmias.

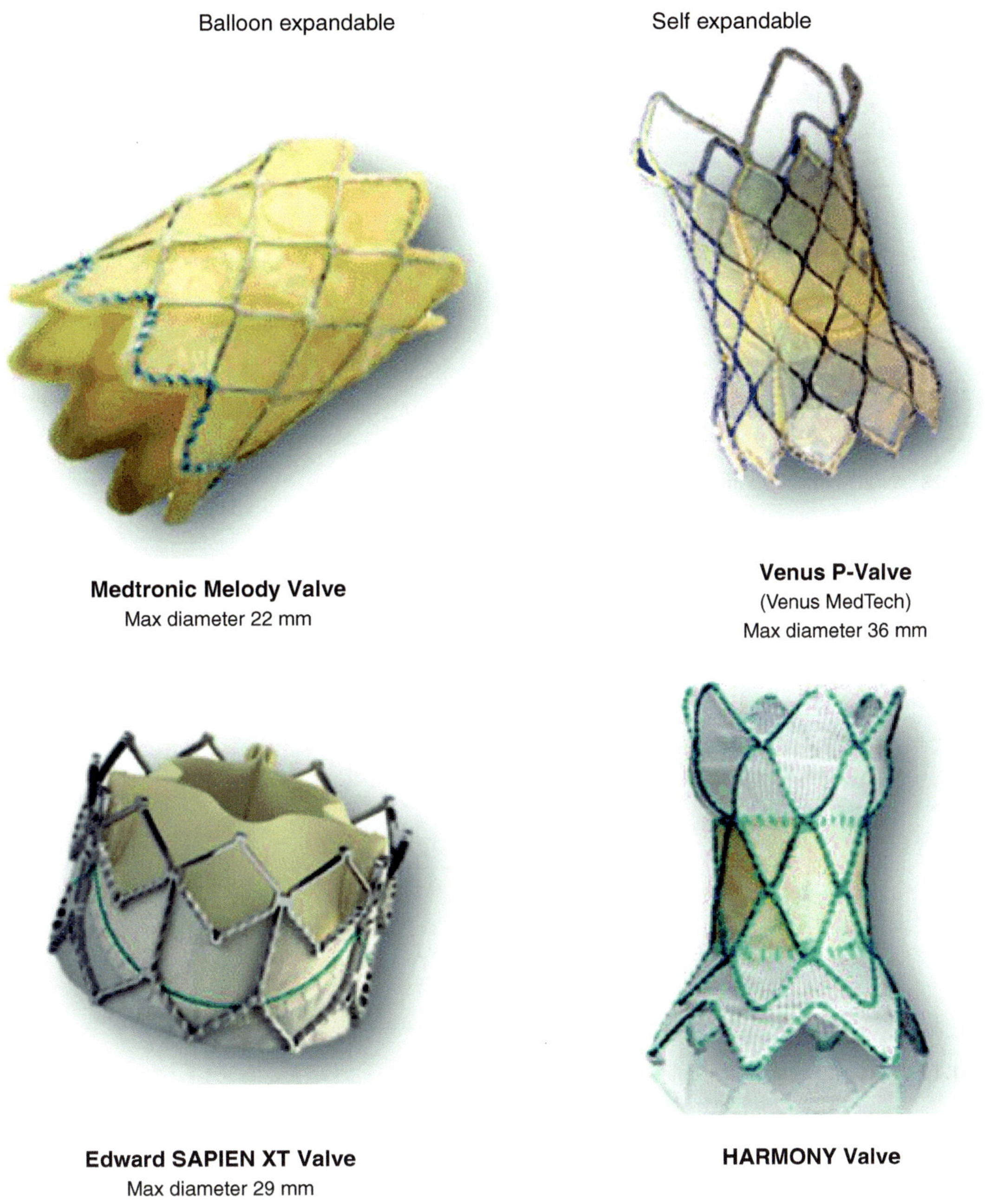

Fig. 1.27 Transcutaneous pulmonary valve replacements

1.7 Cardiomyopathy

Hypertrophic cardiomyopathy (HCM) is a genetic disease characterized by asymmetric septal hypertrophy and the obstructive variety of HCM (HOCM) shows systolic anterior motion (SAM) of anterior mitral valve and the late peaking gradient in the left ventricular outflow tract. Patient presents with exertional shortness of breath due to diastolic dysfunction, chest pain, dizziness, and intermittent episodes of palpitations. Examination reveals jerky pulse, heaving heart with non-displaced apex, s4, and parasternal ejection systolic murmur which increases on

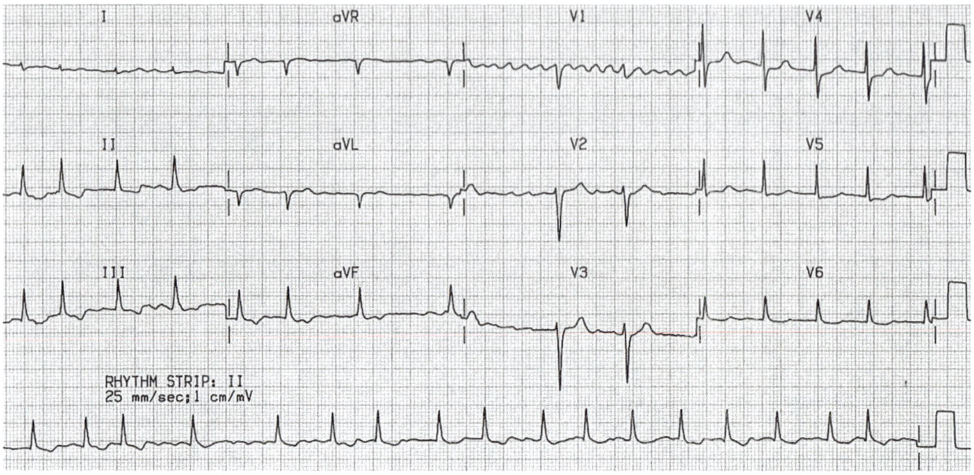

Fig. 1.28 Atrial fibrillation with fast ventricular rate

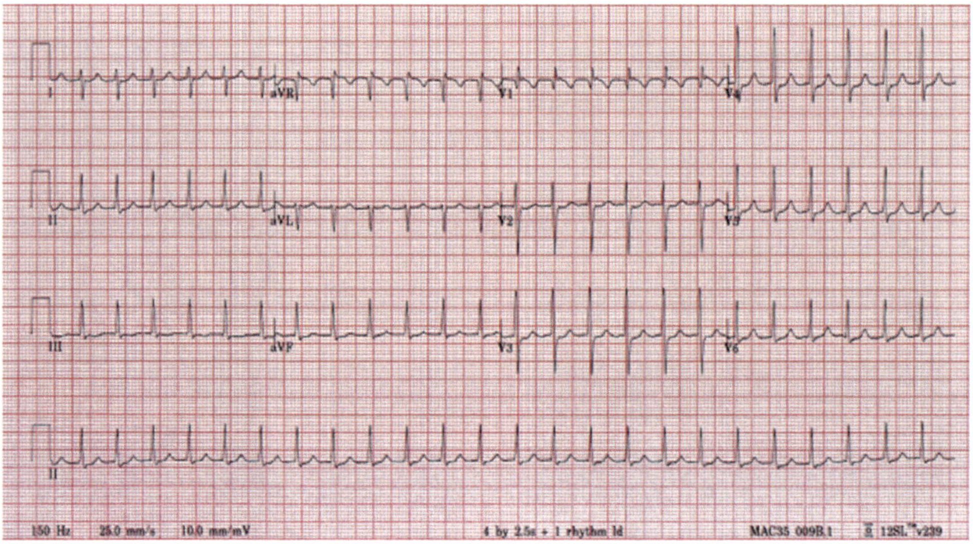

Fig. 1.29 AV nodal reentry tachycardia

standing. ECG in HOCM shows symmetric deep T wave inversions along with features of left ventricular hypertrophy (Fig. 1.37). Treatment for HOCM is beta-blockers or calcium channel blockers and to avoid diuretics, vasodilators, and digoxin. Definitive treatment for HOCM is septal reduction therapy which can be achieved by alcohol septal ablation percutaneously or by surgical myomectomy [44]. To prevent sudden cardiac death due to ventricular arrhythmia, Intracardiac Defibrillator (ICD) is indicated in patients of HOCM with high-risk features (Fig. 1.38).

Restrictive cardiomyopathy could be metabolic or genetic and is characterized by exertional shortness of breath, features of systemic venous congestion with elevated JVP and s4. Leading causes of RCMP are amyloidosis (Fig. 1.39) in elderly, carcinoid in middle age group, and endomyocardial fibrosis (EMF) in children and sarcoidosis in all age group. It is of utmost important to rule out restrictive cardiomyopathy by echocardiography and catheter study, as, prognosis of RCMP is worse than constrictive pericarditis and often no definitive therapy is available.

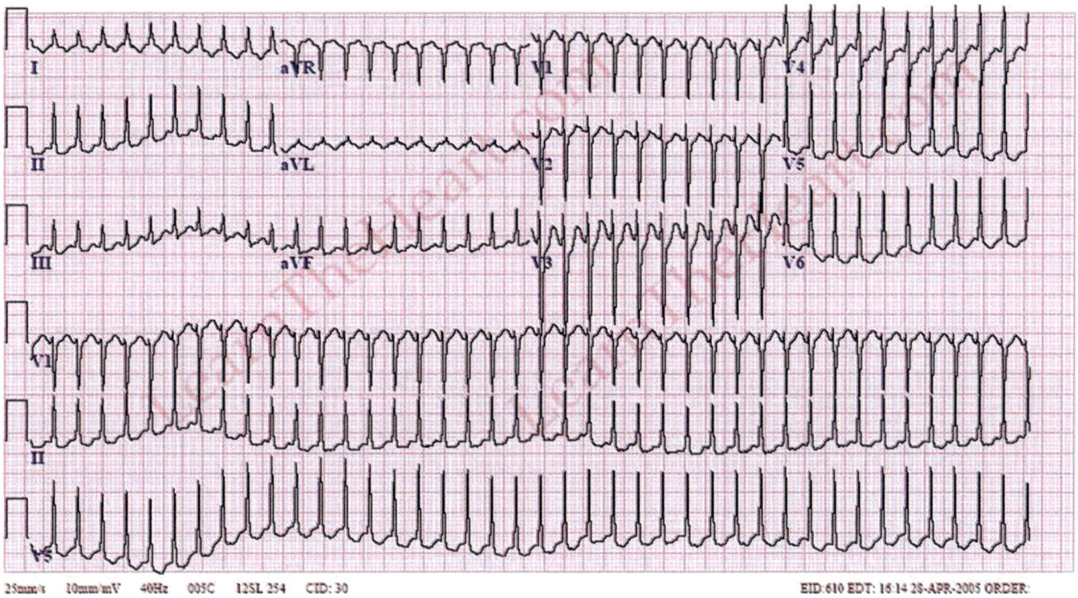

Fig. 1.30 AV reentry tachycardia

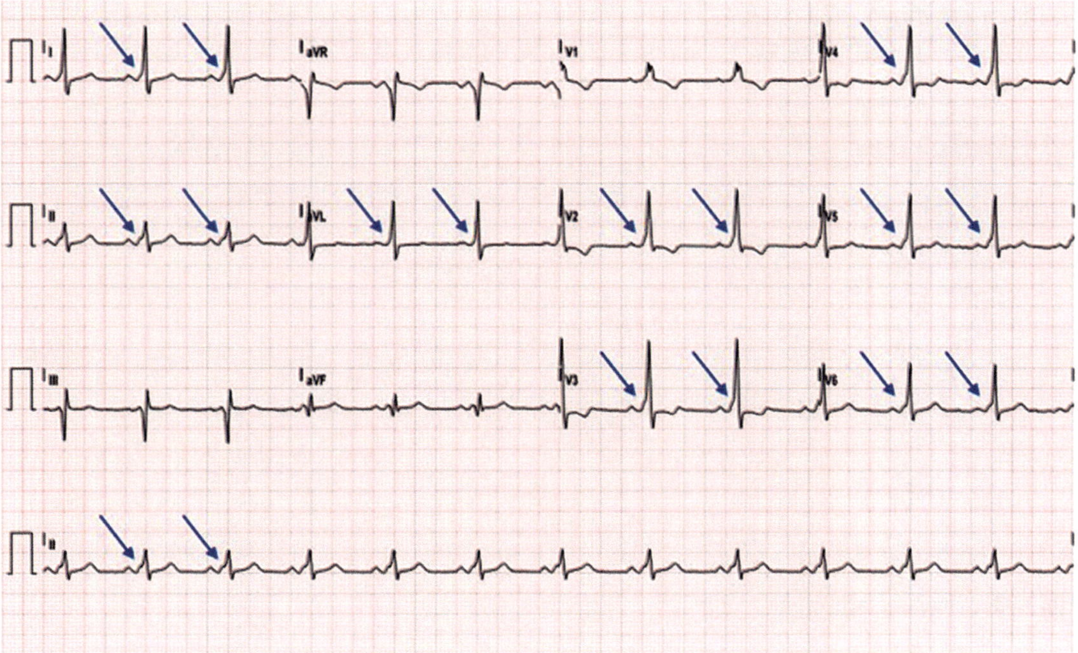

Fig. 1.31 Wolff-Parkinson-White (WPW) syndrome is characterized by short PR interval and delta wave

Dilated cardiomyopathy (DCMP) can be ischemic (suggested by history of myocardial infarction and angiographic evidence of significant coronary artery disease) or non-ischemic (without angiographic evidence of significant coronary artery disease). DCM patients are characterized by low voltage in limb leads, high voltage in chest leads, and poor progression of R waves in precordial leads (Fig. 1.40). DCMP patients present with uni or biventricular failure

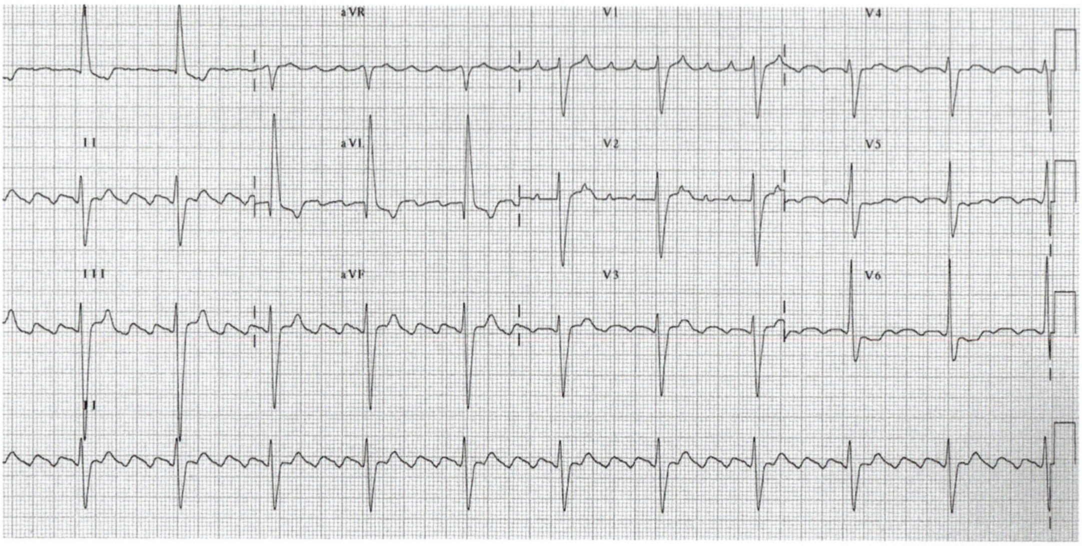

Fig. 1.32 Atrial flutter

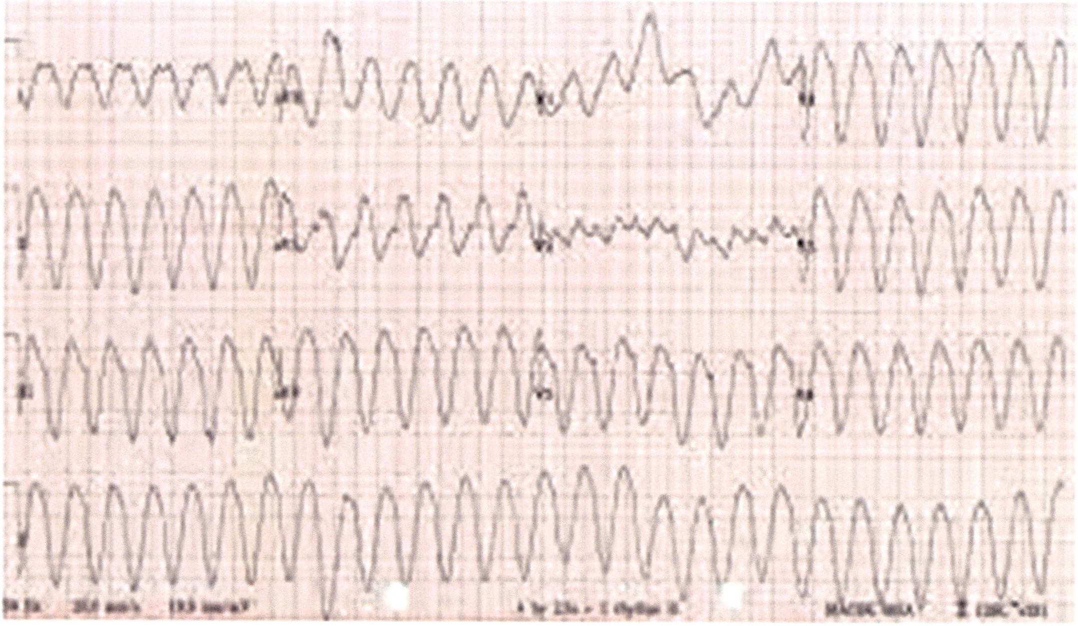

Fig. 1.33 Ventricular tachycardia

and are often difficult to manage with conventional anti-failure therapies which include diuretics, beta-blockers, and ACEI/ARB. Role of digoxin is still debatable. Newer drugs like ivabradine have been found to be beneficial if beta-blockers are contraindicated [45]. Angiotensin receptor and neprilysin inhibitors (ARNI) like sacubitril + valsartan are the class I indication in heart failure and found to be changing the natural history of the patients in heart failure with dramatic change in symptoms, mortality and hospital admissions [45]. Cardiac re-synchronizing therapy (CRT) is indicated in DCM with low ejection fraction (<35%) with LBBB morphology in patients with NYHA I-IVa and has been found to reverse LV remodeling

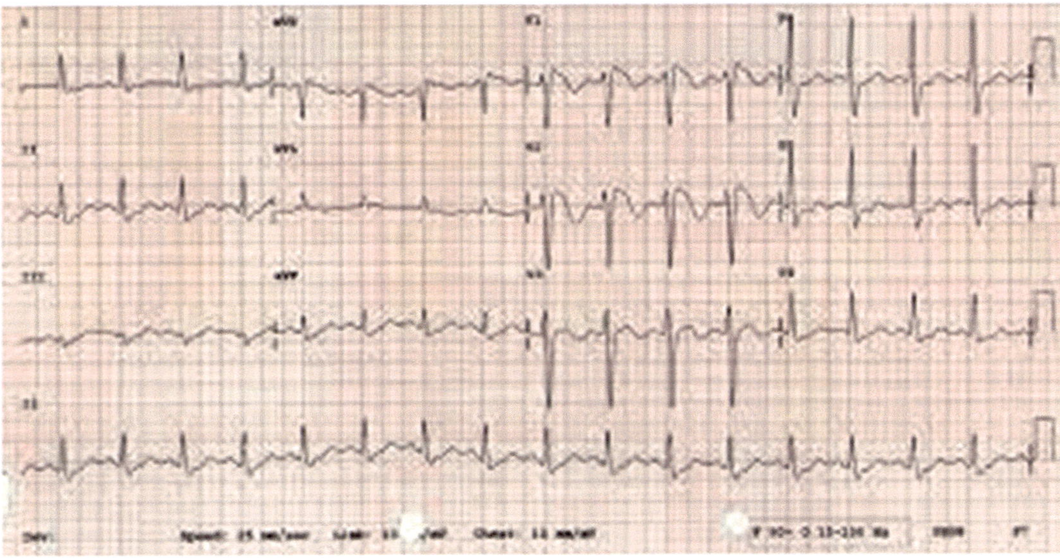

Fig. 1.34 Brugada syndrome

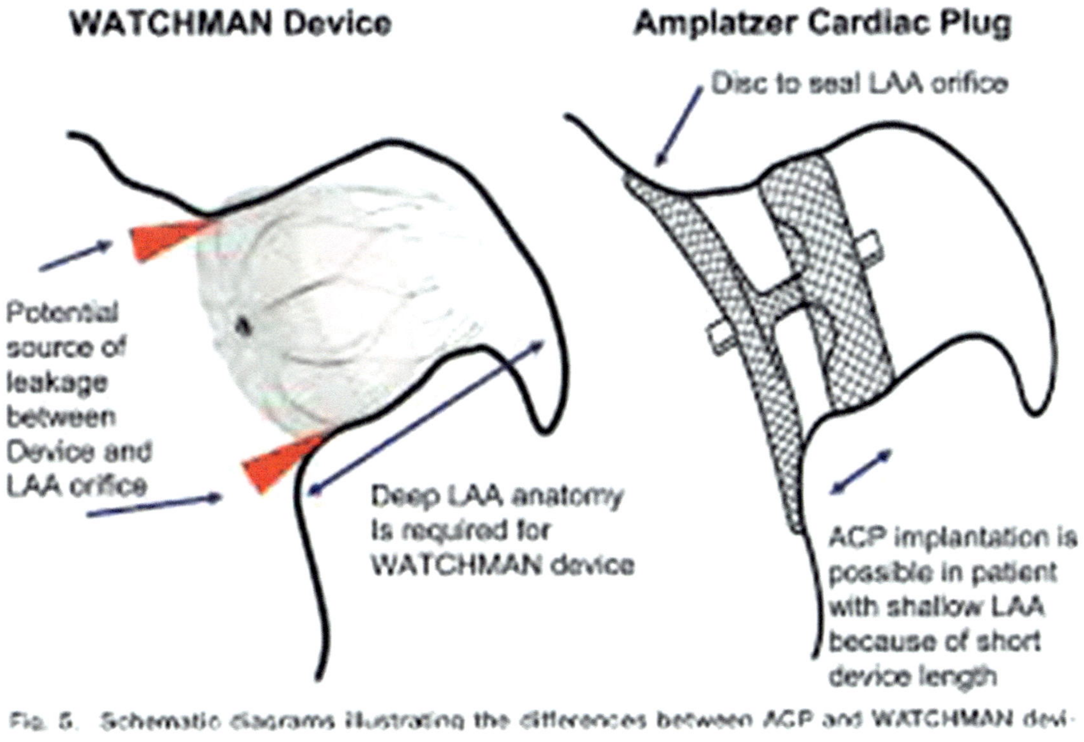

Fig. 1.35 LAA occluder devices

along with improvement of symptoms (Fig. 1.41). However, as high as one-third of CRT recipients could be non-responders and thus adaptive CRT programming is being evaluated [46]. His bundle pacing is also emerging as an alternative to LV pacing in patients with heart failure, especially with non-LBBB morphology (Fig. 1.41) [47].

Reversible cardiomyopathy is a relevant entity and is often seen with the background of hypothyroidism, vitamin deficiency, peripartum car-

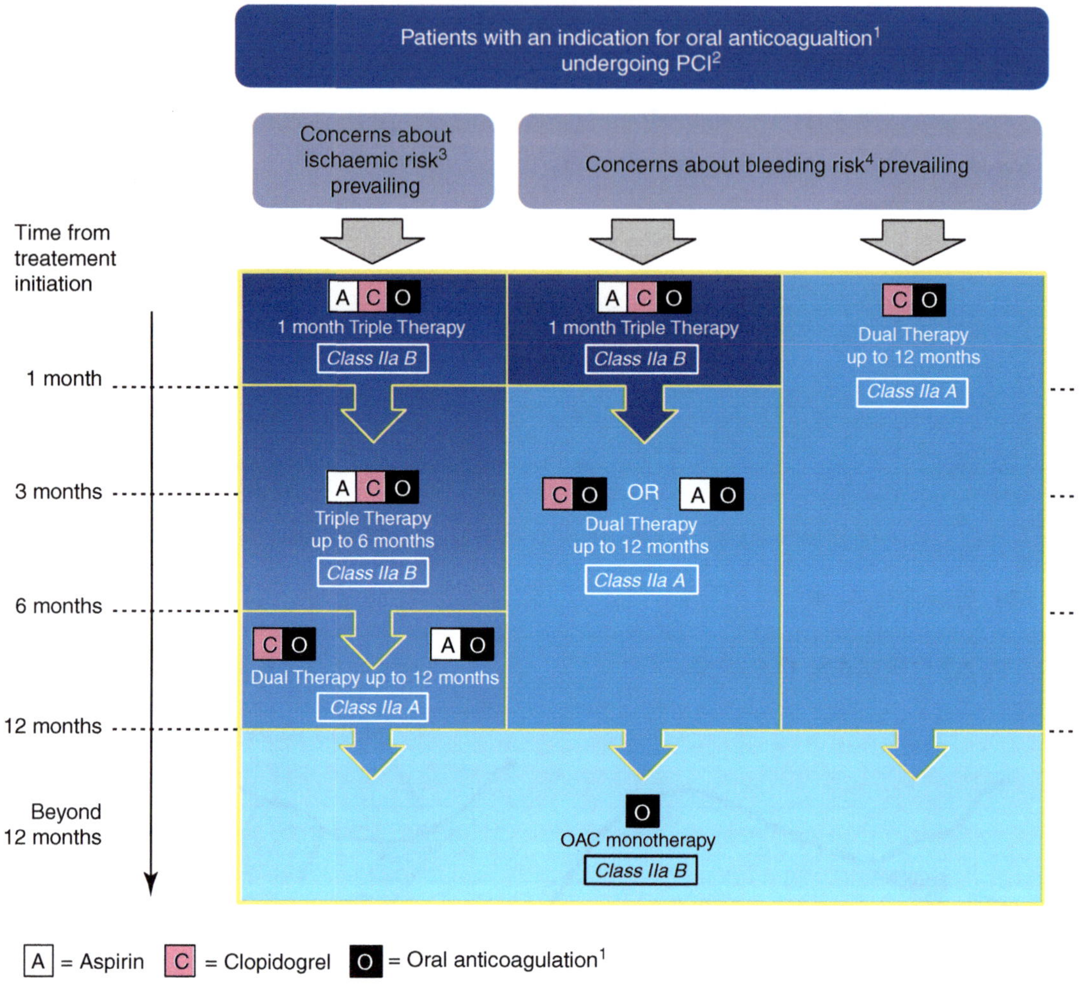

Fig. 1.36 Anticoagulation in patients undergoing angioplasty

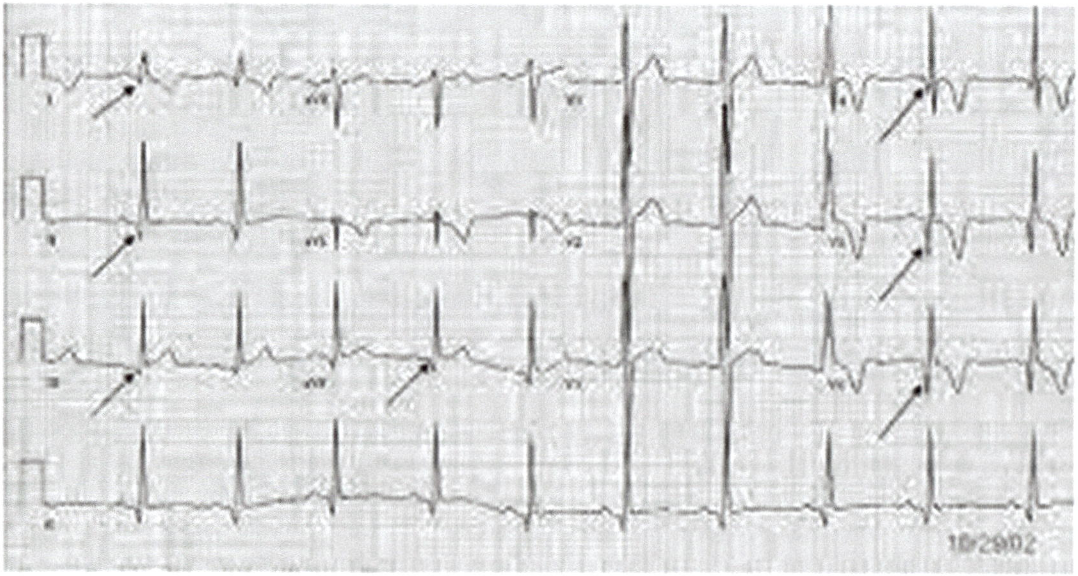

Fig. 1.37 ECG of hypertrophic obstructive cardiomyopathy

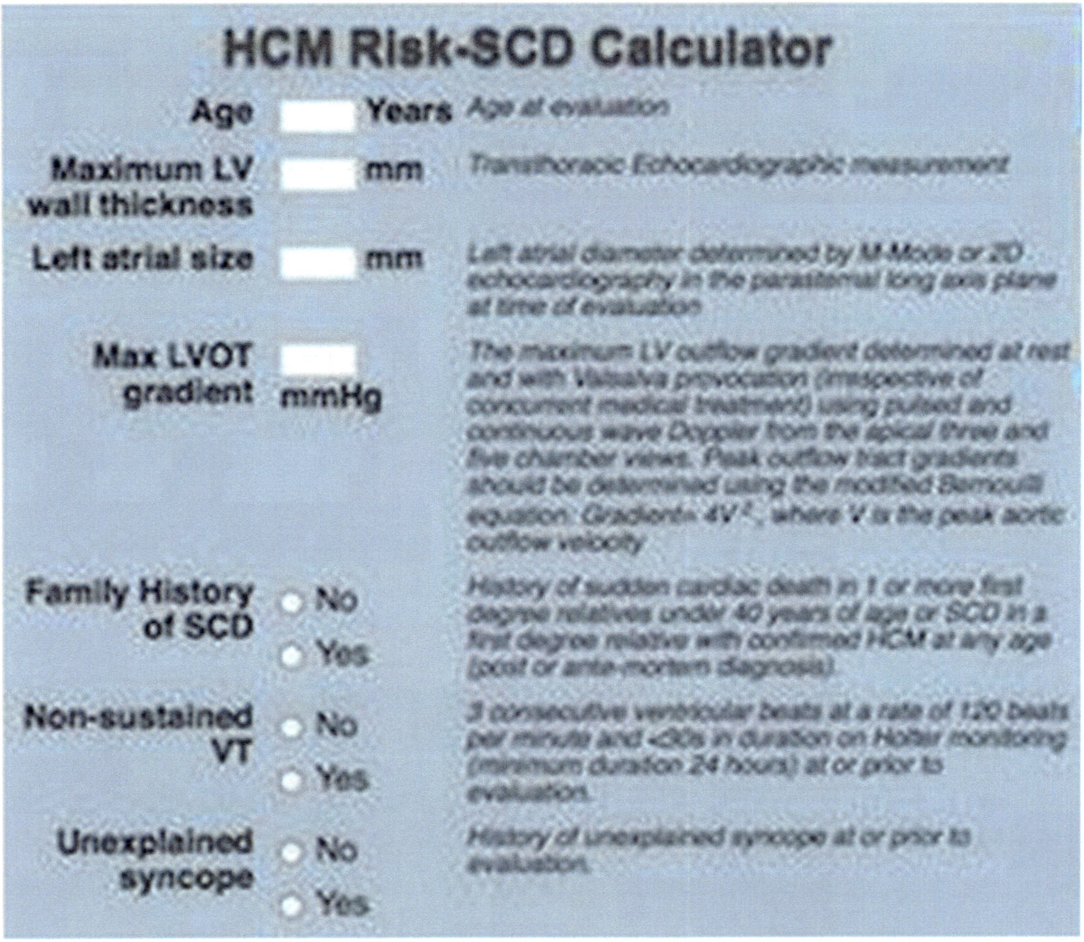

Fig. 1.38 Secondary prevention of sudden cardiac death with intracardiac defibrillator in patients with HOCM

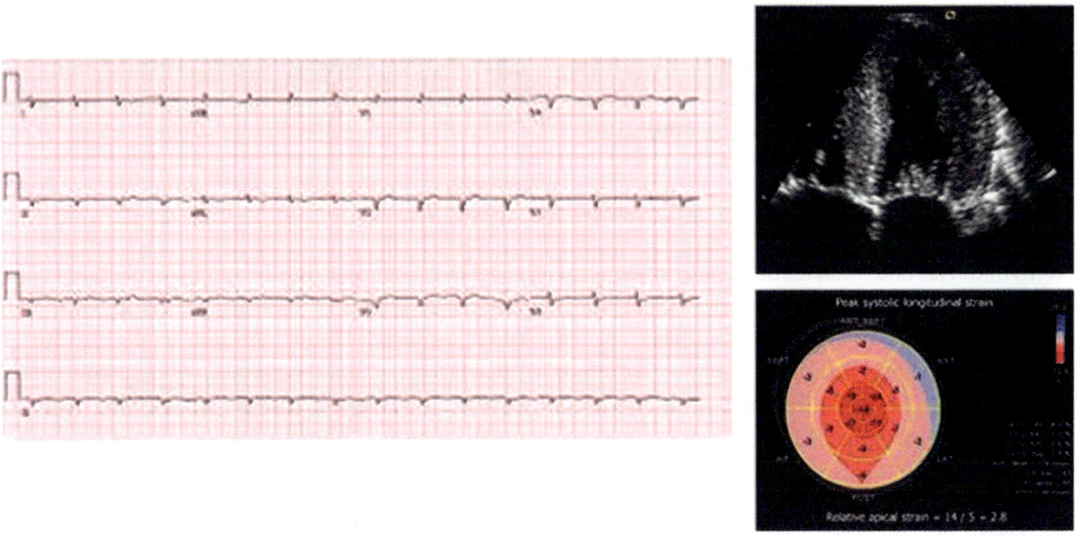

Fig. 1.39 Amyloidosis, ECG shows low voltage complexes and Echocardiography shows left ventricular hypertrophy with speckled pattern

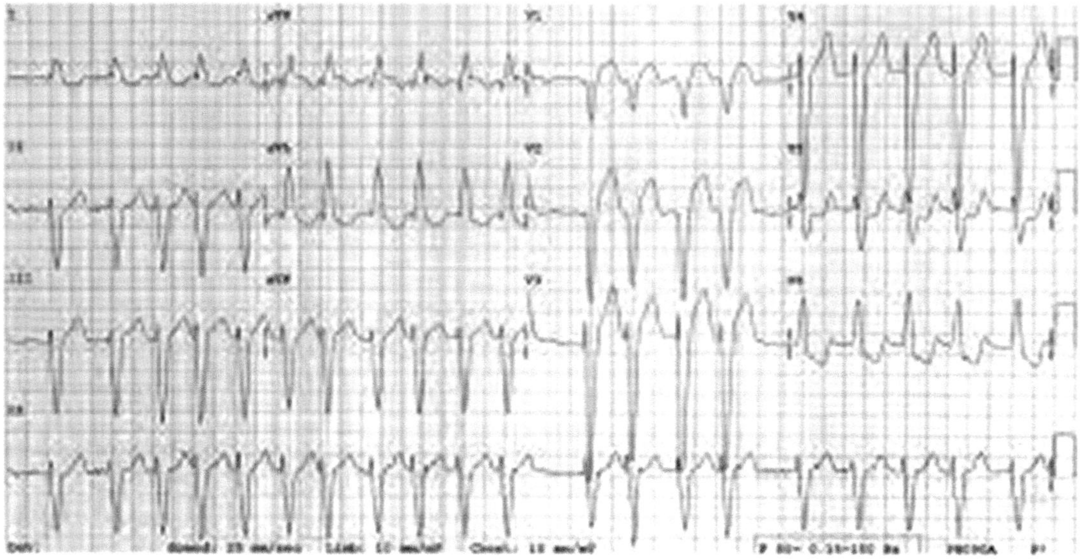

Fig. 1.40 ECG of dilated cardiomyopathy (DCM)

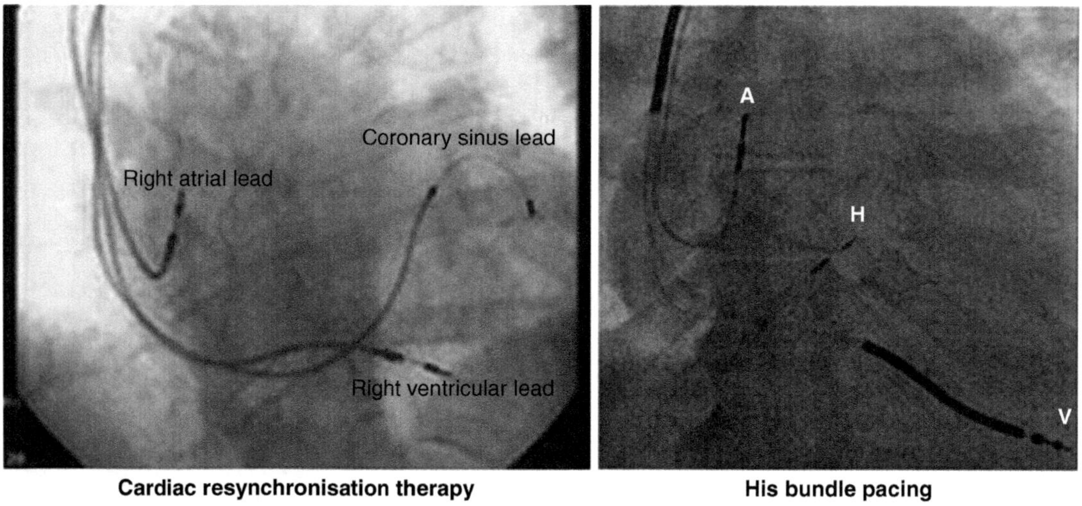

Fig. 1.41 CRT and His bundle pacing

diomyopathy, and takotsubo cardiomyopathy. Gadolinium-enhanced Cardiac MRI is an important investigation in this setting where site of LGE can be a useful marker to diagnose different disease entities and also the total area of LGE is an important prognostic marker for recovery (Fig. 1.42).

Acute pericarditis is mostly viral and often due to uremia in chronic kidney disease patients (CKD). Pericardial rub is a very evanescent phenomenon, which is a superficial scratchy sound, often triphasic. Chest pain due to pericarditis is often lateralized and is more in lying position and patient get relief on sitting and stooping forward position. In the setting of acute coronary syndrome (ACS), pain radiating to the back, classically, to the left trapezius, is suggestive of pericarditis, and escalating dose of aspirin is the treatment.

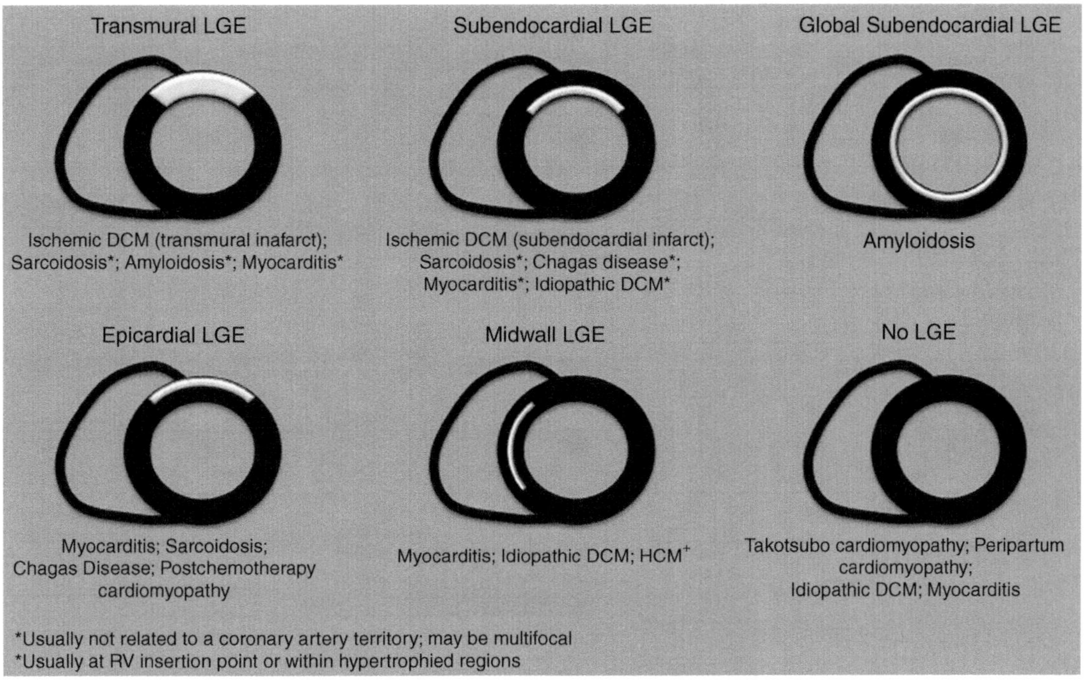

Fig. 1.42 CMRI distribution of late gadolinium enhancement in different cardiomyopathies

1.8 Heart Failure

Heart failure with reduced ejection fraction (EF < 50%) can be ischemic (suggested by history of myocardial infarction and angiographic evidence of significant coronary artery disease) or non-ischemic (without angiographic evidence of significant coronary artery disease). HFrEF patients' presents are often difficult to manage with conventional anti-failure therapies which include diuretics (including potassium-sparing loop diuretics), beta-blockers, and ACEI/ARB. Role of digoxin is still debatable. Newer drugs like ivabradine have been found to be beneficial if beta-blockers are contraindicated. Angiotensin receptor and neprilysin inhibitors (ARNI) like sacubitril + valsartan are the class I indication in heart failure and found to be changing the natural history of the patients in heart failure with dramatic change in symptoms, mortality and hospital admissions (Fig. 1.43) [45]. Cardiac re-synchronizing therapy (CRT) is indicated in DCM with low ejection fraction (<35%) with LBBB morphology in patients with NYHA I-IVa and has been found to reverse LV remodeling along with improvement of symptoms [46]. However, as high as one-third of CRT recipients could be non-responders and thus adaptive CRT programing is being evaluated. His bundle pacing is also emerging as an alternative to LV pacing in patients with heart failure [47]. Vaccination with annual influenza vaccine and five-yearly pneumococcal vaccine is important for patients with heart failure.

The burden of heart failure with preserved ejection fraction (EF > 50%) is increasing along with increase in hypertension, diabetes mellitus, obstructive sleep apnea, metabolic syndrome, atrial fibrillation, and age [48]. No conventional treatments for heart failure has been found to be beneficial in HFpEF patients. ARNI is being investigated in HFpEF patients in PARAGON HF trial [49]. Recent trials showed the role of transcatheter inter-atrial shunt devices in reducing pulmonary capillary wedge pressure (PCWP) in HFpEF patients [50]. Chapter 25 describes the role of yoga in heart Failure.

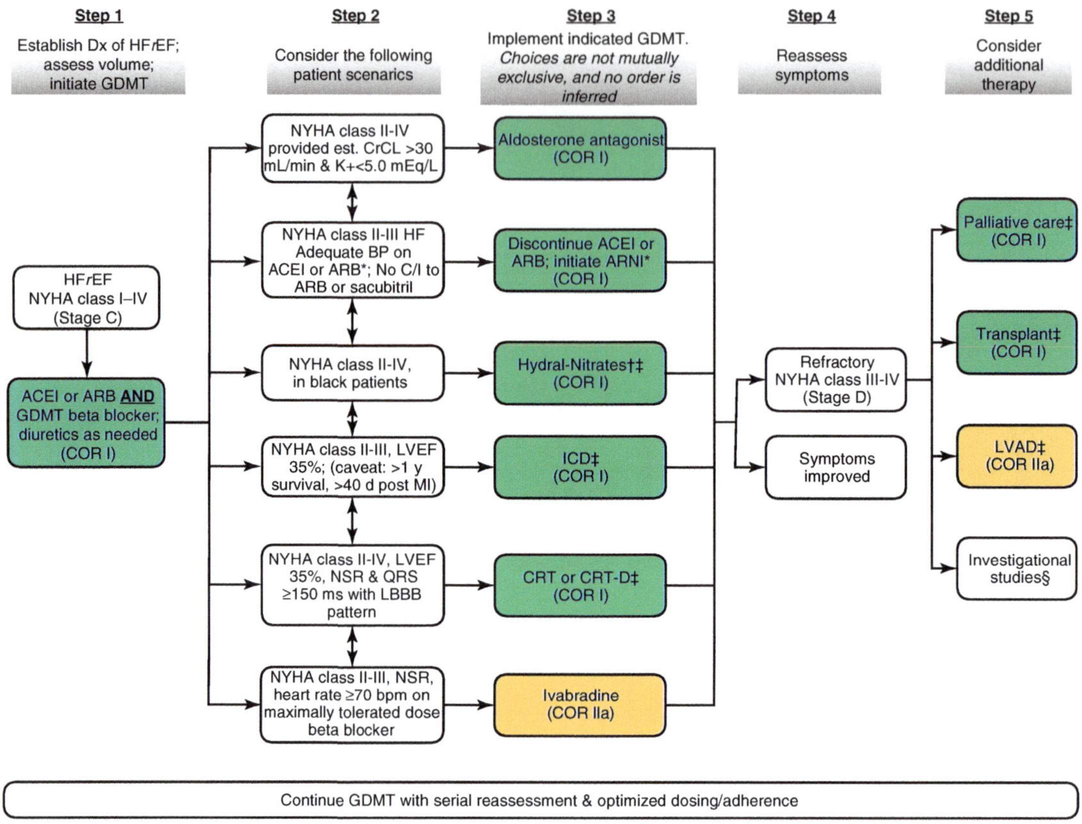

Fig. 1.43 Heart failure guidelines

1.9 Congenital Heart Disease

Congenital heart disease (CHD) can be of acyanotic and cyanotic nature. Acyanotic CHD (ACHD) can be obstructive or shunt lesions. Obstructive congenital heart disease like pulmonary stenosis or aortic stenosis presents at birth with murmur whereas shunt lesions present with murmur after 6 weeks when pulmonary vascular resistance (PVR) drops. Symptomatic severe obstructive lesions like AS or PS can be treated with balloon aortic valvotomy (BAV) or balloon pulmonary valvotomy (BPV) respectively. Shunt lesions can be present at pre-tricuspid or post-tricuspid levels. Atrial septal defect (ASD) is the prototype of pre-tricuspid shunt and is the commonest CHD to be present at birth. Post-tricuspid shunts can be of ventricular septal defect (VSD), patent ductus arteriosus (PDA), and aortopulmonary window (APW). Children with pre-tricuspid shunt present earlier during infancy and their mothers complain of increased precordial activity along with suck-rest-suck cycle and failure to thrive whereas pre-tricuspid shunt patients present in the adult life due to diastolic left-right shunt. In VSD pulmonary artery is exposed to systolic volume overload; diastolic as well as systolic volume overload in PDA (as connection is with descending aorta to left pulmonary artery); as well as systolic volume and pressure overload in APW (as connection is with ascending aorta to main pulmonary artery) and thus intuitively APW presents with Eisenmengerization within the first year of life, in first decade in PDA, second decade in large VSD, and in third decade in ASD. Early Eisenmengerization in ASD is often seen in presence of mitral stenosis (Lutembeche's syndrome), high altitude, anomalous pulmonary venous connections, OP-ASD, associated PAH due to non-cardiac cause. On clinical examination, right ventricular (RV) apex with pulmonary ejection systolic murmur (PESM) and wide fixed S2 split are classical of OS-ASD whereas left ventricular apex (LV) points toward VSD or PDA. Holosystolic murmur with audible P2 is suggestive of VSD and continuous murmur with S2 drowned within the murmur is suggestive of PDA along with high volume pulse. Large left to right shunts with symptoms are an indication of closure in ASD, VSD, and PDA [51]. In suitable cases, percutaneous device closure can be undertaken. Otherwise, surgical closure of shunts is recommended. Once irreversible Eisenmengerization state is achieved, repair of shunt is no more helpful. In shunt lesions with severe PAH and bidirectional shunt exercise-induced drop of SPO2 is a reliable sign of irreversibility, however, cath studies with results of high flow oxygen are indicated to assess operability.

Coarctation of aorta is another obstructive lesion, often presented in the adult life where patients present with upper limb hypertension and lower limb fatigue and characterized by prominent suprasternal pulse, feeble femoral pulse, palpable collaterals in the back (Suzman's sign) with three sign and bilateral notching of third to ninth ribs in the outer and lower parts with sclerosis. Treatments include percutaneous coarctoplasty or surgical repair. Presence of bicuspid aortic valve with AS, PDA, and VSD is not uncommon in COA patients and a thorough clinical and echocardiographic search is necessary.

Cyanotic congenital heart disease (CCHD) can be of four physiological types: right to left shunt (e.g., Tetralogy of Fallot and double outlet right ventricle), admixture physiology (e.g., single ventricle and tricuspid atresia), transposition physiology (transposition of great ventricles), Eisenmengerization (discussed above) and miscellaneous (e.g., Total anomalous pulmonary venous return, Ebstein's anomaly, and pulmonary arteriovenous fistula). Commonest cyanotic congenital heart disease is tetralogy of Fallot is a constellation of infundibular pulmonary stenosis, right ventricular hypertrophy, non-restrictive VSD, and over-riding of aorta and is clinically characterized by the presence of all the following: late-onset cyanosis, normal JVP, no cardiomegaly with RV apex, single loud S2 (A2), short and soft pulmonary ESM, and silent diastole. Cyanosis at birth is usually present in transposition and atresia/aplasia physiology and they present with heart failure in childhood. JVP is elevated in tricuspid atresia. Cardiomegaly is found in transposition physiology and often LV apex signifies absence of pulmonary stenosis physiology or the presence of extensive collaterals in aplasia physiology. The latter group of patients often presents with hemoptysis. Longer and louder pulmonary ESM is often found in ASD/PS physiology (Trilogy and Pentalogy of Fallot) and often in DORV. Diastole is typically silent in TOF and having diastolic murmur may point toward truncus arteriosus in presence of LV apex, collapsing pulse, and cyanosis since birth. CCHD living up to adulthood is commonly seen in Pink Tetralogy, Trilogy, Ebstein, and Eisenmengerization. Since RV impulse is found in both, the key difference is to differentiate PS from PAH and the key finding is dull percussion note over pulmonary area denotes dilated pulmonary artery with banging P2 signifies Eisenmenger's (PAH) and resonant note and prominent suprasternal pulsation with single loud A2 signifies PS physiology (e.g., Tetralogy). Listening to a wide fixed split will clinch the diagnosis of trilogy and more than four heart sounds suggests a diagnosis of Ebstein where RV impulse is dramatically absent. However, echocardiography is the cornerstone in the diagnosis of CCHD.

Treatment of TOF remains intra-cardiac repair (ICR). However, modified Blalock Taussig

Shunt (MBTS) is done in TOF with very small child (weight < 2.5Kg), muscular VSD unamenable to repair, unmanageable recurrent cyanotic spell, and unfavorable coronary artery anomaly [51]. In recent days, RVOT stenting is becoming a choice in neonates with TOF to buy time before ICR and which can be achieved percutaneously without hazard of cardio-pulmonary bypass, midline sternotomy, or prolonged hospital stay [52]. During ICR, BT shunt can be taken down surgically or can be closed by percutaneous device during a hybrid approach. In transposition physiology, switch operation is the treatment of choice but before that Pulmonary artery banding is often necessary to raise the PVR before switch. In single ventricular physiology, where VSD is not routable to any of the great arteries, first step of surgery is to grow pulmonary artery by MBTS and then bidirectional Glenn shunt (BDGS) is done to connect SVC to right pulmonary artery (RPA) and later Fontan procedure is done by connecting IVC to RPA with a fenestration to unload left ventricle. Fontan's ten commandments have been of historical importance and the most important is to have a low PVR to allow passive blood flow thru total cavopulmonary connection (TCPC). Fontan failure is not uncommon where patients present with systemic venous congestion, protein losing enteropathy and deepening of cyanosis, and low cardiac output and a challenge to the surgeons to manage.

1.10 Pericardial Disease

Acute onset of shortness of breath with hypotension with clear lung field and elevated jugular venous pulse (JVP) and muffled heart sounds point toward cardiac tamponade and requires urgent echocardiography to confirm and pericardiocentesis. Common etiologies of massive pericardial effusion are malignancy, tuberculosis, and connective tissue disorders.

Constrictive pericarditis is another entity that leads to low output state and prominent JVP, pericardial knock, and features of systemic venous congestions are telltale features. In developing countries like India, tuberculosis is still the leading cause. It is of utmost importance to rule out restrictive cardiomyopathy by echocardiography and catheter study, as, however, dismal is the prognosis, is still amenable to surgical pericardiectomy.

1.11 Infection of Heart

Viral infections like parvovirus B19, adenovirus, coxsackie B can cause acute myocarditis leading to acute heart failure. Lake Louis criteria have been proposed as diagnostic criteria for acute myocarditis in Gd enhanced cMRI [53]. Viral pericarditis has already been discussed before.

In Indian subcontinents, rheumatic fever caused by Group A beta-hemolytic streptococcus (GABHS) infection, causing acute rheumatic fever, is common to cause pan-carditis. Serological markers like ASO, antiDNAase B, CRP are supportive of GABHS infection.

Chagas disease of heart, is uncommon in India but is known to cause dilated heart with conduction abnormalities and patients often need CRT-D implantation.

1.12 Pulmonary Embolism

In emergency, in patients presenting with acute onset non-central chest pain, cough, and shortness of breath with hemoptysis should be suspected for pulmonary embolism and urgent CT pulmonary angiogram (CTPA) is the test of choice. History of deep vein thrombosis, prolonged immobilization or recent flight travel, or family history of coagulopathy and pulmonary embolism poses the patients at high risk of suspicion. Modified Wells score and simplified Geneva score can be used to suspect patients for having pulmonary embo-

Criteria	Points
Clinical signs/symptoms of DVT	3
PE is most likely diagnosis	3
Tachycardia (>100 bpm)	1.5
Immobilization/surgery in previous 4 weeks	1.5
Prior DVT/PE	1.5
Hemoptysis	1
Active malignancy (trt w/in 6 month)	1

Low Risk	Intermediate risk	High risk
< 2 points	2-6 points	>6 points

PE unlikely	PE Likely
0-4 points	>4 points

Modified Well's score

Geneva score	Original	Simplified
Pain on lower limb deep venous palpation and unilateral edema	4	1
Previous PE or DVT	3	1
Heart rate 75-94 bpm ≥95 bpm	3 5	1 2
Unilateral limb pain	3	1
Surgery or fracture within 1 month	2	1
Hemoptysis	2	1
Active cancer	2	1
Age >65 years	1	1
Clinical probability*		
PE unlikely	≤5	≤2
PE likely	>5	>2

Parameter[a,b]	Score
Age > 80 years	1
History of cancer	1
Chronic cardiopulmonary disease	1
Pulse ≥ 110 bpm	1
Systolic blood pressure < 100 mm Hg	1
Arterial oxyhemoglobin saturation level < 90%	1

0 points = 30-day mortality risk 1.0% (95% CI, 0.0%-2.1%).[b]
≥ 1 point(s) = 30-day mortality risk 10.9% (95% CI ,8.5%-13.2%).[b]

sPESI

Clinical setting	Recommendation
First provoked PE/proximal leg DVT	6 mo
First provoked upper extremity DVT or isolated calf DVT	3 mo
Second provoked VTE	12 mo or indefinite duration
Third VTE	Indefinite duration
Cancer	6 mo or indefinite duration

Fig. 1.44 Pulmonary embolism

lism (Fig. 1.44). In low risk of suspicion, D-dimer could be done. However, sudden on right bundle branch block with sinus tachycardia along with right ventricular dilation with low-pressure tricuspid regurgitation could be a useful marker for suspected pulmonary embolism. Treatment revolves around the simplified pulmonary embolism severity index (sPESI) and in severe hypotension thrombolysis is the choice of treatment in the emergency [54]. Newer modalities like catheter- or ultrasound-guided thrombolysis using EKOS device are proved to be better in long-term results in recent studies (Fig. 1.45). In provoked PE, anticoagulation for 3–6 months and an unprovoked PE, anticoagulation for at least 1 year is necessary along with valuation for any existing pro-thrombotic conditions (Fig. 1.44).

1.13 Peripheral Arterial Disease

Peripheral artery disease is to be suspected in patients with a history of intermittent claudication with risk factors like smoking, diabetes, and dyslipidemia. PAD can be diagnosed by ankle-brachial pressure index (ABPI) <0.9 and should be treated with antiplatelets and statins. Clopidogrel is found to be better than aspirin only in a recent study in patients with rest pain and in gangrene, peripheral artery interventions are indicated. In aortoiliac diseases, percutaneous angioplasty with stenting is a class I indication [55].

Device	Mechanism	Technical Considerations	Regulatory Status in United States
EkoSonic	USAT	5-French catheter	510(k) clearance for marketing in acute PE
Unifuse	CDF	4- to 5-French catheter	510(k) clearance for treatment of peripheral vasculature
Cragg-McNamara	CDF	4- to 5-French catheter	510(k) clearance for treatment of peripheral vasculature
Angiovac	Veno-veno bypass. Funnel-shaped inflow tip to engage thrombi	26-French access for inflow, 16 to 20-French access for outflow. Requires perfusion team	510(k) clearance for removal of undersirable intravascular material
Flowtriever	Nitinol discs engage and mechanically retrieve clot with simultaneous aspiration	20-French catheter. Must manage blood loss associated with large bore aspiration	510(k) clearance for peripheral thrombectomy Investigational device exemption study for PE
Indigo System	Mechanical clot engagement with mechanized aspiration	8-French catheter. Large size of some proximal PE renders en bloc aspiration difficult with 8 French device	510(k) clearance for peripheral thrombectomy
AngioJet	Rheolytic thrombectomy with option of thrombotytic vs saline spray	Hypotension and bradycardia	510(k) clearance for peripheral thrombectomy. Black box warning for use in pulmonary arteries

CDF indicates catheter-directed fibrinolysi; PE, pulmonary embolis; and USAT, ultrasound-assisted catheter-directed thrombolysis.

Fig. 1.45 Device therapies for pulmonary embolism

1.14 Conclusion

Cardiology is an ever-changing domain of science and modern cardiology relies a lot on technological advances: from newer wires to open chronic total coronary occlusions to newer generation of polymer-free stents; left ventricular assist devices in cardiogenic shock to heart transplant for end-stage heart failure. The previous decade has seen the rise of primary PCI to win the war of ischemic injury and the new decade is investigating the role of different therapeutic options to prevent reperfusion injury. Electrophysiological interventions like implantation of his bundle pacing and left ventricular pacing and ablation of complex arrhythmia is increasing with the availability of advanced technological support and expertise. However despite massive technological and scientific development in cardiovascular medicine there remain a large gap in treating chronic cardiovascular diseases. Stress, diet and lifestyle issues dominate as the cause of this epidemic that remains the largest killer in the world killing almost twice the number of patients than cancer the second largest killer. It is thus imperative that people providing cardiovascular care think out of the box and integrate therapies like yoga both to prevent and treat cardiovascular diseases that predominantly arise from lifestyle aberration and stress like Hypertension, certain types of cardiomyopathy, diabetes mellitus and related complications etc. Extensive research in the last decade has delineated the role of yoga in reducing stress and decreasing vascular inflammation that is the hall mark of coronary artery diseases, stroke, peripheral artery disease. Lifestyle diseases including hypertension and diabetes also are remedied or better controlled with yoga as it has shown not only to reverse the pathology of vascular inflammation but also reduce stress and improve compliance to both drugs and diet [56]. Part IV has chapters dedicated to the role of yoga in different cardiovascular conditions.

References

1. Regazzoli D, Ancona F, Trevisi N, et al. Left atrial appendage: physiology, pathology, and role as a therapeutic target. Biomed Res Int. 2015; https://doi.org/10.1155/2015/205013.
2. Basu-Ray I, Sudhakar D, Schwing G, et al. Complex left atrial appendage morphology is an independent risk factor for cryptogenic ischemic stroke. Front Cardiovasc Med. 2018;5:131. https://doi.org/10.3389/fcvm.2018.00131.

3. Lunetta M, Costa F, La Gattuta M. Transesophageal contrast echocardiography is not always the gold standard method in the identification of a patent foramen ovale: a clinical case. J Cardiovasc Echogr. 2015;25(3):86–9. https://doi.org/10.4103/2211-4122.166084.
4. Qian ZY, Hou XF, Xu DJ, Yang B, et al. An algorithm to predict the site of origin of focal atrial tachycardia. Pacing Clin Electrophysiol. 2011;34(4):414–21. https://doi.org/10.1111/j.1540-8159.2010.02980.x.
5. De Maria GL, Kassimis G, Raina T, et al. Reconsidering the back door approach by targeting the coronary sinus in ischaemic heart disease. Heart. 2016;102:1263–9. https://doi.org/10.1136/heartjnl-2016-309642.
6. Mocumbi AO, Ferreira MB, Sidi D, et al. A population study of endomyocardial fibrosis in a rural area of Mozambique. N Engl J Med. 2008;359:43–9.
7. Carey RM, Whelton PK. 2017 ACC/AHA/AAPA/ABC/ACPM/AGS/APhA/ASH/ASPC/NMA/PCNA guideline for the prevention, detection, evaluation, and management of high blood pressure in adults: a report of the American College of Cardiology/American Heart Association task force on clinical practice guidelines. J Am Coll Cardiol. 2018;71:e127–248.
8. Carey RM, Calhoun DA. Resistant hypertension: detection, evaluation, and management a scientific statement from the American Heart Association. Hypertension. 2018;72:e53–90. https://doi.org/10.1161/HYP.0000000000000084.
9. Briasoulis A, Bakris GL. Current status of renal denervation in hypertension. Curr Cardiol Rep. 2016;18(11):107. https://doi.org/10.1007/s11886-016-0781-2.
10. Gordin D, Fadl Elmula FEM, Andersson B, et al. The effects of baroreflex activation therapy on blood pressure and sympathetic function in patients with refractory hypertension: the rationale and design of the Nordic BAT study. Blood Press. 2017;26(5):294–302. https://doi.org/10.1080/08037051.2017.1332477.
11. Kapil V, Sobotka PA, Saxena M. Central iliac arteriovenous anastomosis for hypertension: targeting mechanical aspects of the circulation. Curr Hypertens Rep. 2015;17(9):73. https://doi.org/10.1007/s11906-015-0585-6.
12. Thygesen K, Alpert JS, Jaffe AS, et al. European Society of Cardiology (ESC)/American College of Cardiology (ACC)/American Heart Association (AHA)/World Heart Federation (WHF) task force for the universal definition of myocardial infarction. Circulation. 2018;138(20):e618–51. https://doi.org/10.1161/CIR.0000000000000617.
13. Moss AJ, Williams MC, Newby DE, et al. The updated NICE guidelines: cardiac CT as the first-line test for coronary artery disease. Curr Cardiovasc Imaging Rep. 2017;10:15. https://doi.org/10.1007/s12410-017-9412-6.
14. Nakanishi R, Budoff MJ. Noninvasive FFR derived from coronary CT angiography in the management of coronary artery disease: technology and clinical update. Vasc Health Risk Manag. 2016;12:269–78. https://doi.org/10.2147/VHRM.S79632.
15. Timmis A, Roobottom CA. National Institute for health and care excellence updates the stable chest pain guideline with radical changes to the diagnostic paradigm. Heart. 2017;103(13):982–6. https://doi.org/10.1136/heartjnl-2015-308341.
16. Neumann EJ, Sousa-Uva M, Ahlsson A, et al. 2018 ESC/EACTS guidelines on myocardial revascularization the task force on myocardial revascularization of the European Society of Cardiology (ESC) and European Association for Cardio-Thoracic Surgery (EACTS). Eur Heart J. 2018;40:87–165. https://doi.org/10.1093/eurheartj/ehy394.
17. Götberg M, Cook CM, Sen S, et al. The evolving future of instantaneous wave-free ratio and fractional flow reserve. N Engl J Med. 2017;377:1240–9.
18. De Jaegere PP, Arnold AA, Balk AH, et al. Intracranial hemorrhage in association with thrombolytic therapy: incidence and clinical predictive factors. J Am Coll Cardiol. 1992 Feb;19(2):289–94.
19. Guha S, Sethi R, Ray S, et al. Cardiological Society of India: position statement for the management of ST elevation myocardial infarction in India. Indian Heart J. 2017 Apr;69(Suppl 1):S63–97. https://doi.org/10.1016/j.ihj.2017.03.006.
20. Ibanez B, James S, Agewall S, et al. ESC guidelines for the management of acute myocardial infarction in patients presenting with ST-segment elevation: the task force for the management of acute myocardial infarction in patients presenting with ST-segment elevation of the European Society of Cardiology (ESC). Eur Heart J. 2017;2018:119–77. https://doi.org/10.1093/eurheartj/ehx393.
21. Huu AL, Shum-Tim D. Intra-aortic balloon pump: current evidence & future perspectives. Futur Cardiol. 2018;14(4):319–28. https://doi.org/10.2217/fca-2017-0070.
22. Kapur NK, Alkhouli M, DeMartini T, et al. Unloading the left ventricle before reperfusion in patients with anterior ST-segment elevation myocardial infarction. Circulation. 2019;139(3):337–46.
23. Marco Valgimigli M, Bueno H, Byrne RA, et al. Focused update on dual antiplatelet therapy (DAPT). ESC clinical practice guidelines. Eur Heart J. 2018;39(3):213–60. https://doi.org/10.1093/eurheartj/ehx419.
24. Grundy SM, Stone NJ, Bailey AL, et al. 2018 ACC/AHA/AACVPR/AAPA/ABC/ACPM/ADA/AGS/APhA/ASPC/NLA/PCNA guideline on the management of blood cholesterol: a report of the American College of Cardiology Foundation/American Heart Association task force on clinical practice guidelines. J Am Coll Cardiol. 2019;73(24):3168–209.
25. Adams DH, Raphael Rosenhek R, Falk V, et al. Degenerative mitral valve regurgitation: best practice revolution. Eur Heart J. 2010;31(16):1958–66.

26. Manjunath CN, Srinivas P, Ravindranath KS, et al. Incidence and patterns of valvular heart disease in a tertiary care high-volume cardiac center: a single center experience. Indian Heart J. 2014;66(3):320–6. https://doi.org/10.1016/j.ihj.2014.03.010.
27. Nishimura RA, Otto CM, Robert O, et al. 2017 AHA/ACC focused update of the 2014 AHA/ACC guideline for the management of patients with valvular heart disease: a report of the American College of Cardiology/American Heart Association task force on clinical practice guidelines. Circulation. 2017;135:e1159–95.
28. Manjunath CN, Srinivasa KH, Ravindranath KS, et al. Balloon mitral valvotomy in patients with mitral stenosis and left atrial thrombus. Catheter Cardiovasc Interv. 2009;74(4):653–61. https://doi.org/10.1002/ccd.22176.
29. Duggal B, Bajaj M, Prabhu S, Mathew T, et al. The mitral leaflet separation index for assessment of mitral stenosis during percutaneous mitral commissurotomy: validation of the index in the immediate post-PMC period. Echocardiography. 2012;29(10):1143–8. https://doi.org/10.1111/j.1540-8175.2012.01787.x.
30. O'Gara PT, Grayburn PA, Badhwar V, et al. 2017 ACC expert consensus decision pathway on the management of mitral regurgitation. A report of the American College of Cardiology task force on expert consensus decision pathways. J Am Coll Cardiol. 2017;70(19):2421–49. https://doi.org/10.1016/j.jacc.2017.09.019.
31. El Sabbagh A, Reddy V, Nishimura RA, et al. Mitral valve regurgitation in the contemporary era. JACC Cardiovasc Imaging. 2018;11(4):628–43. https://doi.org/10.1016/j.jcmg.2018.01.009.
32. Rodés-Cabau J. Transcatheter mitral valve replacement. J Am Coll Cardiol. 2018;71(1):22–4. https://doi.org/10.1016/j.jacc.2017.11.015.
33. Kusumoto FM, Schoenfeld MH, Barrett C, et al. 2018 ACC/AHA/HRS guideline on the evaluation and management of patients with bradycardia and cardiac conduction delay: a report of the American College of Cardiology/American Heart Association task force on clinical practice guidelines, and the Heart Rhythm Society. J Am Coll Cardiol. 2018; https://doi.org/10.1016/j.jacc.2018.10.043.
34. Zhuang L, Mao Y, Wu L, et al. Effects of right ventricular septum or His-bundle pacing versus right ventricular apical pacing on cardiac function: a systematic review and meta-analysis of randomized controlled trials. J Int Med Res. 2018;46(9):3848–60. https://doi.org/10.1177/0300060518781415.
35. Wilkoff BL. The dual chamber and VVI implantable defibrillator (DAVID) trial: rationale, design, results, clinical implications and lessons for future trials. Card Electrophysiol Rev. 2003;7(4):468–72.
36. Arruda MS, McClelland JH, Wang X, Beckman KJ, et al. Development and validation of an ECG algorithm for identifying accessory pathway ablation site in Wolff-Parkinson-White syndrome. J Cardiovasc Electrophysiol. 1998;9(1):2–12.
37. Qian Z, Hou X. An algorithm to predict the site of origin of focal atrial tachycardia. Pacing Clin Electrophysiol. 2011;34(4):414–21.
38. Turagam MK, Garg J, Whang W, et al. Catheter ablation of atrial fibrillation in patients with heart failure: a meta-analysis of randomized controlled trials. Ann Intern Med. 2018; https://doi.org/10.7326/M18-0992.
39. Brugada J, Pappone C, Berruezo A, et al. Brugada syndrome phenotype elimination by epicardial substrate ablation. Arrhythm Electrophysiol. 2015;8:1373–81.
40. Steffel J, Verhamme P, Potpara TS, et al. The 2018 European Heart Rhythm Association practical guide on the use of non-vitamin K antagonist oral anticoagulants in patients with atrial fibrillation. Eur Heart J. 2018;39(16):1330–93.
41. Yaghi S, Song C, Gray WA, et al. Left atrial appendage function and stroke risk. Stroke. 2015;46(12):3554–9. https://doi.org/10.1161/STROKEAHA.115.011273.
42. Kosturakis R, Price MJ. Current state of left atrial appendage closure. Curr Cardiol Rep. 2018;20(6):42. https://doi.org/10.1007/s11886-018-0981-z.
43. Maron BJ, Rowin EJ, Udelson JE. Clinical spectrum and management of heart failure in hypertrophic cardiomyopathy. JACC Heart Fail. 2018;6(5):353–63. https://doi.org/10.1016/j.jchf.2017.09.011.
44. Prinz C, Farr M, Hering D, Horstkotte D, Faber L. The diagnosis and treatment of hypertrophic cardiomyopathy. Dtsch Arztebl Int. 2011;108(13):209–15. https://doi.org/10.3238/arztebl.2011.0209.
45. Yancy CW, Jessup M, Bozkurt B, et al. 2017 ACC/AHA/HFSA focused update of the 2013 ACCF/AHA guideline for the management of heart failure: a report of the American College of Cardiology/American Heart Association task force on clinical practice guidelines and the Heart Failure Society of America. Circulation. 2017;136:e137–61.
46. Martens P, Verbrugge FH, Nijst P, et al. Incremental benefit of cardiac resynchronisation therapy with versus without a defibrillator. Heart. 2017;103:1977–84.
47. Arnold AD, Shun-Shin MJ, Keene D, et al. His resynchronization versus biventricular pacing in patients with heart failure and left bundle branch block. J Am Coll Cardiol. 2018;72(24):3112–22. https://doi.org/10.1016/j.jacc.2018.09.073.
48. Lam CSP, Voors AA, de Boer RA, et al. Heart failure with preserved ejection fraction: from mechanisms to therapies. Eur Heart J. 2018;39:2780–92. https://doi.org/10.1093/eurheartj/ehy301.
49. Solomon SD, Rizkala AR, Gong J, et al. Angiotensin receptor neprilysin inhibition in heart failure with preserved ejection fraction: rationale and design of the PARAGON-HF trial. JACC Heart Fail. 2017;5(7):471–82. https://doi.org/10.1016/j.jchf.2017.04.013.
50. Feldman T, Mauri L, Kahwash R, et al. Transcatheter interatrial shunt device for the treatment of heart failure with preserved ejection fraction (REDUCE LAP-HF I [reduce elevated left atrial pressure in patients with heart failure])-A phase 2, ran-

domized, sham-controlled trial. Circulation. 2017;137:364–75.
51. Stout KK, Daniels CJ, Aboulhosn JA, et al. 2018 AHA/ACC guideline for the Management of Adults with Congenital Heart Disease: a report of the American College of Cardiology/American Heart Association task force on clinical practice guidelines. J Am Coll Cardiol. 2018; https://doi.org/10.1016/j.jacc.2018.08.1028.
52. Quandt D, Ramchandani B, Penford G, et al. Right ventricular outflow tract stent versus BT shunt palliation in tetralogy of Fallot. Heart. 2017;103(24):1985–91.
53. Friedrich MG, Sechtem U, Schulz-Menger J, et al. Cardiovascular magnetic resonance in myocarditis: a JACC white paper. J Am Coll Cardiol. 2009;53(17):1475–87.
54. Aggarwal V, Nicolais CD, Aaron Lee A, et al. Acute management of pulmonary embolism. JACC expert analysis 2017. American College of Cardiology.
55. Kithcart AP, Beckman JA. ACC/AHA versus ESC guidelines for diagnosis and management of peripheral artery disease. *JACC* guideline comparison. J Am Coll Cardiol. 2018;72(22):2789–801.
56. Dutta A, Aruchunan M, Mukherjee A, et al. Journal of integrative and complementary medicine. https://doi.org/10.1089/jicm.2021.0420.

Addressing the Common Risk Factors for Reducing the Burden of Cardiovascular Diseases: The Impact of Yoga

2

K. Srinath Reddy and Manu Raj Mathur

2.1 Introduction

Health is an integral part of psychosocial well-being and population productivity. However, it is constantly faced with numerous challenges. Of these multifarious health challenges, the challenge posed by the rising burden of non-communicable diseases (NCDs) such as Cardiovascular diseases (CVDs), Diabetes, Chronic Respiratory Diseases, and cancers are the most significant. A comprehensive response is, therefore, urgently required to reverse this rising prevalence of NCDs. This will require both a robust health system response and coordinated multi-sectoral actions on the many determinants of NCDs.

CVDs such as Ischemic Heart Disease (IHD), hypertensive heart disease, rheumatic heart disease, and cerebrovascular disease or stroke [1] are the major contributors of deaths due to NCDs (17.9 million deaths out of 41 million annual NCD deaths). More than one-third of the deaths are confined to low- and middle-income countries [2] (Fig. 2.1). CVDs have a wide range of contributing risk factors, and are mostly preventable. However, a number of effective low-cost prevention strategies are required to be addressed to reduce its current burden. With the current efforts, less than half of the countries will be able to achieve the sustainable development goals (SDG) 2030 target to reduce CVDs burden by one-third [3].

K. S. Reddy (✉) · M. R. Mathur
Public Health Foundation of India,
Gurgaon, Haryana, India
e-mail: Ksrinath.reddy@phfi.org

2.2 The Global Burden of Cardiovascular Diseases

Noncommunicable diseases are currently leading the way in global mortality. A major proportion of this burden is attributable to CVDs (Fig. 2.2). According to the Global Burden of Disease [4], the mortality for CVDs was estimated to be 32% in 2017 remaining constant throughout the entire spectrum of socioeconomic hierarchy (Table 2.1) predominantly occurring in 70 plus years old.

Regionally, mortality due to CVDs is highest in Central Europe, Eastern Europe, and Central Asia (54%), closely followed by North Africa and Middle East (39%). For the age group of 15–49 years the mortality is gradually climbing the ladder; with Central Europe, Eastern Europe (22%) and Central Asia Southeast Asia, East Asia, and Oceania (22%) in 2017 from (20.9%) and (16.22%), respectively, in 1990.

I. Basu-Ray, D. Mehta (eds.), *The Principles and Practice of Yoga in Cardiovascular Medicine*,
https://doi.org/10.1007/978-981-16-6913-2_2

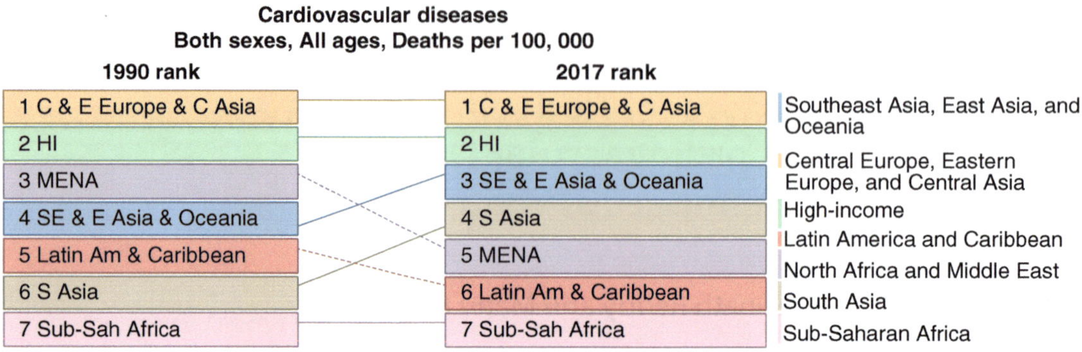

Fig. 2.1 Cardiovascular diseases: regions (both sexes, all ages, deaths per 100 k)

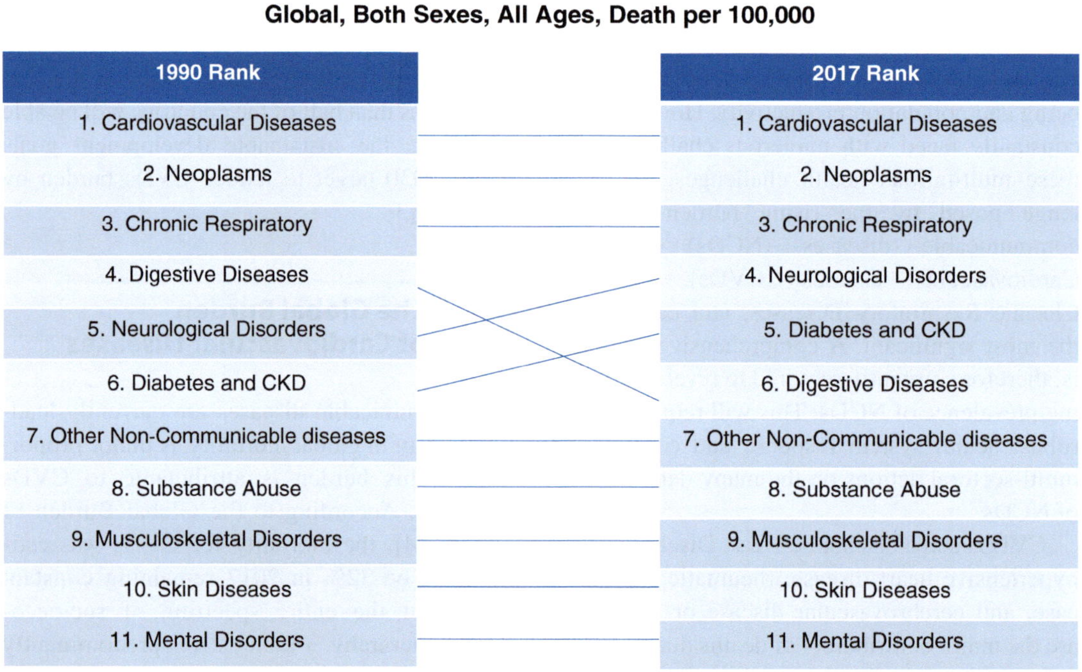

Fig. 2.2 Noncommunicable diseases rank

Table 2.1 CVD summary statistics: globally

Indicator	1990	2005	2017
Deaths (%)	26	28	32
Incidence rate per 100,000	738	834	952
Prevalence rate per 100,000	4914	5458	6356
YLDs rate per 100,000	353	384	467
DALYs rate per 100,000	4946	4761	4788

2.3 Yoga and Cardiovascular Health

An efficient non-pharmacological approach to manage CVD risk factors is "*Yoga*," described by WHO as a "*valuable tool to increase physical activity and decrease noncommunicable dis-*

ease" [5]. Yoga has been particularly seen in the management of NCDs and/or CVDs. "*Adapted everywhere by people of all age groups, irrespective of their socioeconomic status.*" Intervention such as "*Asanas*" (Yoga postures), "*Pranayama*" (Yoga breathing techniques), "*Dhyana*" (meditation), educational gatherings, Yogic diet, and/or Yogic lifestyle have been proven to improve the flexibility and physiological process of the body.

2.4 Epidemiological Evidence: Yoga and Cardiovascular Diseases

The first epidemiological evidence on the favorable effect of Yoga was reported in 1969 from India [6]. Since then studies have associated Yoga with several cardioprotective effects and cardiac rehabilitation [7–9].

One of the first trials on Yoga, "*The Lifestyle Heart Trial*" [10] conducted on 48 participants from 1986 to 1992 with an intervention package including "*aerobic exercise*" concluded "*More regression of coronary atherosclerosis occurred after 5 years than after 1 year in the experimental group.*" The lead author for the said study Dr. Dean Ornish further conducted several studies to test the "*Ornish Programme*" which is a popular phenomenon now. A study done in 2007, by Aldana et al. [11] tested the said regime to conclude an improvement in risk factors.

Observational studies have also determined, reduction in CVD risk factors at yoga retreats [12]. Although, safety of "*Yoga*" interventions is poorly recorded and/or not at all reported in literature [13].

A majority of the systematic reviews and meta-analysis done, for the subject has endorsed the demand for high-quality randomized controlled trials. For example: A systematic review, done in 2014 on the effect of Yoga on CVD risk factors [13] concluded "*the low methodological quality of most of the included studies, future RCTs should ensure rigorous methodology and reporting.*" Another systematic review on the Alternative and Complimentary Therapies for CVD (2016) [14] stated that "*yoga versus at-home yoga versus a control could be of value to measure the benefits of social support for patients at-risk for or diagnosed with cardiovascular disease.*" A review (2018) [15] done on heart failure echoed the same results, the review suggested yoga as a successful addition to the current regime, however, supported the need for high-quality research.

Systematic reviews are done in 2014 [16] and 2015 [17] also concluded that there is moderate evidence on the protective effects of Yoga on diastolic blood pressure, HDL cholesterol and triglycerides, LDL cholesterol, and secondary prevention of coronary heart disease, respectively. Published in 2014, a systematic review highlighted no better effects of meditation as compared to standard treatment in reducing psychological stress [18].

Recognizing the need of the hour, the "*The BABEX Trial*" [19] was conducted in 2016 to recognize, scalable tobacco cessation (risk factor) solutions in a low-cost setting. With approximately 36,000 participants, the trial included an intervention of a single training session of yogic breathing exercises in both the intervention and the control group combined with a single session on quit advice (15 min-intervention group and 1 min-control group). The trial concluded "*substantial effect of a potentially inexpensive, scalable, non-physician-dependent, culturally sensitive intervention to aid cessation of tobacco use in LMIC,*" however, the authors acknowledged the limitation of a small effect size. Another randomized trial in 2018, the "*The Yoga-CaRe trial*" [20] was conceptualized to look at the cardiac rehabilitation after Acute Myocardial Infarction and health benefits of yoga, designed for low-source setting the trial with a sample size of (4014 participants) largest till date, the trial concluded "*numerically fewer outcomes in the Yoga-CaRe group, but not statistically significant.*" However, "*improvement in the self-rated quality of life was significantly greater in the Yoga-CaRe group.*"

A subset of the "*Yoga-CaRe Trial*" and one of the first trials, in geriatric patients after an acute coronary event, the "*Yoga and Cardiovascular Health Trial (YACHT)*" [21] was done in 2019 to test a "*comprehensive approach to measuring cardiovascular clinical and subclinical outcomes in response to a yoga intervention.*" The randomized trial was parallel arm with a sample size of 80 patients (Yoga + Standard Treatment vs Standard Treatment), however, it also estimated no effect in the intervention group.

To summarize, the findings of several studies confirm the beneficial effects of yoga on CVDs. However, a greater part of the evidence has limitations such as small sample size, generalizability, well-defined control group, confounding risk factors, and longer time frame. Well-designed Randomized controlled trials are necessary with precise methodology (sample size, randomization, allocation concealment, intention-to-treat analysis, and blinding) for strong evidence and for perceived side effects.

2.5 Integration of Yoga: Indian Case Study

Yoga has been an integral part of the prevention strategy for India. As a zero-cost health intervention, Yoga has been successfully integrated into the National health stream. The National Health Policy (2017) [22] amalgamates the AYUSH (Ayurveda, Yoga, Unani, Siddha, Homeopathy) as a "*stand-alone to a three-dimensional mainstreaming*" at primary, secondary, and urban levels. The Central Board of Secondary Education (CBSE) in India has also made it mandatory in the curriculum [23], and has also been made compulsory for teacher training by the National Council for Teacher Education (NCTE). In an innovative incorporation, Indian government has also introduced "*Yoga Visas*" to promote yoga education [24].

Emphasizing on the existing strong rationale, the Government of India has also merged AYUSH (Ayurveda, Yoga, Unani, Siddha, Homeopathy) in "*National Programme on Prevention and Control of Diabetes, Cardiovascular diseases and Stroke (NPCDCS)*" at the Primary Health Care (PHC) and Community Health Care (CHC) centers in 2015 [25]. Currently, in its second phase, the program is still ongoing and has been successfully executed in 52 centers (49 CHC and three District Hospital). Interim analysis has shown the reduction and/or discontinuation of the dosage of allopathic medicine after the integration of Ayurveda [26].

2.6 The Future Ahead

The past few years have seen a rejuvenated interest in strengthening primary health care to deliver quality, accessible, and affordable health services for all. The WHO, in 2018, proposed the Declaration of Astana asserting that "*Primary Health Care is a cornerstone of sustainable health system for universal health coverage (UHC) and health-related Sustainable Development Goals.*" With almost one-fifth of the world's population, NCDs are the biggest contributor to the disease burden in India and are still not effectively managed at the PHC level. The achievement of Sustainable Development Goals (SDGs) are also closely linked with reduction of the burden of NCDs [27]. From a health systems perspective, it is easier and economically feasible to detect any chronic disease like cardiovascular diseases in its early stages [28] and employ prevention and rehabilitation strategies at the primary level. CVDs and other NCDs share common risk factors such as diet, physical activity, tobacco use, and alcohol consumption. Yoga programs which promote physical activity, prevention strategies, and recovery as the key interventions are crucial in the effective management of these risk factors in individuals and this contributing to the primordial and primary prevention of CVDs.

2.7 Recommendations

- The primary health care centers must become the focal point for delivering essential yoga-based cardio-interventions. A wide action on the risk factors and deliverance of services by Non-Physician Healthcare Providers (community health workers, nurses, and other allied health professionals) should be empowered and enabled.

- Community based (Peer Group), home based (self-management education), and Internet technology (Mobile Interventions) should be given high priority at the primary health care level.
- Yoga should be an essential component of school and college curriculum, school-based programs focusing on risk factors with emphasis on screening, counselling, and awareness should be executed.

References

1. World Health Organization. Quick facts cardiovascular diseases. 2015.
2. World Heart Federation. Heart fact sheet on cardiovascular diseases. 2015.
3. Barbosa M, Champagne B, Chen D, Gamra H, Harold JG, Josephson S, et al. Sustainable development goals and the future of cardiovascular health: a statement from the global cardiovascular disease taskforce putting the heart into the sustainable development goals. J Am Hear Assoc. 2014;3:504.
4. Institute for Health Metrics and Evaluation. Global burden of disease. 2017.
5. World Health Organization. Yoga is a valuable tool to increase physical activity and decrease noncommunicable disease.2018.
6. Datey KK, Deshmukh SN, Dalvi CP, Vinekar SL. 'Shavasan': a yogic exercise in the management of hypertension. Angiology. 1969;20:325–33.
7. Merritt TA, et al. Intensive lifestyle changes for reversal of coronary heart disease. JAMA. 1998;280:2001–7.
8. Ornish D, Brown SE, Scherwitz LW, Billings JH, Armstrong WT, Ports TA, et al. Can lifestyle changes reverse coronary heart disease? The lifestyle heart trial. Lancet. 1990;336:129–33.
9. Manchanda SC, Narang R, Reddy KS, Sachdeva U, Prabhakaran D, Dharmanand S, et al. Retardation of coronary atherosclerosis with yoga lifestyle intervention. J Assoc Physicians India. 2000;48:687–94.
10. Ornish D, Scherwitz LW, Billings JH, Lance Gould K, Merritt TA, Sparler S, et al. Intensive lifestyle changes for reversal of coronary heart disease. JAMA. 1998;280(23):2001–7.
11. Aldana SG, Greenlaw R, Salberg A, Merrill RM, Hager R, et al. The effects of an intensive lifestyle modification program on carotid artery intima-media thickness: a randomized trial. Am J Health Promot. 2007;21(6):510–6.
12. Schmidt T, Wijga A, Von Zur MA, Brabant G, Wagner TOF. Changes in cardiovascular risk factors and hormones during a comprehensive residential three month kriya yoga training and vegetarian nutrition. Acta Physiolog Scand Suppl. 1997;161:158–62.
13. Cramer H, Lauche R, Haller H, Steckhan N, Michalsen A, Dobos G. Effects of yoga on cardiovascular disease risk factors: a systematic review and meta-analysis. Int J Cardiol. 2014;173(2):170–83.
14. Haider T, Sharma M, Branscum P. Yoga as an alternative and complimentary therapy for cardiovascular disease: a systematic review. J Evid-Based Complement Altern Med. 2017;22:310–6.
15. Pullen P, Seffens W, Thompson W. Yoga for heart failure: a review and future research. Int J Yoga. 2018;11(2):91.
16. Hartley L, Dyakova M, Holmes J, Clarke A, Lee MS, Ernst E, et al. Yoga for the primary prevention of cardiovascular disease. Cochrane Database Syst Rev. 2014;(5):CD010072.
17. Jsw K, Hlc L, KwongJSW CP, Kwong JS, Lam Caren Lau H, Yeung F, et al. Cochrane library cochrane database of systematic reviews yoga for secondary prevention of coronary heart disease (review). 2015. www.cochranelibrary.com. Accessed 21 Apr 2020.
18. Goyal M, Singh S, Sibinga EMS, Gould NF, Rowland-Seymour A, Sharma R, et al. Meditation programs for psychological stress and well-being: a systematic review and meta-analysis. JAMA Intern Med. 2014;174(3):357–68.
19. Sarkar BK, West R, Arora M, Ahluwalia JS, Reddy KS, Shahab L. Effectiveness of a brief community outreach tobacco cessation intervention in India: a cluster-randomised controlled trial (the BABEX trial). Thorax. 2017;72(2):167–73.
20. Chattopadhyay K, Chandrasekaran AM, Praveen PA, Manchanda SC, Madan K, Ajay VS, et al. Development of a yoga-based cardiac rehabilitation (Yoga-CaRe) programme for secondary prevention of myocardial infarction. Evid Based Complement Alternat Med. 2019;2019:7470184.
21. Tillin T, Tuson C, Sowa B, Chattopadhyay K, Sattar N, Welsh P, et al. Yoga and cardiovascular health trial (YACHT): a UK-based randomised mechanistic study of a yoga intervention plus usual care versus usual care alone following an acute coronary event. BMJ Open. 2019;9(11):e030119.
22. Ministry of Health and Family Welfare Goverment of India. National health policy. 2017.
23. Government of India. National curriculum framework. NCERT; 2005.
24. Government of India. What is Indian eVisa for yoga programs? 2019.
25. Ministry of AYUSH, Govt. of India. Research Councils, Central Council for Research in Ayurvedic Sciences, New Delhi. Ministry of AYUSH; 2015.
26. Singh R, LNU B, Rani S, Bhadula A, Sharma R, Shahi VK. Integration of AYUSH (ayurveda and yoga) with national programme for prevention and control of cancer, diabetes, cardiovascular diseases and stroke (NPCDCS): an appraisal of Central Council for Research in Ayurvedic Sciences Research and Development Initiatives. J Res Ayurvedic Sci. 2018;2(1):27–36.
27. World Health Organization. Noncommunicable diseases and development. 2007.
28. World Health Organization. Global status report on noncommunicable diseases. 2010.

3 The Nature, Meaning, and Practice of Yoga: Traditional Base Meets Scientific Rigor

Paul Dallaghan and Indranill Basu-Ray

The long-awaited finale to one of modern media's most critically acclaimed series chose to end with the show's protagonist sitting cross-legged, eyes closed, finally finding peace and uttering the sound of "Om." I refer to none other than MadMen and the wayward life of the classic Don Draper, out of the 1950s into a new social dawn by 1970. It highlights, at the least, the social impact the message of yoga, and the impact of its practices, has had on our modern evolving society. With that, we know the word "yoga" conjures up many preconceived, popularly transmitted, images, typically physical contortions from the bizarre to the more current socially relevant look of cool, healthy, and conscious. However, changing social views and images of yoga do little to inform us of what yoga is exactly. Commercial propaganda speaks of a myriad of benefits but how are these separated from hype and the extreme bias of numerous anecdotal self-reported accounts, especially by "gurus" invested in their outcome? The concern extends into the field of research where the contextual setting for a study population, the specific type and nature of a yoga practice, and its intensity and frequency in implementation are necessary elements of integrity in research coupled with exceptional scientific methods to accurately measure, analyze, and report. Aside from this our modern post-WWII world, coinciding with post-Indian independence, has seen a non-stop interest in yoga and its practices, beyond the survival rate of any fad, where there must be some genuine level of inherent value. Even the White House weighed in 2013 declaring it within its Presidential Active Lifestyle Award (PALA), acknowledging it "crossing many lines of religions and cultures" whereby "[e]very day millions of people practice yoga to improve their health and overall well-being" [1]. With so much attention it warrants scientific assessment to answer if the feel-good factor people claim, along with several anecdotally reported health benefits, can be translated into improved health outcomes, in terms of cardiovascular health, not just for those who practice but even as a prescription to aid those suffering from the different pathophysiological states involving the cardiovascular system.

3.1 Yoga: Nature and Meaning

Yoga is both a process and the culmination of that process in a meditative experience, what we can refer to as an end-state. A clear and experienced

P. Dallaghan
Emory University, Atlanta, GA, USA

I. Basu-Ray (✉)
Memphis VA Medical Center, Memphis, TN, USA

All India Institute of Medical Sciences, Rishikesh, Uttarakhand, India

School of Public Health, University of Memphis, Memphis, TN, USA
e-mail: ibr@ibasuray.com

I. Basu-Ray, D. Mehta (eds.), *The Principles and Practice of Yoga in Cardiovascular Medicine*,
https://doi.org/10.1007/978-981-16-6913-2_3

interpretation of its meaning from both the rich textual literature and the ongoing tradition of practice makes it clear that yoga and meditation are one and the same. The word yoga then becomes a technical term that needs to be unpacked for a scientific audience. Too often yoga is interpreted from a theistic, even religious, point of view which requires a belief structure and the subscription to a doctrine. For both this current scientific review and for the correct understanding of yoga, a clear non-theistic definition and explanation is needed and fortunately exists in some of the oldest of texts. A clear understanding of yoga, its process, and state, the *Pātañjalayogaśāstra*, [2], c. 350 CE, known commonly as the *Pātañjali Yoga Sutras* (PYS heretofore), is the most coherent source of yoga historically available. It illuminates the meaning and process of yoga in a string of sentences that are further elaborated on in its commentary. The opening sutras (short sentences) give a clear explanation of yoga:

> Yoga is the direct experience by you of who you really are, now, in this moment, not who you think or perceive you are (PYS I.1)
> It is experienced when the full force of energy that drives life, from every thought to bodily impulse, is channeled to a complete coherent state of oneness (PYS I.2)
> Upon this experience all that remains to be experienced is your own essence (PYS 1.3)
> When not experiencing your own essence then you are experiencing the multitude of elements that constitute a human life, from every thought to every bodily impulse within a world of elements that we perceive and make contact with. (PYS I.4)

This last statement (PYS I.4) refers to the elements of life we measure and observe in any research study or reported account. In terms of yoga, the PYS I.1-3 explain something that can almost not be measured by the scientific method except in the absence of all the elements referred to in PYS I.4. The nature of all these elements, from body to thought and the phenomenal world, is continuous change, impermanent. We, therefore, explain PYS I.2 as *the management of bodily functions in a healthy and energetic way coupled with a skillful handling of the mental activities, to see them as ongoing functions of a lived life, residing in a balanced, healthy and peaceful state, not caught up in, yet capable of handling, the continuous events of life.* This centered state itself matures till one witnesses the temporary nature of all phenomena and experiences the essence of that which is unchanging, explained as our own true nature (PYS I.3). As scientists, we can then attempt a level of study on aspects of bodily and mental health affected by various techniques of yoga practice. The yoga process is a woven composition of various techniques which are essentially meditative techniques. Thus, the state of yoga, a direct experience, is a state of meditation (PYS I.1-2).

3.2 Yoga: From the Esoteric to Practice for Research

Though the foregoing detail may be of an esoteric nature for some readers it should be understood that within such an original understanding of what yoga stands for arises multiple techniques and their influence on the lives of people, especially on maintenance, and even amelioration, of good cardiovascular health. The market has artificially divided yoga into physical practices and meditation into sitting mental techniques. A correct understanding of yoga reveals that the physical and mental cannot be separated so much so it is less about *what* is done and more about *how* it is done. The physical supports the mental and the mental impacts the physical. A careful read of the original material on yoga reveals a scientific approach to the description and practice of techniques. If such techniques are to reach a standard of therapeutic competency and efficacy then a marriage of the detail described in the original material, which we identify as the traditional base, followed faithfully, with rigorous scientific method, not just in study design and assessment, but in the precise definition and execution of the selected techniques is required.

3.3 Yoga: The Physical and Mental

Every technique of yoga is based within this overarching explanation of yoga as described above. In short, a body position (posture or *āsana*) or a regulated breath technique, are all intended toward optimizing bodily function as well as mental activity, which ideally culminates in good health and a clear mind. If yoga is to aid cardiovascular health in a genuine therapeutic sense, then the science of yoga, through the detail of its techniques, needs to be established first. An examination of the several techniques that make up the process of yoga, which is the process of meditation, would reveal each has its own value and can potentially benefit different aspects of physical, emotional, and mental health. Yet each technique involves a complete merging of both physical and mental aspects. Just as yoga and meditation are one any sitting practice cannot ignore the health of the body and nor can any physically involved practice, be it mild or intense, ignore the mental component.

3.4 Yoga: Mastery over the Senses, Skill in Execution, Mental Equilibrium

One of the very first descriptions of yoga, c 300 BCE, in an early Indian Sanskrit text describes yoga as the mastery over the senses with a completely still mental level[1] [3]. Yoga is thus the experience of "nothing," no thought, no sensation. This is only nihilistic if one considers constant contact with sensory elements as the needed experience of life. Subsequent teachings from the *Bhagavad Gīta* [4], c 200 CE, reveal yoga to be a mastery over how one engages in and carries out any detail or action, which means a mind not caught up in anything other than the task at hand, be it as mundane as wiping down a table to as skilled as performing open-heart surgery.[2] It further adds that to take care of what needs to be done is to be in the moment, not caught up in a selfish agenda and personal desire.[3] To maintain equilibrium at all times, in all situations, with all people, becomes the expression of yoga.[4] The unpacking of these definitions reveals that yoga is an unfolding cultivation of good management of bodily processes, even in the face of continuous decay and senescence, while developing the understanding that leads to a highly regulated emotional and cognitive state. This brings us back then to the various techniques of yoga and how they can be practiced, in what combination, when and where, moderately or intensely, over how long, so as to impact both physical and mental health, to see which techniques will be more beneficial for certain aspects of body and psyche. This is where the modern scientific approach must work with the traditional base to greater understand the separate elements of yoga practice and how and when they can benefit people in different states of bodily and mental health, if at all.

3.5 Yoga: A Plan of Action and a Life-System Approach

The PYS offers a comprehensive understanding of yoga's traditional base. It elucidates that yoga is ultimately an experience of deep inner absorp-

[1] Katha Upanishad: 6.10-11 Yoga as firm restraint of the senses

10. When the five senses, along with the mind, remain still and the intellect is not active, that is known as the highest state.

11. They consider yoga to be firm restraint of the senses. Then one becomes undistracted, for yoga is the arising and passing away.

[2] From the Bhagavad Gīta: *Yoga Karmasukauśālam* – Yoga is Expertise in action, not entangled (2.50)

[3] From the Bhagavad Gīta: *Niṣkāma Karma* – Yoga is Action free from agenda and desire (2.47)

[4] From the Bhagavad Gīta: *Samatvam Yoga Ucyate* – Yoga is to Practice balance, find equilibrium (2.48)

tion, complete inner peace, achieved through constant inner practices, and a non-dependent emotional state. To be this centered involves a mastery over the senses, skill in the execution of what needs to be done, an ability to stay balanced, have equilibrium, in all situations, as referred to above. How is this to be achieved and does it have practical relevance to the state of our health? The PYS offers a method, or way, to achieve such balance but without specific details of techniques, other than the description of a few mental meditative approaches. Instead, what is emphasized is action on the part of the practicing subject, termed as *kriya yoga*, that involves approaches across the body, mind, and, for want of a better term, the open heart, symbolically of course.[5] *Kriya yoga* is essentially an "action plan" to bring balance to our bodily, emotional and mental health. In contrast to the modern market of yoga, this traditional base of work only gives two prefixes to the word yoga, one being "action" (*kriya*), and the other "eight-limbs" (*astānga*), which refers to a mix of auxiliaries (limbs) to an overall life-system approach. Closer examination reveals the elements of *kriya yoga* are further presented as a subset of this life system. Thus, the traditional base of yoga prescribes an initial course of action, that in and of itself is highly effective in terms of transforming the mental, and thus bodily, state, but also offers as its central thesis a system that covers all aspects of a human lived life. This is said to remove all confusion and misunderstanding about what life is and bring a degree of optimal consistency to the body and mind. In a functional life, this means a highly regulated autonomic system. If we take this traditional base to the later described techniques of yoga practice it should be clear that whatever the practice is it is only correctly classified as yoga if it involves an internal focus and effort. This deeper understanding is essential for the scientific process and application to therapeutic health approaches as yoga practices are not a set of physical or mental gymnastics. The two are different and yield different outcomes. Thus, the therapeutic value of yoga involves a mental state attuned to what one is actually engaged in.

3.6 Yoga: Action, Attention, Openness

Over the centuries the practices of yoga have developed per the social need, cultural climate, or environmental setting. The *Bhagavad Gita* opens with a clinical description of anxiety, severe stress, and a confused state of mind accompanied by dejection within its protagonist, Arjuna. It then goes on to deliver the teachings of yoga in a narrative form that essentially highlights the correct understanding and actions for a balanced life, emphasizing the use of the breath and attention to one's inner state beyond sensory input and the endless stream of thoughts. Essentially yoga practice has as its base (1). action to be done, (2). mental attention to it, and (3). a complete open-mindedness, or lack of agenda. This is repeated in Patanjali's *Kriya yoga*, the "action plan." The 8-limb life system implements this action-attention-openness across all relationships, our anatomy and physiology, and the mental absorptive state. Thus, the action of doing a body or breath technique follows the above principles. Numerous prefixes to the word yoga have developed in today's market yet tend to be mostly tag words for yoga as some kind of moving flow. However, in the traditional sense, which is of most importance for science and research, a prefix to the word yoga denotes a specific approach with a set of techniques that are both part of the yogic (meditative) process and bring about meditation, or a state of yoga, awake with an understanding of one's essence. In that respect, *Hatha Yoga* embraces the same principles and teachings as described above in the PYS and gives a *hatha* approach to affect that.

[5] *Pātañjalayogaśāstra* (II.1) *Tapaḥ-svādhyāyeśvara-praṇidhānāni kriyā-yogaḥ*

Yoga through action is penance or austerity, self-study and surrender or trust in the unknown

3.7 Hatha Yoga: Practical Techniques to Do, Research, and Offer as Therapy

The recent spread of yoga is predominantly the proliferation of body practices, known as *āsanas*. *Āsana* is defined in the PYS[6] but is developed as a practice in the tradition of *Hatha Yoga*. Hatha, as yoga, is based on the principles previously defined, with techniques elaborated from tantric tradition. When published studies reference yoga as a set of body, breath, and meditation practices they are loosely referring to elements that are taught publicly from the corpus of *Hatha Yoga*. *Hatha Yoga* makes use of physiological forces and anatomical structure and in so doing becomes very specific in its techniques and methods. One small but important element is the practice of *āsana* (body posture) yet this same element has taken center stage in current yoga approaches, both in the market and in research. In fact, even more erroneously *Hatha Yoga* has been termed in numerous studies and yoga studios worldwide as a mild approach to *āsana*.

3.8 Hatha Yoga: Autonomic Balance, Free from NCD

Hatha Yoga describes, in an original c. 1450 CE text, the *Hathapradipika* [5], four main categories of techniques to bring about a fully functional autonomic nervous system, in balance, which can be inferred as good health and free from non-communicable disease (NCD). In so doing it emphasizes the natural breath cycle and a return to natural breathing as a primary factor that cultivates internal awareness. These four techniques culminate in a meditative experience where the full flow of consciousness is not caught up with any external stimuli but rather deeply absorbed, said to be with an inner sound. It is here the experience of yoga takes over. In this understanding what we commonly term, and research, as yoga is primarily these Hatha techniques, that exist to address physiological imbalances, support the body, and overall augment health over a longer period of time. They are done with a purpose of directing the flow of consciousness inside, leading to greater awareness of what is happening in the body, with the breath, and ultimately the mental state. Yet their function and a successful outcome cannot be separated from the key elements described earlier under the life-system approach of PYS, the attention to one's relationships while managing the body and breath.

3.9 Hatha Yoga: Impact on ANS, Spine and Joints, Neuromuscular System

Hatha Yoga, more specifically, functions to balance the autonomic forces in the body by regulating and managing the function of breath. It pays particular attention to the difference in breath flow across the two nostrils, an area still not properly researched in modern science. To affect this balance it prescribes as its four categories of techniques (1). a selection of bodily postures, *āsanas* divided between one's that train the body and others that one stays in, (2). bodily cleansing practices, *krīyas*, and (3). specific breath retained techniques, *kumbhakas* but known as *prāṇāyāma* in most circles. The fourth (4) technique, mudras, is really a skillful use of retained breath with powerful bodily held positions that require specific pelvic-diaphragm and abdominal control. This means a training in *Hatha Yoga* is not just the executing, often mimicking, of certain bodily positions, but rather the skillful management of the body and breath in various training positions that affect, in order of importance, the autonomic nervous system, the spine and joints, and the neuromuscular system. It is the latter that garners most attention when practicing "yoga" and though important muscular activity needs to be done with an attention to autonomic balance and support of the spine and other joints in the body.

[6] *Pātañjalayogaśāstra* (II.46) *Sthira sukham āsanam*Āsana, referring to the anatomical body, as posture is optimal when supported and free, open, happy

It is within this setting and understanding that the original teachings of *Hatha Yoga* describe practice and the benefits that come from it, benefits we hope to research and apply to CVD.

It is clear that the "yoga" we hope to research and ascribe to certain healing and health maintaining benefits in terms of cardiovascular health and other areas of the body has many elements, diverse techniques, not dissimilar to the division of elements and function in a cell. Yet the latter has been examined in detail by the scientific method while yoga is typically placed non-differentially en-masse into one broad category for inclusion in scientific research studies. Though the research has revealed some interesting results it has still not gone far enough to cross the line and distinctively state how, what, and when will work for which population in both a health maintaining category and in various pathological states. Interestingly the CDC reports that Yoga was the most commonly used complementary health approach among U.S. adults in 2012 (9.5%) and 2017 (14.3%) [6] even though the American Medical Association considers yoga an alternative therapy of "unproven treatments," and calls for "rigorous research to study safety and efficacy" of these therapies [7].

3.10 Āsana as Opposed to Exercise

Yoga is often associated with exercise yet a correct understanding of the practice clearly differentiates the two. The most outstanding marker being that the breath is always managed through the nose, never lost control of, coupled with a focus on internal body processes so a balance across the autonomic nervous system is maintained. Approaches to body posture techniques, the doing of *āsana*, differ. Some are more physical and involve movement, which has triggered the popularity of yoga worldwide, more so than static approaches. The emphasis in *āsana* is on the pose yet the focus in popular practice has gone to the flow and movement. Flow and movement are completely valid functions in and of themselves but if they make up the dominant element in a measured yoga technique then regardless of correct scientific methods we are measuring something other than intended in yoga. Further, if the practice performed shows greater affinity to exercise than actual *yoga āsana*, by a marked increase in sympathetic stimulation due to excessive effort, tension and breathing, then our method measures exercise in the name of yoga. If we apply scientific rigor to the techniques of yoga then we should be able to describe its features in terms of yoga and not other forms of workout, detail how it is executed, and to what aim.

3.11 Āsana Performed Correctly with Integrity

Yoga āsana is managed mainly from the pelvic and trunk muscles and employs the legs and arms to support that. An emphasis on using the legs and arms with a typically excessive grip in the upper abdomen, as is most common, mimics exercise, adds strain to the *āsana*, and increases the sympathetic response. Such an approach is common and why people get injured or receive muscle strain when doing yoga practice. As an example, the doing of a particular set of bodily poses, *āsanas,* are by nature physically challenging. If the focus is on their physical performance, then the breath might be disturbed or even occur through the mouth, the heart rate may go higher than otherwise managed, and excessive muscular tension, particularly in the abdomen, will be added to perform the physical pose. This is in complete contrast to the *Hatha Yoga* prescribed nature of *āsana* whereby the step into the pose should be slow, on a long drawn-out breath, the body managed primarily through a core central support from the base of the pelvis along the spine that avoids unnecessary muscular tension, especially in areas of the body that tend to hold stress such as shoulders and upper abdomen. This manages the load on the heart even though the heart rate increases a little, avoiding sympathetic dominance, thereby giving optimal care to the state of the inner organs, which includes the heart and its vasculature, with key support to the spine without loading other joints of the body. Essentially the *āsana* develops gradually over time. If claims for the therapeutic benefit of (Hatha) Yoga are to be made based on research that mainly tests subjects doing *āsana* then correct detail to what is taught and practiced is required for accurate scientific reporting. Then the science of yoga and its therapeutic value can proceed.

3.12 Yoga Practice: The Scientific Approach

The intrinsic positive effects of a generalized yoga practice plus qualified and capable instructors of yoga practice, who understand it well and can teach in an inspiring and helpful manner, are sufficient to continue the growth of yoga in the recreational market. However, a more scientific approach is needed if the techniques of yoga are to pass to the therapeutic realm. They must be capable of being duplicated by qualified instructors, applicable to a specific state of health or pathology, follow established protocols of techniques, and be delivered at a recommended "dose" level. Studies on exercise tend to be divided between aerobic activity, endurance levels, high-intensity training, resistance strength work, and so on. The marketplace of yoga mainly consists of brand names that are *āsana*-heavy and tend to get confused with yoga traditions. These brand name approaches, as opposed to method-specific approaches, are often used in research studies. As a result, it is difficult to make a standardized claim about specific yoga methods and their effect on aspects of health, a point noted in several meta-analyses on yoga [8–12].

Five elements are recommended to further study the specific effects of yoga practices:

1. Yoga practice techniques: a brand name-free breakdown and categorization
2. Fundamental aspects of techniques: inclusion of the signature points of āsana, the separation of breath levels, and the direction of mental attention
3. Attention to the context and situation of practice especially in light of certain lifestyle factors—gender, health status, socioeconomics, location, intensity, duration, diet
4. Established protocols of yoga practice approaches
5. Experimental "dose" options across time, session, and intensity

It is then possible to adequately differentiate the aspects of practice and match them to the intended condition. Though the trend in research to date has been to apply yoga to certain pathological populations a progressive breakdown of subject bases is first required:

(a) Novice versus experienced at yoga practice, and a further distinction of how experienced and in what actual techniques
(b) Active lifestyle versus sedentary
(c) Reporting as healthy or unhealthy. If unhealthy then treated or nontreated

The first two elements of a brand name-free breakdown and categorization of yoga practice techniques with the inclusion of the signature points of āsana, the separation of breath levels, and the direction of attention as fundamental aspects of yoga practice require a comprehensive study that draws from original textual references of yoga and a scientific description of how to perform such techniques. A tabulated presentation will highlight what breath level is used for which practice technique, the degree of physical effort required, and where attention is directed.

3.13 Yoga Practice: Context and Situation

Context and situation of practice is for the most part largely ignored in both the design and discussion of research studies. The scientific method applied to other fields controls for this as it builds from in vitro to in vivo studies. The study of yoga techniques will, for the most part, take place in living human beings, which are further integrated within a set of lifestyle factors that need to be considered. They involve diet, sleep, and activity level across specifics of where the practice is carried out, a residential setting versus attending an urban class, frequency per week, duration of time in practice, in addition to SES, gender, and health status. The majority of reported practitioners of yoga are female in the age group of 18–44, closely followed by those 45–64 [6]. Given that several studies on ANS and CVD highlight differences between males and females in terms of sympathetic function in the body and between pre- and post-menopausal females, gender and age are crucial to any study involving yoga techniques [13–20]. However, a recent study on aging and cardiac rehabilitation using exercise found that young, old, and very old patients all benefitted from the intervention with the most improvements based on the degree of physical impairments at baseline [21]. In addition, cardiac phenotypes differ between typically sedentary human beings and those that engage in either endurance or resistance physical activity, where marked differences in stroke volume and cardiac output have been noted based on the plasticity in a human left ventricle [22].

Typically studies either have subjects attend a short class two or three times a week over 6–16 weeks or report for a singular event practice to be measured pre- and post-technique. Though a recreational approach to yoga practice involves people attending classes two or three times a week this is at odds with classical descriptions of yoga practice where diet, sleep, and activity are referred to [5] as well as frequency and intensity [2]. Though ecologically valid, rarely is a study carried out in a residential setting, a setting typical of the tradition of practice up to the present time and highly popular in modern times as many choose to practice and learn in a dedicated environment. The primary work on *Hatha Yoga*, *Hathapradipika* [5], explains six obstacles that render a yoga practice useless, that include overeating, over-exertion, over-doing practice, a fickle mind, excessive talking, and social distraction. The same teaching equally offers six elements that support the successful outcome of a yoga practice, such as enthusiasm, courage, perseverance, determination, correct understanding, and making appropriate time and space away from the contact of others to practice. Though certain elements can be statistically controlled for the teachings of yoga are clear that both the attitude and lifestyle factors, as part of the context and situation, play a crucial part in supporting or undermining the effect of an intended set of yoga practice techniques. Given that loneliness and poor patient-reported outcomes and 1-year mortality in both men and women across cardiac diagnoses has been recently observed [23], location, setting, group versus alone, are key contextual factors.

3.14 Yoga Practice: Established Protocols and Recommended "Dose" Options

The research team at Kaivalyadhama Institute, Lonavala, India and Emory University, Atlanta, USA, have developed specific protocols of practice, following the above-mentioned criteria, used in a clinically registered trial on stress and aging biomarkers. These protocols focus on *āsana* approach, breath practices, and mental meditative techniques to be detailed in a separate publication but here identified as:

- SEDA: Slow Engaged Dynamic Āsana
- BREM: Breath Regulated Engaged Meditation
- SHEM: Sound and Heart Engaged Meditation

The scientific literature on yoga for the most part has only referred to "dose" in terms of the number of years subjects self-report to have followed the practice of certain yoga techniques [24]. The PYS refers to a practitioner being either mild, medium, or intense in practice and that the outcome follows the effort and focus put into practice [2]. Regularity and time in practice is of greater importance than the number of years, though the latter denotes a supposed longevity in practice. The amount of time spent in a session, regularity of that session, whether daily or a few times a week, longevity of time, over weeks, months, and years, and the volume of techniques followed in that time all impact the "dose" effect. This will not be obvious in a popular transmission setting where predominantly group classes on flowing *āsana*, a few times a week that vary in length from 45 to 90 min is the norm. This differs from the above-mentioned historical approach, which has become relevant today, where a temporary residence for a period of time in a retreat location to learn and do practice is considered effective [25–27]. This has become quite common today where many people either take a retreat away or engage in a training in a dedicated facility. In addition, the degree to which a practitioner engages with the practice is of vital importance, similar to compliance in any medical approach. The original teachings, specifically in the PYS, highlight the sincerity of the individual as key. Our team has developed a measure for a degree of "engaged participation" by both self-report and teacher-report, following a hypothesis that teacher-reported "engaged participation," not self-reported, will predict the degree of health outcome.

3.15 Conclusion

The description of yoga can be reliably traced back at least 2500 years with a large corpus of texts detailing its meaning and subsequent practices over the centuries. It has been practiced in various forms by renunciants and ancient Indian rulers right up to colonial British India where a new approach of scholarly attention was paid to it leading the way for its explosion on to the intellectual scenes of the USA and Europe from the 1890s onwards [28]. Since the cultural and economic shifts of the 1950s interest in yoga in its more popular physical form has gone from a fringe alternative pastime to a meaningful health and fitness practice to be found in almost every country of the world in the last decade. Though scientific research began on yoga techniques in 1924, initiated by *Sri Kuvalayananda* with the founding of the Kaivalyadhama Institute and the journal *Yoga Mimasa* [29], the rise in the number of studies on yoga has matched yoga's popular spread in the last 10 years. Such an interest in yoga is beyond pop culture and indicates some level of value in terms of health benefits and lifestyle amelioration. The scientific literature has touched on elements of this but for it to move ahead and effectively usher yogic practices into the realm of therapy and prevention, in terms of cardiovascular disease and other pathologies, fundamental studies followed by specific use of techniques detailed in precise terms, accounted for under different populations and settings, in full accord with the description and explanation of practice techniques described in the original texts is still in the making. Though many in the public domain will already claim to know and get benefit from their yoga practice regardless of the science. Yet the science is needed, just as the original texts have served to date, to more clearly explain the nature and effect of techniques and well-developed protocols involving a suite of practices. It is clear that the average yoga practitioner, instructor, or even senior teacher is not able to answer with this level of detail yet. A more organized approach combining the traditional base with the scientific method across protocols and dose in clinically-based trials is underway to help increase the understanding of yoga and improve the methods of practice and their implementation in various settings across lifestyle and health.

References

1. Rajghatta C. Obama White House embraces yoga amid conservative contortions [White House "Yoga Garden For Easter"] [press release]. 2013. http://www.freerepublic.com/focus/news/3002743/posts?page=33
2. Patañjali. Patanjali Yoga Sutras. In: Aranya-Hariharananda, Mukerji PN, Vyasa, editors. Yoga philosophy of Patañjali : containing his yoga aphorisms with Vyasa's commentary in Sanskrit and a translation with annotations including many suggestions for the practice of yoga. Albany: State University of New York Press; 1983. pp. xix, 483 p.
3. Katha Upanishad. In: Nikhilananda S, editor. The upanishads. Kolkata: Advaita Ashrama; 2008.
4. Kauśika AO. Śrīmad Bhagavadgītā. 5th rev. ed. New Delhi: Star Publications; 2000. p. 444.
5. Svatmarama. Hathapradipika: light on the teachings of hatha yoga. The original 13th century classical work on hatha. In: Digambarji S, editor. Kaivalyadhama; 1983.

6. Clarke TC, Barnes PM, Black LI, Stussman BJ, Nahin RL. Data brief no. 325: use of yoga, meditation, and chiropractors among U.S. adults aged 18 and over. Retrieved from National Center for Health Statistics, Centers for Disease Control and Prevention, U.S. Department of Health and Human Services; 2018.
7. Landers SJ. Alternative therapy use documented in new survey: American Medical Association. American Medical News; 2009. https://amednews-com.proxy.library.emory.edu/article/20090113/health/301139999/8. Accessed 15 Dec 2019.
8. Domingues RB. Modern postural yoga as a mental health promoting tool: a systematic review. Complement Ther Clin Pract. 2018;31:248–55. https://doi.org/10.1016/j.ctcp.2018.03.002.
9. Gallegos AM, Crean HF, Pigeon WR, Heffner KL. Meditation and yoga for posttraumatic stress disorder: a meta-analytic review of randomized controlled trials. Clin Psychol Rev. 2017;58:115–24. https://doi.org/10.1016/j.cpr.2017.10.004.
10. Li AW, Goldsmith C-A. The effects of yoga on anxiety and stress. Altern Med Rev. 2012;17:21–35.
11. Luu K, Hall PA. Hatha yoga and executive function: a systematic review. J Altern Complement Med. 2016;22(2):125–33. https://doi.org/10.1089/acm.2014.0091.
12. Ross A, Thomas S. The health benefits of yoga and exercise: a review of comparison studies. J Altern Complement Med. 2010;16(1):3–12. https://doi.org/10.1089/acm.2009.0044.
13. Airaksinen KEJ, Ikäheimo MJ, Linnaluoto M, Tahvanainen KUO, Huikuri HV. Gender difference in autonomic and hemodynamic reactions to abrupt coronary occlusion. J Am Coll Cardiol. 1998;31(2):301–6. https://doi.org/10.1016/s0735-1097(97)00489-0.
14. Argiento P, Vanderpool RR, Mule M, Russo MG, D'Alto M, Bossone E, Chesler NC, Naeije R. Exercise stress echocardiography of the pulmonary circulation: limits of normal and sex differences. Chest. 2012;142(5):1158–65. https://doi.org/10.1378/chest.12-0071.
15. Dart AM, Du X-J, Kingwell BA. Gender, sex hormones and autonomic nervous control of the cardiovascular system. Cardiovasc Res. 2002;53:678–87.
16. Gleim GW, Stachenfeld NS, Coplan NL, Nicholas JA. Gender differences in the systolic blood pressure response to exercise. Am Heart J. 1991;121(2):524–30.
17. Jones PP, Davy KP, Seals DR. Influence of gender on the sympathetic neural adjustments to alterations in systemic oxygen levels in humans. Clin Physiol. 1999;19(2):153–60.
18. Maric-Bilkan C, Manigrasso MB. Sex differences in hypertension: contribution of the renin-angiotensin system. Gend Med. 2012;9(4):287–91. https://doi.org/10.1016/j.genm.2012.06.005.
19. Matsukawa T, Sugiyama Y, Watanabe T, Kobayashi F, Mano T. Gender difference in age-related changes in muscle sympathetic nerve activity in healthy subjects. Am J Phys. 1998;275(5):R1600–4. https://doi.org/10.1152/ajpregu.1998.275.5.R1600.
20. Ng AV, Callister R, Johnson DG, Seals DR. Age and gender influence muscle sympathetic nerve activity at rest in healthy humans. Hypertension. 1993;21(4):498–503.
21. Deley G, Culas C, Blonde MC, Mourey F, Verges B. Physical and psychological effectiveness of cardiac rehabilitation: age is not a limiting factor! Can J Cardiol. 2019;35(10):1353–8. https://doi.org/10.1016/j.cjca.2019.05.038.
22. Shave RE, Lieberman DE, Drane AL, Brown MG, Batterham AM, Worthington S, Atencia R, Feltrer Y, Neary J, Weiner RB, Wasfy MM, Baggish AL. Selection of endurance capabilities and the trade-off between pressure and volume in the evolution of the human heart. Proc Natl Acad Sci U S A. 2019;116(40):19905–10. https://doi.org/10.1073/pnas.1906902116.
23. Christensen AV, Juel K, Ekholm O, Thrysoe L, Thorup CB, Borregaard B, Mols RE, Rasmussen TB, Berg SK. Significantly increased risk of all-cause mortality among cardiac patients feeling lonely. Heart. 2019; https://doi.org/10.1136/heartjnl-2019-315460.
24. Gothe NP, Khan I, Hayes J, Erlenbach E, Damoiseaux JS. Yoga effects on brain health: a systematic review of the current literature. Brain Plast. 2019:1–17. https://doi.org/10.3233/bpl-190084.
25. Conklin Q, King B, Zanesco A, Pokorny J, Hamidi A, Lin J, Epel E, Blackburn E, Saron C. Telomere lengthening after three weeks of an intensive insight meditation retreat. Psychoneuroendocrinology. 2015;61:26–7. https://doi.org/10.1016/j.psyneuen.2015.07.462.
26. Conklin QA, King BG, Zanesco AP, Lin J, Hamidi AB, Pokorny JJ, Álvarez-López MJ, Cosín-Tomás M, Huang C, Kaliman P, Epel ES, Saron CD. Insight meditation and telomere biology: the effects of intensive retreat and the moderating role of personality. Brain Behav Immun. 2018;70:233–45. https://doi.org/10.1016/j.bbi.2018.03.003.
27. Jacobs TL, Epel ES, Lin J, Blackburn EH, Wolkowitz OM, Bridwell DA, Zanesco AP, Aichele SR, Sahdra BK, MacLean KA, King BG, Shaver PR, Rosenberg EL, Ferrer E, Wallace BA, Saron CD. Intensive meditation training, immune cell telomerase activity, and psychological mediators. Psychoneuroendocrinology. 2011;36(5):664–81. https://doi.org/10.1016/j.psyneuen.2010.09.010.
28. White DG. The yoga sutra of Patanjali: a biography. Princeton University Press; 2014.
29. Kuvalayananda, Vinekar SL. Yogic therapy: its basic principles and methods. New Delhi: Central Health Education Bureau; 1963.

4 Yoga in the Management of Cardiovascular Disease: A Brief Introduction

Gregory Fricchione

4.1 Introduction

Mind-body medicine (MBM) is a subdiscipline approach that recognizes that the brain and body are one. It endorses the evidence-based effects of our beliefs, thoughts, and emotions on our overall health promotion. To do this, it employs a variety of researched techniques that purposefully affect mental and physical fitness, including relaxation exercises, meditation, biofeedback, guided imagery, hypnosis, yoga, tai chi, qigong, and autogenic training [1, 2].

The common elements of these techniques characterize MBM, which all elicit the relaxation response (RR). The use of a repetitive phrase, word, or prayer and breaking the train of everyday thoughts and concerns are the two main behavioral features of eliciting the RR. Many distinct methods of enhancing attention and mindfulness can be accessed after first eliciting the RR. The RR itself is a physiological state of decreased stress characterized by diminished heart rate, blood pressure, respiratory rate and oxygen consumption along with peripheral vasodilatation [3].

G. Fricchione (✉)
Department of Psychiatry, Benson-Henry Institute for Mind Body Medicine & The McCance Center for Brain Health, Massachusetts General Hospital, Harvard Medical School, Boston, MA, USA
e-mail: gfricchione@mgh.harvard.edu

4.2 The Health Challenges of the Twenty-First Century

In 2011 a report from the Harvard School of Public Health and commissioned by the World Economic Forum (WEF) focused on the costs of the major classes of non-communicable diseases (NCDs) and projected these costs in terms of the economic burden through 2030 [4]. The results of three different estimate methods project enormous costs over the next two decades, with cardiovascular disease, chronic respiratory disease, cancer, diabetes, and mental health representing a cumulative output loss of $47 T, roughly 75% of the global GDP in 2010. NCDs have thus been recognized as the major health challenge of the twenty-first century. The WEF report adds another layer of concern to the pain and suffering individuals with NCDs face [4].

In 2013, Whiteford and colleagues writing in the Lancet reported that mental and substance use disorders accounted for 183.9 million Disability Adjusted Life Years (DALYs) or 7.4% (6.2–8.6) of all DALYs worldwide. Mental and substance use disorders were the leading cause of Years Lost to Disability (YLDs) worldwide. Depressive disorders accounted for 40.5% (31.7–49.2) of DALYs caused by mental and substance use disorders, with anxiety disorders accounting for 14.6% (11.2–18.4), illicit drug use disorders

I. Basu-Ray, D. Mehta (eds.), *The Principles and Practice of Yoga in Cardiovascular Medicine*,
https://doi.org/10.1007/978-981-16-6913-2_4

for 10.9% (8.9–13.2), alcohol use disorders for 9·6% (7.7–11.8), schizophrenia for 7.4% (5.0–9·8), bipolar disorder for 7·0% (4.4–10.3), pervasive developmental disorders for 4·2% (3.2–5.3), childhood behavioral disorders for 3·4% (2.2–4.7), and eating disorders for 1.2% (0.9–1.5). The burden of mental and substance use disorders increased by 37.6% between 1990 and 2010, which for most disorders was driven by population growth and aging [5].

Neuropsychiatric disorders (NPD) of the type described above are examples of stress-related, chronic non-communicable diseases (NCDs) [6]. These illnesses compound the enormous burden of cardiovascular diseases (CVDs). NCDs constituted more than 36 M deaths (60%) worldwide in 2005 according to the WHO; 80% of deaths occurred in low- and middle-income countries, and CVD alone was responsible for half of these deaths [4, 7]. Depression, which is the most burdensome disease, increases the relative risk of cardiac events even in those without a cardiac disease history [8], so the combination of these two NCDs—CVD and NPD—is devastating to public health around the world.

Stress-related NCDs, including CVDs, chronic respiratory diseases, diabetes, arthritis, and NPD, continue to stymie primary care practitioners all over the world. This accounts for severe morbidity and mortality, leading to great suffering and leads to an explosion of health care costs around the world mentioned above [4]. Long term, NCDs represent the most important global health challenge of the twenty-first century in terms of disease burden and mortality despite the once in a century global COVID-19 pandemic of 2020–2021 [6, 9].

Against this background, we might ask if Yoga can provide the kind of evidence-based, integrated mind-body strategy for global mental health promotion that might be instituted in under-resourced settings to begin to address the enormous public mental health challenge embedded in the common pathogenesis of chronic stress-related NCDs in an effective yet efficient way.

4.3 Stress, Allostatic Load, and NCDs

Stress demands biological, psychological, and social adaptation of the organism. The term "*eustress*" describes the normal physiological performance of the living organism in the setting of normal everyday stress. Homeostatic mechanisms constitute the process of "*eustasis*" reflected statistically as an inverted U-shaped curve with suboptimal responsivity at either end representing poor adaptation [10]. Normal eustress situationally increases into the tolerable stress range when increasing demands occur in one's life. In these circumstances, homeostasis remains effective in maintaining a physiology in the normative range. Toxic *pathogenic stress* or *distress* occurs when homeostasis is persistently threatened in the setting of overwhelming or sustained external and internal stressors with accompanying hyperstimulation of the stress response systems mediated primarily by paraventricular hypothalamic nucleus derived corticotrophin-releasing hormone (CRH), locus coeruleus derived norepinephrine (NE) and a chronic innate immune response. Walter Cannon, in the early 1900s, did seminal research on the autonomic nervous system (ANS) axis of the stress response system [11]. Focusing on the sympathetic nervous system (SNS) and its mediation of "*the flight-fight response*" he was first to use the term *homeostasis.* Hans Selye, another twentieth century stress researcher, focused on the hypothalamus–pituitary–adrenal (HPA) axis [12].

Toxic stress as *distress* disrupts homeostasis [13]. The distressed person's physiological, psychological, and social dimensions are misattuned as a result of the disruptive perception of an external or internal environmental threat that engages the physiological stress response system. Three key factors—stressors, the stress system and the stress response—constitute this process.

The stress response system includes the central nervous system (CNS), the HPA axis, and the immune system. The CNS and the peripheral nervous system (PNS) have sympathetic (SNS) and parasympathetic (PNS) components. This matrix promotes homeostasis through maintenance of bodily functions within a normative range while permitting flexibility of cybernetic physiological responses, thus modulating the distribution and application of energy resources. In this manner, the brain is continually autoregulating through feedback and feed-forward mechanisms. Nevertheless, the brain can become overstimulated by persistent or overwhelming stressors making homeostatic adaptation difficult and ushering in the potential for *distress*.

The stress response activates metabolic functions, cardiac output, vascular tone, respiration, and muscle contraction—heart rate, respiratory rate, oxygen consumption, and brain wave activity all increase. At the same time, the stress response suppresses gastrointestinal, excretory, and reproductive activity [14, 15]. The SNS activates the stress response while the parasympathetic PNS mollifies this effect and restores balance in the ANS [15].

Allostasis, a concept introduced in the field of stress medicine by Sterling and Eyer, refers to the capacity to achieve stability through change [16]. Allostasis involves biological processes that buffer against the threat of toxic stress. This aids the internal balance of homeostasis; however, the stress system can overheat in the setting of overwhelming or persistent stress leading to a state of metabolic wear and tear called *allostatic load*. If left unchecked by chronic stress, this can lead to a variety of diseases. This long-term vulnerability of the physiologic response to chronic stress has been termed *allostatic overload*—the metabolic cost of maintaining allostasis of physiological systems at the cellular level [17]. Allostatic load is attributed to four proposed mechanisms [18]. They include frequent stress or multiple stressors; prolonged exposure to stress and the consequent lack of adaptation; inability to shut off allostatic responses or delay in shutting down after a stressor abates; and an inadequate response, that leads to compensatory overresponse in other systems.

Selye [12] had presaged this understanding with his so-called General Adaptation Syndrome, the final stage of which he called the *state of exhaustion*, in which stress continues for a long time causing the body to function abnormally and organ systems to fail.

Psychosocial stress is processed at the cellular level as *oxidative stress*. This is because mental stress is processed in the brain cortico-striatal-thalamo-cortical circuitry and the mesocortico-limbic system as a challenge or a threat in the face of uncertainty, and threat evolved as a challenge to the organism's allostatic state of "stability through change" [18, 19]. Metabolic brain energy must be expended to maintain physiological parameters within a normative range in response to external and internal environmental stressors leading to the risk of allostatic overload. The brain's stress response systems, consisting of amygdala/lateral hypothalamus SNS overdrive, the excessive output of the HPA axis and a pro-inflammatory state, serve as conduits to the body's end organs. This modulation by a stress hormone and neurotransmitter-induced state, alerts target tissues to their need to adjust metabolism to maintain allostasis. This is satisfactory when a challenge is acute and self-limited, but if the psychosocial stress is chronic, cellular oxidative stress and allostatic overload may lower the threshold for disease [20].

4.4 The "New" Mind-Body Medicine

Our understanding of MBM has benefitted from advances in studies of genomics, epigenetics, and oxidative metabolism. Epel et al. [21] showed that perceived stress or the psychological stress of chronic, highly demanding caregiving were both associated with telomere length shortening and low telomerase activity in peripheral blood mononuclear cell (PBMC) and with oxidative stress measures.

The pro-inflammatory transcription factor NF-kB has been tapped as a possible link between psychosocial stress and cellular oxidative stress [22]. The activation of this transcription factor is known to play a key role in vascular and renal disease. This suggests that activation of NF-kB, evoked by psychosocial stress and causing vascular inflammation, may damage vascular endothelial functioning and present an additional risk factor for cardiovascular, cerebrovascular, and renal disease.

Chronic elevation in psychosocial stress leading to allostatic overload results in downstream complications including overactive NF-kB gene pathway expression and under-activation of anti-viral type I interferon (IFN) pathway genes [23]. This results in an increase in susceptibility to NCDs as well as viral diseases, including coronavirus illnesses. This process is thought to be propelled by the overactivation of immune cell gene expression in the NF-kB activation pathway and the under-activation of gene expression in the IFN pathway. This gene expression profile has become known as "*the conserved transcriptional response to adversity (CTRA).*" [23–25].

Allostatic loading can lead to oxidative stress with the resultant production of free radicals and stress-sensitive heat shock protein (HSP) gene expression/production as a ligand for toll-like 4 receptors. This can be understood as mitochondrial allostatic load (MAL) [26]. Chronic psychosocial stress, through metabolic and neuroendocrine signals, causes adjustments of mitochondrial structure and function, which can lead to MAL and inefficiency of energy processing.

The mitochondrial allostatic load can induce macrophages to produce pro-inflammatory and cytotoxic mediators including inducible Nitric Oxide (iNO), Tumor Necrosis Factor (TNF), and cytokines Il-6 and Il-12 through an inducible Nitric Oxide Synthase (iNOS)/NF-kB / cAMP response element-binding protein (CREB)/COX-2 mechanism [27].

The metabolic syndrome, which includes hypertension, truncal obesity, insulin-resistant diabetes mellitus, and hyperlipidemia, can create a non-pathogen associated molecular pattern (non-PAMP) that activates pro-inflammatory transcription factor NF-kB and can psychologically produce oxidative stress, cytokines, growth factors, angiotensin II, and advanced glycation end-products (AGEs). The translocation of NF-kB into the nucleus then takes place in endothelial, smooth muscle, monocyte/macrophage and renal glomerular and epithelial cells. NF-kB then binds to nuclear DNA, activating transcription of cytokines, coagulation and adhesion factors and AGE receptors (RAGEs). This situation promotes endothelial dysfunction setting the stage for cardiovascular, cerebrovascular disease, and renal disease.

The degree of NF-kB activation in PBMCs correlates with oxidative stress [28]. Immobilization stress in rats activates NF-kB and dependent gene expression [29]. Lymphocyte NF-kB increases in women stressed by breast biopsy [30]. And PBMC NF-kB is activated by psychosocial stress, which correlates with a stress-induced rise in catecholamines and cortisol.

Removing stress in normal circumstances will usually downregulate NF-kB within an hour. However, there is a variability in stress perception that can be translated into prolonged NF-kB activation, perhaps related to a variance in stress-related gene activation. Therapeutic interventions that decrease stress-related oxidative stress can reduce NF-kB activation [28]. Yogic meditation may reverse the pattern of increased NF-κB-related transcription of pro-inflammatory cytokines in healthy individuals confronting a significant life stressor [31].

Psychosocial stress-induced NF-kB activation may be converted into a constant threat of allostatic overload, increasing the risk of a myriad of NCDs, often existing in multi-morbidity. The fact that psychosocial stress-induced NF-kB activation can be measured in accessible PBMCs has, along with single cell analysis of selected cell lines and measurement of genomic alterations, changes in oxidative metabolites and telomere dynamics, helped with research into the stress—NCD pathology link and also into whether mind-body therapies can therapeutically affect cellular activities [32].

Bower and Irwin [33] reviewed seven randomized controlled studies of gene expression effects of mind-body therapies [33]. These trials all showed a decrease in pro-inflammatory gene expression patterns with consistent reductions in

NF-kB activity [33]. These effects were seen with Yoga, Tai Chi, and meditation, and occurred in diverse populations.

Buric et al. [34] reviewed clinical and non-clinical studies using a variety of research designs that have studied gene expression analysis in relaxation response eliciting mind-body interventions (i.e., mindfulness and other meditation techniques, Yoga, Tai Chi, Qigong, and breath regulation). Eighteen relevant studies were analyzed. Overall, the studies indicate that these interventions are associated with a down-regulation of the NF-kB gene ontology pathway. Thus, it appears that mind-body therapies may attenuate the adverse impact that chronic stress has on gene expression, with implications for health promotion and illness prevention, notably among individuals with heightened chronic stress, including marginalized racial or ethnic groups or individuals of low socioeconomic status (SES).

We see in this "new" molecular MBM the opportunity for greater understanding and insight into the pillars of human resiliency—relaxation response eliciting meditation, cognitive skills, social support and the conscious positive expectation that comes with belief in positive psychological principles that often accompany spiritual meaning and purpose in one's life. When lifestyle improvements (sleep hygiene, low glycemic diet, and exercise) are added, even greater effects can be seen. Mindful exercise like Yoga incorporates many of these resilience dimensions in one approach.

4.5 Resilience, Health Promotion, and Illness Prevention

In engineering terms, the word *resilienc*e refers to the ability to bounce back from a stressor or adversity. Resilience infers effective adaptation across personal dimensions in the setting of significant adversity. Resilient people display five major capacities. They show the capacity to experience reward and are motivated by optimism and purpose. They have the capacity to circumscribe fear responsiveness, enabling them to effect needed change despite fear. They have the capacity to use flexible, adaptive behaviors to obtain social support through affiliation and to provide other-regarding support to others. They show the ability to use cognitive skills to reinterpret the meaning of negative stimuli in a more positive light. They integrate a sense of life purpose and meaning in combination with and ethical moral compass and spiritual connectedness [35, 36].

It is increasingly clear that our genetic endowment really is not the sole author of our destiny. The environment is a major contributor through epigenetic influences whereby certain genes are activated, and others inactivated in relation to environmental variables. This realization has revolutionized our understanding not only of mind-body medicine but of medicine in general.

Thus if one perceives a task as stressful, such as taking care of a chronically-ill child, telomeres will show accelerated aging as measured in the number of base pairs lost per year [21]. This effect is tied to the increased production of oxidative metabolites in the face of psychosocial stress. At the same time, as discussed above, we will see the instigation of a chronic pro-inflammatory state that can increase vulnerability to NCDs [25]. Epigenetics studies advance the potential for a new field of medicine, which is being called *enviromimetics* [37]. They also suggest a question. Can naturally salutogenic environmental changes be reliably approximated by mind-body therapies like Yoga to change gene activation and deactivation states resulting in health benefits? This is a ripe area for exploratory research.

4.6 The Mind-Body Medicine Stress to Resilience Ratio

In 1982, the medical sociologist George Albee proposed an interesting ratio [38]. It included a numerator (stress) and a denominator (resilience) that when processed led to a fairly good approximation of future vulnerability to mental illness. This could be considered an Illness Index reflecting propensity to not only to mental illness but to all stress-related NCDs based on allostatic loading. For example, in women with systemic lupus erythematosus, a low social support group (low resilience denominator) had an increased risk of a lupus flare. There are many examples of this Illness Index relationship in the literature [39–45].

In a classic 1984 paper, Ruberman and his colleagues sifted from a cohort of over 2000 men post-MI, a group with a high life stress numerator. Mortality was increased over 36 months. In another group with low social support or high social isolation representing a low denominator, they also found a high mortality rate at 36 months. When subjects with both the high numerator and low denominator signifying a high Illness Index were tracked the 3-year mortality rate was enormously high.

Mind-body Interventions, including RR-based meditative approaches have been known for some time to benefit patients with stress-related disorders [46]. However, research is spotty and study reliability and replicability are often substandard. Methodological issues plague the field. Despite these research challenges, evidence for the efficacy of Mind-Body interventions is increasing, and the biological basis for positive effects is becoming clearer [47].

Astin et al. [48], in their review, found strong to moderate evidence of Mind-Body Intervention efficacy in a variety of stress-related medical conditions including cardiovascular disease, hypertension, insomnia, low back pain, headache, arthritis self-care, incontinence, surgical outcomes and cancer treatment tolerance. Pelletier [49] found strong evidence of benefit for acute pain and fibromyalgia. There is also RCT efficacy data in the management of asthma, allergies, dermatological disorders, diabetes, HIV progression, irritable bowel syndrome, post-stroke rehabilitation, peptic ulcer, pregnancy outcomes, chronic obstructive pulmonary disease, and tinnitus.

Mind-Body Interventions have been shown to be effective in stress-related anxiety and depression [50–53] though these studies have methodological limitations [54, 55]. Thus meditation techniques, such as mindfulness-based stress reduction, have been used for anxiety and depressed mood, but also for cardiovascular complaints, insomnia, premenstrual syndrome, psoriasis, and chronic pain. Hypnosis has been used for the treatment of acute and chronic pain, including surgical interventions; biofeedback can be useful for defecation disorders, enuresis, stroke rehabilitation and many pediatric conditions; and relaxation response therapies are indicated for the adjunctive treatment of sleep dysfunction, hypertension, and headache. Overall there appears to be little specificity in the application of mind-body therapies. Given similar underlying mechanisms of action, e.g., better emotion regulation, if one approach is efficacious, chances are other techniques will also show some efficacy. Personal preference for one approach over another often adds to the potency. More research will be required to explore whether personalized medicine with specific appraisal-based recommendations for certain disorders will become more commonplace [56].

Philosophically meditation can come to focus on the impermanence of all things and on "release from mental fixations," something referred to as non-attachment (*Sanskrit: virāga*) [57] But somewhat paradoxically, meditation creates a relaxed state commensurate with somatic markers reminiscent of what is felt during the solace of secure attachment [58]. The meditative state reminds us of mother-child attunement wherein parasympathetic tone predominates with lower heart rate and blood pressure, a decrease in galvanic skin response, an increase in belly respiratory amplitude, accompanied by decreased respiratory rate and increased high-frequency heart rate variability (HRV) [59, 60].

Mind-body interventions can promote cost-effective self-care. Reports suggest that these approaches can lower outpatient visits, postoperative length of stay, unnecessary procedures and overall medical costs [61–63]. When patient satisfaction and quality of life are queried as part of a cost-effectiveness analysis, mind-body interventions are found to be helpful [64]. In most cases, these therapies are employed as adjunctive aids to conventional medical treatments. There is increasing interest in researching the role mind-body medicine might play in primary prevention and secondary as well as tertiary prevention in light of the important role that stress plays in vulnerability to many diseases and in their exacerbations [65].

4.7 Yoga in Cardiovascular Disease

Yoga is a mindful exercise approach that has been used for thousands of years in the East, and has increasingly been adopted as a preventative and therapeutic tool in the West [66]. The National Health Interview Survey showed that Yoga was the most commonly used complementary health approach among US adults. In 2012, 9.5% of Americans used yoga, and in 2017 that number went up to 14.3%. In 2017, women were more likely to use yoga meditation in the past 12 months then were men [67].

Thus, Yoga is becoming more popular as a complementary approach to stress-related chronic illnesses, including cardiac disease. There is some limited evidence that it can mitigate the CVD risk factors inherent in stress-related metabolic syndrome [68].

4.7.1 Mechanisms of Yoga

Yoga is thought to improve insulin resistance as well as other aspects of metabolic syndrome [68]. The benefits of the physical postures and breathing exercises of Yoga performed with mindful focus and its effects on stimulating the vagal nerve are theorized to promote health.

Along with other forms of RR and mindfulness and mindful exercise, Yoga reduces perceived stress. This stress reduction may connect with three interconnected physiological changes. Yoga can stimulate the vagus nerve imparting a parasympathetic tone. Yoga can also reduce perceived stress through a mindfulness meditative stance that strengthens selective attention on exercise and musculoskeletal stretching. And the kinetics of Yoga itself can adjust connective tissue hormonal messengers and immune factors in connective tissue [69]. The mechanical effects of musculoskeletal stretching achieved through yoga may reduce the innate inflammatory response [68].

Yoga may promote a healthy parasympathetic to sympathetic nervous system ratio. Increases in HRV along with decreased heart rate and blood pressure may ensue. Through these stimulating effects on parasympathetic tone, it is thought that Yoga may decrease anxiety and depressive symptoms and improve restorative sleep. Diminishments in metabolic syndrome (insulin resistance with Type II diabetes risk, truncal obesity, hyperlipidemia, and hypertension) and reductions in body mass index can also be seen [68].

These three physiological changes of Yoga may produce downstream improvements in coagulation and inflammatory states. Enhancing fibrinolysis and reducing oxidative stress may reduce atherosclerosis as the product of a chronic inflammatory state driven by macrophages.

There is also some research, which is in its infancy, suggesting that Yoga can improve brachial artery reactivity in coronary artery disease patients as the effect of an increased parasympathetic to sympathetic ratio with benefits for arterial function. Yoga researchers are also studying baroreflex sensitivity improvements and reductions in terminal pro-B-atrial natriuretic peptide (BNP) as a result of Yoga interventions [70].

4.7.2 Yoga and Heart Rate Variability

Heart rate variability (HRV), as a reflection of the balance between sympathetic and parasympathetic nervous system functioning, serves as a marker for health and fitness. The HRV measure can also be thought of as a reflection of resilience to chronic or overwhelming stress, in other words, as a version of the stress to resilience Illness Index. Tyagi et al. [71] published a comprehensive literature review on Yoga and HRV. Fifteen studies were RCTs, and they suggested that Yoga can affect autonomic regulation of the heart and increase HRV. Yoga practicing subjects showed increased vagal tone at rest compared to non-Yoga subjects. However, the authors stressed that these studies were generally of poor quality with limitations in methodology and sample size.

In 2018, Praveena et al., in a prospective and longitudinal study of 67 women who were studied within 5 years post-menopause, showed cardiovascular protection after 3 months of Yoga practice [72]. Yoga increased HRV leading the authors to suggest that such improving HRV with Yoga practice can potentially reduce cardiovascular disease risk in postmenopausal women.

Sullivan et al. [73] have suggested that the *gunas* of Yoga map onto neural platforms associated with the polyvagal theory [74]. This theory states that the autonomic nervous system (ANS) evolved in stages in order to enhance and refine our defensive strategies against stress. The first evolvement is said to have been the dorsal vagal complex (DVC) associated with diminished activation, heart rate and blood pressure, along with an avoidance approach that disconnects the person from the stressor. The authors suggest this might align with the *tamas* state of the Yoga practitioner. Next to evolve was the SNS responsible for a physiology marked by increases in norepinephrine and epinephrine along with decreased HRV, increased heart rate and blood pressure. This state leads to anxiety and fear in the face of uncertainty and threat and bears a resemblance to the Yogic state of *rajas*. Finally, the ventral vagal complex (VVC) came on line, expressed as increased respiratory sinus arrhythmia, decreased blood pressure and decreased catecholamines, associated with subjective experiences such as calm, equanimity, and connection that practitioners describe as *sattva?*

4.7.3 Yoga and Heart Failure

Stable heart failure patients are considered candidates for cardiac rehabilitation programs with the hope of improving exercise tolerance and quality of life while providing some tertiary prevention of future cardiovascular events. Public insurance in the USA supports cardiac rehabilitation for heart failure patients. However, there are presently no multicenter clinical trials studying Yoga for heart failure.

In an RCT that looked at the effects of Yoga therapy on cardiac function and terminal pro-BNP in heart failure patients, Krishna et al. [75] found improvement in left ventricular ejection fraction and a reduction in pro-BNP.

Pullen et al. [76] studied 19 New York Heart Association Class I-III HF patients with a mean ejection fraction of 25% who were randomized to either yoga treatment ($n = 9$) or standard medical therapy ($n = 10$). These researchers performed graded exercise tests and collected biomarkers, including interleukin-6 (IL-6), C-reactive protein (CRP), and superoxide dismutase (SOD). They also used the Minnesota Living with Heart Failure Questionnaire (MLHFQ) to study the quality of life (QOL) changes. The Yoga treatment cohort showed significantly improved exercise tolerance. In addition, IL-6 and CRP levels were significantly reduced while the anti-oxidant SOD was significantly increased in Yoga group. The QOL scores improved by 25.7% in the Yoga group compared to a 2.9% increase in the medical therapy group. The authors concluded that Yoga may increase exercise tolerance while lowering inflammation and improving QOL and call for longitudinal research with larger sample sizes [69].

4.7.4 Yoga and Arrhythmia

The Yoga My Heart study studied patients with paroxysmal atrial fibrillation (AF) using a single-center pre-post design [77]. A three-month non-interventional observational phase was followed by twice weekly one-hour Yoga sessions for the next 3 months. The frequency of atrial fibrillation episodes was recorded along with SF 36 anxiety and depression scales. Yoga practice significantly reduced symptomatic and asymptomatic AF episodes as well as depression and anxiety. Quality of life measures of physical functioning and general health vitality and social activity all significantly improved. In addition, heart rate and systolic and diastolic blood pressure all decreased. The researchers suggest that Yoga can improve atrial arrhythmia symptoms and health burden along with symptoms of anxiety and depression and quality of life in patients with AF. More studies to replicate these findings will be important [78].

4.7.5 Yoga and Cardiac Rehabilitation

Yoga offers a primary, secondary, and tertiary prevention modality. Yadav et al. [79] looked at short-term yoga-based lifestyle interventions using Framingham risk score to estimate 10-year cardiovascular risk in a single-arm pre-post study of 386 subjects, 252 of whom were females. Results indicated a significant reduction in estimated cardiovascular risk in the Yoga intervention group. In November 2018 at the American Heart Association meetings in Chicago, a multicenter RCT study of a Yoga-based cardiac rehabilitation (Yoga-CaRe) program was presented as an example of tertiary prevention. The study from India looked at 1989 standard cardiac rehabilitation patients and 1970 Yoga cardiac rehabilitation subjects [80]. While mortality, stroke rate and admissions for cardiac emergencies were comparable in both cohorts, secondary outcomes at 3 months showed better health status, tobacco cessation and compliance with medication in the intention to treat group analysis.

In a prospective single-blind study, 250 male post coronary artery bypass grafting (CABG) patients were randomized into two groups—a Yoga group and a treatment as usual group [81]. Significant findings in the Yoga group included a lowering of blood glucose at 1 year in those with pre-study elevated fasting blood sugars, improvement in HDL levels, and improvements in positive affect. There were also improvements in anxiety, depression, and negative affect. The researchers suggest that supplementing traditional cardiac rehabilitation with Yoga therapy can potentially enhance tertiary prevention in this population.

4.8 Yoga Side Effects

Yoga has a low risk of side effects when performed in moderation. Yoga should be performed with proper training and guidance [66]. Hyperactive and sudden changes in yoga postures may be stressful and should be avoided, especially in the elderly or people with high ocular pressure disorders. A number of cardiovascular side effects, such as occasional reports of vertebral artery occlusion after neck manipulations during yoga practice, have been noted. Shoulder standing exercises that flex the neck should be avoided in patients with hypertension and CHD to avoid neck arterial damage. Patients with cardiac or pulmonary conditions should avoid painful or stressful exercises. Yoga is not a substitute for allopathic medical care and should be viewed as a complementary approach [66].

4.9 Conclusion

The stress-related NCDs are the most significant challenges to health around the world. Cardiovascular diseases account for 30% of the deaths and create a significant burden of disease as well, especially when comorbid with depression. Yoga and meditation are safe, inexpensive adjunctive approaches to the treatment of cardiovascular disease that can help us address this public health crisis. The research will need to be more methodologically rigorous before these complementary approaches are more widely accepted.

References

1. NCCAM National Institutes of Health. Mind-body medicine: an overview. 2007. http://nccam.nih.gov/health/backgrounds/mindbody.htm. Accessed 26 Feb 2008.
2. NCCIH National Institutes of Health. Mind and body practices. 2017. https://www.nccih.nih.gov/health/mind-and-body-practices
3. Benson H. The relaxation response. New York: Avon Books; 1976.
4. Bloom DE, Cafiero ET, Jané-Llopis E, Abrahams-Gessel S, Bloom LR, Fathima S, Feigl AB, Gaziano T, Mowafi M, Pandya A, Prettner K, Rosenberg L, Seligman B, Stein A, Weinstein C. The global economic burden of non-communicable diseases. Geneva: World Economic Forum; 2011.
5. Whiteford HA, Degenhardt L, Rehm J, Baxter AJ, Ferrari AJ, Erskine HE, Charlson FJ, Norman RE, Flaxman AD, Johns N, Burstein R, Murray CJ, Vos T. Global burden of disease attributable to mental and substance use disorders: findings from the global burden of disease study 2010. Lancet. 2013;9382(9904):1575–86.
6. Fricchione GL. The science of mind body medicine and the public health challenges of today. S Afr J Psychol. 2014;44(4):404–15.
7. WHO. Preventing chronic diseases: a vital investment. WHO global report. Geneva: WHO; 2005.
8. Hare DL, Toukhsati SR, Johansson P, Jaarsma T. Depression and cardiovascular disease: a clinical review. Eur Heart J. 2014;35(21):1365–72.
9. Narayan KM, Ali MK, Koplan JP. Global noncommunicable diseases--where worlds meet. N Engl J Med. 2010;363(13):1196–8.
10. Chrousos GP. Stress and disorders of the stress system. Nat Rev Endocrinol. 2009;5:374–81. https://doi.org/10.1038/nrendo.2009.106.
11. Cannon W. Bodily changes in pain, hunger, fear, and rage. New York: Appleton; 1929.
12. Selye H. The general adaptation syndrome. J Clin Endocrinol. 1946;6:177.
13. Chrousos GP, Gold PW. The concepts of stress and stress system disorders. Overview of physical and behavioral homeostasis. JAMA. 1992;267:1244–52.
14. Tsigos C, Chrousos GP. Hypothalamic-pituitary-adrenal axis, neuroendocrine factors and stress. J Psychosom Res. 2002;53:865–71.
15. Chrousos GP. Organization and integration of the endocrine system. Sleep Med Clin. 2007;2:125–45.
16. Sterling P, Eyer J. Allostasis: a new paradigm to explain arousal pathology. In: Fisher S, Reason J, editors. Handbook of life stress, cognition and health. New York: Wiley; 1988.
17. McEwen BS, Stellar E. Stress and the individual. Mechanisms leading to disease. Arch Intern Med. 1993;153:2093–101.
18. McEwen BS. Protective and damaging effects of stress mediators. N Engl J Med. 1998;338:171–9.
19. McEwen BS, Seeman T. Protective and damaging effects of mediators of stress. Elaborating and testing the concepts of allostasis and allostatic load. Ann N Y Acad Sci. 1999;896:30–47.
20. Epel ES, Lin J, Wilhelm FH, Wolkowitz OM, Cawthon R, Adler NE, Dolbier C, Mendes WB, Blackburn EH. Cell aging in relation to stress arousal and cardiovascular disease risk factors. Psychoneuroendocrinology. 2006;31:277–87.
21. Epel ES, Blackburn EH, Lin J, Dhabhar FS, Adler NE, Morrow JD, Cawthon RM. Accelerated telomere shortening in response to life stress. Proc Natl Acad Sci U S A. 2004;101:17312–5.
22. Bierhaus A, Humpert PM, Nawroth PP. NF-kappaB as a molecular link between psychosocial stress and organ dysfunction. Pediatr Nephrol. 2004;19:1189–91.
23. Cole SW. The conserved transcriptional response to adversity. Curr Opin Behav Sci. 2019;28:31–7.
24. Gelaye B, Foster S, Bhasin M, Tawakol A, Fricchione G. SARS-CoV-2 morbidity and mortality in racial/ethnic minority populations: a window into the stress related inflammatory basis of health disparities? Brain Behav Immun Health. 2020;9:100158.
25. Cole SW. Human social genomics. PLoS Genet. 2014;10:e1004601.
26. Picard M, McEwen BS. Psychosocial stress and mitochondria. A conceptual framework. Psychosom Med. 2018;80(2):126–40.
27. Billack B, Heck DE, Mariano TM, Gardner CR, Sur R, Laskin DL, Laskin JD. Induction of cyclooxygenase-2 by heat shock protein 60 in macrophages and endothelial cells. Am J Physiol Cell Physiol. 2002;283:C1267–77.
28. Hofmann MA, Schiekofer S, Isermann B, Kanitz M, Henkels M, Joswig M, Treusch A, Morcos M, Weiss T, Borcea V, Abdel Khalek AK, Amiral J, Tritschler H, Ritz E, Wahl P, Ziegler R, Bierhaus A, Nawroth PP. Peripheral blood mononuclear cells isolated from patients with diabetic nephropathy show increased activation of the oxidative-stress sensitive transcription factor NF-kappaB. Diabetologia. 1999;42(2):222–32.
29. Madrigal JL, Hurtado O, Moro MA, Lizasoain I, Lorenzo P, Castrillo A, Boscá L, Leza JC. The increase in TNFalpha levels is implicated in NF-kappaB activation and inducible nitric oxide synthase expression in brain cortex after immobilization stress. Neuropsychopharmacology. 2002;26(2):155–63.
30. Nagabhushan M, Mathews HL, Witek-Janusek L. Aberrant nuclear expression of AP-1 and NFkappaB in lymphocytes of women stressed by the experience of breast biopsy. Brain Behav Immun. 2001;15:78–84.
31. Black DS, Cole SW, Irwin MR, Breen E, St Cyr NM, Nazarian N, Khalsa DS, Lavretsky H. Yogic meditation reverses NF-κB and IRF-related transcriptome dynamics in leukocytes of family dementia caregivers in a randomized controlled trial. Psychoneuroendocrinology. 2013;38(3):348–55.

32. Bierhaus A, Wolf J, Andrassy M, Rohleder N, Humpert PM, Petrov D, Ferstl R, von Eynatten M, Wendt T, Rudofsky G, Joswig M, Morcos M, Schwaninger M, McEwen B, Kirschbaum C, Nawroth PP. A mechanism converting psychosocial stress into mononuclear cell activation. Proc Natl Acad Sci U S A. 2003;100(4):1920–5.
33. Bower JE, Irwin MR. Mind-body therapies and control of inflammatory biology: a descriptive review. Brain Behav Immun. 2016;51:1–11.
34. Buric I, Farias M, Jong J, Mee C, Brazil IA. What is the molecular signature of mind-body interventions? A systematic review of gene expression changes induced by meditation and related practices. Front Immunol. 2017;8:670.
35. Feder A, Nestler EJ, Charney DS. Psychobiology and molecular genetics of resilience. Nat Rev Neurosci. 2009;10:446–57.
36. Southwick SM, Vythilingam M, Charney DS. The psychobiology of depression and resilience to stress: implications for prevention and treatment. Annu Rev Clin Psychol. 2005;1:255–91.
37. McOmish CE, Hannan AJ. Enviromimetics: exploring gene environment interactions to identify therapeutic targets for brain disorders. Expert Opin Ther Targets. 2007;11:899–913.
38. Albee GW. Preventing psychopathology and promoting human potential. Am Psychol. 1982;37:1043–50.
39. Ward MM, Lotstein DS, Bush TM, Lambert RE, van Vollenhoven R, Neuwelt CM. Psychosocial correlates of morbidity in women with systemic lupus erythematosus. J Rheumatol. 1999;26:2153–8.
40. Sutcliffe N, Clarke AE, Levinton C, Frost C, Gordon C, Isenberg DA. Associates of health status in patients with systemic lupus erythematosus. J Rheumatol. 1999;26:2352–6.
41. Sewitch MJ, Abrahamowicz M, Bitton A, Daly D, Wild GE, Cohen A, Katz S, Szego PL, Dobkin PL. Psychological distress, social support, and disease activity in patients with inflammatory bowel disease. Am J Gastroenterol. 2001;96:1470–9.
42. Seeman TE. Health promoting effects of friends and family on health outcomes in older adults. Am J Health Promot. 2000;14:362–70.
43. Case RB, Moss AJ, Case N, McDermott M, Eberly S. Living alone after myocardial infarction. Impact on prognosis. JAMA. 1992;267:515–9.
44. Horsten M, Mittleman MA, Wamala SP, Schenck-Gustafsson K, Orth-Gomér K. Depressive symptoms and lack of social integration in relation to prognosis of CHD in middle-aged women. The Stockholm Female Coronary Risk Study. Eur Heart J. 2000;21:1072–80.
45. Ruberman W, Weinblatt E, Goldberg JD, Chaudhary BS. Psychosocial influences on mortality after myocardial infarction. N Engl J Med. 1984;311:552–9.
46. Mandle CL, Jacobs SC, Arcari PM, Domar AD. The efficacy of relaxation response interventions with adult patients: a review of the literature. J Cardiovasc Nurs. 1996;10:4–26.
47. Ernst E, Pittler MH, Wider B, Boddy K. Mind-body therapies: are the trial data getting stronger? Altern Ther Health Med. 2007;13:62–4.
48. Astin JA, Shapiro SL, Eisenberg DM, Forys KL. Mind-body medicine: state of the science, implications for practice. J Am Board Fam Pract. 2003;16:131–47.
49. Pelletier KR. Mind-body medicine in ambulatory care: an evidence-based assessment. J Ambul Care Manage. 2004;27:25–42.
50. Benson H, Frankel FH, Apfel R, Daniels MD, Schniewind HE, Nemiah JC, Sifneos PE, Crassweller KD, Greenwood MM, Kotch JB, Arns PA, Rosner B. Treatment of anxiety: a comparison of the usefulness of self-hypnosis and a meditational relaxation technique. An overview. Psychother Psychosom. 1978;30:229–42.
51. Kabat-Zinn J, Massion AO, Kristeller J, Peterson LG, Fletcher KE, Pbert L, Lenderking WR, Santorelli SF. Effectiveness of a meditation-based stress reduction program in the treatment of anxiety disorders. Am J Psychiatry. 1992;149:936–43.
52. Esch T, Stefano GB, Fricchione GL, Benson H. The role of stress in neurodegenerative diseases and mental disorders. Neuro Endocrinol Lett. 2002;23:199–208.
53. Swaab DF, Bao AM, Lucassen PJ. The stress system in the human brain in depression and neurodegeneration. Ageing Res Rev. 2005;4:141–94.
54. Pilkington K, Kirkwood G, Rampes H, Richardson J. Yoga for depression: the research evidence. J Affect Disord. 2005;89:13–24.
55. Toneatto T, Nguyen L. Does mindfulness meditation improve anxiety and mood symptoms? A review of the controlled research. Can J Psychiatr. 2007;52:260–6.
56. Barrows KA, Jacobs BP. Mind-body medicine. An introduction and review of the literature. Med Clin North Am. 2002;86:11–31.
57. Sahdra BK, Shaver PR, Brown KW. A scale to measure nonattachment: a Buddhist complement to Western research on attachment and adaptive functioning. J Pers Assess. 2010;92(2):116–27.
58. Fricchione GL. Compassion and healing in medicine and society: on the nature and use of attachment solutions to separation challenges. Johns Hopkins University Press; 2011.
59. Tang YY, Ma Y, Fan Y, Feng H, Wang J, Feng S, Lu Q, Hu B, Lin Y, Li J, Zhang Y, Wang Y, Zhou L, Fan M. Central and autonomic nervous system interaction is altered by short-term meditation. Proc Natl Acad Sci U S A. 2009;106(22):8865–70.
60. Craigmyle NA. The beneficial effects of meditation: contribution of the anterior cingulate and locus coeruleus. Front Psychol. 2013;4:731. https://doi.org/10.3389/fpsyg.2013.00731.
61. Benson H, Beary JF, Carol MP. The relaxation response. Psychiatry. 1974;37:37–46.
62. Sobel DS. The cost-effectiveness of mind-body medicine interventions. Prog Brain Res. 2000;122:393–412.
63. Stahl JE, Dossett ML, LaJoie AS, Denninger JW, Mehta DH, Goldman R, Fricchione GL, Benson H. Relaxation response and resiliency training and its

effect on healthcare resource utilization. PLoS One. 2015;10(10):e0140212. https://doi.org/10.1371/journal.pone.0140212.
64. Sobel DS. Rethinking medicine: improving health outcomes with cost-effective psychosocial interventions. Psychosom Med. 1995;57:234–44.
65. Astin JA. Mind-body therapies for the management of pain. Clin J Pain. 2004;20:27–32.
66. Mehta JL, Mehta P, Balakrishna VP. Yoga and cardiovascular disease. J Yoga Physiother. 2017;3(1):555604. https://doi.org/10.19080/JYP.2017.02.555603.
67. NCCIH. Use of yoga and meditation. US adult age 18 and over, 2012 and 2017. National Health Interview Survey; 2017.
68. Manchanda SC, Madan K. Yoga and meditation in cardiovascular disease. Clin Res Cardiol. 2014;103(9):675–80. Erratum in: Clin Res Cardiol. 2014;103(9):763. https://doi.org/10.1007/s00392-014-0663-9.
69. Pullen PR, Seffens WS, Thompson WR. Yoga for heart failure: a review and future research. Int J Yoga. 2018;11(2):91–8.
70. Bhagat OL, Kharya C, Jaryal A, Deepak KK. Acute effects on cardiovascular oscillations during controlled slow yogic breathing. Indian J Med Res. 2017;145(4):503–12.
71. Tyagi A, Cohen M. Yoga and heart rate variability: a comprehensive review of the literature. Int J Yoga. 2016;9(2):97–113.
72. Praveena SM, Asha G, Sunita M, Anju J, Ratna B. Yoga offers cardiovascular protection in early postmenopausal women. Int J Yoga. 2018;11(1):37–43.
73. Sullivan MB, Erb M, Schmalzl L, Moonaz S, Noggle Taylor J, Porges SW. Yoga therapy and polyvagal theory: the convergence of traditional wisdom and contemporary neuroscience for self-regulation and resilience. Front Hum Neurosci. 2018;12:67. https://doi.org/10.3389/fnhum.2018.00067.
74. Porges SW. The polyvagal theory: phylogenetic contributions to social behavior. Physiol Behav. 2003;79:503–13. https://doi.org/10.1016/s0031-9384(03)00156-2.
75. Krishna BH, Pal P, Pal G, et al. A randomized controlled trial to study the effect of yoga therapy on cardiac function and N terminal pro BNP in heart failure. Integr Med Insights. 2014;9:1–6. https://doi.org/10.4137/IMI.S13939.
76. Pullen PR, Nagamia SH, Mehta PK, Thompson WR, Benardot D, Hammoud R, Parrott JM, Sola S, Khan BV. Effects of yoga on inflammation and exercise capacity in patients with chronic heart failure. J Card Fail. 2008;14(5):407–13.
77. Lakkireddy D, Atkins D, Pillarisetti J, Ryschon K, Bommana S, Drisko J, Vanga S, Dawn B. Effect of yoga on arrhythmia burden, anxiety, depression, and quality of life in paroxysmal atrial fibrillation: the YOGA my heart study. J Am Coll Cardiol. 2013;61(11):1177–82.
78. Akella K, Kanuri SH, Murtaza G, Della Rocca D, Kodwani N, Turagam M, Shenthar J, Padmanabhan D, Basu Ray I, Natale A, Gopinathannair R, Lakkireddy D. Impact of yoga on cardiac autonomic function and arrhythmias. J Atr Fibrillation. 2020;13(1):2408. https://doi.org/10.4022/jafib.2408.
79. Yadav R, Yadav RK, Sarvottam K, Netam R. Framingham risk score and estimated 10-year cardiovascular disease risk reduction by a short-term yoga-based lifeStyle intervention. J Altern Complement Med. 2017;23(9):730–7.
80. Prabhakaran D. Effectiveness of a yoga-based cardiac rehabilitation (Yoga-CaRe) program: a multi-centre randomised controlled trial of patients with acute myocardial infarction from India. Presented at: AHA 2018. November 10, 2018. Chicago, IL.
81. Raghuram N, Parachuri VR, Swarnagowri MV, et al. Yoga based cardiac rehabilitation after coronary artery bypass surgery: one-year results on LVEF, lipid profile and psychological states--a randomized controlled study. Indian Heart J. 2014;66(5):490–502.

Part II

Pathophysiology

5 Mechanistic Model for Yoga as a Therapeutic Modality in Cardiovascular Disease

Indranill Basu-Ray

5.1 Introduction

Yoga is an ancient Indian technique of healthy living. It is a combination of practices: asana (structured physical exercises), pranayama (breathing techniques), dharana (mindfulness), and dhyana (meditation). Numerous studies have corroborated the beneficial effects of yoga, which include a favorable influence on cardiac autonomic function and the alleviation of negative emotions and stress.

Today, we face a growing burden of noncommunicable diseases. Cardiovascular disease is the number one killer worldwide [1], with a fatality rate that is double that of cancer, the second largest killer. The number of patients with coronary artery disease, heart failure, or atrial fibrillation is on the rise due to a sedentary lifestyle, unhealthy food habits, and stress. Extensive research in the last few decades has revealed the critical role that yoga can play to eradicate stress, laying the foundation for a scientific understanding that stress-induced diseases can be alleviated or eliminated with a yogic lifestyle. This, in turn, has accentuated the relevance of yoga as a powerful preventive intervention in many other conditions and noncommunicable diseases, including heart disease, cancer, and rheumatological disorders—not only to ameliorate risk but also to modify neurohormonal causes that potentiate vascular inflammation that results in disease. The precise mechanism by which yoga induces such beneficial changes is yet to be delineated. However, a plethora of pointers indicates that neural, endocrine, immunological, cellular, genetic, and epigenetic mechanisms are at play [2].

This chapter attempts to cobble together the existing research to delineate a mechanistic model for a 5000-year-old practice from India. This is imperative, as a mechanistic hypothesis of this ancient but complex system would enable a more comprehensive understanding of its mechanism and reveal its yet-undiscovered positive health effects.

5.2 The Brain

The use of functional magnetic resonance imaging, computed tomography, and radioactive targeting to discern neuronal activity, neurotransmitter concentration, blood flow, and other physiological correlates have revealed a staggering amount of information about the yoga's effect on the brain. Yoga practice of varied lengths has been correlated with many changes, including increased cortical thickness and gray

I. Basu-Ray (✉)
Memphis VA Medical Center, Memphis, TN, USA

The University of Memphis, Memphis, TN, USA

All India Institute of Medical Sciences, Rishikesh, Uttarakhand, India
e-mail: ibr@ibasuray.com

I. Basu-Ray, D. Mehta (eds.), *The Principles and Practice of Yoga in Cardiovascular Medicine*,
https://doi.org/10.1007/978-981-16-6913-2_5

matter concentration in brain areas associated with arousal, mood, and memory [3, 4]. Areas related to negative emotional processing, including the amygdala, are attenuated in their function by yoga, while amplifications in other sites positively influence the cognitive part of the brain [5]. Changes in brain chemistry and selective neuronal firing propagate elevated mood by an enhanced release of neurotransmitters like serotonin and norepinephrine. Decreased stimulation of brain basal areas associated with negative emotions and stress could ensure reduced activation of the hypothalamic–pituitary–adrenal (HPA) axis, which fosters sympathetic discharges that release a cascade of hormones that initiate the "fight-or-flight" response.

The increased somatic sympathetic tone associated with these responses results in a plethora of aberrant pathological effects, such as vascular inflammation that leads to cardiovascular disease, dangerous arrhythmias, and sudden cardiac death. In fact, all chronic stress is associated with this response and, unfortunately, is a harbinger of cardiovascular disease. Direct damage to the heart leading to cardiomyopathy and arrhythmias have also been reported in this setting [6], although angina and other forms of chest pain syndrome are more common [7]. Coronary artery spasm that decreases nutritional flow to the cardiac musculature also has been documented, resulting in ischemia and type 2 Myocardial Infarction [8].

Electroencephalographic brain-wave recordings have shown increased theta, and alpha frequency ranges among yoga practitioners. Considerable evidence indicates that a global increase in alpha activity fosters an increased feeling of calm and positive affect, appropriately attenuating anxiety. Higher-frequency gamma activation (>30 Hz) also has been reported, particularly in long-term meditation practitioners [9]. Gamma frequency appears to be associated with various cognitive functions, and it has been proposed that gamma activity may facilitate the neural mechanisms underlying attention [9–11].

Yoga and meditation have also been found to influence medulla oblongata, a brain-stem structure that contains a central vagal relay station with thousands of neurons. This neuronal station is instrumental in regulating heart rate and respiration and is modulated by parasympathetic discharges that are evidenced in long-term yoga practitioners [4]. Even so, the details of neural pathways involved in many of these effects are yet to be delineated. Yoga elevates mammalian (or mechanistic) target of rapamycin (mTOR) signaling, which promotes the synthesis of proteins necessary for synapse formation and maturation; mTOR-dependent translational cascade may be the final pathway representing neurogenesis and neuroplasticity [12, 13].

Yoga has also been found to influence the sirtuin 1 signaling pathway [12]. Potential underlying molecular mechanisms for enhancing neuroplasticity and alleviating depression by increasing sirtuin 1 include promotion of mTOR signaling, reduction of methylation in brain-derived neurotrophic factor (BDNF) transcription, and regulation of circadian rhythm by inhibiting CLOCK protein, a histone acetyltransferase [12, 14].

5.3 The Autonomic Nervous System

Humans are a dominant species today because of the fight-or-flight mechanism, which prompted our forefathers to either escape from or kill the saber-toothed tiger that had entered the cave. Fight-or-flight is a primal behavior pattern that has enabled humans to deal with emergencies. Although we no longer live in caves or face such primal threats, when we are stressed due to anxiety, depression, or difficult situations such as economic downturns and pandemics, we generate the same fight-or-flight response, which is severely detrimental to the health of the cardiovascular system. Accentuated sympathetic nervous system (SNS) activity unleashed by psychological stress (Fig. 5.1) can induce and propagate heart failure, leading to end-stage heart disease and death. The SNS increases heart rate and works in conjunction with the HPA axis to switch on the inflammatory cascade. Atrial fibrillation and ventricular tachycardia, both associated

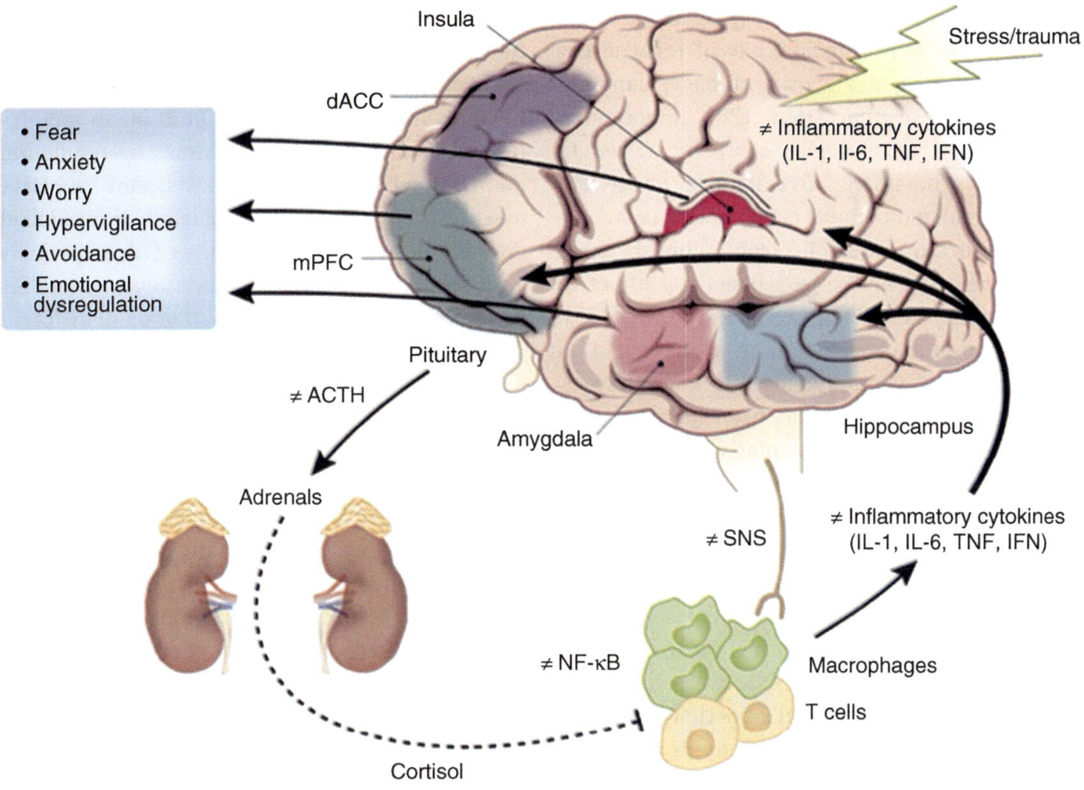

Fig. 5.1 Mechanisms and consequences of inflammation in fear- and anxiety-based disorders. Exposure to acute stressors in individuals with anxiety may facilitate increased immune activity in both the periphery and the central nervous system via stress and trauma effects on neuroendocrine systems and the sympathetic nervous system (SNS). Overactivity of the SNS and decreased activity of the parasympathetic nervous system promote pro-inflammatory cytokine release. The suppressed ability of glucocorticoids to inhibit inflammatory processes in these chronic stress states also contributes to a pro-inflammatory state that can influence neurotransmitter systems, neurocircuitry, and affective behavior. Cytokines may contribute to the maintenance of anxiety by affecting the activity and connections of related brain regions, including the amygdala, hippocampus, insula, medial prefrontal cortex (mPFC), and the anterior cingulate (ACC). Figure adapted from Felger et al. (2016) and reproduced by permission of Oxford University Press (http://global.oup.com/?cc=us). Michopoulos V, Powers A, Gillespie CF, Ressler KJ, Jovanovic T. Inflammation in fear- and anxiety-based disorders: PTSD, GAD, and beyond. Neuropsychopharmacology. 2017;42(1):254–70. Reprinted by permission

with considerable morbidity and mortality, are induced and sustained by an activated SNS [15, 16]. Sudden cardiac death is a syndrome of ventricular tachycardia and ventricular fibrillation that can be induced by a sympathetic surge [17]; it is responsible for half of all heart disease deaths. Indeed, sudden cardiac death is the largest cause of natural death in the USA, causing 325,000 adult deaths each year. Atrial fibrillation affects more than 33 million people worldwide. The parasympathetic nervous system (PNS) also is essential for regulating heart rate variability, which, when pronounced, can be detrimental [18].

Modern medicine uses many modalities to decrease SNS activity, such as beta-blockers and even sympathectomy in refractory cases. In refractory hypertension, the patient's blood pressure is not amenable to five or more drugs, and high SNS activity is believed to be the cause. Renal artery denervation and baroreceptor stimulation techniques are being investigated in these subsets of patients to reduce sympathetic drive [19–21]; however, clinical trials of renal artery denervation have not shown efficacy, damping enthusiasm to a great extent [22]. Importantly, although new technologies are being tested to attenuate sympathetic overactivity, most are experimental and come at considerable cost.

In contrast, research from almost three decades ago showed yoga's beneficial effect in accentuating the PNS over the SNS [23]. Pranayam, an ancient breathing exercise and an inherent part of yoga practice, is known to regulate the PNS [24]. Yoga has been found to tone down SNS activity, particularly in long-term practitioners, and can achieve better cardiac health [19]. By effectively attenuating SNS overactivity, yoga reduces heart rate and achieves a better quality of life for patients with atrial fibrillation, the most common arrhythmia seen in clinical practice [25, 26]. Yoga has been shown to help patients with discrete SNS overactivity that results in poorly controlled hypertension. Yoga reduces wear and tear on the body produced by chronic stress [27] by lessening sympathetic overactivity and improving parasympathetic tone, as evidenced by oxygen consumption level, heart rate, and the high-frequency component of heart rate variability [28].

5.4 Psychological Effects

Aberrant psychological states, including anxiety and depression, foster organic changes in the body and can influence mortality and morbidity [29]. Cardiac changes can include the development of severe heart failure due to heart muscle damage and the occurrence of rapid cardiac rhythms, such as atrial fibrillation. Acute triggers, such as anxiety, despair, and anger, may be risk factors for new symptomatic atrial fibrillation [30]. Heart failure with low cardiac function is known to precipitate sudden cardiac death.

Various clinical trials have indicated that yoga could play a significant role in reducing depression and related factors [31]. In times of stress, yoga helps its practitioners to develop a positive attitude, to become more self-aware, and to cope more effectively. Asana, pranayama, and meditation techniques enhance calm, mindfulness, and self-control [32]. Hatha yoga (a variation that includes only postures, with little or no meditation) hastens recovery from stress by regulating autonomic balance, homeostasis, and the HPA axis [33]. Yoga has been associated with reduced depression and improved quality of life in patients with atrial fibrillation [26]. Additional research is needed to examine the effects of yoga in different clinical cardiovascular diseases.

5.5 Endocrine Effects

Chronic stress perpetuates blood glucocorticosteroid (GCS) elevation with feedback-mediated glucocorticoid receptor downregulation. Modulation of the glucocorticoids, which are a slew of powerful hormones, occurs through the HPA axis (Fig. 5.2). Whereas acute GCS elevation is a survival mechanism that underlies the fight-or-flight response, chronic GCS elevation is counterproductive and could produce a plethora of cardiovascular pathologies, including endothelial dysfunction and vascular inflammation. This in turn accelerates the development of atherosclerosis, leading to stroke, myocardial infarction, and peripheral arterial disease. Persistent GCS elevation also activates the inflammatory cascade by activating the nuclear factor (NF)-κB pathway and heralds conserved transcriptional response to adversity (CTRA), as discussed below [34–37]. It is also apparent that GCS acts in the "neural alarm system" of the brain, which is related to anxiety, stress, and depression: high levels of GCS have been found in patients with depression [38, 39]. This connection may have other ramifications. It probably potentiates the vicious cycle of psychological anomalies potentiating endocrine changes that in turn intensify brain signals to potentiate further psychological aberrations. Potentiated GCS may also inhibit neuroplasticity, although the mechanism is yet not clearly delineated; lowering BDNF has been suggested as one possible mechanism [12, 35]. Dehydroepiandrosterone (DHEA), another hormone released by the adrenal glands, affects

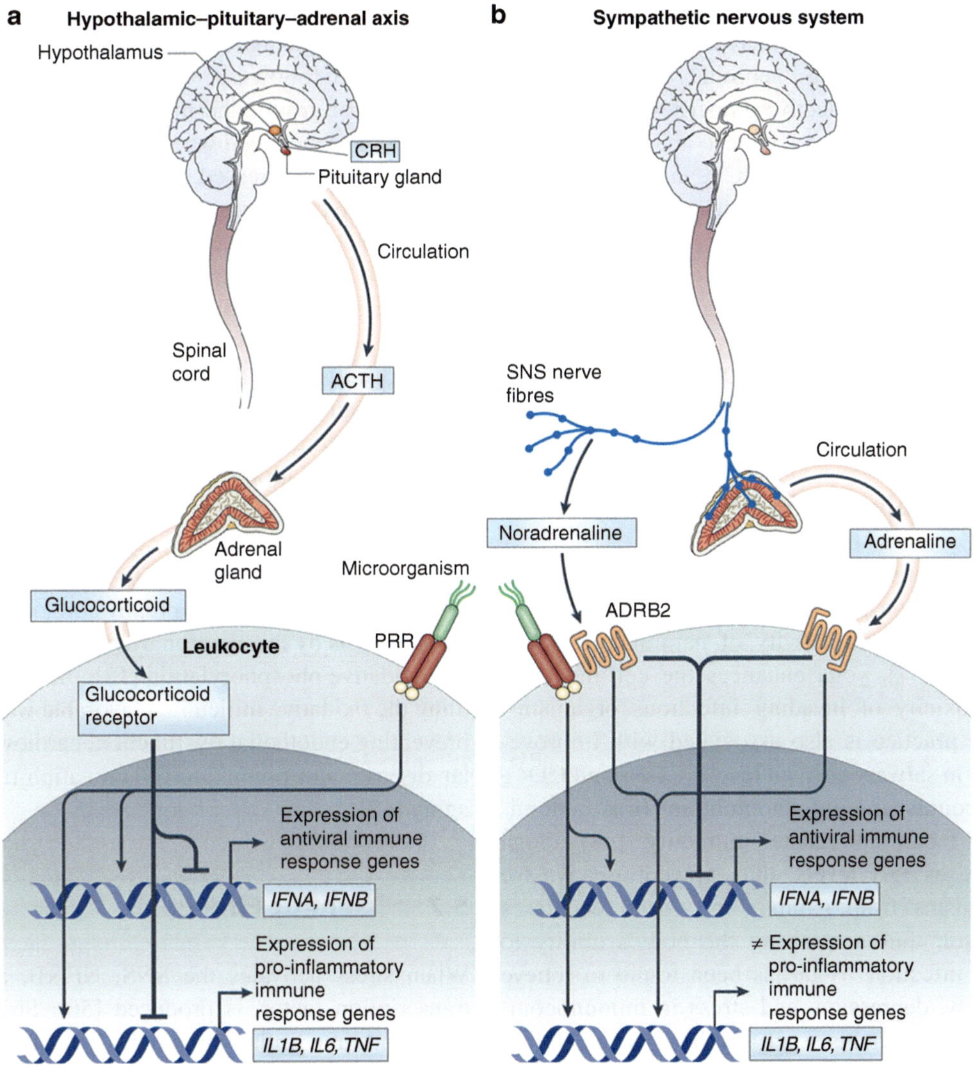

Fig. 5.2 Central nervous system regulation of innate immune response gene programs. (**a**) The HPA axis distributes glucocorticoid hormones through the blood to regulate gene expression in virtually every cell of the body. Hormone activation of the glucocorticoid receptor in leukocytes results in profound suppression of both pro-inflammatory gene networks (for example, NF-κB-mediated transcription of pro-inflammatory cytokine genes, such as *IL1β, IL6* and *TNF*) and antiviral gene programs (for example, IRF-mediated transcription of type I interferon (IFN) genes, such as *IFNA* and *IFNB*). Activation of cytokine receptors in the hypothalamus triggers the production of glucocorticoids by the HPA axis. This constitutes the body's primary systemic mechanism for negative feedback control of pro-inflammatory gene expression triggered by microbial pattern recognition receptors (PRRs). (**b**) During fight-or-flight responses and acute injury, nerve fibers from the sympathetic nervous system (SNS) release the neurotransmitter noradrenaline into primary and secondary lymphoid organs, all other major organ systems (including the vasculature and perivascular tissues) and many peripheral tissues in which pro-inflammatory reactions occur. SNS nerve fibers can also stimulate the adrenal glands to release stored adrenaline into the systemic circulation. Both of these neuromediators regulate vascular function and stimulate leukocyte adrenergic receptors (for example, ADRB2) to activate transcription factors such as CREB and GATA family factors. SNS-induced transcriptional alterations can modulate hematopoiesis, redeploy leukocytes between tissue and blood, and repress IRF-mediated antiviral immune response gene programs while enhancing many NF-κB-mediated pro-inflammatory programs. *ACTH* adrenocorticotropic hormone, *ADRB2* β2-adrenergic receptor, *CRH* corticotropin-releasing hormone, *HPA* hypothalamic–pituitary–adrenal, *IL* interleukin, *IRF* interferon regulatory factor, *NF-κB* nuclear factor-κB, *TNF* tumor necrosis factor. Irwin MR, Cole SW. Reciprocal regulation of the neural and innate immune systems. Nat Rev. Immunol. 2011;11(9):625–32. Reprinted by permission

several neurotransmitter systems within the central nervous system by increasing neuronal excitability, modulating neuronal plasticity, and exerting neuroprotective properties [40].

Growing evidence suggests that yoga acts on the HPA axis, decreases GCS, and increases glucocorticoid receptors and thus can reverse or prevent the deleterious effects of chronic stress. The cumulative effect is decreased cardiovascular disease in particular and decreased aging in general [41]. Yoga has been acknowledged both to increase the secretion of DHEA sulfate and to limit its destruction [42].

5.6 Cellular Effects

Yoga positively affects the immune system and inflammation pathways [43–45]. By increasing the number and activity of natural killer cells [32, 46, 47], yoga enhances the cell-mediated cytotoxicity of invading infectious organisms. Yoga practice is also associated with improvement in salivary cortisol levels, CD3+ and CD4+ cell counts, and immunoglobulin (Ig)A, a dominant factor in innate immunity [48]. Yoga increases IgA levels, thus preventing invasive organisms from gaining entry, and decreases cortisol, thus amplifying the body's ability to fight infection. Yoga has been found to relieve anxiety, depression, and stress in immunocompromised patients, such as those with HIV or cancer, thus enhancing immunity by improving CD+ cell counts [43, 46, 49].

Multiple studies have documented yoga's beneficial role in attenuating the immunological dysfunction that results in the overproduction of powerful pro-inflammatory cytokines and chemokines [50]. Yoga practice has been shown to downregulate an array of initiators and modulators of chronic inflammation, including interleukin (IL)-6, IL-1β, and tumor necrosis factor (TNF)-α [51, 52], including in randomized controlled trials [53]. One randomized trial found that IL-6, IL-1β, and TNF-α secretion were significantly lower in healthy individuals after yoga practice and in cultured blood challenged with a toll-like receptor agonist [54] (Fig. 5.3). Another study found that breast cancer patients who practiced yoga had a significant reduction in IL-6 at the 3-month follow-up, compared with a non-yoga control group, and that this reduction was even more pronounced when the amount of yoga practice was increased, suggesting a dose-response effect [55].

Markers for cellular recovery (such as the eukaryotic translation in initiation factor 2 alpha) are higher in yoga practitioners, which is an adaptive response to integrated stress response [12]. Yoga also was found to reduce the activity of the transcription factor cAMP response element-binding protein (CREB), suggesting SNS downregulation [13]. Previous studies have shown that mind-body interventions such as yoga improve mitochondrial integrity, as evident from increased cyclo-oxygenase (COX) activity [12]. This aids in reducing supraphysiological free radical levels by the electron transport chain during oxidative phosphorylation [12], thereby handling the oxidative milieu in a favorable way and preventing endothelial dysfunction, cardiovascular disease, and premature inflammation-related aging [42].

5.7 Genetic Effects

When stress activates the SNS, NF-κB, a key transcription factor, is produced [56]. Stress is translated into inflammation by the action of NF-κB to change the expression of genes that code for inflammatory cytokines [57] (Fig. 5.2). Yoga and other mind-body interventions directly inhibit the NF-κB pathway and thus reduce the expression of inflammatory genes. In one study, significant silencing of the pro-inflammatory genes *RIPK2* and *COX2* was noted among long-term yoga practitioners [13].

Epigenetic alterations among yoga practitioners are an important mechanism of favorable genetic modification achieved by yoga. Yoga decreases methylation of the *BDNF* gene, augmenting its activity and in turn enhancing neuroplasticity and cortical growth. Meditation is also seen to be associated with a significant reduction in methylation of the glucocorticoid

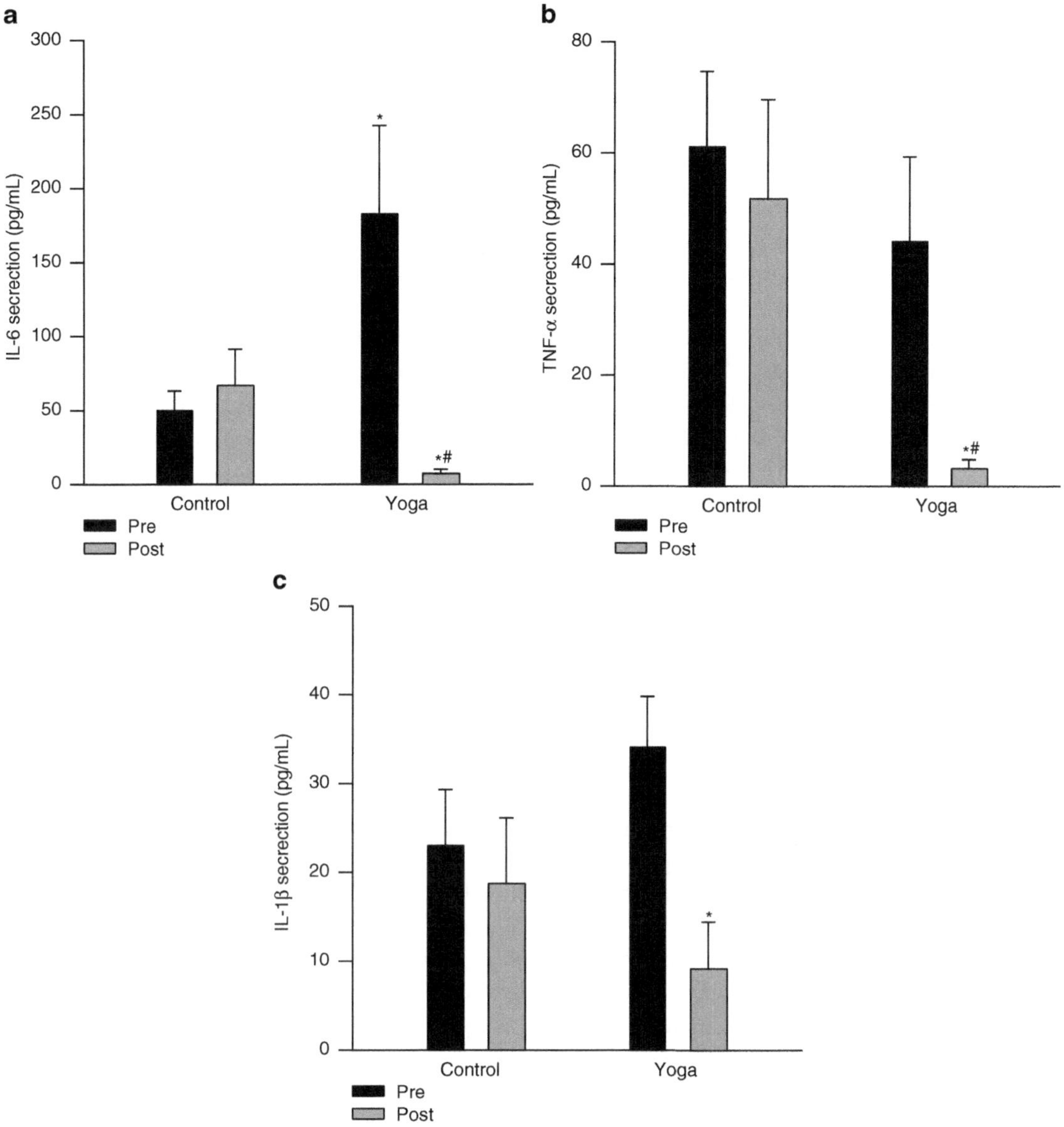

Fig. 5.3 Reduced secretion of (**a**) IL-6, (**b**) TNF-α, and (**c**) IL-1β from cultured whole blood ex vivo after yoga training. Whole blood was collected from 15 healthy participants at baseline and after yoga. Collected blood was diluted and cultured in 24-well plates under identical culture conditions. Supernatants were centrifuged and collected at 24 h for the measurement of IL-6, TNF-α, and IL-1β secretion via ELISA. Significant reduction in IL-6, TNF-α, and IL-1β secretion was seen after yoga, compared with the pre-yoga condition. Data are presented as mean + SEM. *$P < 0.05$ versus pre-yoga training condition within the same treatment; #$P < 0.05$ versus control group at the baseline level. Chen N, Xia X, Qin L, Luo L, Han S, Wang G, et al. Effects of 8-week Hatha yoga training on metabolic and inflammatory markers in healthy, female Chinese subjects: a randomized clinical trial. Biomed Res Int. 2016;2016:5387258. Reprinted by permission

receptor gene (*NR3C1* exon 1F and the co-chaperone FKBP5) and thus is related to a decrease in cortisol activity and stress levels. Global modification of histones (H4ac and H3K4me3) and the silencing of several histone deacetylase genes (HDAC 2, 3, and 9) have been noted in practitioners of yoga and meditation [13, 58].

Telomerase activity has been a major talked-about mechanism in mind-body intervention studies, as it is associated with premature aging and inflammation. However, results from these studies have been mixed, and most were short-term observational studies that failed to show reasonable improvement in telomerase activity. One study in hypertensive individuals did suggest that a combination of lifestyle modification techniques improves telomere maintenance, including increases in Gar1 and HnRNPA1, which encode proteins that bind telomerase RNA and telomeric DNA [59]. However, we are far from knowing what the truth is, as many more randomized trials are required to have a better understanding of yoga's role in this regard.

Recent evidence suggests that yoga and meditation could reduce oxidative stress in apparently healthy people by increasing total antioxidant capacity, reducing inflammation and improving mitochondrial DNA integrity [12, 60]. Oxidative stress-mediated DNA damage and defective sperm function leading to infertility has been shown to be attenuated by yoga [61].

Yoga has been credited with dampening the activation of CTRA [13], the primary characteristic of which is the upregulation of pro-inflammatory genes that produce major inflammation at the cellular level. Whereas acute inflammation is a short-lived, adaptive response that increases the activity of the immune system to fight injury or infection, chronic inflammation is maladaptive because it persists when no actual threat to the body exists [14]. Chronic inflammation is associated with increased risk for certain cancers, degenerative diseases, neurodegenerative diseases, cardiovascular diseases, and psychiatric diseases. The secondary characteristic of CTRA is the downregulation of antiviral and antibody-related genes, which is associated with susceptibility to viral infections. As a result, CTRA is considered a molecular signature of chronic stress [13, 55, 62, 63]. Yoga has been conclusively documented to lessen chronic stress, thus preventing the widespread activation of a pathophysiological state that garners chronic inflammation perpetuated by CTRA activation. Blocking activation of the CTRA genes has been suggested as a prime mechanism of yoga's anti-inflammatory effects [13].

5.8 Conclusions

Yoga reduces inflammation by inhibiting the NF-κB pathway, moderating epigenetic alteration, and preserving telomerase length, which in turn reduces GCS level and increases glucocorticoid receptor sensitivity. Yoga also augments neuroplasticity by promoting the mTOR pathway and enhancing gene expressions for BDNF, leading to increased cortical thickness in parts of the brain related to mood, awareness, and cognition. Yoga also depresses SNS and improves PNS activity, which is relevant to battling stress and maintaining a healthy cardiovascular profile. This appropriately may attenuate the initiation and perpetuation of multiple cardiovascular pathologies, including heart failure and atrial fibrillation, among others. Yoga has been found to reduce oxidative stress and prevent endothelial dysfunction, thus preventing premature atherosclerosis and coronary artery disease. Yoga's role in reducing arrhythmia burden in atrial fibrillation by inducing PNS activity and reversing atrial remodeling has been described in multiple studies. Newer studies in yoga practitioners that explore proteomic and genomic sequencing, along with advanced neural imaging, will lead us further toward deciphering the yet-unretrieved mechanism of the brain-heart axis that mediates aberrant cardiovascular pathophysiology.

Even more important, yoga fills the need of the hour as a low-investment, readily available, and effective therapeutic alternative from both the individual and public health perspectives [64].

References

1. Patel NJ, Atti V, Mitrani RD, Viles-Gonzalez JF, Goldberger JJ. Global rising trends of atrial fibrillation: a major public health concern. Heart. 2018;104:1989–90. https://doi.org/10.1136/heartjnl-2018-313350.
2. Lazar SW, Kerr CE, Wasserman RH, Gray JR, Greve DN, Treadway MT, et al. Meditation

experience is associated with increased cortical thickness. Neuroreport. 2005;16:1893–7. https://doi.org/10.1097/01.wnr.0000186598.66243.19.
3. Hölzel BK, Carmody J, Vangel M, Congleton C, Yerramsetti SM, Gard T, et al. Mindfulness practice leads to increases in regional brain gray matter density. Psychiatry Res. 2011;191:36–43. https://doi.org/10.1016/j.pscychresns.2010.08.006.
4. Vestergaard-Poulsen P, van Beek M, Skewes J, Bjarkam CR, Stubberup M, Bertelsen J, et al. Long-term meditation is associated with increased gray matter density in the brain stem. Neuroreport. 2009;20:170–4. https://doi.org/10.1097/WNR.0b013e328320012a.
5. Gianaros PJ, Jennings JR, Sheu LK, Greer PJ, Kuller LH, Matthews KA. Prospective reports of chronic life stress predict decreased grey matter volume in the hippocampus. NeuroImage. 2007;35:795–803. https://doi.org/10.1016/j.neuroimage.2006.10.045.
6. Liang JJ, Cha YM, Oh JK, Prasad A. Sudden cardiac death: an increasingly recognized presentation of apical ballooning syndrome (takotsubo cardiomyopathy). Heart Lung. 2013;42:270–2. https://doi.org/10.1016/j.hrtlng.2013.04.003.
7. Kraynak TE, Marsland AL, Gianaros PJ. Neural mechanisms linking emotion with cardiovascular disease. Curr Cardiol Rep. 2018;20:128. https://doi.org/10.1007/s11886-018-1071-y.
8. Wei J, Rooks C, Ramadan R, Shah AJ, Bremner JD, Quyyumi AA, et al. Meta-analysis of mental stress-induced myocardial ischemia and subsequent cardiac events in patients with coronary artery disease. Am J Cardiol. 2014;114:187–92. https://doi.org/10.1016/j.amjcard.2014.04.022.
9. Brandmeyer T, Delorme A, Wahbeh H. The neuroscience of meditation: classification, phenomenology, correlates, and mechanisms. Prog Brain Res. 2019;244:1–29. https://doi.org/10.1016/bs.pbr.2018.10.020.
10. Li AW, Goldsmith CA. The effects of yoga on anxiety and stress. Altern Med Rev. 2012;17:21–35.
11. Gaillard R, Dehaene S, Adam C, Clémenceau S, Hasboun D, Baulac M, et al. Converging intracranial markers of conscious access. PLoS Biol. 2009;7:e61. https://doi.org/10.1371/journal.pbio.1000061.
12. Tolahunase MR, Sagar R, Faiq M, Dada R. Yoga- and meditation-based lifestyle intervention increases neuroplasticity and reduces severity of major depressive disorder: a randomized controlled trial. Restor Neurol Neurosci. 2018;36:423–42. https://doi.org/10.3233/RNN-170810.
13. Buric I, Farias M, Jong J, Mee C, Brazil IA. What is the molecular signature of mind-body interventions? A systematic review of gene expression changes induced by meditation and related practices. Front Immunol. 2017;8:670. https://doi.org/10.3389/fimmu.2017.00670.
14. Ravnik-Glavač M, Hrašovec S, Bon J, Dreo J, Glavač D. Genome-wide expression changes in a higher state of consciousness. Conscious Cogn. 2012;21:1322–44. https://doi.org/10.1016/j.concog.2012.06.003.
15. Patterson E, Lazzara R, Szabo B, Liu H, Tang D, Li YH, et al. Sodium-calcium exchange initiated by the Ca2+ transient: an arrhythmia trigger within pulmonary veins. J Am Coll Cardiol. 2006;47:1196–206. https://doi.org/10.1016/j.jacc.2005.12.023.
16. Sharifov OF, Fedorov VV, Beloshapko GG, Glukhov AV, Yushmanova AV, Rosenshtraukh LV. Roles of adrenergic and cholinergic stimulation in spontaneous atrial fibrillation in dogs. J Am Coll Cardiol. 2004;43:483–90. https://doi.org/10.1016/j.jacc.2003.09.030.
17. Dunbar SB, Kimble LP, Jenkins LS, Hawthorne M, Dudley W, Slemmons M, et al. Association of mood disturbance and arrhythmia events in patients after cardioverter defibrillator implantation. Depress Anxiety. 1999;9:163–8. https://doi.org/10.1002/(sici)1520-6394(1999)9:4<163::aid--da3>3.0.co;2-b.
18. Khattab K, Khattab AA, Ortak J, Richardt G, Bonnemeier H. Iyengar yoga increases cardiac parasympathetic nervous modulation among healthy yoga practitioners. Evid Based Complement Alternat Med. 2007;4:511–7. https://doi.org/10.1093/ecam/nem087.
19. Cohen DL, Bloedon LT, Rothman RL, Farrar JT, Galantino ML, Volger S, et al. Iyengar yoga versus enhanced usual care on blood pressure in patients with prehypertension to stage I hypertension: a randomized controlled trial. Evid Based Complement Alternat Med. 2011;2011:546428. https://doi.org/10.1093/ecam/nep130.
20. Mizuno J, Monteiro HL. An assessment of a sequence of yoga exercises to patients with arterial hypertension. J Bodyw Mov Ther. 2013;17:35–41. https://doi.org/10.1016/j.jbmt.2012.10.007.
21. Miles SC, Chun-Chung C, Hsin-Fu L, Hunter SD, Dhindsa M, Nualnim N, et al. Arterial blood pressure and cardiovascular responses to yoga practice. Altern Ther Health Med. 2013;19:38–45.
22. Bakris GL, Townsend RR, Flack JM, Brar S, Cohen SA, D'Agostino R, et al. 12-month blood pressure results of catheter-based renal artery denervation for resistant hypertension: the SYMPLICITY HTN-3 trial. J Am Coll Cardiol. 2015;65:1314–21. https://doi.org/10.1016/j.jacc.2015.01.037.
23. Murugesan M, Taylor AG. Effect of yoga on the autonomic nervous system: clinical implications in the management of atrial fibrillation. J Yoga Physiother. 2017;3:555601. https://doi.org/10.19080/JYP.2017.03.555602.
24. Pramanik T, Sharma HO, Mishra S, Mishra A, Prajapati R, Singh S. Immediate effect of slow pace bhastrika pranayama on blood pressure and heart rate. J Altern Complement Med. 2009;15:293–5. https://doi.org/10.1089/acm.2008.0440.
25. Santaella DF, Devesa CR, Rojo MR, Amato MB, Drager LF, Casali KR, et al. Yoga respiratory training improves respiratory function and cardiac sympathovagal balance in elderly subjects: a randomised controlled trial. BMJ Open. 2011;1:e000085. https://doi.org/10.1136/bmjopen-2011-000085.

26. Lakkireddy D, Atkins D, Pillarisetti J, Ryschon K, Bommana S, Drisko J, et al. Effect of yoga on arrhythmia burden, anxiety, depression, and quality of life in paroxysmal atrial fibrillation: the YOGA my heart study. J Am Coll Cardiol. 2013;61:1177–82. https://doi.org/10.1016/j.jacc.2012.11.060.
27. Streeter CC, Gerbarg PL, Saper RB, Ciraulo DA, Brown RP. Effects of yoga on the autonomic nervous system, gamma-aminobutyric-acid, and allostasis in epilepsy, depression, and post-traumatic stress disorder. Med Hypotheses. 2012;78:571–9. https://doi.org/10.1016/j.mehy.2012.01.021.
28. Vempati RP, Telles S. Yoga-based guided relaxation reduces sympathetic activity judged from baseline levels. Psychol Rep. 2002;90:487–94. https://doi.org/10.2466/pr0.2002.90.2.487.
29. van den Broek KC, Tekle FB, Habibović M, Alings M, van der Voort PH, Denollet J. Emotional distress, positive affect, and mortality in patients with an implantable cardioverter defibrillator. Int J Cardiol. 2013;165:327–32. https://doi.org/10.1016/j.ijcard.2011.08.071.
30. Lampert R, Jamner L, Burg M, Dziura J, Brandt C, Liu H, et al. Triggering of symptomatic atrial fibrillation by negative emotion. J Am Coll Cardiol. 2014;64:1533–4. https://doi.org/10.1016/j.jacc.2014.07.959.
31. Basu Ray I, Metri K, Khanra D, Chinnaiyan KM, Nagarathna R, Misra MC, et al. Yoga: a potential intervention for augmenting immunomodulation and mental health in COVID-19. Front Med. 2020. submitted.
32. Cook-Cottone CP. Mindfulness and yoga for self-regulation: a primer for mental health professionals. New York: Springer Publishing Company; 2015. 322 p
33. Patil SG, Aithala MR, Naregal GV, Shanmukhe AG, Chopade SS. Effect of yoga on cardiac autonomic dysfunction and insulin resistance in non-diabetic offspring of type-2-diabetes parents: a randomized controlled study. Complement Ther Clin Pract. 2019;34:288–93. https://doi.org/10.1016/j.ctcp.2019.01.003.
34. Tost H, Champagne FA, Meyer-Lindenberg A. Environmental influence in the brain, human welfare and mental health. Nat Neurosci. 2015;18:1421–31. https://doi.org/10.1038/nn.4108.
35. Cole SW, Hawkley LC, Arevalo JM, Sung CY, Rose RM, Cacioppo JT. Social regulation of gene expression in human leukocytes. Genome Biol. 2007;8:R189. https://doi.org/10.1186/gb-2007-8-9-r189.
36. O'Donovan A, Sun B, Cole S, Rempel H, Lenoci M, Pulliam L, et al. Transcriptional control of monocyte gene expression in post-traumatic stress disorder. Dis Markers. 2011;30:123–32. https://doi.org/10.3233/DMA-2011-0768.
37. Miller GE, Chen E, Fok AK, Walker H, Lim A, Nicholls EF, et al. Low early-life social class leaves a biological residue manifested by decreased glucocorticoid and increased proinflammatory signaling. Proc Natl Acad Sci U S A. 2009;106:14716–21. https://doi.org/10.1073/pnas.0902971106.
38. Bottaccioli AG, Bottaccioli F, Minelli A. Stress and the psyche-brain-immune network in psychiatric diseases based on psychoneuroendocrineimmunology: a concise review. Ann N Y Acad Sci. 2019;1437:31–42. https://doi.org/10.1111/nyas.13728.
39. Weber MD, Godbout JP, Sheridan JF. Repeated social defeat, neuroinflammation, and behavior: monocytes carry the signal. Neuropsychopharmacology. 2017;42:46–61. https://doi.org/10.1038/npp.2016.102.
40. Lhullier FL, Nicolaidis R, Riera NG, Cipriani F, Junqueira D, Dahm KC, et al. Dehydroepiandrosterone increases synaptosomal glutamate release and improves the performance in inhibitory avoidance task. Pharmacol Biochem Behav. 2004;77:601–6. https://doi.org/10.1016/j.pbb.2003.12.015.
41. Thirthalli J, Naveen GH, Rao MG, Varambally S, Christopher R, Gangadhar BN. Cortisol and antidepressant effects of yoga. Indian J Psychiatry. 2013;55:S405–8. https://doi.org/10.4103/0019-5545.116315.
42. Chatterjee S, Mondal S. Effect of regular yogic training on growth hormone and dehydroepiandrosterone sulfate as an endocrine marker of aging. Evid Based Complement Alternat Med. 2014;2014:240581. https://doi.org/10.1155/2014/240581.
43. Naoroibam R, Metri KG, Bhargav H, Nagaratna R, Nagendra HR. Effect of integrated yoga (IY) on psychological states and CD4 counts of HIV-1 infected patients: a randomized controlled pilot study. Int J Yoga. 2016;9:57–61. https://doi.org/10.4103/0973-6131.171723.
44. Gopal A, Mondal S, Gandhi A, Arora S, Bhattacharjee J. Effect of integrated yoga practices on immune responses in examination stress - a preliminary study. Int J Yoga. 2011;4:26–32. https://doi.org/10.4103/0973-6131.78178.
45. Hari Chandra BP, Ramesh MN, Nagendra HR. Effect of yoga on immune parameters, cognitive functions, and quality of life among HIV-positive children/adolescents: a pilot study. Int J Yoga. 2019;12:132–8. https://doi.org/10.4103/ijoy.IJOY_51_18.
46. Rao RM, Nagendra HR, Raghuram N, Vinay C, Chandrashekara S, Gopinath KS, et al. Influence of yoga on mood states, distress, quality of life and immune outcomes in early stage breast cancer patients undergoing surgery. Int J Yoga. 2008;1:11–20. https://doi.org/10.4103/0973-6131.36789.
47. Vijayaraghava A, Doreswamy V, Narasipur OS, Kunnavil R, Srinivasamurthy N. Effect of yoga practice on levels of inflammatory markers after moderate and strenuous exercise. J Clin Diagn Res. 2015;9:CC08–12. https://doi.org/10.7860/JCDR/2015/12851.6021.
48. Chen PJ, Yang L, Chou CC, Li CC, Chang YC, Liaw JJ. Effects of prenatal yoga on women's stress and immune function across pregnancy: a

randomized controlled trial. Complement Ther Med. 2017;31:109–17. https://doi.org/10.1016/j.ctim.2017.03.003.
49. Kiloor A, Kumari S, Metri K. Impact of yoga on psychopathologies and QoLin persons with HIV: a randomized controlled study. J Bodyw Mov Ther. 2019;23:P278–83. https://doi.org/10.1016/j.jbmt.2018.10.005.
50. Nagarathna R, Nagendra H, Majumdar V. A perspective on yoga as a preventive strategy for coronavirus disease 2019. Int J Yoga. 2020;13:89–98. https://doi.org/10.4103/ijoy.IJOY_22_20.
51. Yadav RK, Magan D, Mehta N, Sharma R, Mahapatra SC. Efficacy of a short-term yoga-based lifestyle intervention in reducing stress and inflammation: preliminary results. J Altern Complement Med. 2012;18:662–7. https://doi.org/10.1089/acm.2011.0265.
52. Kiecolt-Glaser JK, Bennett JM, Andridge R, Peng J, Shapiro CL, Malarkey WB, et al. Yoga's impact on inflammation, mood, and fatigue in breast cancer survivors: a randomized controlled trial. J Clin Oncol. 2014;32:1040–9. https://doi.org/10.1200/JCO.2013.51.8860.
53. Pullen PR, Thompson WR, Benardot D, Brandon LJ, Mehta PK, Rifai L, et al. Benefits of yoga for African American heart failure patients. Med Sci Sports Exerc. 2010;42:651–7. https://doi.org/10.1249/MSS.0b013e3181bf24c4.
54. Chen N, Xia X, Qin L, Luo L, Han S, Wang G, et al. Effects of 8-week hatha yoga training on metabolic and inflammatory markers in healthy, female Chinese subjects: a randomized clinical trial. Biomed Res Int. 2016;2016:5387258. https://doi.org/10.1155/2016/5387258.
55. Bower JE, Greendale G, Crosswell AD, Garet D, Sternlieb B, Ganz PA, et al. Yoga reduces inflammatory signaling in fatigued breast cancer survivors: a randomized controlled trial. Psychoneuroendocrinology. 2014;43:20–9. https://doi.org/10.1016/j.psyneuen.2014.01.019.
56. Bierhaus A, Wolf J, Andrassy M, Rohleder N, Humpert PM, Petrov D, et al. A mechanism converting psychosocial stress into mononuclear cell activation. Proc Natl Acad Sci U S A. 2003;100:1920–5. https://doi.org/10.1073/pnas.0438019100.
57. Liang Y, Zhou Y, Shen P. NF-kappaB and its regulation on the immune system. Cell Mol Immunol. 2004;1:343–50.
58. Kaliman P, Alvarez-López MJ, Cosín-Tomás M, Rosenkranz MA, Lutz A, Davidson RJ. Rapid changes in histone deacetylases and inflammatory gene expression in expert meditators. Psychoneuroendocrinology. 2014;40:96–107. https://doi.org/10.1016/j.psyneuen.2013.11.004.
59. Duraimani S, Schneider RH, Randall OS, Nidich SI, Xu S, Ketete M, et al. Effects of lifestyle modification on telomerase gene expression in hypertensive patients: a pilot trial of stress reduction and health education programs in African Americans. PLoS One. 2015;10:e0142689. https://doi.org/10.1371/journal.pone.0142689.
60. Bhasin MK, Dusek JA, Chang BH, Joseph MG, Denninger JW, Fricchione GL, et al. Relaxation response induces temporal transcriptome changes in energy metabolism, insulin secretion and inflammatory pathways. PLoS One. 2013;8:e62817. https://doi.org/10.1371/journal.pone.0062817.
61. Bisht S, Faiq M, Tolahunase M, Dada R. Oxidative stress and male infertility. Nat Rev Urol. 2017;14:470–85. https://doi.org/10.1038/nrurol.2017.69.
62. Irwin MR, Olmstead R, Breen EC, Witarama T, Carrillo C, Sadeghi N, et al. Tai chi, cellular inflammation, and transcriptome dynamics in breast cancer survivors with insomnia: a randomized controlled trial. J Natl Cancer Inst Monogr. 2014;2014:295–301. https://doi.org/10.1093/jncimonographs/lgu028.
63. Bower JE, Crosswell AD, Stanton AL, Crespi CM, Winston D, Arevalo J, et al. Mindfulness meditation for younger breast cancer survivors: a randomized controlled trial. Cancer. 2015;121:1231–40. https://doi.org/10.1002/cncr.29194.
64. Dutta A, Aruchunan M, Mukherjee A, Metri KG, Ghosh K, and Basu-Ray I. Journal of integrative and complementary medicine. Ahead of print. https://doi.org/10.1089/jicm.2021.0420.

The Anatomical, Physiological and Neurochemical Correlates of Yoga

6

Mrithunjay Rathore

Cardiovascular disorders (CVDs) are a significant source of morbidity and mortality globally. Much of this can be attributed to an unhealthy lifestyle including poor nutrition, stress, lack of physical activity, and smoking. While there have been significant advances in the treatment of CVDs, the prevalence continues to increase, and there is tremendous economic burden, especially in developing countries.

Asanas, pranayama, and meditation may provide additional treatment options in the primary and secondary prevention of CVDs, which will be reviewed in this section.

6.1 Introduction

CVDs are the primary source of mortality and dysfunction worldwide, considering 17.3 million deaths every year, which anticipated to expand to beyond 23.6 million by 2030. As stated by WHO, 293 million dysfunction-modify life spans (DALYs) were lost due to CVDs in 2008, considering 11% of all DALYs lost (Mendis et al. 2011). In developed western nations CVD remains the number one killer. Whereas in many developing countries like India there has been an alarming rise in CVD. The disease has been malignant in India and occurs at an early age with considerable morbidity and mortality, resulting in a substantial financial burden. India expended approximately 243 billion dollars from 2005 to 2015 for cardiac disease, stroke, and diabetes mellitus [1]. While there has been enormous advances in cardiology the disease continues to proliferate in an epidemic proportion all over the world. This is particularly so in ill-affording poor nations.

It has been illustrated in various research that yoga has several cardioprotective outcomes [2, 3] (Manchanda et al. 2014). Asanas, pranayama, and meditation are used as therapeutic interventions work at different levels such as anatomical, physiological, and psychological in the CVDs.

M. Rathore (✉)
AIIMS, Raipur, India

I. Basu-Ray, D. Mehta (eds.), *The Principles and Practice of Yoga in Cardiovascular Medicine*,
https://doi.org/10.1007/978-981-16-6913-2_6

6.2 Anatomical Aspect of Asanas in Cardiovascular Disorders

Cardiac tissue has its own rhythm, which is regulated by innervations from both the sympathetic and the parasympathetic divisions of the autonomic nervous system. Modulation of this rhythm is know as heart rate variability (HRV), and it is the subject of ongoing research. Variation in HRV patterns is seen in heart disorders such as hypertension, ischemia, sudden cardiac death, and cardiac failure.

Asanas (Yoga postures) are an essential part of contemporary yoga practice. Specific asanas are accomplished in slow, consecutive patterns and blended with the practitioner's breathing. There are four types of asanas: standing asanas, supine asanas, prone, and sitting asana. There is very little scientific literatureon the effect of various yoga postures on HRV. Asanas for CVD:

Asanas for the cardiovascular disorders
• Corpse pose
• Ardha chakrasana
• Vakrasana (right side)
• Bhujangasana
• Inversion posture

The research studies have shown that the forward head and kyphotic posture are related to depression [4]. Depression escalates the risk of ischemic heart disease and congestive cardiac failure [5]. In this connection, the back-bending yoga posture such as *Ardhachakrasana bhujangasana and ustrasana* reverse the postural path mechanics.

A study from Bhavanani et al. (2014) showed the effects of cardiovascular rhythm during and after the practice of different yogic postures. And result showed remarkable changes in heart rate (HR) and blood pressure both immediately after the yogic posture as well as during the recovery interval. In the recovery period, there were noteworthy intergroup differences from 2 min onward in both systolic pressure (SP) and diastolic pressure (DP). The decrease of SP after *Vakrasana (right side) (VA-R)* was significantly greater than *Shavasana* (fourth, sixth, and eighth min) and *Janusirasasana (left side) (JSA-L)* at sixth and eighth min. DP reduced remarkably after performing JSA-L compared to VA-R at the sixth and eighth mi. Post-postural HR and BP both down below the initial values during the went recovery period and this was consequently seen to be even lower than the responses to supine relaxation in *Shavasana*. It was noticed that the impact of supine relaxation is more noticeable after practice of the asanas, as compared to just relaxing in *shavasana*. This may be allocated to a standardization and equilibrium effect occurring due to a greater, healthier deactivation of autonomic nervous system occurring due to the presence of prior activation. One of the remarkable findings of that study is the report of subtle variance between right- and left-sided practices of *vakrasana* and *janusirasasana* that may take place due to the variation of inside architectures like muscles and nerve fibres including ganglions that get activated or inactivated.

Marian et al. [6] indicate their pilot research on the effect of the inversion posture and after the 8-week study period, results indicate a remarkable enhancement in the HRV of subjects. High HRV is viewed as a sign of a healthier cardiac condition; high HRV stipulates greater parasympathetic control, which in turn demonstrates a restorative effect on the autonomic nervous system, an increased vagal tone, and reduced sympathetic activity in the heart.

Possible Mechanism of Asanas in Cardiovascular Disorders

- Balance of autonomic nervous system with increased parasympathetic and decreased sympathetic activity.
- Overactivity of gamma-aminobutyric acid (GABA), the primary inhibitory neurotransmitter system.

The aforesaid observation demonstrated that the performance of *Ardha chakrasana, Bhujangasana*, etc. could improve the cardiovagal status, decrease the sympathetic overactivity, and enhance the equilibrium between the sympathetic and parasympathetic nervous system. It is important to understand that sympathetic dominance is one of the root cause for Insulin resistance as well as the development of atherosclerosis. Increasing stress increase allostatic afterload that leads also to decreased GABA in the brain [7]. Asanas boost GABA levels in the thalamus on functional magnetic resonance imaging [8]. These enhancements are associated with mood improvement. This is probably the neurobiological mechanism as to how yoga activates the GABAergic system inside the brain. It may be recalled that many adverse psychological situations including stress, depression and anxiety has been directly responsible for decreasing GABA in the braub.

6.3 Physiological Aspect of Pranayama in Cardiovascular Disorders

The word pranayama gets from two Sanskrit words, namely, prana, which anticipates "life force" or "vital energy." Furthermore, Yama, which means "to extend." Hence, pranayama techniques involve voluntarily slowing down and prolonging breathing. Respiration is a fundamental physiological process for endurance as it is the only means to transport oxygen to the tissues to generate energy. Bhavanani et al. (2014) demonstrated the reduction in systolic and diastolic blood pressure after alternate nostrils yoga breathing and a decrease in systolic and mean blood pressure after *Chandra bhedana pranayama (CBP).* CBP is left nasal breathing.

In an earlier study, *Nadishodhana pranayama* (NSP*)* illustrates that after performing NSP for 4 weeks, volunteers remarked a reduction in Heart rate (H.R.) and systolic blood pressure (SBP) both at rest, and they held their breath until breaking point. NSP resembles reducing sympathetic activation in the presence of a physical stressor (i.e., breath holding) [9]. There is also an indication that NSP improved the vagal modulation of the cardiac rhythm [10]. Another study explained that *slow-paced bhastrika pranayama* could decrease systolic and diastolic blood pressure (Pramanik et al. 2009).

Pranayama for the Cardiovascular Disorders

- *Chandra bhedana pranayama*
- *Nadishodhana pranayama*
- *Bhramari pranayama*
- *Slow Kapalbhati pranayama*
- *Sukha pranayama*

Bhavanani et al. [11] showed they analyzed the immediate effect of *sukha pranayama* (S.P.) on a cardiovascular variable in hypertension patients. Post-intervention statistical analysis revealed a remarkable (*p* 0.05) decrease in H.R. and a highly impressive (*p* 0.001) reduction in systolic pressure, pulse pressure, mean arterial pressure, rate-pressure product, and double product with a negligible fall in diastolic pressure, it stipulates normalization of autonomic cardiovascular rhythm as a consequence of enhanced vagal modulation and decreased sympathetic activity and to improve baroreflex sensitivity. Slow breathing beyond tidal volume inhalation may activate pulmonary stretch receptors (as in Hering Bruer reflex), causing the withdrawal of sympathetic tone leading to widespread vasodilatation and thus decreasing the diastolic blood pressure (Pramanik et al. 2009). Further, baroreceptor sensitivity could be magnified by slow breathing as supported by a slight reduction in the heart rate observed during slow breathing and in a decrease in both systolic and diastolic pressures.

Exercising bhramari pranayama *(Bhp)* training every day for 10 min and 20 min of left and NSP over 8 weeks lowered anxiety symptoms in subjects diagnosed with stress neurosis (Crisan 1984). Moreover, these changes are indicative of reduced sympathetic nervous system activity. A study on healthy adolescents informed that the heart rate, pulse pressure, mean arterial pressure, rate pressure product, and double product declined significantly after 45 min of practicing *Bhp* [12]. Another research inscribed a decrease in diastolic and mean blood pressure after 5 min of practicing *Bhp* [13]. A Pilot Study on the result of bhramari pranayama on heart rate variability and hemodynamics (Sujan et al. 2005) showed that during the practice of pranayama, there was a notable increase in LF/HF ratio ($t = -5.1$; $p = 0.000$) when compared to a baseline recording. But following pranayama practice there is shift toward parasympathetic activity and decreased LF/HF ratio ($t = 5.6$, $p = 0.000$) compared to during practice and baseline LF/HF ($t = 4.2$, $p = 0.000$). There was reduction in SBP ($t = 3.2$, $p = 0.004$), DBP ($t = 5.7$, $p = 0.000$), and HR ($t = 1.3$, $p = 0.185$).

Another important breathing technique is *kapalbhati* (kapala = forehead, and bhati = shining in Sanskrit) (K.B.) name explained to mean that K.B. practice is mentally stimulating. An analogous result was reported when 12 experienced practitioners practiced K.B. and NSP for 1 min on separate days. A frequency-domain analysis was carried out [14]. To understand the results it is important to understand that the heart rate variability (HRV) is an indicator of the cardiac autonomic control. Two spectral components are usually recorded, viz. high frequency [HF] (0.15–0.50 Hz), which is due to vagal efferent activity and a low frequency component [LF] (0.05–0.15 Hz), due to sympathetic activity. Thus HF dominance indicates parasympatheic or vagal dominance whereas LF indicated sympathetic stimulation. They observed a significant increase in the low frequency and the LF/HF ratio, while the H.F. power was significantly lower following K.B. The results suggest that K.B. modifies the autonomic status by increasing sympathetic activity with reduced vagal activity. There was no significant change after NSP. Telles et al. (2011) studied heart rate variability changes during high-frequency yoga breathing (HFYB) and breath awareness, the result showed a significant decrease in NN50, p NN50 and the mean RR interval during and after HFYB and after breath awareness, compared to the respective 'pre' values ($p < 0.05$) (repeated measures ANOVA followed by post-hoc analysis). The LF power increased and HF power decreased during and after breath awareness and LF/HF ratio increased after breath awareness ($p < 0.05$). Moreover, the results suggest reduced parasympathetic modulation during and after HFYB and increased sympathetic modulation with reduced parasympathetic modulation during and after breath awareness.

> **Possible Mechanism of Pranayama in Cardiovascular Disorders**
> - Decreased sympathetic system
> - Decreased heart rate and blood pressure
> - Decreased activation of HPA axis
> - Increased heart rate variability
> - Increased baroreflex sensitivity and insulin sensitivity

So, the conclusion of the various studies postulated two interconnected pathways by which yoga decreases the risk of cardiovascular diseases through the mechanisms of parasympathetic activation coupled with reduced reactivity of the sympathoadrenal system and the hypothalamic–pituitary–adrenal (HPA) axis. Low heart rate variability and baroreflex sensitivity indicate impaired cardiovagal adaptability and suggest low parasympathetic tone. These alterations are, in turn, strong independent predictors of cardiovascular morbidity and mortality. In contrast, high HRV and baroreflex sensitivity are generally considered to indicate good cardiovagal adaptations and sympathovagal balance, permitting greater sensitivity to alterations in environmental demands.

6.4 Psychological Aspect of Meditation in Cardiovascular Disorders

The impact of acute psychological stress on heart disease is an emerging public wellness concern. Brain regions implicated in regulating psychological stress-related variances in heart rate variability include the prefrontal cortex, anterior cingulate, insula, and amygdala [15]. Shah et al. (2019) observed the brain relates stress-induced peripheral vasoconstriction in the CVDs; consequences have shown that stress-induced vasoreactivity is correlated with changes in brain responses to stress in areas implicated in emotion, including the medial prefrontal cortex (m PFC) and insula.

Meditation for the Cardiovascular Disorders
- Mindfulness meditation or focused attention meditation
- Transcendental meditation

Meditation has been used as a tool to train the mind for thousands of years. A systematic review and meta-analysis [16] showed that meditation programs can institute stress reduction and also ameliorate other adverse emotions including anxiety and depression.

Research studies have shown that Focused attention meditation (FAM) has been shown to decrease activity in the ventral medial prefrontal cortex (vmPFC) and posterior cingulate cortex (PCC)/precuneus, which are core hubs of the DMN. In neuroscience, the default mode network (DMN), also known as the default network, default state network, or anatomically the medial fronto-parietal network (M-FPN), is a large-scale brain network primarily composed of the medial prefrontal cortex, posterior cingulate cortex/precuneus and angular gyrus. It is best known for being active when a person is not focused on the outside world and the brain is at wakeful rest, such as during daydreaming and mind-wandering. There is indication that meditation can decrease activity in the DMN. In contrast, prolonged activation was observed in brain regions involved in the ventral and dorsal attention network, including the frontal eye field (FEF), visual cortex, dorsolateral prefrontal cortex (dlPFC), and anterior insula.

Meditation is a component of many mindfulness-based interventions and has been credited with a reduction in hypertension [17]. Derioush et al. [18] study the effectiveness of mindfulness-based stress reduction enforcement on the quality of life in CVDs. Their result concluded that the quality of life of CVDs patients could be improved by implementing mindfulness stress reduction programs.

A systematic review and meta-analysis research [19] on the impact of transcendental meditation (TM) on depressive symptoms and blood pressure in adults with the cardiovascular disease showed that TM was associated with within-group (but not between groups) improvements in BP. There were no changes in depressive symptoms for TM or control participants. In a randomized observation of stress reduction in 201 black men and women with angiographically proven coronary artery disease randomized to TM or health advocacy, 5.4-year follow-up observed a 4.9 mm Hg lower systolic blood pressure, in the TM group rather than the health education group (Schneider 2012).

Possible Mechanism of Meditation in Cardiovascular Disorders
- Regulation of ventromedial prefrontal cortex and Insular cortex activity
- Enhanced the psychological profile

Insula, plays a significant role in regulating peripheral cardiovascular responses to stress [20]. Increased insula activity leads to sympathetic activation and parasympathetic deactivation. Moreover, the insula has connections with the anterior cingulate cortex, amygdala, prefrontal cortex, superior temporal gyrus, hippocampus, and other brain areas that accentuate emotional and physiological responses to stress. Brain areas that revealed similar deactivation in peripheral vasoconstrictors involved the m PFC (anterior cingulate). The m PFC, which consists of several related areas, including the orbitofrontal cortex, anterior cingulate and subcallosal gyrus, and anterior prefrontal cortex, have inhibitory inputs to the amygdala. Inhibition of the amygdala by the m PFC represents the mechanism of extinction of fear memories, and a failure in function in this area is associated with an increases in fear and stress responses.

6.5 Biochemical Aspect of Yoga in Cardiovascular Disorders

Free radicals play a vital role in the pathogenesis of atherosclerosis, diabetes, and vascular disease. Antioxidants scavenge free radicals and are believed to decrease oxidative stress and inflammation. Several antioxidants such as malondialdehyde (MDA), superoxide dismutase (SOD), glutathione, are recognized for their anti-oxidative role and have been used as surrogate markers in cardiovascular disease, the effect of yoga on these biomarkers has been studied by few investigators. Bhattacharya et al., in a prospective age- and sex-matched study, enrolled 30 young male participants between 18 and 21 years of age who were given training in yogic breathing exercises and relaxation techniques for 30 min daily for 10 weeks [21]. The lipid peroxide MDA content decreased significantly, from 9.57 + 0.56 mmol/L to 8.21 + 0.76 mmol/L (p < . Ol), in the yoga group whereas the control group showed no change, suggesting that there was a decrease in the production of free radicals following yoga practice; Similarly, Singh et al. [22] in patients with T2DM, showed a significant decrease in MDA and HbAIC levels after 40 days of training in several yoga asanas [22]. Jatuporn et al. [23] observed that in an RCT of 44 patients with CHD, 4 months of a yoga-based intensive lifestyle program resulted in a statistically significant increase in plasma total antioxidants, plasma vitamin E, and erythrocyte glutathione (GSH) compared to controls. Procoagulant changes caused by oxidative stress have a pivotal role in the development and progression of CVD, metabolic syndrome, and diabetes [24]. In two uncontrolled studies in healthy adults, it was observed that 12–16 weeks of yoga practices resulted in a significant decline in fibrinogen and an increase in fibrinolytic activity [25] suggesting that yoga may foster beneficial changes in the coagulation and fibrinogen systems. However, the studies were not randomized. In another important study 10 days of daily yoga intervention, the researchers observed a significant reduction in BMI (body mass index), a significant reduction in plasma IL-6, and an increase in plasma adiponectin, suggesting that even a short-term yoga-based program may reduce the risk 1 for CVD as indicated by weight loss and decrease in inflammatory markers [26].

Biochemical of Yoga in Cardiovascular Disorders

- Decrease the Oxidative stress
- Decrease the inflammatory cytokine
- Improved the lipid profile and telomere length

Shorter Telomere Length (TL) has predicted higher mortality risk and disease of aging, including cardiovascular (Blackburn et al. 2015). Khoa D. Le Nguyen [27] wanted to delineate the effect multiple meditation practices have to reduce the attrition of telomeres, the protective caps of chromosomes (Carlson et al., 2015). Here, they probed the distinct effects on telomere length (TL) of mindfulness meditation (MM) and loving-kindness meditation (LKM). Midlife adults (N = 142) were randomized to be in a waitlist control condition or to learn either MM or LKM in a 6-week workshop. Telomere length was assessed 2 weeks before the start of the workshops and 3 weeks after their termination. After controlling for appropriate demographic covariates and baseline TL, we found TL decreased significantly in the MM group and the control group, but not in the LKM group. There was also significantly less TL attrition in the LKM group than the control group. The MM group showed changes in TL that were intermediate between the LKM and control groups yet not significantly different from either. Self-reported emotions and practice intensity (duration and frequency) did not mediate these observed group differences. This study is the first to disentangle the effects of LKM and MM on TL and suggests that LKM may buffer telomere attrition. Accumulating data suggest that inflammation contributes to the causation and progression of CVDs [26]. In addition, inflammatory mediators may trigger rupture of atherosclerotic plaque, resulting in coronary thrombosis and acute ischemia. The key inflammatory markers that have gained recognition include IL-6, fibrinogen, C-reactive protein, and TNF-alpha, all of which have been considered as independent predictors of CVDs. Adiponectin, an important regulator of endothelial nitric oxide synthase, is a key determinant of endothelial function and is cardioprotective. Evidence is accumulating that yoga can not only decrease IL6 and other inflammatory mediators but increase adiponectin and other vascular protective entities.

References

1. Tunstall-Pedoe H. Preventing chronic diseases. A vital investment: WHO global report. Geneva: World Health Organization; 2006.
2. Jayasinghe SR. Yoga in cardiac health (a review). Eur J Cardiovasc Prev Rehabil. 2004;11(5):369–75.
3. Raub JA. Psychophysiologic effects of Hatha Yoga on musculoskeletal and cardiopulmonary function: a literature review. J Altern Complement Med (NY). 2002;8(6):797–812.
4. Asghari A, Imanzadeh M. Relationship between kyphosis and depression anxiety in athlete and non-athlete male students in selected universities of Tehran. World Appl Sci J. 2009;7(10):1311–6.
5. Dhar AK, Barton DA. Depression and link with cardiovascular disease. J Front Psychiatr. 2016;7:33.
6. Papp ME, Lindfors P, Storck N. Blood pressure from eight weeks of hatha yoga – a pilot study. BMC Res Notes. 2013;6:59.
7. Black PH, Garbutt LD. Stress, inflammation and cardiovascular disease. J Psychosom Res. 2002;52(1):1–23.
8. Streeter CC, Gerbarg PL, Saper RB, Ciraulo DA, Brown RP. Effects of yoga on the autonomic nervous system, gamma-aminobutyric-acid, and allostasis in epilepsy, depression, and post-traumatic stress disorder. Med Hypotheses. 2012;78(5):571–9.
9. Bhargava R, Gogate MG, Mascarenhas JF. Autonomic responses to breath holding and its' variations following pranayama. Indian J Physiol Pharmacol. 1998;32:257–64.
10. Subramanian RK, Devaki PR, Saikumar P. Alternate nostril breathing at different rates and its influence on heart rate variability in non-practitioners of yoga. J Clin Diagn Res. 2016;10(1):CMO1–02.
11. Bhavanani AB, Sanjay Z, Madanmohan. Immediate effect of sukha pranayama on cardiovascular variable in patients of hypertension. Int J Yoga Ther. 2011;21(1):73–6.
12. Kuppusamy M, Kamaldeen D, Pitani R, Shanmugam P. Effect of Bhramari pranayama on health- a systematic review. J Tradit Complement Med. 2017;8(1):11–6.
13. Rajesh SK, Ilavarasu J, Srinivassn TM. Effect of Bhramari Pranayama on response inhibition: evidence from the stop signal task. Int J Yoga. 2014;7(2):138–41.
14. Raghuraj P, Ramakrishnan AG, Nagendra HR, Telles S. Effect of two selected yogic breathing techniques of heart rate variability. Indian J Physiol Pharmacol. 1998;42(4):467–72.
15. Thayer JF, Hansen AL, Saus-Rose E, Johnsen BH. Heart rate variability, prefrontal neural function, and cognitive performance: the neurovisceral integration perspective on self-regulation, adaptation, and health. Ann Behav Med. 2009;37(2):141–53.
16. Goyal M, Singh S, Sibinga EMS, Gould NF. Meditation programs for psychological stress and well-being: a systematic review and meta-analysis. JAMA Intern Med. 2014;174(3):357–68.
17. Schneider RH, Alexander CH, Staggers F, Barnes VA. Impact of transcendental meditation on mortality in older African Americans with hypertension—eight-year follow-up. J Soc Behav Pers. 2005;17:201–16.
18. Jalali D, Abdolazimi M, Alaei Z. Effectiveness of mindfulness-based stress reduction program on quality of life in cardiovascular disease patients. Int J Cardiol Heart Vasc. 2019;12:23.
19. Gathright EC, Blotche ES, DeCosta J. The impact of transcendental meditation on depressive symptoms and blood pressure in adults with cardiovascular disease: a systematic review and meta-analysis. Complement Ther Med. 2019;46:172–9.
20. De Morree HM, Szabo BM, Rutten GJ, Kop WJ. Central nervous system involvement in the autonomic responses to psychological distress. Neth Hear J. 2013;21:64–9.
21. Bhattacharya S, Pandey US, Verma NS. Improvement in oxidative status with yogic breathing in young healthy males. Indian J Physiol Pharmacol. 2002;46(3):349–54.
22. Singh S, Malhotra V, Singh KP, Sharma SB, Madhu SV, Tandon OP. A preliminary report on the role of yoga asanas on oxidative stress in non-insulin dependent diabetes mellitus. Indian J Clin Biochem. 2001;16(2):216–20.
23. Jatuporn S, Sangwatanaroj S, Saengsiri AO, Rattanapruks S, Srimahachota S, Uthayachalerm W. Shorter on lipid effects of an intensive lifestyle modification program on lipid peroxidation and antioxidant systems in patients with coronary artery disease. Clin Hemorheol Microcirc. 2003;29(3-4):429–36.
24. Ceriello A, Motz E. Is oxidative stress the pathogenic mechanism underlying insulin resistance, diabetes, and cardiovascular disease? The common soil hypothesis revisited. Arterioscler Thromb Biol. 2004;24(5):816–23.
25. Chohan IS, Nayar HS, Thomas P, Geetha NS. Influence of yoga on blood coagulation. Thromb Haemost. 1984;51(2):196–7.
26. Sarvottam K, Magan D, Yadav RK, Mehta N, Mahapatra SC. Adiponectin, interleukin-6, and cardiovascular disease risk factors are modified by a short-term yoga-based lifestyle intervention in overweight and obese men. J Altern Complement Med. 2013;19(5):397–402.
27. Le Nguyen KD. Loving-kindness meditation slows biological aging in novices: evidence from a 12-week randomized controlled trial. Psychoneuroendocrinology. 2019;108:20–7.

Cardiovascular Influence of Yoga Assessed with Heart Rate Variability Measures

7

Inbaraj Ganagarajan, Kaviraja Udupa, and T. N. Sathyaprabha

7.1 Introduction

Yoga, an ancient system of Indian medicine known to bestow good health, is widely used globally as a form of mind–body medicine. It has numerous health benefits, which help improve well-being, promote good health, enhance psycho-physiological balance and prevent illnesses [1]. There has been an increased interest in exploring the physiological benefits of yoga in the last few decades resulting in a wide range of scientific studies. In addition, yoga has received considerable attention for its therapeutic benefits in effectively addressing chronic illnesses such as stress, anxiety, depression, hypertension, diabetes, obesity, anxiety, insomnia, back pain, neurodegenerative diseases, and coronary artery disease [2]. Cardiovascular disease (CVD) is the leading cause of mortality and disability worldwide, even though 90% of CVDs are preventable. Preventing CVDs implies treating risk factors associated with CVDs [3]. Considering the therapeutic benefits of yoga and its possible ability to prevent or minimize the incidences of CVDs, heart rate variability assessment in yoga-based interventions can be invaluable.

7.2 Cardiovascular Disease

Cardiovascular diseases affect the heart and blood vessels of the body and are the leading cause of global mortality, which is of high relevance in developing countries owing to its increased prevalence. The underlying pathology for a large proportion of CVD is due to atherosclerosis and systemic inflammation, the leading cause of coronary artery disease (CAD) and cerebrovascular disease (stroke). The Framingham Heart Study has shown that CVD is associated with several risk factors, which detrimentally affect cardiac health [4]. Studies indicate that chronic work-related stress, unhealthy diet and, sedentary lifestyle represents the most important and independent risk factor for CVDs [5].

Cardiovascular diseases are known to be associated with adverse changes in autonomic function with elevated sympathetic activity for a prolonged period along with parasympathetic withdrawal. This rise in the sympathetic nervous system (SNS) activity mediates modification in the neuroendocrine system through the hypothalamic–pituitary–adrenal (HPA) axis. This, in turn, brings a change in the level of stress hormones (e.g., adrenaline, aldosterone, cortisol, and norepinephrine), leading to an increase in heart rate, blood pressure, and concentrations of blood glucose and lipids. This mechanism contributes to the

I. Ganagarajan · K. Udupa · T. N. Sathyaprabha (✉)
Department of Neurophysiology, National Institute of Mental Health and Neuro Sciences (NIMHANS), Bangalore, India

I. Basu-Ray, D. Mehta (eds.), *The Principles and Practice of Yoga in Cardiovascular Medicine*,
https://doi.org/10.1007/978-981-16-6913-2_7

advancement of atherosclerosis and CVDs, especially in people with chronic stress and a sedentary lifestyle [6].

7.3 Heart Rate Variability

Changes in autonomic function can be assessed using various techniques. Heart rate variability (HRV) assessment is considered to be of prime importance owing to its ability to accurately evaluate ANS regulation. HRV reflects changes in body physiology, endocrine, and psycho-emotional balance. It is also an independent mortality predictor in patients and healthy individuals [7].

HRV is a simple and noninvasive method of measuring the variation in the time interval between successive heartbeats. The other term used for HRV is "RR variability." It is a measure of the autonomic influence on the cardiovascular system and is carried out by recording with a standard electrocardiography (ECG) device and appropriate software processing. HRV is measured in two ways, Time-domain (using brief electrocardiographic periods) and Frequency domain (using 24-h or short-term recorded signal processing).

The time-domain method is the simplest way to measure HRV, analyzed based on calculating the mean R–R interval and variations of the standard deviation of heart rate over time as the unit of analysis. The smaller standard deviation of R–R intervals indicates reduced HRV. These time-domain measures include SDNN (Standard deviation of all NN (normal to normal RR) intervals, RMSSD (root mean square of successive differences between adjacent NN intervals), NN50 & pNN50 (Count and percentage of the number of pairs of NN intervals differing by more than 50 ms), and Triangular index of NN interval (TINN) [8].

The frequency-domain method is used to determine the frequency content of the signal using spectral analysis. With short- and long-term ECG recordings, power spectral analyses can be calculated. The important frequency domain measures are total power (TP), low frequency (0.04–0.15 Hz, LF), high frequency (0.15–0.4 Hz, HF), and sympathovagal balance (SVB = LF/HF power) [8].

The time and frequency domain measures are related to each other. HF corresponds to the square root of the mean square differences of successive NN intervals, and LF and VLF are comparable to the standard deviation of the NN interval (SDNN). Very low frequency (VLF), low frequency (LF), High frequency (HF), and LF/HF are usually, the parameters for evaluating ANS activity. The HF and LF parameters are also represented in normalized units (HFnu and LFnu). The LFnu and reduced LF/HF ratio of HRV represent sympathetic modulation and HFnu represents parasympathetic modulation [9]. These analyses are used to determine power at various frequencies, helping to differentiate the PNS and SNS contribution to heart rate variability. The HF component in HRV is associated with respiratory sinus arrhythmias and is attributed to PNS. The LF/HF ratio is a sympathetic/vagal balance index. An increased LF/HF value represents higher sympathetic cardiac modulation, lower parasympathetic modulation, or both [8].

7.4 Heart Rate Variability a Marker for Stress

Studying the heart gives us an enormous amount of knowledge about the body. The heart rate varies constantly from beats to beats, to meet the needs of the body. Heart rate variability (HRV) refers to the variation in time between successive heartbeats. It is recognized unanimously as a noninvasive marker of autonomic nervous system (ANS) activity. HRV is influenced by several physiological manifestations which include respiration, physical activity, posture, cognitive processing, stress, and emotional reactions. Heart rate variability increases during relaxing activities and decreases during stress.

Long-term stress has become one of the most common health hazards in society today. Stress a maladaptive state of mind cause acute or chronic physical, psychological, and behavioral impairments [10]. To date, the search for stress biomarkers remained challenging for researchers and there is no universally recognized standard for stress evaluation. In recent years research studies using HRV as a marker for stress are increasing in frequency.

7.4.1 Autonomic Regulation of Psychological Stress

The hypothalamic–pituitary–adrenal (HPA) axis and sympathetic nervous system (SNS) are the two major mechanisms that affect the body through psychological stress [11]. The ANS and HPA axis are well-coordinated and interlinked. The ANS promotes physiological changes rapidly through SNS and parasympathetic nervous system (PNS). In particular, PNS plays a major role in alleviating an individual's stress reactions through the inhibition of the SNS and HPA axis. There is a growing body of evidence that physiological and psychological stress impedes autonomic balance and is associated with several somatic and mental illnesses. These autonomous imbalances are mirrored in HRV assessments reflected in the form of reduced R–R intervals. In addition, psychological stress was significantly associated with an increase in the LF/HF ratio, suggesting an increase in SNS activity and a decrease in parasympathetic activity, exhibited in the form of reduction in HF and an increase in LF in HRV during stress [12].

7.4.2 Effect of Yoga on Stress

A growing body of research evidence supports the conviction that certain yoga strategies can reduce stress by downregulating the HPA axis and SNS activity. Although the mechanism through which yoga affects the autonomic activity is poorly understood, some yogic approaches seem to stimulate distinctly the vagus nerve and enhance parasympathetic activity leading to enhanced cardiac function, mood, and reduced stress [13].

Research has shown that yoga reverses the negative impact of stress on the immune system by raising the levels of natural killer cells and immunoglobulin A. Practicing yoga is also found to reduce sensitivity to C-reactive protein and inflammatory cytokines such as interleukin-6 and lymphocyte-1B. Although the exact mechanism of action has not been established, it has been speculated that yoga leads to a shift toward dominance in the parasympathetic nervous system [13].

Studies on yoga for stress assessed using HRV have shown modulatory effect on ANS by exhibiting reduced LF nu and increased HF nu mainly with the practice of meditation (Dhyana), focus (Dharana), no meditative thinking (ekagrata), and random thinking (cancatla) [14]. All major yoga practices including asana, pranayama, meditation, and relaxation techniques shown to improve autonomic regulation and enhanced vagal dominance reflected in HRV measures.

7.5 Yoga and Cardiovascular Disease

Yoga which involves a wide range of practices, has numerous health benefits, significantly reducing the risk associated with CVD. The neurohumoral mechanism which is found to be dysregulated in CVD can be favorably modulated through yoga, by reducing serum cortisol, aldosterone, and catecholamine levels. Moreover, the regular practice of yoga is known to improve nitric oxide bioavailability leading to reduced oxidative stress and enhanced endothelial function [15]. In addition, yoga reduces the rate pressure product (a measure of myocardial oxygen consumption and cardiac load), lipid profiles, and even atherosclerosis regression when combined with dietary and other lifestyle changes [16]. Systemic inflammation has been considered a strong predictor of mortality in CVD. Yoga has also shown to reduce inflammation by reducing pro-inflammatory response genes and reverse the nuclear factor-κB-related transcription of pro-inflammatory cytokines [17]. Thus, providing relief from the effect of stress-induced CVD's and promoting a sense of well-being.

7.6 Efficacy of Yoga on HRV in Patients with CVD

In addition to the conventional risk factors of CVD, cardiac autonomic dysfunction is an independent predictor of mortality. This is evidenced by decreased HRV and baroreflex sensitivity which correlates well with associated hypertension, diabetic neuropathy, cerebrovascular disease, congestive heart failure, lethal arrhythmias, and acute myocardial infarction. Psychosocial factors such as stress, anxiety, and panic disease are also associated with reduced HRV [18]. Lower HRV in populations without a known CVD is associated with a 32–45 percent higher risk of a first cardiovascular event. An increase of SDNN by 1% will reduce the risk of fatal CVD by 1% [19]. Moreover, several studies have shown the beneficial effect of yoga on the cardiovascular system evaluated using HRV measures [8] (Fig. 7.1).

A study by Huang et al. has shown that the practice of hatha yoga can reduce perceived stress and salivary cortisol, a major effector of SNS and HPA pathways, and enhance cardiometabolic health. Besides, the author also claims that even a single hatha yoga session (90 min) can significantly increase the HF power component of HRV. A 12-week yoga study by Hari Krishna et al. showed that yoga in addition to standard medical treatment had significant improvement in parasympathetic activity and decreased sympathetic activity in patients with heart failure. In another study by Muralikrishnan et al., Isha yoga practitioners had balanced positive vagal efferent activity and improved HRV while resting and breathing deeply compared to non-yoga practitioners. A study by Patil et al. on elderly subjects with arterial stiffness has shown that yoga helps in reducing arterial stiffness along with a reduction in blood pressure when compared to brisk walking. The author has also shown that yoga helps to reduce sympathetic activity and enhance endothelial function with increased Nitro Oxide bioavailability. Even in resting conditions, regular yoga practitioners have increased vagal tone compared to non-yoga practitioners. These changes in autonomic balance coupled with positive changes in the HPA axis, endothelial functions, and oxidative stress mechanisms possibly protect an individual from cardiovascular morbidities. Thus, by improving cardio-vagal activity and reducing sympathetic function, yoga modulates neurocardiac regulation and reduces the risk of CVDs (Fig. 7.2).

Thus, yoga reduces the effect of stress and improves cardiovascular function in patients with various cardiac and other medical conditions.

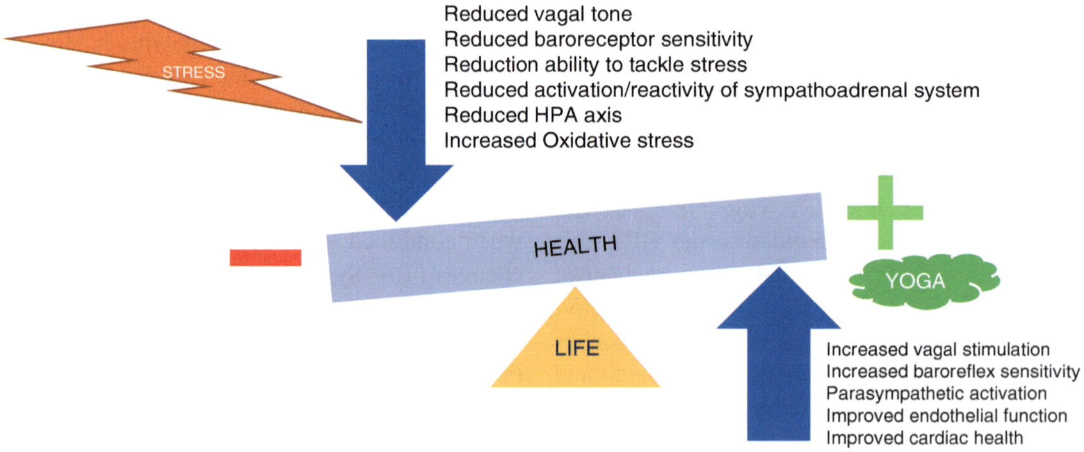

Fig. 7.1 Improved vagal stimulation through yoga offsets stress-induced sympathetic activation

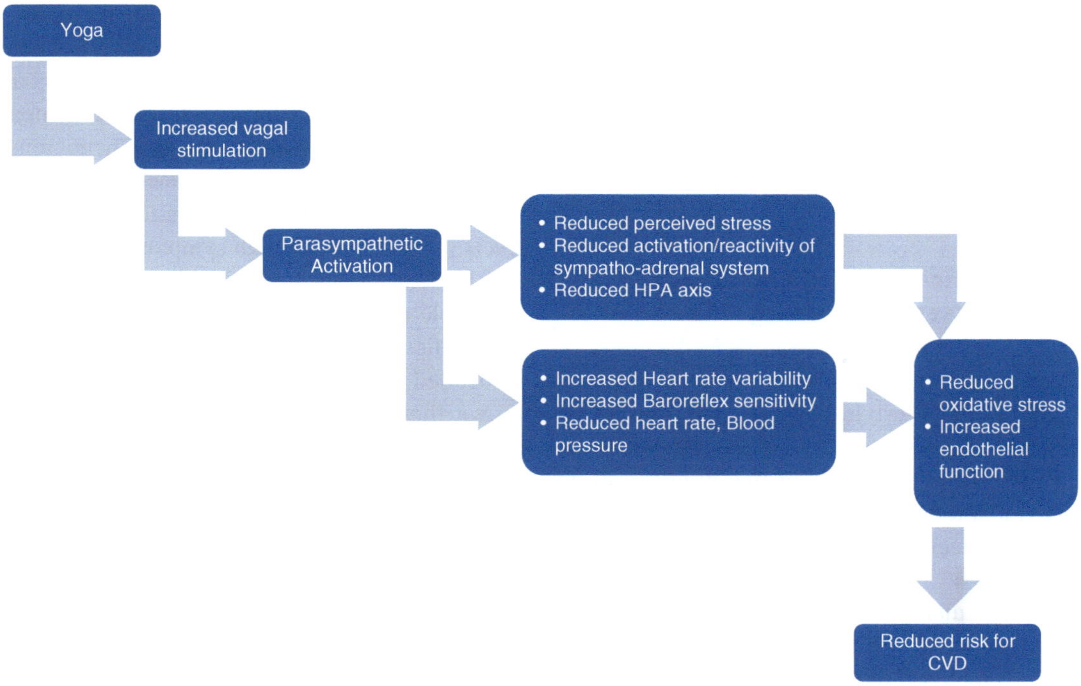

Fig. 7.2 Mechanisms of cardiovascular improvement by yoga

7.7 Yoga for CVD Risk Factors

A wide range of risk factors is known to be associated with CVDs. The most common of which are of metabolic (hypertension, diabetes, obesity, and dyslipidemia) and behavioral (smoking, sedentary lifestyle, and diet) origin [20]. The best strategy in preventing CVD is probably a multifactorial approach, one that takes into account all the risk factors. Yoga was beneficial in this aspect, as several studies on yoga have shown its efficacy in reducing the risk factors associated with CVD [21]. This section discusses the risk variables in which yoga was found to be effective in management assessed using HRV.

7.7.1 Efficacy of Yoga on Hypertension Assessed by Using HRV

Hypertension is one of the most significant risk factors in nearly all different kinds of CVDs acquired during the lifetime, including coronary artery disease, stroke, ventricular hypertrophy, valvular disease, arrhythmias, and renal failure [22]. Prehypertensive individuals also have an increased risk of developing cardiovascular diseases. There is a strong association between the incidence of hypertension and diabetes mellitus as well as high BMI [8]. Interestingly, this hypertension is linked to autonomic nervous system dysregulation [23]. It has been postulated that yoga practices such as relaxation and pranayama were found to be more effective in reducing blood pressure. This induces slow proprioceptive and exteroceptive rhythms thereby reducing the adrenergic peripheral activity and enhancing autonomic balance. This, in turn, reduces chemoreceptor responses and enhances baroreflex sensitivity [24]. A 12-week yoga study has shown that yoga helps in modulating HRV by improving the parasympathetic tone and reducing the sympathetic tone and reducing BP [25]. Yoga is helpful in the management of ischemic heart disease. However these benefits are not only limited to preventing ischemic heart disease, but also include managing signs, changing the risk factors, and regressing atherosclerotic plaques in diseased arteries [26]. Thus, yoga improves cardiovascular functioning, and prevents the likelihood of the cardiovascular system from developing any morbidity.

7.7.2 Efficacy of Yoga on Obesity Assessed by Using HRV

People are generally obese due to a blend of heredity and lifestyle changes that consists of low physical exercise and overconsumption of calories. Obesity is a factor that predisposes an individual to the development of CVD. The bioactive molecules synthesized by tissue adipocytes have a detrimental effect on the cardiovascular system and influence the risk factors associated with CVD. These bioactive molecules include adiponectin, resistin, leptin, plasminogen activator inhibitor-1, tumor necrosis factor-α, and interleukin-6 [27]. Obesity has been associated with reduced heart rate variability. The associated link between blood leptin and resistin concentration has been postulated as a cause for this ANS disturbance [28]. Yoga helps with weight loss by enhancing energy expenditure during the session, improving body flexibility by reducing back and joint pain, reducing stress, thereby reducing food intake, allowing people to feel more linked to their bodies, leading to increased awareness of satiety and preventing overeating. Moreover, consumption of proper food habits and involvement in other positive lifestyle changes makes a person more active and energetic than lazy or sober, which is the root cause of lifestyle-induced cardiovascular disorders [29].

7.7.3 Efficacy of Yoga on Depression Assessed by Using HRV

Multiple studies have shown that depression and associated symptoms are major risk factors for the development of CVD. Major depression and depressive symptoms are frequently underdiagnosed and undertreated in patients with cardiovascular disease (CVD). We have shown the association of depression with altered cardiac autonomic function toward increased sympathetic tone and reduced parasympathetic tone. The practice of yoga helps enhance parasympathetic activity and lower depression and stress levels in patients with high symptoms of depression [30].

Ample research evidence suggests that yoga is beneficial in managing depression and its associated comorbidities. It has been previously shown that regular practice of yoga for about 3 months had a beneficial effect on depression by showing improvement in plasma brain-derived neurotrophic factor (BDNF) and reduced cortisol levels [31]. Yoga has also shown a significant increase in HF, reduction in LF, and a reduction in LF/HF ratio. Yogic breathing adjusts the imbalances in the autonomic nervous system and influences a broad range of mental health conditions. It was shown that controlled respiratory patterns in the course of yoga exercise could modify the cardiac autonomic nervous system and boost HRV imbalances [32]. It is hypothesized that the increase in HRV after yoga training can be attributed to the stimulation of dermal or subdermal pressure receptors and stretch receptors in the cardiorespiratory system which are innervated by parasympathetic afferent fibers. Thus, yoga helps resolve clinical depression, thereby reducing cardiovascular morbidity due to impaired neurocardiac regulation.

7.7.4 Efficacy of Yoga on Epilepsy Assessed Using HRV

Studies have shown that patients with epilepsy are at greater risk developing myocardial infarction (MI) and subsequent stroke than non-epileptics. The use of anti-epileptic drugs (AED) may also carry various risks for cardiovascular and cerebral diseases. A study in South Carolina, USA has shown that epileptic patients aged more than 18 years are vulnerable to MI [33].

HRV has been researched for over 30 years in patients with epilepsy and, generally, they exhibit modified HRV, indicating a change in autonomic equilibrium toward sympathetic dominance. This autonomic demodulation appears to be more severe in those with temporal lobe epilepsy and drug-resistant epilepsy, exhibiting a reduction in both time-domain (SDNN, RMSSD, pNN50), frequency domains (VLF, LF, HF, TP), and nonlinear (SD1, SD2) parameters of HRV as compared to healthy controls [34].

It was found that individuals who practiced yoga had a significant reduction in recurrence of seizures, as well as AED dosage requirements including their side effects. In addition, we have previously shown that a multi-week (10 weeks daily) yoga intervention led to a significant decline in seizure frequency scores and also better performance in autonomic function testing by enhancing parasympathetic activity [35]. Thus, practicing yoga helps in reducing seizure frequency and reducing AED dosage, thereby leading to enhanced cardiac function and preventing CVD.

7.8 Conclusion

There has been a rapid rise in publications in yoga and cardiovascular health. The pharmacological therapy used to treat CVDs has limited effectiveness and serious adverse effects. Therefore, patients choose other approaches for a healthy lifestyle and stress management to enhance health-related quality of life and minimize recurrent diseases. Yoga shows promise as a practical lifestyle intervention integrated into cardiovascular disease management strategies. Given the scientific evidence discussed to date, it is reasonable to say that yoga can help reduce the incidence of cardiovascular disease and can play a primary or complementary role in managing CVD. The practice of yoga is postulated to trigger neurohormonal mechanisms that provide health benefits through suppression of sympathetic nervous system activity and enhancement of parasympathetic activity. Thus, the regular practice of yoga is definitely a boon and a cost-effective measure for managing and reversing the symptoms associated with CVDs.

References

1. Posadzki P, Kuzdzal A, Lee MS, Ernst E. Yoga for heart rate variability: a systematic review and meta-analysis of randomized clinical trials. Appl Psychophysiol Biofeedback. 2015;40(3):239–49.
2. Mohammad A, Thakur P, Kumar R, Kaur S, Saini RV, Saini AK. Biological markers for the effects of yoga as a complementary and alternative medicine. J Complement Integr Med. 2019;16(1) http://www.ncbi.nlm.nih.gov/pubmed/30735481
3. Razavi M, Fournier S, Shepard DS, Ritter G, Strickler GK, Stason WB. Effects of lifestyle modification programs on cardiac risk factors. PLoS One. 2014;9(12):e114772. http://www.ncbi.nlm.nih.gov/pubmed/25490202
4. Anderson KM, Odell PM, Wilson PWF, Kannel WB, Framingham MPH. Cardiovascular disease risk profiles. Am Heart J. 1991;121(1):293–8.
5. Cheema BS, Marshall PW, Chang D, Colagiuri B, MacHliss B. Effect of an office worksite-based yoga program on heart rate variability: a randomized controlled trial. BMC Public Health. 2011;11(1):578. http://www.biomedcentral.com/1471-2458/11/578
6. Chrousos GP. The role of stress and the hypothalamic-pituitary-adrenal axis in the pathogenesis of the metabolic syndrome: neuro-endocrine and target tissue-related causes. Int J Obes Relat Metab Disord. 2000;24(Suppl 2):S50–5. http://www.ncbi.nlm.nih.gov/pubmed/10997609
7. Nunan D, Sandercock GRH, Brodie DA. A quantitative systematic review of normal values for short-term heart rate variability in healthy adults. Pacing Clin Electrophysiol. 2010;33(11):1407–17. http://www.ncbi.nlm.nih.gov/pubmed/20663071
8. Terathongkum S, Pickler RH. Relationships among heart rate variability, hypertension, and relaxation techniques. J Vasc Nurs. 2004;22(3):78–82; quiz 83–4. http://www.ncbi.nlm.nih.gov/pubmed/15371972
9. Abhishekh HA, Nisarga P, Kisan R, Meghana A, Chandran S, Raju T, et al. Influence of age and gender on autonomic regulation of heart. J Clin Monit Comput. 2013;27(3):259–64.
10. Gottlieb NH, Mullen PD. Stress management in primary care: physicians' beliefs and patterns of practice. Am J Prev Med. 1987;3(5):267–70. http://www.ncbi.nlm.nih.gov/pubmed/3452365
11. Marques AH, Silverman MN, Sternberg EM. Evaluation of stress systems by applying noninvasive methodologies: measurements of neuroimmune biomarkers in the sweat, heart rate variability and salivary cortisol.

Neuroimmunomodulation. 2010;17(3):205–8. http://www.ncbi.nlm.nih.gov/pubmed/20134204
12. Sloan RP, Shapiro PA, Bagiella E, Boni SM, Paik M, Bigger JT, et al. Effect of mental stress throughout the day on cardiac autonomic control. Biol Psychol. 1994;37(2):89–99. http://www.ncbi.nlm.nih.gov/pubmed/8003592
13. Innes KE, Bourguignon C, Taylor AG. Risk indices associated with the insulin resistance syndrome, cardiovascular disease, and possible protection with yoga: a systematic review. J Am Board Fam Pract. 2005;18(6):491–519. http://www.ncbi.nlm.nih.gov/pubmed/16322413
14. Telles S, Raghavendra BR, Naveen KV, Manjunath NK, Kumar S, Subramanya P. Changes in autonomic variables following two meditative states described in yoga texts. J Altern Complement Med. 2013;19(1):35–42. http://www.ncbi.nlm.nih.gov/pubmed/22946453
15. Patil SG, Aithala MR, Das KK. Effect of yoga on arterial stiffness in elderly subjects with increased pulse pressure: a randomized controlled study. Complement Ther Med. 2015;23(4):562–9. https://doi.org/10.1016/j.ctim.2015.06.002.
16. Ornish D, Scherwitz LW, Doody RS, Kesten D, McLanahan SM, Brown SE, et al. Effects of stress management training and dietary changes in treating ischemic heart disease. JAMA. 1983;249(1):54–9. http://www.ncbi.nlm.nih.gov/pubmed/6336794
17. Black DS, Cole SW, Irwin MR, Breen E, St Cyr NM, Nazarian N, et al. Yogic meditation reverses NF-κB and IRF-related transcriptome dynamics in leukocytes of family dementia caregivers in a randomized controlled trial. Psychoneuroendocrinology. 2013;38(3):348–55. http://www.ncbi.nlm.nih.gov/pubmed/22795617
18. Vrijkotte TG, van Doornen LJ, de Geus EJ. Effects of work stress on ambulatory blood pressure, heart rate, and heart rate variability. Hypertens (Dallas, Tex 1979). 2000;35(4):880–6. http://www.ncbi.nlm.nih.gov/pubmed/10775555
19. Hillebrand S, Gast KB, De Mutsert R, Swenne CA, Jukema JW, Middeldorp S, et al. Heart rate variability and first cardiovascular event in populations without known cardiovascular disease: meta-analysis and dose-response meta-regression. Europace. 2013;15(5):742–9.
20. Thomas H, Diamond J, Vieco A, Chaudhuri S, Shinnar E, Cromer S, et al. Global atlas of cardiovascular disease 2000-2016: the path to prevention and control. Glob Heart. 2018;13(3):143–63.
21. Guddeti RR, Dang G, Williams MA, Alla VM. Role of yoga in cardiac disease and rehabilitation. J Cardiopulm Rehabil Prev. 2019;39(3):146–52.
22. Kjeldsen SE. Hypertension and cardiovascular risk: general aspects. Pharmacol Res. 2018;129:95–9. http://www.ncbi.nlm.nih.gov/pubmed/29127059
23. Schroeder EB, Liao D, Chambless LE, Prineas RJ, Evans GW, Heiss G. Hypertension, blood pressure, and heart rate variability: the atherosclerosis risk in communities (ARIC) study. Hypertension. 2003;42(6):1106–11.
24. Bernardi L, Gabutti A, Porta C, Spicuzza L. Slow breathing reduces chemoreflex response to hypoxia and hypercapnia, and increases baroreflex sensitivity. J Hypertens. 2001;19(12):2221–9.
25. Punita P, Trakroo M, Palamalai SR, Subramanian SK, Bhavanani AB, Madhavan C. Randomized controlled trial of 12-week yoga therapy as lifestyle intervention in patients of essential hypertension and cardiac autonomic function tests. Natl J Physiol Pharm Pharmacol. 2016;6(1):19–26.
26. Yogendra J, Yogendra HJ, Ambardekar S, Lele RD, Shetty S, Dave M, et al. Beneficial effects of yoga lifestyle on reversibility of ischaemic heart disease: caring heart project of International Board of Yoga. J Assoc Physicians India. 2004;52:283–9. http://www.ncbi.nlm.nih.gov/pubmed/15636328
27. Sowers JR. Obesity as a cardiovascular risk factor. Am J Med. 2003;115(8 SUPPL. 1):37–41.
28. Piestrzeniewicz K, Łuczak K, Lelonek M, Wranicz JK, Goch JH. Obesity and heart rate variability in men with myocardial infarction. Cardiol J. 2008;15(1):43–9. http://www.ncbi.nlm.nih.gov/pubmed/18651384
29. Bernstein AM, Bar J, Ehrman JP, Golubic M, Roizen MF. Yoga in the management of overweight and obesity. Am J Lifestyle Med. 2014;8(1):33–41.
30. Udupa K, Sathyaprabha TN, Thirthalli J, Kishore KR, Lavekar GS, Raju TR, et al. Alteration of cardiac autonomic functions in patients with major depression: a study using heart rate variability measures. J Affect Disord. 2007;100:137–41.
31. Naveen GH, Varambally S, Thirthalli J, Rao M, Christopher R, Gangadhar BN. Serum cortisol and BDNF in patients with major depression-effect of yoga. Int Rev Psychiatry. 2016;28(3):273–8. http://www.ncbi.nlm.nih.gov/pubmed/27174729
32. Sovik R. The science of breathing - the yogic view. Prog Brain Res. 2000;122:491–505.
33. Brigo F, Lochner P, Nardone R, Manganotti P, Lattanzi S. Increased risk of stroke and myocardial infarction in patients with epilepsy: a systematic review of population-based cohort studies. Epilepsy Behav. 2020;104:106307. https://doi.org/10.1016/j.yebeh.2019.05.005.
34. Liu H, Yang Z, Huang L, Qu W, Hao H, Li L. Heart-rate variability indices as predictors of the response to vagus nerve stimulation in patients with drug-resistant epilepsy. Epilepsia. 2017;58(6):1015–22. http://www.ncbi.nlm.nih.gov/pubmed/28440954
35. Sathyaprabha TN, Satishchandra P, Pradhan C, Sinha S, Kaveri B, Thennarasu K, et al. Modulation of cardiac autonomic balance with adjuvant yoga therapy in patients with refractory epilepsy. Epilepsy Behav. 2008;12(2):245–52. http://www.ncbi.nlm.nih.gov/pubmed/18024208

8 Mechanisms and Biomarkers to Understand Impacts of Yoga in Cardiovascular Diseases

Chainika Khatana, Neeraj K. Saini, Priyanka Thakur, Reena V. Saini, and Adesh K. Saini

8.1 Biomarkers to Understand the Impact of Yoga

Biomarkers in cardiovascular events have evolved as potent therapeutic targets lately. Precisely, a plethora of novel biomarkers, increasing evidences and marks behind the use of natriuretic peptides, and amplified prominence on targeting therapies toward pathophysiological diseases have all contributed to expanded use of a biomarker in heart failure clinical trials [1]. These biomarkers could be useful in identifying the impacts of yoga on CVD patients. These include biomarkers for inflammation, oxidative stress, lifestyle, or depression.

C. Khatana · P. Thakur · R. V. Saini
Center of Research for Himalayan Studies and Development, Shoolini University, Solan, Himachal Pradesh, India

N. K. Saini
School of Biotechnology, Jawaharlal Nehru University, New Delhi, India

A. K. Saini (✉)
Department of Biotechnology, Maharishi Markandeshwar (Deemed to be University), Mullana, Ambala, Haryana, India

8.1.1 Inflammation Markers

Multiple lines of evidence suggest a crucial role of inflammation in the development and progression of CVDs [2]. Depression and stress have been demonstrated to be associated with inflammation, explicitly with the increase in three markers; a) C-reactive protein (CRP10–12), a hallmark of inflammation [3], b) the action of inflammatory cytokines interleukin-6 (IL-6) [4], and c) tumor necrosis factor (TNF6–9) [4]. TNF6–9 has been considered a potential target for heart failure therapy [5, 6]. In an 8-week yoga-based program in patients with systolic heart failure, another marker called extracellular superoxide dismutase (EC-SOD) which is linked with oxidative stress-induced endothelial dysfunction and flow-dependent vasodilatation, showed significant improvement [7, 8]. Yoga may reduce oxidative stress, hence inflammatory cytokines and improve disease symptoms by reducing inflammation. Modifications in the anti-inflammatory factors have been seen with the intervention of yoga practices. Biochemical studies indicated that practicing yoga is allied to reducing inflammatory responses associated with depression and stress [9]. However, the exact molecular mechanism behind the modulatory effects of yoga still remains to be comprehensively explored [10].

I. Basu-Ray, D. Mehta (eds.), *The Principles and Practice of Yoga in Cardiovascular Medicine*,
https://doi.org/10.1007/978-981-16-6913-2_8

8.1.2 Depression

Depression is a major health disorder found to be strongly associated with a variety of cardiovascular events [11]. In particular, this association is likely bidirectional and multifaceted. People with mental depression, anxiety or bipolar disorder, and schizophrenia, are more prone to cardiovascular diseases as compared to the general population [12]. Likewise, mental depression is frequent in patients with coronary heart disease and history of heart failure events. Several studies have documented depressive diseases as important risk factors for CVDs not only in patients with heart diseases but also in people with no clinical symptoms of cardiac events [13]. Depression and CVDS are also observed in the clinical manifestations of the central autonomic nervous system [9], multiple sclerosis [14], hypercoagulable state [15], endothelial dysfunction [16], inflammation [17], and platelet activation [18]. Mind–body medical interventions can be used to abate depression and CVDs. Notably, yoga is considered one of the most effective mind–body interventions [19]. Preceding literature pinpoints central neurotransmitter, gamma-aminobutyric acid to be involved in the plethora of depression dynamics [20].

Breast cancer patients reportedly experience a high level of psychosocial stress and emotional dysfunction, with fear of disease progression being the primary stressor. Additionally, cortisol dysregulation is suggested to influence inflammation that may promote depression, fatigue, and cancer [19]. Several prospective studies have demonstrated beneficial effects of meditative type of yoga in physiological and physical functioning along with a significant stress and salivary cortisol level reduction [21]. A notable improvement in emotional well-being and fatigue scores were reported in a study of a yoga group ($n = 84$) compared to the control group ($n = 44$). The yoga session included meditative types of practices for a period of 12 weeks [22]. A study on women undergoing radiation therapy encountered the effect of yoga sessions on DNA damage. Yoga practices for 6 weeks improved stress and physiological function yoga practices for 6 weeks improved stress and physiological function scores and attenuated DNA damage [23].

Atrial fibrillation, a frequent cardiac arrhythmia has been reported to impair quality of life imposing a significant psychosocial burden involving anxiety and depression. In a study designed by Lakkireddy revealed that yoga trainings like Iyengar, pranayamas, and asanas performed at least twice a week may prevent atrial fibrillation initiation and perpetuation [24].

8.1.3 Oxidative Stress

High reactive oxygen species (ROS) production and inadequate cellular and dietary antioxidant levels lead to the milieu of oxidative stress (Fig. 8.1). Major reactive oxygen species are superoxide radicals, hydrogen peroxide, and hydroxyl radical, generated mostly in the mitochondria. Major reactive species are shown in Table 8.1. A failed machinery to neutralize ROS may implicate deleterious effect on DNA, RNA, lipids, and proteins. Oxidative stress has also been reported to inactivate nitric oxide (required for the endothelial functions) resulting in increased blood pressure and hypertension [25]. Former evidence into the line demonstrated a strong association between oxidative stress, blood pressure and hypertension [26].

Superoxide dismutase, glutathione, catalase, vitamin C, and E are some major antioxidants, which contribute the first line of defense against deleterious effects of ROS on the biomolecules. A decline in the amount of these antioxidants may also elevate oxidative stress and eventually, complications like hypertension, atherosclerosis, and stroke. Incorporation of yoga has

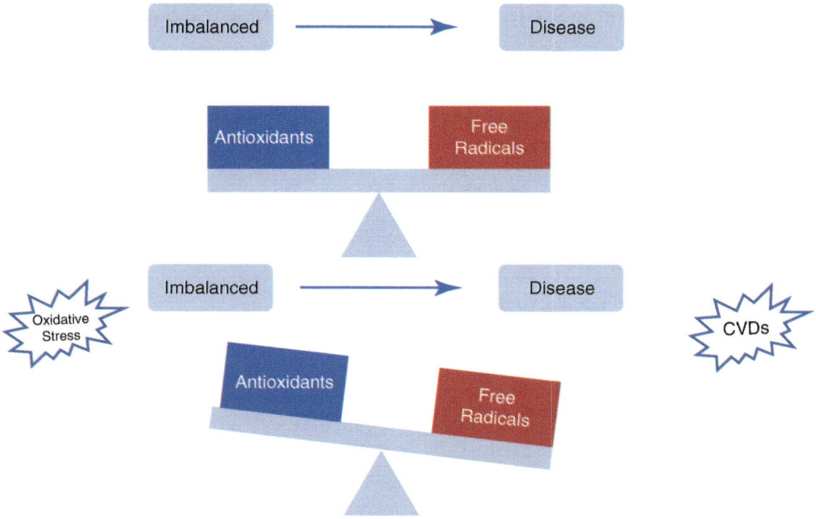

Fig. 8.1 Imbalance between antioxidants and free radicals leads to oxidative stress resulting in CVDs

Table 8.1 Major reactive species

Reactive species	Free radicals	Non-radicals
ROS (Reactive oxygen species)	Superoxide anion radical ($O_2^{\bullet-}$) Hydroxyl radical (•OH) Alkoxyl radical (RO•) Peroxyl radical (ROO•)	Hydrogen peroxide (H_2O_2) Organic hydroperoxide (ROOH) Singlet molecular oxygen ($O_2 1\Delta g$) Electronically excited carbonyls (RCO)a
RNS (Reactive nitrogen species)	Nitric oxide (NO•) Nitrogen dioxide (NO_2•)	Nitrite (NO_2^-) Nitroxyl anion (NO^-) Peroxynitrite ($ONOO^-$) Peroxynitrate (O_2NOO^-) Nitrosuperoxycarbonate ($ONOOCO_2^-$)

been indicated to improve antioxidant status in human and animal models [27, 28]. Yoga induced SOD level is also demonstrated to prevent the production of peroxynitrite, an oxidant and nitrating agent aiding to reduce the possibility of nitrosative stress.

Oxidative stress damages polyunsaturated fatty acid (PUFA) producing malonaldehyde (MDA), a biomarker for lipid peroxidation. Hypertensive patients usually have elevated levels of MDA in the serum [29]. A substantial reduction in serum MDA levels was observed in yoga practitioner in which a yoga and control group consisting of 30 patients with a hypertension history were selected for a 3 month period. Yoga training module involved yoga practices like breathing (hands in and out, ankle and lumber stretch, and straight leg raise), various postures, meditation, and relaxation techniques. The control group was provided with flexibility or stretching practices followed by walking for 6 days a week. After 3 months of this training, serum MDA level ($p < 0.001$) was reduced in yoga practitioners, whereas it was significantly elevated ($p = 0.04$) in the non-yoga practitioners. Antioxidant capacity, SOD, vitamin C and glutathione level ($p = 0.002$) were significantly increased in the yoga group whereas no such change was noted in the control group [30]. Hence concluded that the reduced MDA level is an outcome of low oxygen consumption, which is generally associated with yoga asanas and posture practices [31] (Table 8.2).

Table 8.2 Effect of yoga intervention on risk factors for CVDs where increase is shown with ↑ and decrease is shown with ↓

S. no.	Risk factors	Markers	Helpful yoga practices	References
1.	Anti-inflammatory	·Interleukin – 6 ·C reactive protein ·Tumor necrosis factor ·Leptin } ↓ ·Adiponectin↑	Yogasanas, meditation and pranayama (including standard medical therapy and relaxation phase	[3, 4]
2.	Immune system	·CD4 + T cell activity ·Antibody levels ·Telomere activity } ↑ ·Neutrophil count↓	Asnas, pranayama and shavasana, kirtan kriya or listening to relaxation and meditation	[32]
3.	Autonomic nervous system	·Baroreflex sensitivity ·Parasympathetic sensitivity ·Heart rate variability } ↑ ·Sympathetic activation↓	Meditation and pranayama with breathing and relaxation techniques	[33, 34]
4.	Neuroendocrine system	·Serum cortisol ·Serum aldosterone ·Serum adrenaline } ↓ ·Endorphin↑	Meditation and pranayama with breathing and relaxation techniques	[21]
5.	Metabolism	·Total cholesterol ·LDL, MDA ·TG } ↓ ·Improves BP	Meditation and pranayama along with diet control	[27, 35]
6.	Oxidative stress and antioxidants	·SOD ·GSH ·GSH / GSSG ratio ·GST ·GR ·Glucose 6 phosphate ·Vitamin C, E ·Total antioxidant status ·Catalase ·Nitric oxide } ↑ ·GSSH ·GPx ·MDA ·Protein oxidation } ↓	Yogasana, shavasana, hatha yoga, and pranayama with breathing technique	[27, 36]

Table 8.2 (continued)

S. no.	Risk factors	Markers	Helpful yoga practices	References
7.	Cardiovascular	·Heart Rate ·Systolic BP ·Diastolic BP ·Rate pressure product ·Normalized Low Frequency power ·N terminal pro b – type natriuretic peptide } ↓ ·Normalized High Frequency power↑	Meditation and pranayama with standard medical therapy	[37, 38]
8.	Aging	·Peripheral blood leukocyte telomere length ·Telomerase activity ·β – endorphin ·Sirtuin – 1 ·Brain – derived neurotrophic factor ·Cortisol } ↑ ·Oxidative DNA damage↓	Asnas, pranayama and shavasana, kirtan kriya or listening to relaxation music along with a healthy lifestyle intervention	[39]

8.2 Conclusion

Taken together, these studies implicate that yoga as a lifestyle intervention has become an important factor that can be used as an effective lifestyle modality to reduce oxidative stress, enhance antioxidant defense, retard progression, and increase regression of coronary atherosclerosis in patients with severe coronary artery disease. Furthermore, it is essential to improve symptomatic status, functional class, and risk factor profile. Yoga practices like slow breathing, meditation, relaxation, postures, and integrated practices, appear to improve overall cardiovascular health. Although, more rigorous and specific studies are required to elucidate molecular mechanisms behind its clinical and autonomic role and cure. Further, studies of yoga must include a detailed reporting of the yoga practices used with a wider number of patients. Mechanistic studies and therapeutic targets must be explored for a better understanding and treatment of CVDs.

Acknowledgment CK and PT are supported by the Department of Science and Technology, Government of India, Grant No. DST/INSPIRE Fellowship/[IF180523] and [IF170502].

Conflicts of Interest Authors declared no conflicts of interest.

References

1. Ibrahim NE, Gaggin HK, Konstam MA, Januzzi JL Jr. Established and emerging roles of biomarkers in heart failure clinical trials. Circ Heart Fail. 2016;9(9):1–11.
2. Seta Y, Shan K, Bozkurt B, Oral H, Mann DL. Basic mechanisms in heart failure: the cytokine hypothesis. J Card Fail. 1996;2(3):243–9.
3. Jabs WJ, Theissing E, Nitschke M, Bechtel JM, Duchrow M, Mohamed S, Jahrbeck B, Sievers HH, Steinhoff J, Bartels C. Local generation of C-reactive protein in diseased coronary artery venous bypass grafts and normal vascular tissue. Circulation. 2003;108(12):1428–31.
4. Genth-Zotz S, Blankenberg S. Immunactivation in chronic heart failure. Inflammatory mediators. Clin Res Cardiol. 2004;93(4):24–30.
5. Writing Group Members, Lloyd-Jones D, Adams R, Carnethon M, De Simone G, Ferguson TB, Flegal K, Ford E, Furie K, Go A, Greenlund K. Heart disease and stroke statistics—2009 update: a report from the American Heart Association sStatistics Committee and Stroke Statistics Subcommittee. Circulation. 2009;119(3):480–6.
6. Braunwald E. Biomarkers in heart failure. N Engl J Med. 2008;358(20):2148–59.
7. Lozano R, Naghavi M, Foreman K, Lim S, Shibuya K, Aboyans V, Abraham J, Adair T, Aggarwal R, Ahn SY,

AlMazroa MA. Global and regional mortality from 235 causes of death for 20 age groups in 1990 and 2010: a systematic analysis for the global burden of disease study 2010. Lancet. 2012;380(9859):2095–128.
8. Pullen PR, Nagamia SH, Mehta PK, Thompson WR, Benardot D, Hammoud R, Parrott JM, Sola S, Khan BV. Effects of yoga on inflammation and exercise capacity in patients with chronic heart failure. J Card Fail. 2008;14(5):407–13.
9. Matthews SC, Nelesen RA, Dimsdale JE. Depressive symptoms are associated with increased systemic vascular resistance to stress. Psychosom Med. 2005;67(4):509–13.
10. Brown KM, Hui Q, Huang Y, Taylor JY, Prescott L, Barcelona de Mendoza V, Crusto C, Sun YV. Association between stress and coping with DNA methylation of blood pressure-related genes among African American women. Chronic Stress. 2019;3:1–9.
11. Janszky I, Ahnve S, Lundberg I, Hemmingsson T. Early-onset depression, anxiety, and risk of subsequent coronary heart disease: 37-year follow-up of 49,321 young Swedish men. J Am Coll Cardiol. 2010;56(1):31–7.
12. Rozanski A, Bairey CN, Krantz DS, Friedman J, Resser KJ, Morell M, Hilton-Chalfen S, Hestrin L, Bietendorf J, Berman DS. Mental stress and the induction of silent myocardial ischemia in patients with coronary artery disease. N Engl J Med. 1988;318(16):1005–12.
13. Januzzi JL, Stern TA, Pasternak RC, DeSanctis RW. The influence of anxiety and depression on outcomes of patients with coronary artery disease. Arch Intern Med. 2000;160(13):1913–21.
14. Thakur P, Mohammad A, Rastogi YR, Saini RV, Saini AK. Yoga as an intervention to manage multiple sclerosis symptoms. J Ayurveda Integr Med. 2020;11(2):114–7.
15. Geiser F, Meier C, Wegener I, Imbierowicz K, Conrad R, Liedtke R, Oldenburg J, Harbrecht U. Association between anxiety and factors of coagulation and fibrinolysis. Psychother Psychosom. 2008;77(6):377–83.
16. Lippi G, Montagnana M, Favaloro EJ, Franchini M. Mental depression and cardiovascular disease: a multifaceted, bidirectional association. Semin Thromb Hemost. 2009;35(03):325–36.
17. Petersen JW, Felker GM. Inflammatory biomarkers in heart failure. Congest Heart Fail. 2006;12(6):324–8.
18. Nemeroff CB, Musselman DL. Are platelets the link between depression and ischemic heart disease? Am Heart J. 2000;140(4):S57–62.
19. Cramer H, Lauche R, Langhorst J, Dobos G. Yoga for depression: a systematic review and meta-analysis. Depress Anxiety. 2013;30(11):1068–83.
20. Kalueff A, Nutt D. Role of GABA in anxiety and depression. Depress Anxiety. 2007;24:495–517.
21. Banasik J, Williams H, Haberman M, Blank SE, Bendel R. Effect of Iyengar yoga practice on fatigue and diurnal salivary cortisol concentration in breast cancer survivors. J Am Acad Nurse Pract. 2011;23(3):135–42.
22. Moadel AB, Shah C, Wylie-Rosett J, Harris MS, Patel SR, Hall CB, Sparano JA. Randomized controlled trial of yoga among a multiethnic sample of breast cancer patients: effects on quality of life. J Clin Oncol. 2007;25(28):4387–95.
23. Banerjee B, Vadiraj HS, Ram A, Rao R, Jayapal M, Gopinath KS, Ramesh BS, Rao N, Kumar A, Raghuram N, Hegde S. Effects of an integrated yoga program in modulating psychological stress and radiation-induced genotoxic stress in breast cancer patients undergoing radiotherapy. Integr Cancer Ther. 2007;6(3):242–50.
24. Lakkireddy D, Atkins D, Pillarisetti J, Ryschon K, Bommana S, Drisko J, Vanga S, Dawn B. Effect of yoga on arrhythmia burden, anxiety, depression, and quality of life in paroxysmal atrial fibrillation: the YOGA my heart study. J Am Coll Cardiol. 2013;61(11):1177–82.
25. Jin RC, Loscalzo J. Vascular nitric oxide: formation and function. J Blood Med. 2010;1:147.
26. Rodrigo R, Prat H, Passalacqua W, Araya J, Guichard C, Bächler JP. Relationship between oxidative stress and essential hypertension. Hypertens Res. 2007;30(12):1159.
27. Gordon L, McGrowder DA, Pena YT, Cabrera E, Lawrence-Wright MB. Effect of yoga exercise therapy on oxidative stress indicators with end-stage renal disease on hemodialysis. Int J Yoga. 2013;6(1):31.
28. Dai Kim J, Yu BP, McCarter RJ, Lee SY, Herlihy JT. Exercise and diet modulate cardiac lipid peroxidation and antioxidant defenses. Free Radic Biol Med. 1996;20(1):83–8.
29. Yavuzer H, Yavuzer S, Cengiz M, Erman H, Doventas A, Balci H, Erdincler DS, Uzun H. Biomarkers of lipid peroxidation related to hypertension in aging. Hypertens Res. 2016;39(5):342.
30. Patil SG, Dhanakshirur GB, Aithala MR, Naregal G, Das KK. Effect of yoga on oxidative stress in elderly with grade-I hypertension: a randomized controlled study. J Clin Diagn Res. 2014;8(7):BC04.
31. Radak Z, Chung HY, Goto S. Exercise and hormesis: oxidative stress-related adaptation for successful aging. Biogerontology. 2005;6(1):71–5.
32. Serhan CN. Pro-resolving lipid mediators are leads for resolution physiology. Nature. 2014;510(7503):92–101.
33. Bär KJ, Schuhmacher A, Höfels S, Schulz S, Voss A, Yeragani VK, Maier W, Zobel A. Reduced cardio-respiratory coupling after treatment with nortriptyline in contrast to S-citalopram. J Affect Disord. 2010;127(1–3):266–73.
34. Birdee GS, Legedza AT, Saper RB, Bertisch SM, Eisenberg DM, Phillips RS. Characteristics of yoga users: results of a national survey. J Gen Intern Med. 2008;23(10):1653–8.
35. Reaven PD, Witztum JL. Oxidized low density lipoproteins in atherogenesis: role of dietary modification. Annu Rev Nutr. 1996;16(1):51–71.

36. Sivasankaran S, Pollard-Quintner S, Sachdeva R, Pugeda J, Hoq SM, Zarich SW. The effect of a six-week program of yoga and meditation on brachial artery reactivity: do psychosocial interventions affect vascular tone? Clin Cardiol. 2006;29(9):393–8.
37. Mohammad A, Thakur P, Kumar R, Kaur S, Saini RV, Saini AK. Biological markers for the effects of yoga as a complementary and alternative medicine. J Complement Integr Med. 2019;16(1) https://doi.org/10.1515/jcim-2018-0094.
38. Krishna BH, Pal P, Pal GK, Balachander J, Jayasettiaseelon E, Sreekanth Y, Sridhar MG, Gaur GS. Effect of yoga therapy on heart rate, blood pressure and cardiac autonomic function in heart failure. J Clin Diagn Res. 2014;8(1):14–6.
39. Gautam S, Kumar M, Dada R. Yoga and meditation: the holistic way to decrease incidence of childhood cancer. Clin Oncol. 2018;3:1404.

Stress and the Autonomic Nervous System: Implication of Yoga

9

Kaviraja Udupa, Ananda Balayogi Bhavanani, and Meena Ramanathan

Contents

K. Udupa
Department of Neurophysiology, National Institute of Mental Health and Neuro Sciences (NIMHANS), Bangalore, India

A. B. Bhavanani (✉) · M. Ramanathan
Centre for Yoga Therapy, Education and Research (CYTER), Sri Balaji Vidyapeeth, MGMC & RI, Pondicherry, India
e-mail: yoga@mgmcri.ac.in

9.1 Modern Day Stress

Stress is an inevitable part of modern day lifestyle and this has been implicated in various medical disorders including psychosomatic, cardiovascular, psychiatric, and neurological conditions. All these non-communicable disorders (NCD) are constantly on an upscale (CVD is the most common cause of mortality and disability, WHO 2011) after the effective control of communicable disorders with antibiotics and hygiene practices. The increasing stress could be attributed to "competitive" modern day life, the perception of this stress and its subsequent biological effects on various systems and this has been investigated ever since the days of Cannon. He provided the classic 3 F's response to stress in terms of fright (having fear and other emotions to decide on subsequent course of action) which would be either flight (moving away from the threat) or fight (face the threat) and face that challenge effectively. Thus stress could be any challenge to well-being or homeostasis of the system which the individual would face or run away based on the level of threat and his ability to face the challenge effectively that would lead to the consequences of stress. As per the vascular prediction model the metabolic requirement to face the stress would lead to derangement in the system. Individuals who react in an exaggerated manner show increase in heart rate and blood pressure up to 30 units to face any challenge

I. Basu-Ray, D. Mehta (eds.), *The Principles and Practice of Yoga in Cardiovascular Medicine*,
https://doi.org/10.1007/978-981-16-6913-2_9

normally but under such situations it would go beyond 50 units. These individuals whose response is hyper-reactive to stress are prone to develop cardiovascular morbidity and this vulnerability has been attributed to hyperactivity of amygdala [1]. Brain imaging studies have demonstrated that individuals who have shown hyperactivity of cardiovascular response to stress have shown increased activity in the regions of anterior cingulate cortex, hippocampus, amygdala, insula, and pons [2]. Behavioral activation may relate to both withdrawal and approach and trait stress reactivity is influenced by such behavior activation and cardiac vagal activity.

9.2 Autonomic Nervous System (ANS)

ANS is an extensive neural network involved in regulating the human internal environment by controlling homeostasis and visceral functions. This is important for the maintenance of optimal environment for cells, tissues, and organs so as to enable continuous adjustments to the varying internal and external demands on the body. The word "autonomic" was coined by JN Langley in 1898 and he proposed that this word implied independent action but exercised under control of higher power. The functions of heart muscle, smooth muscle, secretory glands, and hormone secretions are regulated by ANS thus maintaining these homeostatic functions essential for existence of life [3].

Langley divided ANS into sympathetic, parasympathetic, and enteric nervous systems primarily based on anatomic considerations. Craniosacral outflow constituted the parasympathetic division, thoracolumbar outflow formed the sympathetic division, whereas the enteric nervous system was intrinsically present in the wall of the gastrointestinal tract through its interconnecting plexus. Functionally, the sympathetic and parasympathetic nervous systems are complementary to each other and maintain balance in tonic activities of visceral structures and organs. Sympathetic division—prepares the body for strenuous physical activity in stressful situations. This response is often referred to as the "fight-or-flight" response because the sympathetic division prepares the body to fight against or flee from a threat. Parasympathetic division—regulates important body functions such as digestion and "slows down" the body ("rest and digest") after a "flight-or-flight" response [3].

The major factor in vasomotor sympathetic tone is generated mainly by the activity of rostral ventrolateral medullary (RVLM) sympathoexcitatory neurons. Increase in RVLM neuronal activity results in release of catecholamines and vasopressin that increases the blood pressure and heart rate. These neurons innervate the intermediolateral cell column of the spinal cord thoracolumbar region from which sympathetic preganglionic fibers emerge. The hypothalamus has been claimed to be the most important ANS organ, as it integrates autonomic and neuroendocrine functions and serves as an important homeostatic center. In addition to controlling all the visceral functions, paraventricular nucleus, dorsomedial nucleus, and lateral hypothalamic nuclei innervate preganglionic sympathetic and parasympathetic neurons widespread in insula and amygdala. Thus hypothalamus integrates responses to stress and regulates cardiovascular function, energy metabolism and maintains the homeostasis.

9.3 Cardiovascular Autonomic Control: Anatomical Aspects

Heart tissues have special properties to generate its own rhythmicity known as automaticity. But this function is significantly modulated by innervations from both the sympathetic and parasympathetic divisions of ANS. The parasympathetic innervation of the heart originates in the cardiovagal motoneurons in the nucleus ambiguus and the dorsal vagal nucleus passes through two sets of cardiac nerves arising from each vagus nerve. The cardiac branches of the vagus nerve separate in the thorax and innervate several cardiac ganglion cells. The postganglionic fiber is very short as the parasympathetic autonomic ganglion (cardiac ganglion) is situated very close to the end organ (heart). This property makes fast conducting myelinated preganglionic fiber to form majority of the parasympathetic pathways making conduction velocity faster than sympathetic system of innervations. This concept was supported by Levy et al. [4] who have demonstrated maximal response of HR within 400 ms of stimulation of vagus in animal studies. On the other hand, Furnival et al. [5] have shown that response to sympathetic stimulation starts after a latency of 5 s and the maximal response is reached only after 20–30 s. The left and right vagi are distributed differentially, with the left vagus nerve inhibiting AV conduction tissue and the right vagus nerve affecting predominantly the sinus node. This anatomico-functional separation in innervations enables the CNS to selectively influence the sinoatrial (SA) and AV conduction tissue [6].

Sympathetic neurons influencing positive chronotropic and ionotropic activity of the heart are originated from intermediolateral cell columns of the upper thoracic segments of the spinal cord (T1–T4). Parasympathetic and sympathetic nerves interconnect to form ventral and dorsal cardiopulmonary plexuses, from which relatively large and discrete cardiac nerves emerge to supply the ventricles: the right and left coronary cardiac nerves and the left lateral cardiac nerves. A number of smaller nerves also supply the heart and there are many anatomic variations among individuals with regard to the precise "wiring diagram" of the heart. Similar to the parasympathetic system, sympathetic innervations of the heart also function in a lateralized manner. Cowley [7] has demonstrated that the right sympathetic pathway predominantly excites the SA node, increasing heart rate, whereas the left sympathetic pathways predominantly innervate the AV node and the ventricles, resulting in increased AV conduction, cardiac contractility, and oxygen consumption [3].

Once within the substance of the myocardium, sympathetic fibers tend to remain on the epicardial surface, and vagal fibers penetrate deeper into the subendocardium, although both cross the surface of the heart during part of their course. The right-sided sympathetic nerves usually supply the anterior surface of the ventricle, while the left-sided sympathetic nerves supply the posterior surface. In addition to these cardiac afferents heart is richly innervated by other cardiac afferents, which are involved in bringing out various reflexes, which in turn are involved in maintaining the milieu interior [3].

9.4 Physiology of Cardiovascular Autonomic Control

Regulation of the cardiovascular system can be explained under auto regulation, humeral and neural regulatory mechanisms. These three mechanisms with a constant interplay between them regulate cardiac output, systemic vascular resistance, and local organ blood flow to regulate mean arterial pressure marinating the homeostasis. Details about cardiovascular regulation are given elsewhere. The fact that heart and blood vessels are under the control of ANS is shown by dynamic fluctuations in the HR and BP in response to physiological changes [8]. Neural regulation is thus operated through the interaction between sympathetic and parasympathetic limbs of ANS which generally act in a reciprocal manner. This neurocardiac control thus enables beat-to-beat modulation of cardiac activity and vascular tone in response to internal or external stimuli, stresses, and emotional changes and maintains the homeostasis [3].

To study the dynamic nature of neurocardiac regulation, we can consider an example of baroreflex mechanism, which is involved in the short-term regulation of BP [9]. The arterial baroreceptors and the cardiopulmonary receptors with vagal afferents tonically inhibit the vasomotor centers, the firing rate from the receptors increases directly with increased pressure. The primary site of interaction of these afferents within CNS is at the level of NTS. As a consequence, the sympathetic activity is modified selectively to adjust appropriately the performance of the cardiovascular system. Thus the inhibition of sympathetic activity decreases the heart rate and cardiac contractility, relaxes the resistance vessels, and increases capacitance in the splanchnic vascular bed. As a consequence, systemic vascular resistance and cardiac filling pressure are adjusted to maintain arterial BP at an appropriate level [3].

In healthy individuals, HR at rest is dominated by parasympathetic innervations. Either pharmacologically blocking both the divisions of ANS or surgically denervating the heart to study the effects of ANS on heart can experimentally demonstrate this fact. The "intrinsic" HR thus obtained by denervating the heart is more than the resting HR. This demonstrates the fact that the heart is under cardio inhibitory control of the vagus during rest. The inhibitory effects of inspiration on cardiovagal motor-neurons in the nucleus ambiguus and dorsal vagal nucleus cause short-term periodic fluctuations in heart rate the oscillations of which have a close relationship with respiration. The increase in HR in inspiration and decrease in expiration is called respiratory sinus arrhythmia (RSA), which is considered an important clinical index of vagal innervations of the heart. The physiological significance of this oscillation is to provide better oxygenation of blood [10].

Measurement of autonomic nervous system function: ANS functions can be evaluated using following battery of tests (Table 9.1).

9.5 Conventional Cardiac Autonomic Function Tests

The cardiovascular autonomic function tests, involving continuous HR, BP, and respiratory monitoring to define circulatory responses under standardized conditions, provide information about both sympathetic and parasympathetic cardiovascular autonomic regulation [11]. The following commonly used tests are known as "Ewing's tests" [12].

9.5.1 Deep Breathing Test

This is a test of parasympathetic influence on cardiovascular function and it is abolished by atropine. In this test, a subject is asked to breathe slowly and almost fully to their vital capacity taking 5 s for inspiration and 5 s for expiration. Deep breathing difference (DBD) was calculated from the mean of the differences between maximum heart rate during inspiration and minimum heart rate during expiration of six such cycles. DBD

Table 9.1 Battery of autonomic function tests [3]

Test domain	Systems tested	Tests
Physiological	Cardiovascular	HR and BP response to deep breathing, orthostatic test, tilt-table test, Valsalva maneuver, isometric exercise, mental arithmetic, cold pressor test, carotid sinus massage, and exercise test
Biochemical	General	Plasma noradrenaline, renin activity, aldosterone, and urinary catecholamines
Pharmacological	General	Using different agonists and antagonists of various receptor types involved in autonomic pharmacology
Sudomotor	Sweat glands	Thermoregulatory sweat test, quantitative sudomotor axon reflex test, localized sweat test, and sympathetic sweat response
Gastrointestinal (Radiodiagnostic)	Gastrointestinal tract	Barium studies, videocinefluoroscopy, endoscopy, and gastric emptying tests
Urodynamics	Renal function tests	Urine output, Na+/K+ excretion, urodynamic studies, intravenous urography, ultrasound study, and sphincter electromyography
Sexual	Reproductive	Penile plethysmography and intracavernosal papaverine
Respiratory	Lungs and respiratory tract	Laryngoscopy, sleep studies to assess oxygen saturation/apnea
Ophthalmological	Vision	Schirmer' s test, physiological and pharmacological pupillary functions

tends to decrease with age, the value being around 15–20 beats/min in persons of 20 years of age and 5–10 over the age of 60 years [3].

9.5.2 Valsalva Maneuver

In this test, subject is asked to blow out and maintain the intrathoracic pressure at 45 mm of Hg for 15 s. It has to be made sure that the subject is blowing out forcefully and maintaining the high intrathoracic pressure and not merely blowing through cheeks by keeping an air leak in the apparatus. The longest RR interval immediately after the blow out and minimum RR interval during the blow are recorded and highest of three such trials is taken as Valsalva ratio. This response assesses the integrity of the afferent limb (vagus), central processing (central autonomic network), and efferent limb of the baroreceptor reflex. There are four phases of changes in the heart rate and blood pressure which are as shown below in Table 9.2.

9.5.3 Orthostatic Test

Subjects are asked to stand upright from supine position and the change in heart rate and blood pressure is recorded immediately and at first, second, and fifth minutes after standing. The maximum: minimum (M: m) ratio is calculated as the ratio of longest RR interval around 30th second and the minimum RR interval around 15th second after standing up.

9.5.3.1 Physiological Background of the Orthostatic Test

Change in position from supine to standing produces changes in gravitational forces. This creates a head to foot hydrostatic pressure gradient within the cardiovascular system. The hydrostatic gradient causes a redistribution of blood into the compliant veins of the lower limbs creating a lower body negative pressure. Venous pooling ensues resulting in the sequential reductions in central venous pressure, end diastolic pressure (cardiac filling), stroke volume, and cardiac output. Overall, lying to standing creates a change in blood volume redistribution in the venous system. It is the lack of sensitivity responses to various reflex components (sympathetic and parasympathetic responses) of the cardiovascular system to maintain arterial pressure, which is of great importance. Dehydration, stress, illness, and overstraining will affect orthostatic tolerance. It appears that the RR interval mode can provide greater information in the form of HRV responses to the change in blood pressure. The supine position is believed to be dominated by the parasympathetic nervous system along with sympathetic nervous system withdrawal, but once the patient stands suddenly, the sympathetic nervous system will snap into action to compensate for the change in blood pressure and redistribution of blood volume. This can measure

Table 9.2 Different phases of Valsalva maneuver

Phase	Maneuver	Heart rate	Blood pressure
I	Onset of expiration against the partially closed glottis	Rises due to aortic compression	Decreases
II early	Continued expiration	Falls due to decreased venous return	Increases
II late	Continued expiration	Increased sympathetic discharge causing increased total peripheral vascular resistance	Increases at slower rate
III	End of expiration	Falls due to increased capacitance of pulmonary bed	Increases further
IV	Recovery	Increases (overshoot) due to vasoconstriction and increased cardiac output	Compensatory bradycardia

the input from the autonomic nervous system during the overall period and the changes can be tracked [3].

9.5.4 Isometric Handgrip Test

In this test, subjects' diastolic pressure response for an isometric task is measured. The generalized increase in sympathetic activity produced by the isometric exercise causes sympathetically mediated vasoconstriction which in turn causes increase in diastolic pressure. Subject will be asked to maintain the handgrip at one-third of maximal voluntary contraction and the heart rate and blood pressure change at pre-release is compared with the baseline values.

9.6 Heart Rate Variability (HRV) Analysis

HRV is a physiological phenomenon defined as variation in the normal-to-normal RR intervals during normal sinus rhythm. It reflects the effects of the ANS and other physiological control mechanisms on cardiac function. It can be easily analyzed from 5 min or more electrocardiographic (ECG) recordings. These non-invasive and easily performed assessments of HR variability have now attained widespread use in diverse disciplines. With the advent of effective data acquisition and storage devices have resulted in an array of measures of HRV.

The measurement of HRV is non-invasive and has high intra- and inter-individual reproducibility [13], which has led to its popularity in assessing neuroautonomic control of the heart. The traditional methods of HR variability analysis include time and frequency domain analysis, often referred to as linear methods. In the time domain measures of HRV, HR fluctuation is assessed by calculating measures based on statistical operations (means and variance) on R-R intervals. The most widely used time domain measures are average HR and standard deviation of all normal-to-normal R-R intervals (SDNN) which is the square root of variance and is considered to reflect both parasympathetic and sympathetic influences on the heart. The details and the physiological significance of other time domain measures like RMSSD, pNN50, and triangular index are given in Table 9.3.

In frequency domain analysis, the variation of heart rate is divided into different frequency components, which in turn contributed, by different regulatory mechanisms. For this purpose complicated mathematical algorithm, namely power spectral density has to be applied. This power spectral analysis decomposes the heart rate signal into frequency components and quantifies the relative intensity as individual "power" [14]. Fast Fourier transformation and autoregressive analysis are the most commonly used methods providing frequency specific information of HR variability. The spectrum is usually divided into four different frequency bands. The frequency range and the physiological significance of the most commonly used bands as explained by Task force report [15] are given in table of frequency domain measures (Table 9.4). HF power is considered to reflect mainly cardiovagal modulation and the inspiratory inhibition of vagal tone, while LF power is affected by both sympathetic and parasympathetic activity. This fact is based on the observation that vagal stimulation increased HRV power over all frequencies with the pronounced effect in the HF component [16] and large doses of atropine virtually abolished HF fluctuations [10, 17]. On the other hand, sympathetic stimulation has been shown to increase LF component which is further enhanced with add on vagal stimulation [16]. The ratio of LF power to HF power (LF/HF ratio) has been proposed as a measure of sympathovagal balance [18, 19]. Fluctuations in the VLF region have been suggested to reflect thermoregulation and peripheral vascular resistance [17, 20]. ULF represents diurnal variation of long-term regulatory mechanisms, effective calculation of which requires longer-term (say 24 h) ECG-Holter recordings [3].

Table 9.3 Time domain HRV measures

Time domain parameters			
Parameter	Unit	Description	Physiologic correlates
SDNN	ms	Standard deviation of all (normal to normal) NN intervals	Sensitive to all sources of variation, e.g.: respiratory, baroreceptor, thermoregulation, and activity
SDANN	ms	Standard deviation of all NN intervals in all 5-min segments of the entire recording	More sensitive to lowest frequencies, posture, activity, and the basic day-night change in heart rate. This measure basically shows how much heart rate differs during each 5-min period from the overall day-long mean heart rate
RMSSD	ms	The square root of the mean of the sum of squares of differences between adjacent NN intervals	Both RMSSD and pNN50 indices are most sensitive to the highest frequency components. They select the changes that occur from one QRS cycle to the very next. Evidences suggest that these time domain measures are the best predictors of parasympathetic activity
NN50	Count	Count of number of pairs of NN (Normal-to-normal RR) intervals differing by >50 ms	
pNN50	%	NN50 divided by total number of all NN intervals	
TINN	ms	Triangular index of NN interval	Estimate overall HRV

Table 9.4 Frequency domain HRV measures

Frequency domain parameters			
Power	Unit	Frequency range/ equation	Physiologic correlates
Total power	ms^2	0–0.4 Hz	Sensitive to all sources of variation
Ultra low frequency (ULF) power	ms^2	0–0.003 Hz	Postural changes, daily activity, Parasympathetic tone?
Very low frequency (VLF) power	ms^2	0.003–0.04 Hz	Thermoregulation? Renin–angiotensin–aldosterone system (RAAS)?
Low frequency (LF) power	ms^2	0.04–0.15 Hz	Sympathetic and parasympathetic tone
High frequency	ms^2	0.15–0.4 Hz	Parasympathetic tone
(HF) power			Respiration
LF nu	Normalized units	LF/(LF + HF)*100	Sympathetic and parasympathetic tone
HF nu	Normalized units	HF/(LF + HF)*100	Parasympathetic tone, Respiration
LF/HF ratio	Ratio	LF/HF	Sympathovagal balance

9.7 Clinical Utility of HRV

HRV analysis has been applied in many clinical conditions associated with cardiac autonomic disturbances. To site some examples, HRV has been used to study the risk of cardiac electrical instability after myocardial infarction [21], to diagnose diabetic neuropathy [22], to assess re-innervations after cardiac transplantation [23], and to evaluate exercise training [24]. Reduced HRV is a powerful and independent predictor of an adverse prognosis in patients with heart disease and in the general population. The HRV is largely determined by vagally mediated beat-to-beat variability, conventionally known as RSA. Thus, HRV is primarily an indicator of cardiac vagal control. It is still unclear whether the relationship between measures of cardiac vagal control and mortality is causative or mere association. Possible mechanisms by which cardiac vagal activity might beneficially influence prognosis include a decrease in myocardial oxygen demand, a reduction in sympathetic activity, and a decreased susceptibility of the ventricular myocardium to lethal arrhythmia. In animals, augmentation of cardiac vagal control by nerve stimulation or by drugs is associated with a reduction in sudden death in susceptible models. In humans a number of drugs, which have been shown to reduce mortality and sudden death in large randomized trials, can also be demonstrated to increase HRV. As a result of this evidence, it has been suggested that the effect of drugs or other therapeutic maneuvers on HRV might be used to predict clinical efficacy [3].

9.8 Yoga

Yoga is a philosophical, cultural, and social gift of ancient India and potential antidote to the stressful lifestyle of modern world. The word "yoga" is derived from "*yuj*" meaning to "unite." This union can be inferred at various levels: different systems of the human bodily functions; body and mind; ultimately the individual existence (*atma*) and the Divine experience (*paramatma*). With regard to the ANS and its two components, viz., sympathetic and parasympathetic, that act in a reciprocal manner, Yoga can be inferred to "yoke" them together, creating and maintaining a state of dynamic balance manifesting as physiological homeostasis (*samatvam yoga uchyate*, Bhagavad Gita).

9.9 Studies Exploring Effect of Yoga on AFTs

Over the last two decades many studies have explored the physiological benefits of yoga in healthy volunteers and patients with various psychosomatic disorders such as diabetes mellitus, hypertension, epilepsy, irritable bowel syndrome, depression, and other mental health disorders. Salient findings from these studies will be summarized in subsequent sections. Yoga is a comprehensive discipline comprising eight different limbs (ashtanga yoga), but scientific studies mostly concentrate either on asanas and pranayamas or both. It is interesting to note that a study compared the effect of these two limbs asanas and pranayamas and found that all good effects (changes in sympathovagal balance and cognitive performance) were found only in pranayama group and not in yogasana group [25]. Accordingly, we shall restrict to the discussion on the effects of these two limbs (asanas and pranayamas) of yoga on autonomic and other physiological functions. Further these studies can be broadly divided into ones studying the acute (immediate effect of a session of yoga practice) effects and chronic effects of long-term (practice for daily minutes to hours, sometimes under supervision for few weeks to months) practice. Effects might be different in fact quite opposite to each other in these broad categories of acute and chronic practice of yoga. Ideally yoga being practiced as a lifestyle and expertise developed over years or lifetime of dedicated practice over all the limbs of yoga. Thus the real scientific effects could only be studied in few individuals who achieved this state. However, majority of these studies utilized short-term practice in naïve individuals (healthy volunteers and patients with various disorders). Hence the results should always be interpreted carefully in concluding the effects of yoga on autonomic functions. Further, majority of these studies incorporated only cardiac autonomic functions and not involved other autonomic functions involving other systems of the body. Most of these studies showed increase in parasympathetic tone and decrease in sympathetic activity in long-term practitioners of yoga. However, the acute effect of any of these practices could be quite different [26].

9.9.1 Pranayama (Breathing Exercises or Alternate Nostril Breathing)

Tells et al. [27] showed significant increase in baseline oxygen consumption in "right nostril pranayama" group. They suggested these changes could be due to increased sympathetic discharge to the adrenal medulla. They also showed an increase in volar galvanic skin resistance, interpreted as a reduction in sympathetic nervous system activity supplying the sweat glands in "left nostril Pranayama." Khalsa [28] reviewed this technique with others and reported that unilateral forced nostril breathing employing forced breathing through only one nostril while closing off the other; selectively activate the ipsilateral branch of the sympathetic nervous system with a possible compensation effect leading to contralateral vagal nerve stimulation. Their earlier studies [29] showed that right forced nostril breathing selectively causes more increase in the heart rate and verbal cognitive functions [cf: left nostril breathing improving spatial tasks which effect was confirmed later [30]]. Thus unilateral nostril selectively alters autonomic and cognitive functions. In another study [31] showed that immediate effect of alternate nostril breathing exercise for 5 min would be quite different from chronic effects of pranayama. Acute effects increased sympathetic activity and reducing parasympathetic activity whereas chronic effects are just opposite of that as shown by many studies [3].

Further studies by Raghuraj et al. [32] have shown that nadi shuddhi pranayama (slow alternate nostril breathing) decreases the sympathetic activity compared to the kapalabhati (fast and forceful abdominal contractions) which increases the sympathetic functions. Thus the stress alters the milieu interior or homeostasis of various systems of the body. Yoga modulates all these factors to maintain the homeostasis of physiological system. This not only facilitates the individual to face the stress effectively but also, reduces the impact of stress in development of any disorders. Further, if the individual is already suffering from any of the medical condition, yoga improves the clinical condition and modulates the pathogenesis of that specific disorders induced by stress and other etiologies.

References

1. Tawakol A, Ishai A, Takx RA, Figueroa AL, Ali A, Kaiser Y, Truong QA, Solomon CJ, Calcagno C, Mani V, Tang CY, Mulder WJ, Murrough JW, Hoffmann U, Nahrendorf M, Shin LM, Fayad ZA, Pitman RK. Relation between resting amygdalar activity and cardiovascular events: a longitudinal and cohort study. Lancet. 2017;25;389(10071):834–45. https://doi.org/10.1016/S0140-6736(16)31714-7.
2. Ginty AT, Krayank TE, Fischer JP, Gianoros PJ. Cardiovascular and autonomic reactivity to psychological stress: neurophysiological substrates and links to cardiovascular disease. Auton Neurosci Basic Clin. 2017;207:2–9.
3. Udupa K, Sathyaprabha TN. Influence of yoga on the autonomic nervous system. In: Telles S, Singh N, editors. Research-based perspectives on the psychophysiology of yoga. Hershey, PA: IGI Global; 2017. p. 67–85.
4. Levy MN, Martin PJ, Iano T. Effects of single vagal stimuli on heart rate and atrioventricular conduction. Am J Physiol. 1970;218:1256–62.
5. Furnival CM, Linden RJ, Snow HM. Chronotropic and ionotropic effects on the dog heart of stimulating the efferent cardiac sympathetic nerves. J Physiol. 1973;230:137–53.
6. Zipes DP. Influence of myocardial ischemia and infarction on autonomic innervations of heart. Circulation. 1990;82(4):1095–105.
7. Cowley AW Jr. Long-term control of arterial blood pressure. Physiol Rev. 1992;72:231–300.
8. Joyner MJ, Shepherd JT. Autonomic regulation of the circulation. In: Low PA, editor. Clinical autonomic disorders. Philadelphia: Lippincott-Raven Publishers; 1997.
9. Hainsworth R, Ledsome JR, Carswell F. Reflex response from aortic baroreceptors. Am J Physiol. 1970;218:423–9.
10. Eckberg DL. Human sinus arrhythmia as an index of vagal cardiac outflow. J Appl Physiol. 1983;54:961–6.
11. Hohnloser SH, Klingenheben T. Basic autonomic tests. In: Malik M, editor. Clinical guide to cardiac autonomic tests. Dordrecht: Kluwer Academic Publishers; 1998.
12. Mathias CJ, Bannister R. A textbook of clinical disorders of the autonomic nervous system. Oxford: Oxford University Press; 1999.
13. Huikuri HV, Makikallio T, Airaksinen KE, et al. Measurement of heart rate variability: a clinical tool or a research toy? J Am Coll Cardiol. 1999;34(7):1878–83.
14. Hartikainen JEK, Tahvanainen KUO, Kuusela TA. Short-term measurement of heart rate variability. In: Malik M, editor. Clinical guide to cardiac autonomic tests. Dordrecht: Kluwer Academic Publishers; 1998.
15. Task Force of the European Society of Cardiology and the North American Society of Pacing and Electro Physiology. Heart rate variability. Standards of measurement, physiological interpretation and clinical use. Circulation. 1996;93:1043–65.
16. Headman AE, Tahavanainen KU, Hartikainen JE, Hakumäki MO. Effect of sympathetic modulation and sympathovagal interaction on heart rate variability in anaesthetized dogs. Acta Physiol Scand. 1995;39:801–5.
17. Akselrod S, Gordon D, Ubel FA, Shannon DC, Berger AC, Cohen RJ. Power spectrum analysis of heart rate fluctuation: a quantitative probe of beat-to-beat cardiovascular control. Science. 1981;213:220–2.
18. Malliani A, Pagani M, Lombardi F, Cerutti S. Cardiovascular neural regulation explored in the frequency domain. Circulation. 1991;84:482–92.
19. Pagani M, Lombardi F, Guzzetti S, Rimoldi O, Furlan R, et al. Power spectral analysis of heart rate and arterial pressure variabilities as a marker of sympathovagal interaction in man and conscious dog. Circ Res. 1986;59:178–93.
20. Dwain L, Eckberg DL. Sympathovagal balance; a critical appraisal. Circulation. 1997;96:3224–32.
21. Bigger JT Jr, Fleiss JL, Rolnitzky LM, Steinman RC, Schneider WJ. Time course of recovery of heart period variability after myocardial infarction. J Am Coll Cardiol. 1991;18(7):1643–9.
22. Pagani M, Malfatto G, Pierini S, Casati R, Masu AM, et al. Spectral analysis of heart rate variability in the assessment of autonomic diabetic neuropathy. J Auton Nerv Syst. 1988;23(2):143–53.
23. Sands KE, Appel ML, Lilly LS, Schoen FJ, Mudge GH Jr, Cohen RJ. Power spectrum analysis of heart rate variability in human cardiac transplant recipients. Circulation. 1989;79(1):76–82.
24. Perini R, Veicsteinas A. Heart rate variability and autonomic activity at rest and during exercise in various physiological conditions. Eur J Appl Physiol. 2003;90(3–4):317–25.
25. Chandla SS, Sood S, Dogra R, Das S, Shukla SK, Gupta S. Effect of short-term practice of pranayamic breathing exercises on cognition, anxiety, general well being and heart rate variability. J Indian Med Assoc. 2013;111(10):662–5.

26. Benvenutti MJ, Alves EDS, Michael S, Ding D, Stamatakis E, Edwards KM. A single session of hatha yoga improves stress reactivity and recovery after an acute psychological stress task-A counterbalanced, randomized-crossover trial in healthy individuals. Complement Ther Med. 2017;35:120–6.
27. Telles S, Nagarathna R, Nagendra HR. Breathing through a particular nostril can alter metabolism and autonomic activities. Indian J Physiol Pharmacol. 1994;38(2):133–7.
28. Shannahoff-Khalsa DS. Selective unilateral autonomic activation: implications for psychiatry. CNS Spectr. 2007;12(8):625–364.
29. Shannahoff-Khalsa DS, Kennedy B. The effects of unilateral forced nostril breathing on the heart. Int J Neurosci. 1993;73(1–2):47–60.
30. Joshi M, Telles S. Immediate effects of right and left nostril breathing on verbal and spatial scores. Indian J Physiol Pharmacol. 2008;52(2):197–200.
31. Subramanian RK, Devaki PR, Saikumar PS. Alternate nostril breathing at different rates and its influence on heart rate variability in non practitioners of yoga. J Clin Diagn Res. 2016;10(1):CM01–2.
32. Raghuraj P, Ramakrishnan AG, Nagendra HR, Telles S. Effect of two selected yogic breathing techniques of heart rate variability. Indian J Physiol Pharmacol. 1998;42(4):467–72.

Neurobiological Effects of Yoga on Stress Reactivity

10

Michaela C. Pascoe, David R. Thompson, and Chantal F. Ski

10.1 Yoga

Yoga aims to achieve a union of mind, body and spirit and originated thousands of years ago in India. Yoga has eight limbs, which are breathing, rules of conduct, ethical disciplines, control of the senses, postures, concentration of the mind, meditation, and merging one with eternity [1]. In the West, yoga asana, or the practice of yoga postures, is commonly used as a stress management approach [2], with approximately 10% of the American population practicing in 2012 [3]. Medical practitioners often recommend yoga to their patients [4], as shown by a survey showing that approximately 75% of Australian practitioners referred patients to a yoga therapist [5]. Despite yoga asana commonly being used as a stress management approach, its neurobiological effects on stress reactivity are still being explored. This chapter explores the impact of yoga asana practice on stress reactivity.

10.2 The Stress Response

Organisms maintain a homeostasis balance and respond to adverse events or stressors. Stressors can be perceived or actual threats and activate the "fight-or-flight" response, controlled by the autonomic nervous system (ANS) [6]. The ANS comprises the sympathetic nervous system (SNS) and the parasympathetic nervous system (PNS) [7], which together control involuntary body functions including, but not limited to, blood vessel dilation or constriction, blood pressure, respiration, and heartbeat.

The SNS contributes to survival changes by providing energy to the body in dangerous situations [7]. This occurs when the sensory organs relay information to the amygdala, where it is interpreted and from where a signal is sent to the hypothalamus. The SNS is activated via autonomic nerves to the adrenal glands, which release the hormone epinephrine (adrenaline) to the bloodstream. This initiates physiological changes known as the "fight-flight" response and which include increases in heart rate increases, respiration, and blood pressure. Epinephrine triggers blood sugar (glucose) and fat release into the bloodstream for energy [6, 8]. Once the threat has passed, the PNS [9] returns the body to

M. C. Pascoe (✉)
Institute of Sport, Exercise and Active Living, Victoria University, Melbourne, Australia
e-mail: Michaela.pascoe@vu.edu.au

D. R. Thompson
Department of Psychiatry, University of Melbourne, Melbourne, Australia

School of Nursing and Midwifery, Queen's University Belfast, Belfast, UK

C. F. Ski
Integrated Care Academy, University of Suffolk, Ipswich, UK

I. Basu-Ray, D. Mehta (eds.), *The Principles and Practice of Yoga in Cardiovascular Medicine*,
https://doi.org/10.1007/978-981-16-6913-2_10

homeostasis. The stress response balances responding to perceived threats and returning to homeostasis [10, 11].

10.2.1 Hypothalamic–Pituitary–Adrenal Axis

The hypothalamus activates the hypothalamic–pituitary–adrenal (HPA) axis, consisting of the hypothalamus, adrenal glands, and pituitary gland [12]. The hypothalamus releases corticotropin-releasing hormone (CRH), a peptide hormone, which triggers adrenocorticotropic hormone (ACTH) release and the downstream release of the glucocorticoid steroid hormone cortisol [8, 12, 13]. One function of cortisol is to maintain steady supplies of blood sugar by releasing glucose from the liver for energy to cope with prolonged stressors [14].

10.3 The Impact of Persistent Stress

The HPA system is regulated via a feedback loops, which are designed to maintain hormone levels and homeostasis in order to protect against prolonged activity [8]. Cortisol is released in response to stressors and, at a certain blood concentration levels, binds to low-affinity glucocorticoid receptors [15]. This terminates the stress response [13], ensuring that ACTH and cortisol levels are maintained within a relatively narrow bandwidth. This is important is too much or too little cortisol exposure can be detrimental to health and well-being [14, 16].

Frequent or persistent stress, including psychological stress, can result in regular activation of the "fight-or-flight" response [10, 11, 17], and too much exposure to stressful events can disrupt the delicate negative feedback control mechanism [8, 18]. They can become hypersensitive to ACTH and therefore amplify the glucocorticoid response to stressors [19]. High levels of cortisol exposure can impair the function of glucocorticoid receptors (such as via reduced expression, downregulation, nuclear translocation) [20–22] in brain regions such as the prefrontal cortex (as well as the paraventricular nucleus) and hippocampus [23, 24] disrupt glucocorticoid feedback control of the HPA axis [25–27]. Baseline glucocorticoid release increases [19, 28] which can damage the hippocampus (regulation of mood [29]) and prefrontal cortex (executive function, working memory, self-regulatory behaviors) [30], and amygdala [29] (regulation of emotion [31]). People with mood disorders such as depression show changes in the function and structure of these regions [29], demonstrating why activation of the "fight-or-flight" response might be associated with psychiatric disorders [17, 32, 33], charactered by an increase in inflammatory state [34–36].

10.4 Yoga Asana and Stress Regulation

yoga asana practice can decrease stress reactivity and stress and this is associated with better well-being [37]. Yoga asana practices often incorporate elements of the other seven components of yoga, including philosophical teachings and the teaching of psychological skills as well as breathing or meditative techniques [38–40]. Therefore, yoga asana practice may influence psychological, physiological, and neurobiological processes. In this chapter, we explore the impact of yoga asana on stress-related physiological changes.

10.5 Yoga Asana and Autonomic Measures

10.5.1 Blood Pressure

Yoga clearly has beneficial effects on blood pressure (BP). A Meta-Analysis of randomized controlled trials (RCTs) comparing yoga asana to the time/attention control group in diverse populations shows decreases in resting diastolic blood pressure (DBP) of 3.66 millimeters of mercury (mmHg) and systolic blood pressure (SBP) by 5.34 mmHg following yoga [41]. In seven of the primary studies measuring SPB and included in this Meta-Analysis, the control group was an exercise intervention, and therefore yoga decreased resting SBP more than other forms of exercise [41]. Reductions in BP of 2 mmHg decrease the incidence of cardiovascular disease in both normotensive and hypertensive people [42, 43]; thus yoga-related reductions in BP are likely to be clinically beneficial.

10.5.2 Heart Rate

Similar to heart rate, yoga asana can decrease heart rate. In a Meta-Analysis of 15 RCTs comprising 879 participants, yoga decreased heart rate by 3.2 beats per minute, compared to a time/attention control group [41]. Another Meta-Analysis has previously reported that aerobic exercise reducing the heart rate by 5 beats per minute, and therefore, yoga can reduce heart rate in a manner similar to aerobic exercise [44].

10.5.3 Heart Rate Variability

Heart rate variability (HRV), or the time variation interval between heartbeats, is also influenced by yoga practice. A systematic review reported that yoga increased vagal dominance and HRV, which indicates increased PNS, in 59 studies comprising of 2358 participants. This review reported that yoga practitioners had increased vagus nerve activity at rest compared to non-practitioners [45], as the vagus nerve is a major contributor to PNS activity and an antagonist of SNS activity and efferent nerve [46]. Another systematic review found that 10 of 14 RCTs reviewed reported the benefits of yoga asana on HRV in healthy individuals or patients with any medical condition, compared to any type of control intervention [47].

HRV is also reported according to the frequency domain, with heart rate (HR) oscillations divided into low-frequency (LF) and high-frequency (HF) bands [48]. Increased HF-HRV is commonly interpreted to reflect increased PNS, while LF-HRV represents both PNS branches but is thought to be SNS dominant [49–51]. However, the interpretation may oversimplify the complex interactions between the PNS and SNS [49, 52]. Meta-Analysis reports that yoga asana increases LF-HRV and HF-HRV compared to other forms of exercise, indicating the effects cannot be attributed to the exercise-related impacts of yoga asanas [41].

10.6 Cytokines

Cytokines, cell signaling protein molecules that regulate inflammation and immunity [53], are induced by stressors [49–51]. A feedback loop between cytokines and cortisol is central for HPA axis functioning and maintaining homeostasis of the immune system [52, 54]. Stress-induced cytokines, including interleukin-6 [IL-6], tumor necrosis factor-alpha [TNF-α] and interleukin (IL-10), activate the HPA axis and release cortisol [52, 55], which then suppress further cytokines upregulation [52, 56–58]. However, excessive cortisol can result in glucocorticoid receptor abnormalities and reduce the immune system's reactivity to cortisol. This results in sustained cortisol and cytokine release [56, 57, 59], which has been linked to adverse health outcomes, such as coronary artery disease [60].

In a systematic review focusing on adults with chronic inflammatory-related disorders, 11 of 15 studies were found to report a beneficial impact on yoga asana on inflammatory biomarkers, including IL-6 (n = 11 studies), and TNF-α (n = 8 studies), and C-reactive protein (CRP—a protein whose circulating concentrations rise in response to inflammation) (n = 10 studies) [61]. This systematic review also reported that having practiced yoga asana for a longer period of time was associated with greater changes in inflammatory markers [61]. This is somewhat consistent with a Meta-Analysis showing decreases IL-6 following a mindfulness-based stress reduction (MBSR) intervention (n = 3 studies), but no effect on IL-6 following a non-MBSR-based yoga intervention (n = 2 studies). This Meta-Analysis also found no significant effect of yoga on CRP or interleukin-8, however, only four and two studies were included in the analysis, and these studies differed significantly in their methods as some assessed cytokine levels at intervention completion while others assessed cytokine levels at follow up [41].

10.7 Cortisol

Increased ANS activity and dysregulation can be reflected in increased cortisol [62, 63]. Yoga asana has been shown to decrease waking cortisol levels in salvia in five studies of 386 individuals as well as to decrease evening cortisol levels in five studies of 385 individuals, as reported by Meta-Analysis [41].

Yoga programs incorporating aspects from all the eight limbs of yoga appear to impact cortisol more than yoga programs focused on asana only. This is demonstrated by an RCT in which university students with depression and anxiety symptoms or high self-reported stress were randomized one of three groups: (1) yoga program incorporating teachings from multiple limbs of yoga; (2) yoga asana only; or (3) a control group who completed surveys. Both yoga interventions decreased depression symptoms and subjective stress levels, and the yoga program incorporating teachings from multiple limbs of yoga also decreased anxiety symptoms and cortisol levels [64]. This suggests that the observed impacts of yoga on the stress response likely result from the combined effect of the various limbs of yoga, including mindfulness practices, philosophical teachings, meditation techniques, breathing exercises and physical postures.

10.8 Concluding Remarks

Yoga influences the stress response in diverse populations. Yoga can likely be of benefit for individuals with chronic inflammatory conditions. Some people may find yoga to be an appealing stress management approach as it enables individuals to be actively engaged in therapy and can be used ad libitum during stressful periods, enabling self-management.

Grant Support There is no funding to report.

References

1. Iyengar BKS. Light on yoga. New York, NY: Schocken Books; 1994.
2. Penman S, et al. Yoga in Australia: results of a national survey. Int J Yoga. 2012;5(2):92–101.
3. Clarke TC, et al. Trends in the use of complementary health approaches among adults: United States, 2002-2012. Natl Health Stat Report. 2015;(79):1–16.
4. Nerurkar A, et al. When conventional medical providers recommend unconventional medicine: results of a national study. Arch Intern Med. 2011;171(9):862–4.
5. Wardle J, Adams J, Sibbritt D. Referral to yoga therapists in rural primary health care: a survey of general practitioners in rural and regional New South Wales, Australia. Int J Yoga. 2014;7(1):9–16.
6. Charmandari E, Tsigos C, Chrousos G. Endocrinology of the stress response. Annu Rev Physiol. 2005;67:259–84.
7. Nesse RM, Bhatnagar S, Ellis B. Evolutionary origins and functions of the stress response system. In: Stress: concepts, cognition, emotion, and behavior handbook of stress series. Academic Press; 2016. p. 95–101.
8. Herman JP, et al. Regulation of the hypothalamic-pituitary-adrenocortical stress response. Compr Physiol. 2016;6(2):603–21.
9. Olshansky B, et al. Parasympathetic nervous system and heart failure: pathophysiology and potential implications for therapy. Circulation. 2008;118(8):863–71.
10. Mendes WB. Autonomic nervous system. In: Harmon-Jones E, Beer J, editors. Methods in the neurobiology of social and personality psychology. Guilford Press; 2009.
11. Buijs RM. The autonomic nervous system: a balancing act. Handb Clin Neurol. 2013;117:1–11.
12. Ortiga-Carvalho TM, et al. Hypothalamus-pituitary-thyroid axis. Compr Physiol. 2016;6(3):1387–428.
13. Myers B, McKlveen JM, Herman JP. Neural regulation of the stress response: the many faces of feedback. Cell Mol Neurobiol. 2012; https://doi.org/10.1007/s10571-012-9801-y.
14. Hiller-Sturmhofel S, Bartke A. The endocrine system: an overview. Alcohol Health Res World. 1998;22(3):153–64.
15. De Kloet ER, et al. Brain corticosteroid receptor balance in health and disease. Endocr Rev. 1998;19(3):269–301.
16. Stephens MA, Wand G. Stress and the HPA axis: role of glucocorticoids in alcohol dependence. Alcohol Res. 2012;34(4):468–83.
17. Iwata M, Ota KT, Duman RS. The inflammasome: pathways linking psychological stress, depression, and systemic illnesses. Brain Behav Immun. 2013;31:105–14.

18. Varghese FP, Brown ES. The hypothalamic-pituitary-adrenal axis in major depressive disorder: a brief primer for primary care physicians. Prim Care Companion J Clin Psychiatry. 2001;3(4):151–5.
19. Ulrich-Lai YM, et al. Chronic stress induces adrenal hyperplasia and hypertrophy in a subregion-specific manner. Am J Physiol Endocrinol Metab. 2006;291(5):E965–73.
20. Silverman MN, Sternberg EM. Glucocorticoid regulation of inflammation and its functional correlates: from HPA axis to glucocorticoid receptor dysfunction. Ann N Y Acad Sci. 2012;1261:55–63.
21. Kunz-Ebrecht SR, et al. Differences in cortisol awakening response on work days and weekends in women and men from the Whitehall II cohort. Psychoneuroendocrinology. 2004;29(4):516–28.
22. Mackin P. The role of cortisol and depression: exploring new opportunities for treatments. Psychiatr Times. 2004;21(6):92.
23. Cohen S, et al. Chronic stress, glucocorticoid receptor resistance, inflammation, and disease risk. Proc Natl Acad Sci. 2012;109(16):5995–9.
24. Gądek-Michalska A, et al. Influence of chronic stress on brain corticosteroid receptors and HPA axis activity. Pharmacol Rep. 2013;65(5):1163–75.
25. Herman JP, Watson SJ, Spencer RL. Defense of adrenocorticosteroid receptor expression in rat hippocampus: effects of stress and strain. Endocrinology. 1999;140(9):3981–91.
26. Gómez F, et al. Hypothalamic-pituitary-adrenal response to chronic stress in five inbred rat strains: differential responses are mainly located at the adrenocortical level. Neuroendocrinology. 1996;63(4):327–37.
27. Herman JP, Adams D, Prewitt C. Regulatory changes in neuroendocrine stress-integrative circuitry produced by a variable stress paradigm. Neuroendocrinology. 1995;61(2):180–90.
28. Gray M, Bingham B, Viau V. A comparison of two repeated restraint stress paradigms on hypothalamic-pituitary-adrenal axis habituation, gonadal status and central neuropeptide expression in adult male rats. J Neuroendocrinol. 2010;22(2):92–101.
29. McEwen BS, Nasca C, Gray JD. Stress effects on neuronal structure: hippocampus, amygdala, and prefrontal cortex. Neuropsychopharmacology. 2016;41(1):3.
30. McEwen BS, Morrison JH. The brain on stress: vulnerability and plasticity of the prefrontal cortex over the life course. Neuron. 2013;79(1):16–29.
31. LeDoux J. The amygdala. Curr Biol. 2007;17(20):R868–74.
32. Ventriglio A, et al. Early-life stress and psychiatric disorders: epidemiology, neurobiology and innovative pharmacological targets. Curr Pharm Des. 2015;21(11):1379–87.
33. Herbert J. Cortisol and depression: three questions for psychiatry. Psychol Med. 2013;43(3):449–69.
34. Raison CL, Capuron L, Miller AH. Cytokines sing the blues: inflammation and the pathogenesis of depression. Trends Immunol. 2006;27(1):24–31.
35. Berk M, et al. So depression is an inflammatory disease, but where does the inflammation come from? BMC Med. 2013;11:200.
36. Dantzer R. Depression and inflammation: an intricate relationship. Biol Psychiatry. 2012;71(1):4–5.
37. Riley KE, Park CL. How does yoga reduce stress? A systematic review of mechanisms of change and guide to future inquiry. Health Psychol Rev. 2015;9(3):379–96.
38. Farmer J. Yoga body: the origins of modern posture practice. Rev Am Hist. 2012;40(1):145–58.
39. Pflueger LW. Yoga body: the origins of modern posture practice. Relig Stud Rev. 2011;37(3):235.
40. Travis F, Pearson C. Pure consciousness: distinct phenomenological and physiological correlates of "consciousness itself". Int J Neurosci. 2000;100(1-4):77–89.
41. Pascoe MC, Thompson DR, Ski CF. Yoga, mindfulness-based stress reduction and stress-related physiological measures: a meta-analysis. Psychoneuroendocrinology. 2017;86:152–68.
42. Wong GW, Wright JM. Blood pressure lowering efficacy of nonselective beta-blockers for primary hypertension. Cochrane Database Syst Rev. 2014;2:CD007452.
43. Turnbull F, Blood Pressure C, Lowering Treatment Trialists. Effects of different blood-pressure-lowering regimens on major cardiovascular events: results of prospectively-designed overviews of randomised trials. Lancet. 2003;362(9395):1527–35.
44. Kelley GA, Kelley KA, Tran ZV. Aerobic exercise and resting blood pressure: a meta-analytic review of randomized, controlled trials. Prev Cardiol. 2001;4(2):73–80.
45. Tyagi A, Cohen M. Yoga and heart rate variability: a comprehensive review of the literature. Int J Yoga. 2016;9(2):97.
46. Breit S, et al. Vagus nerve as modulator of the brain–gut axis in psychiatric and inflammatory disorders. Front Psych. 2018;9:44.
47. Posadzki P, et al. Yoga for heart rate variability: a systematic review and meta-analysis of randomized clinical trials. Appl Psychophysiol Biofeedback. 2015;40(3):239–49.
48. Shaffer F, Ginsberg J. An overview of heart rate variability metrics and norms. Front Public Health. 2017;5:258.
49. Ruzek MC, et al. Characterization of early cytokine responses and an interleukin (IL)-6–dependent pathway of endogenous glucocorticoid induction during murine cytomegalovirus infection. J Exp Med. 1997;185(7):1185–92.
50. Lemay LG, Vander AJ, Kluger MJ. The effects of psychological stress on plasma interleukin-6 activity in rats. Physiol Behav. 1990;47(5):957–61.
51. Dhabhar FS, et al. Stress-induced changes in blood leukocyte distribution. Role of adrenal steroid hormones. J Immunol. 1996;157(4):1638–44.
52. Turnbull AV, Rivier CL. Regulation of the hypothalamic-pituitary-adrenal axis by cytokines:

actions and mechanisms of action. Physiol Rev. 1999;79(1):1–71.
53. Salim S, Chugh G, Asghar M. Inflammation in anxiety. Adv Protein Chem Struct Biol. 2012;88:1–25.
54. Petrovsky N. Towards a unified model of neuroendocrine–immune interaction. Immunol Cell Biol. 2001;79(4):350–7.
55. Steensberg A, et al. IL-6 enhances plasma IL-1ra, IL-10, and cortisol in humans. Am J Physiol Endocrinol Metab. 2003;285(2):E433–7.
56. Elenkov IJ, Chrousos GP. Stress hormones, Th1/Th2 patterns, pro/anti-inflammatory cytokines and susceptibility to disease. Trends Endocrinol Metab. 1999;10(9):359–68.
57. Chrousos GP. The hypothalamic–pituitary–adrenal axis and immune-mediated inflammation. N Engl J Med. 1995;332(20):1351–63.
58. Reichlin S. Neuroendocrine-immune interactions. N Engl J Med. 1993;329(17):1246–53.
59. Miller GE, Cohen S, Ritchey AK. Chronic psychological stress and the regulation of pro-inflammatory cytokines: a glucocorticoid-resistance model. Health Psychol. 2002;21(6):531.
60. Nijm J, Jonasson L. Inflammation and cortisol response in coronary artery disease. Ann Med. 2009;41(3):224–33.
61. Djalilova DM, et al. Impact of yoga on inflammatory biomarkers: a systematic review. Biol Res Nurs. 2019;21(2):198–209.
62. Barker ET, et al. Daily stress and cortisol patterns in parents of adult children with a serious mental illness. Health Psychol. 2012;31(1):130–4.
63. Staufenbiel SM, et al. Hair cortisol, stress exposure, and mental health in humans: a systematic review. Psychoneuroendocrinology. 2013;38(8):1220–35.
64. Smith JA, et al. Is there more to yoga than exercise? Altern Ther Health Med. 2011;17(3):22–9.

11 Mind and Cardiovascular Disease: Mechanism of Interrelationship

Sanjay S. Phadke and Leena S. Phadke

11.1 Cardiology and Psychology Interface

Obraztsov and Strazhesko are credited with the first observation of negative emotions and coronary thrombosis in 1910 [1]. Subsequently, since the time that cardiologists Friedman and Rosenman described the "Type A Behaviour Pattern" of time pressure and easily aroused anger and its association with increased risk of cardiovascular disease in 1959 [2], and the Whitehall I study of British civil servants of late 1960s which pointed out association of lower employment grade with cardiovascular risk [3] large body of epidemiological and experimental research has uncovered an intimate link between the mind and heart in health and pathology. The linkage is enriching the overall understanding of cardiovascular disease (CVD), from genesis to management.

While the risk associated with "negative" psychological states and traits such as depression, anxiety, anger, hostility, and stress was the focus of initial studies, attention subsequently shifted to explore protective factors like Positive Psychological Wellbeing (PPWB) and optimism. American Heart Association (AHA) formulated the concept of *cardiovascular health* in 2010 which has behavior change at its core [4, 5], and "promotion of healthy lifestyle throughout life" is the first take-home message of 2019 ACC/AHA Guideline on the Primary Prevention of Cardiovascular Disease [6]. Conceptualization of cardiovascular health as a bio-behavioral construct paves the way for experimenting with and developing integrative models of care to suit the needs of populations at different levels of risk, which are cost-effective and scalable so as to achieve ambitious public health goals such as the AHA 2020 Impact Goals.

11.2 Epidemiology of Cardiovascular Disease and Cardiovascular Health

11.2.1 Depression and Cardiovascular Disease

Frasure-Smith et al.'s research published in 1993 identified depression as a significant predictor of mortality following myocardial infarction (MI) in patients with coronary artery disease (CAD) [7]. Since this initial research, epidemiological

S. S. Phadke (✉)
Center for Behavioural Medicine, Jenhangir Hospital and Deenanath Mangeshkar Hospital & Research Center, Pune, India

Indian Psychiatric Society's Task Force on Mind-Body Medicine, Pune, India

L. S. Phadke
Central Research Laboratory, SKN Medical College, Pune, India

I. Basu-Ray, D. Mehta (eds.), *The Principles and Practice of Yoga in Cardiovascular Medicine*,
https://doi.org/10.1007/978-981-16-6913-2_11

studies have explored various facets of relationship between depression and cardiovascular disease which encompass the role of depression as a risk factor in the onset and complications of CVD, contribution of depression to sudden cardiac death, and to all-cause mortality, and additional contribution to risk indirectly through unhealthy lifestyle and poor treatment adherence. Depression is also a consequence of cardiovascular disease and the relationship is therefore bidirectional.

Many meta-analyses established that the prevalence of depression ranges from 15% to 30% in coronary artery disease, which is two- to three-folds higher than in the general population [8], and the occurrence is twice as common in women [9]. Studies exploring depression and incidence of coronary artery disease have frequently demonstrated a dose–response relationship, i.e., higher level of depression symptoms being associated with higher risk of CAD [10]. Depression is also associated with other CAD risk factors such as smoking and physical inactivity. It is noteworthy that depression remains an independent risk factor even after adjusting for other risk factors. A meta-analysis that included 30 prospective cohort studies of 893,850 participants who were initially free of CAD concluded that depression was associated with a 30% increased risk of coronary events during the follow-up that ranged from 2 to 37 years [11]. Depression after acute coronary syndrome is a risk factor for cardiac and all-cause mortality, and also the risk factor for composite outcomes including non-fatal cardiac events [8]. The evidence prompted American Heart Association to assign depression the status of a risk factor for adverse medical outcomes in patients with acute coronary syndrome [12].

In addition to its contribution to the risk, depression has a profound effect on the lives of patients with CAD. Depression has emerged as the strongest predictor of poor Quality of Life (QoL) in CAD and its impact is even more than any symptom directly linked to the severity of heart disease like dyspnoea, angina, or functional impairment [13, 14]. Depressive symptoms are also associated with worse QoL and more physical limitations after Myocardial Infarction (MI) and predict new angina during follow-up, which improves with improvement in depression [15, 16]. In fact, depression is a stronger predictor of angina than severity of CAD or any other traditional risk factors [17]. Negative emotions are known to trigger Atrial Fibrillation (AF) episodes in paroxysmal AF, and depression has been found to be associated with a threefold increase in the risk of recurrence of AF after successful cardiac electroversion [18, 19].

Health behaviors are also impacted adversely by negative emotional states. Depression has been associated with increased risk of becoming a new smoker, increased daily smoking in existing smokers, and reduced probability of quitting smoking [20, 21]. Depression is also associated with excessive drinking, physical inactivity, overeating, overweight and obesity, and a higher risk of Type 2 diabetes; some of these associations are bidirectional [22–24].

11.2.2 Anxiety, Anger, Hostility, Distressed Personality (Personality D), and CVD

A recent meta-analysis of 37 studies in which 1,565,699 individuals were followed up over 1 to 24 years observed that anxiety was associated with 52% increased incidence of CVD, and the risk being independent of traditional risk factors as well as depression [25]. Another meta-analysis of 46 cohort studies of 2,017,276 participants also attested to the association of anxiety disorders with increased risk of a range of cardiovascular events [26].

Research findings show that other negative emotional states and traits like anger, hostility, and Type D personality traits may also play a crucial role in the pathogenesis of CAD. In a meta-analysis of studies which included 25 studies of Coronary Heart Disease (CHD) outcomes in initially healthy people and 19 studies of patients with existing CHD, anger and hostility were associated with increased CHD events in the healthy population and poor prognosis in the CHD patients. Even in those studies which controlled fully for the basal disease status and treatment, an association of anger and hostility with poor prognosis persisted. The harmful effect of anger and hostility on CHD events in healthy populations was greater in men than in women [27]. A subsequent review and meta-analysis regarding outbursts of anger as a trigger of acute cardiovascular events found that there was a higher rate of cardiovascular events in the immediate 2 h period following outbursts of anger [28].

The pioneering work of Friedman and Rosenman on personality factors in CVD subsequently evolved into a description of Distressed (Type D) personality, which is characterized by two stable traits: negative affectivity and social inhibition. A recent review of Type D personality and the mechanisms through which it affects disease progression and prognosis pointed out that nearly 25% of CAD patients have type D personality [29] and the contribution may be directly through physiological mechanisms, and indirectly through unhealthy lifestyle.

Long-term stress, both during early life and in adulthood, has been linked to a 1.5-fold increased risk of CHD. However, it is often confounded by adverse health behaviors, and independent association of psychosocial stress with CVD depends on the degree and duration of stress as well as individual response to the stressor [30, 31]. The stress cardiomyopathy syndrome or Takotsubo cardiomyopathy which predominantly affects elderly women is often preceded by an acute emotional trigger like bereavement or separation.

Two large cohort studies which investigated the relationship of sleep duration and sleep quality with the risk of coronary heart disease have shown that both short duration of sleep and poor quality of sleep are linked to increased risk of CVD. One of these studies found a U-shaped association, i.e., the risk was more in those who slept either less than 4 hours per night or more than 8 hours per night [32, 33].

The risk of CVD is however not limited to common psychological conditions of stress, depression, and anxiety but extends to the entire spectrum of psychiatric disorders including severe mental illness viz. schizophrenia, bipolar disorder, and major depression signifying a deep association of mind and cardiovascular health. A comprehensive meta-analysis of CVD risk in people with severe mental illness (SMI) which included 3,211,768 patients and 113,383,368 controls revealed that SMI patients as a group have significantly increased risk, which is 51% higher in cross-sectional studies and 54% higher in longitudinal studies [34].

11.2.3 Positive Psychological Well-Being (PPWB) and CVD

Similar to the conceptualization of physical health, the traditional conceptualization of psychological health was also in terms of the absence of illness, i.e., the absence of emotional distress or psychiatric symptoms. However, a growing body of research has made it increasingly clear that the absence of psychological distress does not automatically imply the presence of psychological well-being and led to conceptualization of a broad multidimensional construct that includes aspects like one's satisfaction with life, happiness, engagement with others, personal growth, and meaningfulness in life.

Technically speaking, the positive psychological well-being construct consists of two perspectives viz. subjective well-being or hedonic perspective and the eudaimonic perspective. Hedonic perspective is the emotional and cognitive interpretation of the quality of one's life, as assessed by the level of one's happiness, affect, and satisfaction with life. Eudaimonia, on the other hand, is a deeper form of well-being concerned with meaningfulness and realization of an individual's true potential, e.g., purpose in life and personal growth. Other well-being constructs such as optimism and emotional vitality have also been researched in the context of cardiovascular outcomes [35].

Research studies suggest that PPWB is consistently and independently protective against CVD. The protective action includes a lower incidence of CVD in healthy populations as well as reduced risk of adverse outcomes in patients with existing CVD. A meta-analysis of ten prospective studies which had 136,265 participants uncovered a significant association between having a higher purpose in life and reduced all-cause mortality and cardiovascular events [36]. Optimism has been most robustly associated with a reduced risk of cardiovascular events. A latest meta-analysis of 15 studies involving 229,391 participants posited that optimism is associated with a lower risk of cardiovascular events and all-cause mortality [37]. In general, PPWB was found to be positively associated with restorative health behaviors [38].

11.2.4 Ideal Cardiovascular Health

Health behaviors have significant and substantial associations with greater longevity and CVD-free survival. While reviewing the progress of the Impact Goal for 2010 that focused primarily on *reducing* the prevalence of risk factors and CHD and stroke death rates, AHA's Special Report notes that "the implicit assumption was this would improve health. However, it is increasingly evident that health is a broader, more positive construct than just the absence of clinically evident disease." Consequently, while setting national goals for Cardiovascular Health Promotion and Disease Reduction (The American Heart Association's Strategic Impact Goal Through 2020 and Beyond), AHA opted for the construct of Ideal Cardiovascular Health. The committee defined a total of 7 health behaviors and health factors critical to the definition of ideal cardiovascular health. Abundant evidence supports the ideal cardiovascular health construct with respect to longevity, disease-free survival, quality of life, and healthcare costs [4].

Subsequently, several population-based studies examined the prevalence of the AHA's ideal cardiovascular health (CVH) metrics and their association with cardiovascular disease (CVD) related morbidity and mortality, and also non-CVD outcomes. A recent review reported that all 6 mortality studies found a graded inverse association between the increasing number of ideal CVH metrics and CVD-related and all-cause mortality risk. Twelve out of 13 studies found a similar inverse relationship between ideal CVH metrics and incident cardiovascular events. An increasing number of ideal CVH metrics was found beneficial not only for cardiac health but has also been associated with lower prevalence and incidence of non-CVD outcomes such as cancer, depression, and cognitive impairment. Low proportions of persons however achieved 6 or more ideal CVH metrics in both US and non-US populations, and the review concluded that "considering the strong association of CVH metrics with both CVD and non-CVD outcomes, a coordinated global effort for improving CVH should be considered a priority" [39].

Findings from the Coronary Artery Risk Development in Young Adults (CARDIA) study which assessed the long-term impact of healthy behaviors demonstrated that young adults aged 18 to 30 years with healthy behaviors grow up to adulthood with lower risk. 60% of those who practiced all of 5 healthy lifestyle behaviors in young adulthood had all ideal cardiovascular biomarkers in middle age, which is in sharp contrast to fewer than 5% attaining ideal biomarkers in middle age amongst those who practiced none of these healthy behaviors as young adults. The promise of behavior change is highlighted by the fact that those who did not have a healthy lifestyle to start with but took up practising healthy behaviors later in life still had higher rates of ideal cardiovascular biomarkers than those who never adopted healthy behaviors. Thus, regardless of the timing, the adoption of healthy behaviors has value for cardiovascular health [40].

11.3 Mechanisms Linking Psychological States and CVD/CAD

Recent research linking systems such as the amygdala and other stress-responsive brain areas, autonomic nervous system (ANS), endocrine system especially the Hypothalamic–Pituitary–Adrenal (HPA) axis, hematopoietic system, and inflammation with CVD has helped change the simplistic view of CAD as a passive atherosclerotic process resulting from lipid storage to a complex multifactorial process of plaque formation and destabilization in which psycho-neuro-immuno-endocrine (PNIE) interactions play a key role, and has contributed substantially to advance understanding of the role of stress and negative psychological states in CVD.

11.3.1 Neurocardiology

Complex dynamic control networks exist between the heart and the brain. In 1985, Natelson coined the term neurocardiology to describe the interdisciplinary field of research which examines the interaction between the cardiovascular and autonomic nervous system (ANS) in pathological states [41]. ANS is responsible for maintaining homeostasis in response to normal physiological challenges as well as in response to stressful and pathological conditions. Chronic dysregulation of ANS characterized by an imbalance between the sympathetic and parasympathetic components is thought to be a key mechanism linking depression to cardiovascular risk and adverse outcomes [42]. Neuroadrenergic hypothesis of hypertension emphasizes that general sympathetic overdrive is the common underlying mechanism responsible for the development of the spectrum of diseases contributing to CV risk viz. hypertension, metabolic syndrome, and Type 2 diabetes [43]. Reduced Heart Rate Variability (HRV), which is a quantitative measure of cardiac autonomic function, is a predictor of morbidity and mortality in general population as well as in stable CVD patients, and also a predictor of mortality after myocardial infarction [44–46]. HRV is found to be lower in CAD patients with depression than those without depression [10, 42]. It has been experimentally observed that sympathetic stimulation triggers cardiac arrhythmias, reduces atrial and ventricular arrhythmic thresholds, and induces ECG changes in the repolarization phase [47]. In patients with implantable defibrillators, mental stress can induce T wave changes at lower heart rates [48].

11.3.2 Neurocardiac Axis

Neuroimaging data has unraveled a complex set of afferent, efferent, and local circuit neural interactions termed the neurocardiac axis which coordinates cardiac properties, and also involve brain and spine regions associated with autonomic control viz. the insular cortex, anterior cingulate cortex, prefrontal cortex, amygdala, hypothalamic nuclei, medulla, and spinal cord [49]. Amygdala research has provided novel insight into the mechanisms through which emotional stressors can lead to cardiovascular disease. A research that measured metabolic activity of amygdale through18F-fluorodeoxyglucose positron emission tomography (^{18}F-FDG-PET/CT) made the interesting discovery that amygdalar activity independently and robustly predicted cardiovascular disease events in the longitudinal study involving 293 patients [50]. The association seemed to be mediated by a serial pathway of increased amygdala activity, increased bone-marrow activity, and arterial inflammation. Another recent study which assessed the metabolic activity of the amygdale, hematopoietic tissue activity, and adiposity volumes in 246 patients in whom imaging was repeated ~1 year later demonstrated that amygdalar metabolic activity is independently associated with progression of visceral adiposity, and suggested a neurobiological pathway involving the amygdala and bone marrow which links psychosocial stress to adiposity [51].

Investigation into psychological stress-induced myocardial ischemia unraveled activation in more brain areas involved in the stress response and autonomic regulation of the cardiovascular system like anterior cingulate, inferior frontal gyrus, and parietal cortex [52]. Previous studies have shown that ischemic damage to the insular cortex is associated with arrhythmia, disrupted diurnal blood pressure variation, myocardial injury, and breathing disorders during sleep [53].

11.3.3 Psycho-Neuro-Endocrine Axis

Paralleling the dysregulation in the ANS endocrine changes in depression involves prominent dysregulation in the HPA (Hypothalamic–Pituitary–Adrenal) axis which includes alterations in corticotropin-releasing factor (CRF) and adrenocorticotropic hormone (ACTH), and elevated circulating cortisol levels. These changes affect immune functioning as well. A close relationship has been observed between high levels of cortisol and increased risk of ischaemic heart disease and cardiovascular mortality [54, 55].

11.3.4 Psycho-Immunology Axis

Depression has been known to be associated with chronic inflammation as manifested by increased levels of C-reactive protein and cytokines such as TNF-a, IL-1b, and IL-6. Chronic inflammation is a known risk factor for the development of atherosclerosis and CAD and is hypothesized to be contributory to increased risk of CHD associated with depression [56].

Other mechanisms involved in the depression-CAD shared relationship are endothelial dysfunction in which sympathetic activation also seems to play a role, and increased platelet activity [57, 58]. Plasminogen activator inhibitor-1 inhibits the formation of brain-derived neurotrophic factor (BDNF) and decreased BDNF levels are the potential link to thrombosis [59]. The complex psycho-neuro-immuno-endocrine interactions which form the bio-behavioral basis of CVD are depicted in Fig. 11.1.

A common genetic vulnerability has emerged through twin studies and it is suggested that shared, genetically influenced biological pathways underlie the association between depression and CHD that involve autonomic function, inflammation, and the serotoninergic system [60].

11.4 Cardiovascular Health and Yoga-Based Intervention

Considering the bio-behavioral nature of CVD, the application of mind–body intervention like Yoga is logical. Though in its classical form yoga comprises of eightfold body–mind meditative activity as espoused in the *Ashtang Yoga of Patanjali*, its application in clinical studies has been limited mostly to the physical postures (*Yoga-asana*) with the occasional addition of the breath regulation part (*pranayama*), and it is often unclear whether cardinal principals enshrined in other folds were followed. Therefore use of the term *yoga-based intervention* rather than yoga appears to be more apt a label. Despite the constraints of lack of uniformity of practice on one hand and methodological limitations of the intervention studies on the other, generation of positive signal both in terms of efficacy and safety is noteworthy. A recent bibliometric analysis on cardiovascular health noted that an upward trend is evident in the overall research in this area [61].

11.4.1 Yoga-Based Intervention and Neurobiology

Depression, as the prototype of psychological distress, has a significant role in the onset and prognosis of CVD and therefore the evidence linking yoga-based intervention to improvement in known neurobiology of depression is vital. Depression is known to be associated with elevated levels of serum cortisol, which is also a marker of stress. Depression is also associated with low serum brain-derived neurotrophic factor (BDNF) which is known to play important role in neuroplasticity and with low Gamma-Aminobutyric Acid (GABA) the inhibitory neurotransmitter that plays important role in the regulation of activity of brain networks. Recent studies which investigated these neurobiological markers report that the antidepressant effects of Yoga-based practices have been associated with a reduction in serum cortisol, increase in serum BDNF and increase in thalamic GABA [62, 63].

Increased amygdala activity has been shown to be a marker of several CVD risk factors viz. negative emotional, inflammatory, and adiposity factors, all of which pose risk to the heart. The Rotterdam study found that the practice of meditation and Yoga is associated with smaller right amygdala volume [64].

Chronic dysregulation of ANS including sympathetic overdrive links depression with CV outcome. Yoga practice is a known modulator of the autonomic nervous system [65–67] effective in increasing parasympathetic tone and reducing depressive symptoms and perceived stress [68]. Description of the inflammatory reflex explained the role of vagal activity in counteracting sympathetic hyperactivation-induced inflammation [69]. A recent neuroimaging study demonstrated that years of yoga practice

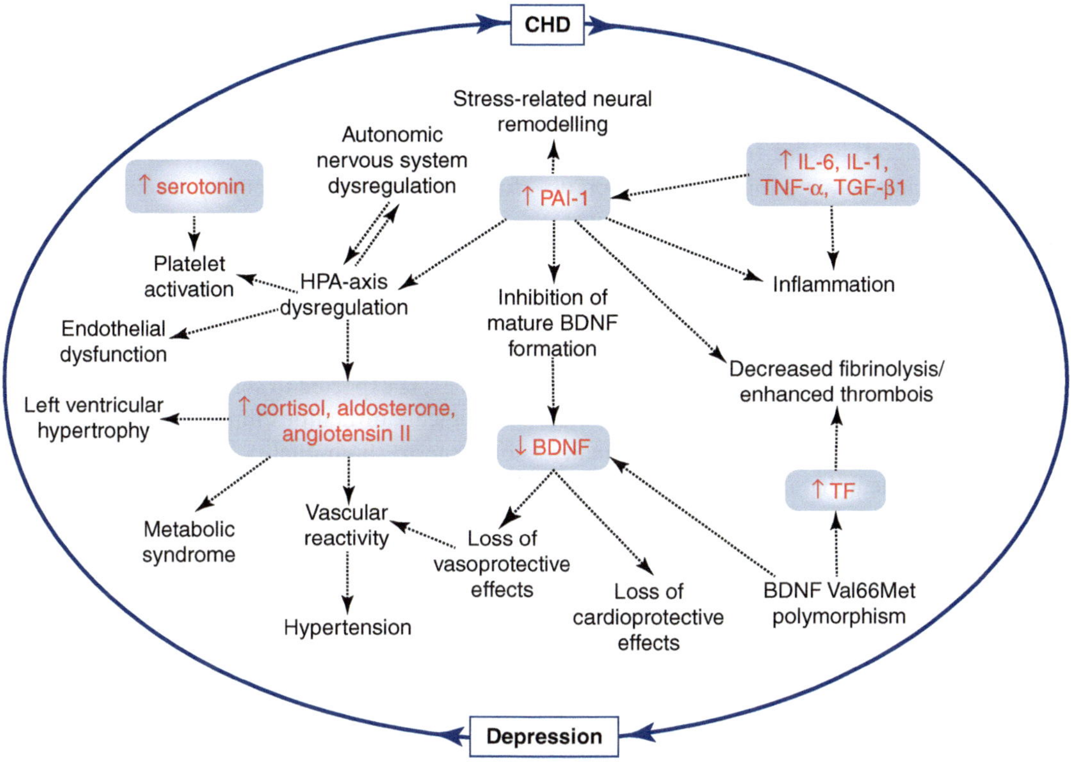

Fig. 11.1 PNIE links between depression, autonomic dysregulation, inflammation, endothelial dysfunction, and thrombosis. BDNF, brain-derived neurotrophic factor; CHD, coronary heart disease; HPA, hypothalamic–pituitary–adrenal axis; IL, interleukin; PAI, plasminogen activator inhibitor; TGF, transforming growth factor; TNF, tumor necrosis factor [with permission from Viola Vaccarino, Lina Badimon, J. Douglas Bremner, Edina Cenko, Judit Cubedo, Maria Dorobantu, Dirk J. Duncker, Akos Koller, Olivia Manfrini, Davor Milicic, Teresa Padro, Axel R. Pries, Arshed A. Quyyumi, Dimitris Tousoulis, Danijela Trifunovic, Zorana Vasiljevic, Cor de Wit, Raffaele Bugiardini. Depression and coronary heart disease: 2018. ESC position paper of the working group of coronary pathophysiology and microcirculation developed under the auspices of the ESC Committee for Practice Guidelines. European Heart Journal (2019) 0, 1–15]

experience correlated mostly with gray matter volume differences in the left hemisphere (insula, frontal operculum, and orbitofrontal cortex) suggesting that yoga tunes the brain toward a parasympatically driven mode and positive states [70]. It is noteworthy that autonomic nervous-based therapeutics have shown great potential in the management of atrial fibrillation, ventricular arrhythmia, and myocardial remodeling.

11.4.2 Yoga-Based Intervention and Cardio-Metabolic Health

The significance of positive psychology is well established in the context of cardiovascular health. A meta-analysis that included 32 studies and took a dual perspective of depression and positive well-being (emotional well-being, psychological well-being, and social-well being) showed that yoga intervention has effects not only on the reduction of depression but also on positive functioning of a person [71].

Yoga-based intervention finds role as an add-on intervention in SMI (severe mental illness), which is a known risk factor for CVD, in the NICE Guideline on Treatment and Management of Psychosis and Schizophrenia in Adults [72].

A meta-analysis that focused on cardiovascular disease (CVD) and metabolic syndrome risk factors generated promising evidence of yoga intervention on improving cardio-metabolic health. It included 37 RCTs in the systematic review and 32 studies in the meta-analysis and compared asana-based yoga to non-exercise controls. Yoga group showed significant improvement in body mass index, systolic blood pressure, low-density lipoprotein (LDL) cholesterol, and high-density lipoprotein (HDL) cholesterol. Significant changes were also seen in body weight, diastolic blood pressure, total cholesterol, triglycerides, and heart rate, but not on fasting blood glucose or glycosylated hemoglobin. Effects of yoga and physical exercise were comparable. One study found an impact on smoking abstinence. The limiting factors were small trial sample sizes, heterogeneity, and moderate quality of RCTs. It is evident that individuals who cannot or prefer not to perform traditional aerobic exercise might still achieve similar benefits in cardiovascular risk reduction [73].

Another meta-analysis that included 44 RCTs with a total of 3168 participants also revealed evidence for clinically important effects of yoga intervention on several cardiovascular disease risk factors in the general population and in the high-risk disease groups. Compared to usual care or no intervention, yoga improved systolic and diastolic blood pressure, heart rate, respiratory rate, waist circumference, waist/hip ratio, total cholesterol, HDL, VLDL, triglycerides, HbA1c, and insulin resistance. Relative to exercise, yoga improved HDL. The risk of bias was high or unclear for most RCTs. The meta-analysis concluded that despite methodological drawbacks of the included studies, yoga can be considered as an ancillary intervention for the general population and for patients with increased risk of cardiovascular disease [74].

11.4.3 Yoga-Based Intervention and Cardiac Rehabilitation

A recent multicentric study that recruited 4014 patients after the occurrence of Acute Myocardial Infarction (AMI) and compared yoga intervention with enhanced standard care, which included educational sessions, reported that improvement in the self-rated quality of life was significantly greater in the Yoga intervention group. There were fewer major adverse cardiovascular events in the yoga intervention group, which however did not reach statistical significance as the study was not powered adequately. Yoga intervention has the potential to be an alternative to conventional cardiac rehabilitation programs and address the unmet needs of cardiac rehabilitation for patients in resource-constrained settings [75].

Overall, it can be concluded that the mind–body integration, which is also the essence of Yoga, is a relatively young but promising enterprise in medicine both in terms of understanding the biological mechanisms and designing interventions, is expected to sort out the current methodological difficulties/limitations and deliver longer-term, high-quality trials for establishing firmly the effectiveness of yoga-based intervention for CVD including prevention [76].

References

1. Obraztsov VP, Strazhesko ND. The symptomatology and diagnosis of coronary thrombosis. In: Vorobeva VA, Konchalovski MP, editors. Works of the First Congress of Russian Therapists. Moscow: Comradeship Typography of A.E. Mamontov; 1910. p. 26–43.
2. Friedman M, Rosenman RH. Association of specific overt behaviour pattern with blood and cardiovascular findings: blood cholesterol level, blood clotting time, incidence of acrus senilis, and clinical coronary artery disease. J Am Med Assoc. 1959;169:1286–96.
3. Marmot MG, Rose G, Shipley M, Hamilton PJS. Employment grade and coronary heart disease in British civil servants. J Epidemiol Commun Health. 1978;32:244–9. https://doi.org/10.1136/jech.32.4.244.
4. Lloyd-Jones DM, Hong Y, Labarthe D, Mozaffarian D, Appel LJ, Van Horn L, Greenlund K, Daniels S, Nichol G, Tomaselli GF, Arnett DK, Fonarow GC, Ho PM, Lauer MS, Masoudi FA, Robertson RM, Roger V, Schwamm LH, Sorlie P, Yancy CW, Rosamond WD. Defining and setting national goals for cardiovascular health promotion and disease reduction: the American Heart Association's strategic impact goal through 2020 and beyond. Circulation. 2010;121:586–613.
5. Spring B, Ockene JK, Gidding SS, Mozaffarian D, Moore S, Rosal MC, Brown MD, Vafiadis DK, Cohen DL, Burke LE, Lloyd-Jones D. Better population health through behavior change in adults a call to action. Circulation. 2013;128:2169–76.
6. Arnett DK, Blumenthal RS, Albert MA, Buroker AB, Goldberger ZD, Hahn EJ, Himmelfarb CD, Khera A, Lloyd-Jones D, McEvoy JW, Michos ED, Miedema MD, Muñoz D, Smith SC Jr, Virani SS, Williams KA Sr, Yeboah J, Ziaeian B. 2019 ACC/AHA guideline

on the primary prevention of cardiovascular disease: a report of the American College of Cardiology/ American Heart Association Task Force on clinical practice guidelines. Circulation. 2019;140:e596–646. https://doi.org/10.1161/CIR.0000000000000678.
7. Frasure-Smith N, Lespérance F, Talajic M. Depression following myocardial infarction. Impact on 6-month survival. JAMA. 1993;270:1819–25.
8. Lichtman JH, Froelicher ES, Blumenthal JA, Carney RM, Doering LV, Frasure-Smith N, Freedland KE, Jaffe AS, Leifheit-Limson EC, Sheps DS, Vaccarino V, Wulsin L, American Heart Association Statistics Committee of the Council on Epidemiology and Prevention and the Council on Cardiovascular and Stroke Nursing. Depression as a risk factor for poor prognosis among patients with acute coronary syndrome: systematic review and recommendations: a scientific statement from the American Heart Association. Circulation. 2014;129:1350–69.
9. Vaccarino V, Bremner JD. Behavioral, emotional and neurobiological determinants of coronary heart disease risk in women. Neurosci Biobehav Rev. 2017;74:297–309.
10. Carney RM, Freedland KE. Depression and coronary heart disease. Nat Rev Cardiol. 2017;14:145–55.
11. Gan Y, Gong Y, Tong X, Sun H, Cong Y, Dong X, Wang Y, Xu X, Yin X, Deng J, Li L, Cao S, Lu Z. Depression and the risk of coronary heart disease: a metaanalysis of prospective cohort studies. BMC Psychiatry. 2014;14:371.
12. Lichtman JH, Froelicher ES, Blumenthal JA, Carney RM, Doering LV, Frasure-Smith N, Freedland KE, Jaffe AS, Leifheit-Limson EC, Sheps DS, Vaccarino V, Wulsin L. Depression as a risk factor for poor prognosis among patients with acute coronary syndrome: systematic review and recommendations. A scientific statement from the American Heart Association. Circulation. 2014;129:1350–69.
13. Lane D, Carroll D, Ring C, Beevers DG, Lip GY. Effects of depression and anxiety on mortality and quality-of-life 4 months after myocardial infarction. J Psychosom Res. 2000;49:229–38.
14. Müller-Tasch T, Peters-Klimm F, Schellberg D, Holzapfel N, Barth A, Junger J, Szecsenyi J, Herzog W. Depression is a major determinant of quality of life in patients with chronic systolic heart failure in general practice. J Card Fail. 2007;13:818–24.
15. Dickens CM, McGowan L, Percival C, Tomenson B, Cotter L, Heagerty A, Creed FH. Contribution of depression and anxiety to impaired health-related quality of life following first myocardial infarction. Br J Psychiatry. 2006;189:367–72.
16. Parashar S, Rumsfeld JS, Spertus JA, Reid KJ, Wenger NK, Krumholz HM, Amin A, Weintraub WS, Lichtman J, Dawood N, Vaccarino V. Time course of depression and outcome of myocardial infarction. Arch Intern Med. 2006;166:2035–43.
17. Hayek SS, Ko YA, Awad M, Del Mar SA, Ahmed H, Patel K, Yuan M, Maddox S, Gray B, Hajjari J, Sperling L, Shah A, Vaccarino V, Quyyumi AA. Depression and chest pain in patients with coronary artery disease. Int J Cardiol. 2017;230:420–6.
18. Lampert R, Jamner L, Burg M, Dziura J, Brandt C, Liu H, Li F, Donovan T, Soufer R. Triggering of symptomatic atrial fibrillation by negative emotion. J Am Coll Cardiol. 2014;64:1533–4.
19. Lange HW, Herrmann-Lingen C. Depressive symptoms predict recurrence of atrial fibrillation after cardioversion. J Psychosom Res. 2007;63:509–13.
20. Fergusson DM, Goodwin RD, Horwood LJ. Major depression and cigarette smoking: results of a 21-year longitudinal study. Psychol Med. 2003;33:1357–67.
21. Anda RF, Williamson DF, Escobedo LG, Mast EE, Giovino GA, Remington PL. Depression and the dynamics of smoking. A national perspective. JAMA. 1990;264:1541–5.
22. Levola J, Holopainen A, Aalto M. Depression and heavy drinking occasions: a cross-sectional general population study. Addict Behav. 2011;36:375–80.
23. Bruch H. Psychological aspects of overeating and obesity. Psychosomatics. 1964;5:269–74.
24. Kawakami N, Takatsuka N, Shimizu H, Ishibashi H. Depressive symptoms and occurrence of type 2 diabetes among Japanese men. Diabetes Care. 1999;22:1071–6.
25. Batelaan NM, et al. Anxiety and new onset of cardiovascular disease: critical review and meta-analysis. Br J Psychiatry. 2016;208:223–31. https://doi.org/10.1192/bjp.bp.114.156554.
26. Emdin CA, Odutayo A, Wong CX, Tran J, Hsiao AJ, Hunn BH. Meta-analysis of anxiety as a risk factor for cardiovascular disease. Am J Cardiol. 2016 Aug 15;118(4):511–9. https://doi.org/10.1016/j.amjcard.2016.05.041.
27. Chida Y, Steptoe A. The association of anger and hostility with future coronary heart disease. A meta-analytic review of prospective evidence. J Am Coll Cardiol. 2009;53(11):936. https://doi.org/10.1016/j.jacc.2008.11.044.
28. Mostofsky E. Elizabeth Anne Penner, and Murray A. Mittleman. Outbursts of anger as a trigger of acute cardiovascular events: a systematic review and meta-analysis. Eur Heart J. 2014;35:1404–10. https://doi.org/10.1093/eurheartj/ehu033.
29. Kupper N, Denollet J. Type D personality as a risk factor in coronary heart disease: a review of current evidence. Curr Cardiol Rep. 2018;20:104. https://doi.org/10.1007/s11886-018-1048-x.
30. Steptoe A, Kivimäki M. Stress and cardiovascular disease: an update on current knowledge. Annu Rev Public Health. 2013;34:337–54.
31. Dar T, Radfar A, Abohashem S, Pitman RK, Tawakol A, Osborne MT. Psychosocial stress and cardiovascular disease. Curr Treat Options Cardiovasc Med. 2019 Apr 26;21(5):23. https://doi.org/10.1007/s11936-019-0724-5.
32. Strand LB, Tsai MK, Gunnell D, Janszky I, Wen CP, Chang SS. Self-reported sleep duration and coronary heart disease mortality: a large cohort study of 400,000 Taiwanese adults. Int J Cardiol.

2016 Mar 15;207:246–51. https://doi.org/10.1016/j.ijcard.2016.01.044.
33. Lao XQ, Liu X, Deng HB, Chan TC, Ho KF, Wang F, Vermeulen R, Tam T, Wong MC, Tse LA, Chang LY, Yeoh EK. Sleep quality, sleep duration, and the risk of coronary heart disease: a prospective cohort study with 60,586 adults. J Clin Sleep Med. 2018;14(1):109–17.
34. Correll CU, Solmi M, Veronese N, et al. Prevalence, incidence and mortality from cardiovascular disease in patients with pooled and specific severe mental illness: a large-scale meta-analysis of 3,211,768 patients and 113,383,368 controls. World Psychiatry. 2017;16(2):163–80.
35. Sin NL. The protective role of positive Well-being in cardiovascular disease: review of current evidence, mechanisms, and clinical implications. Curr Cardiol Rep. 2016 November;18(11):106. https://doi.org/10.1007/s11886-016-0792-z.
36. Cohen R, Bavishi C, Rozanski A. Purpose in life and its relationship to all-cause mortality and cardiovascular events: a meta-analysis. Psychosom Med. 2016 Feb–Mar;78(2):122–33. https://doi.org/10.1097/PSY.0000000000000274.
37. Alan Rozanski MD, Chirag Bavishi MD, Kubzansky LD, Cohen R. Association of optimism with cardiovascular events and all-cause mortality. A systematic review and meta-analysis. JAMA Network Open. 2019;2(9):e1912200. https://doi.org/10.1001/jamanetworkopen.2019.12200.
38. Boehm JK, Kubzansky LD. The heart's content: The association between positive psychological well-being and cardiovascular health. Psychol Bull. July 2012;138(4):655–91.
39. Younus A, Aneni EC, Spatz ES, Osondu CU, Roberson L, Ogunmoroti O, Malik R, Ali SS, Aziz M, Feldman T, Virani SS, Maziak W, Agatston AS, Veledar E, Nasir K. A systematic review of the prevalence and outcomes of ideal cardiovascular health in US and non-US populations. Mayo Clin Proc. 2016;91(5):649–70.
40. Liu K, Daviglus ML, Loria CM, Colangelo LA, Spring B, Moller AC, Lloyd-Jones DM. Healthy lifestyle through young adulthood and the presence of low cardiovascular disease risk profile in middle age: the coronary artery risk development in (young) adults (CARDIA) study. Circulation. 2012;125:996–1004.
41. Natelson BH. Neurocardiology: an interdisciplinary area for the 80s. Arch Neurol. 1985;42(2):178–84.
42. Penninx BW. Depression and cardiovascular disease: epidemiological evidence on their linking mechanisms. Neurosci Biobehav Rev. 2017;74:277–86.
43. Grassi G, Seravalle G, Quarti-Trevano F. The 'neuroadrenergic hypothesis' in hypertension: current evidence. Exp Physiol. 2010 May;95(5):581–6. https://doi.org/10.1113/expphysiol.2009.047381.
44. Nunan D, Sandercock GRH, Brodie DA. A quantitative systematic review of Normal values for short-term heart rate variability in healthy adults. Pacing Clin Electrophysiol. 2010;33(11):1407–17.
45. Dekker JM, Crow RS, Folsom AR, Hannan PJ, Liao D, Swenne CA, Schouten EG. Low heart rate variability in a 2-minute rhythm strip predicts risk of coronary heart disease and mortality from several causes: the ARIC study. Atherosclerosis risk in communities. Circulation. 2000;102:1239–44.
46. Huikuri HV, Stein PK. Clinical application of heart rate variability after acute myocardial infarction. Front Physiol. 2012;3:41. https://doi.org/10.3389/fphys.2012.00041.
47. Shen MJ, Zipes DP. Role of the autonomic nervous system in modulation cardiac arrhythmias. Circ Res. 2014;114:1004–21. https://doi.org/10.1161/CIRCRESAHA.113.302549.
48. Kop W, Krantz D, Nearing B, Gottdiener J, Quigley J, O'Callahan M. Effects of acute mental stress and exercise on T-wave altemans in patients with implantable cardioverter defibrillators and controls. Circulation. 2004;109:1864–9. https://doi.org/10.1161/01.CIR.0000124726.72615.60.
49. Zou R, Shi W, Tao J, Li H, Lin X, Yang S, et al. Neurocardiology: cardiovascular changes and specific brain region infarcts. Bio Med Res Int. 2017;2017:5646348. https://doi.org/10.1155/2017/5646348.
50. Tawakol A, Ishai A, Takx RA, Figueroa AL, Ali A, Kaiser Y, Truong QA, Solomon CJ, Calcagno C, Mani V, Tang CY, Mulder WJ, Murrough JW, Hoffmann U, Nahrendorf M, Shin LM, Fayad ZA, Pitman RK. Relation between resting amygdalar activity and cardiovascular events: a longitudinal and cohort study. Lancet. 2017;389:834–45.
51. Ishai A, Osborne MT, Tung B, Wang Y, Hammad B, Patrich T, Oberfeld B, Fayad ZA, Giles JT, Lo J, Shin LM, Grinspoon SK, Koenen KC, Pitman RK, Tawakol A. Amygdalar metabolic activity independently associates with progression of visceral adiposity. J Clin Endocrinol Metab. 2019 Apr 1;104(4):1029–38. https://doi.org/10.1210/jc.2018-01456.
52. Bremner JD, Campanella C, Khan Z, Shah M, Hammadah M, Wilmot K, Al Mheid I, Lima BB, Garcia EV, Nye J, Ward L, Kutner MH, Raggi P, Pearce BD, Shah AJ, Quyyumi AA, Vaccarino V. Brain correlates of mental stress-induced myocardial ischemia. Psychosom Med. 2018;80:515–25.
53. Oppenheimer S, Cechetto D. The insular cortex and the regulation of cardiac function. Compr Physiol. 2016;6(2):1081–133.
54. Reynolds RM, Labad J, Strachan MWJ, Braun A, Fowkes FGR, Lee AJ, et al. Elevated fasting plasma cortisol is associated with ischemic heart disease and its risk factors in people with type2 diabetes: the Edinburgh type 2 diabetes study. J Clin Endocrinol Metab. 2010;2010:1602–8. https://doi.org/10.1210/jc.2009-2112.
55. Vogelzangs N, Beekman ATF, Milaneschi Y, Bandinelli S, Ferrucci L, Penninx BWJ. Urinary cortisol and six-year risk of all-cause and cardiovascular mortality. J Clin Endocrinol Metab. 2010;95:4959–64. https://doi.org/10.1210/jc.2010-0192.
56. Mason JC, Libby P. Cardiovascular disease in patients with chronic inflammation: mechanisms underlying

premature cardiovascular events in rheumatologic conditions. Eur Heart J. 2015;36:482–9.
57. Sherwood A, Hinderliter AL, Watkins LL, Waugh RA, Blumenthal JA. Impaired endothelial function in coronary heart disease patients with depressive symptomatology. J Am Coll Cardiol. 2005;46:656–9.
58. Laghrissi-Thode F, Wagner WR, Pollock BG, Johnson PC, Finkel MS. Elevated platelet factor 4 and beta-thromboglobulin plasma levels in depressed patients with ischemic heart disease. Biol Psychiatry. 1997;42:290–5.
59. Amadio P, Colombo GI, Tarantino E, Gianellini S, Ieraci A, Brioschi M, Banfi C, Werba JP, Parolari A, Lee FS, Tremoli E, Barbieri SS. BDNFVal66met polymorphism: a potential bridge between depression and thrombosis. Eur Heart J. 2017;38:1426–35.
60. Su S, Lampert R, Lee F, Bremner JD, Snieder H, Jones L, Murrah NV, Goldberg J, Vaccarino V. Common genes contribute to depressive symptoms and heart rate variability: the Twins Heart Study. Twin Res Hum Genet. 2010;13:1–9.
61. Srihari Sharma KN, Choudhary NR, Subramanya P. Evidence base of yoga studies on cardiovascular health: a bibliometric analysis. Int J Yoga. 2019;12:162–71.
62. Naveen GH, Varambally S, Thirthalli J, Rao M, Christopher R, Gangadhar BN. Serum cortisol and BDNF in patients with major depression-effect of yoga. Int Rev Psychiatry. 2016 Jun;28(3):273–8. https://doi.org/10.1080/09540261.2016.1175419.
63. Streeter C, Gerbarg PL, Nielsen GH, Brown RP, Jensen JE, Silveri M. Effects of yoga on thalamic gamma-aminobutyric acid, mood and depression: analysis of two randomized controlled trials. Neuropsychiatry (London). 2018;8(6):1923–39.
64. Gotink RA, Vernooij MW, Ikram MA, Niessen WJ, Krestin GP, Hofman A, Tiemeier H, Myriam Hunink MG. Meditation and yoga practice are associated with smaller right amygdala volume: the Rotterdam study. Brain Imaging Behav. 2018;12:1631–9. https://doi.org/10.1007/s11682-018-9826-z.
65. Khattab K, Khattab AA, Ortak J, Richardt G, Bonnemeier H. Iyengar yoga increases cardiac parasympathetic nervous modulation among healthy yoga practitioners. Evid Based Complement Alternat Med. 2007;4(4):511–7.
66. Phadke L, Phadke S, Boegle R, Bhavsar SN, Dandare KM, Patki N. Differential modulation of sympathetic and parasympathetic influences during different yoga asanas: understanding the ‘process’. Int J Basic Appl Physiol. 2012;1(1):271.
67. Tajane K, Pitale R, Phadke LS, Joshi A, Umale J. Characteristics of HRV patterns for different yoga postures. 2014 Annual IEEE India Conference (INDICON). 2014; https://doi.org/10.1109/INDICON.2014.7030672.
68. I-Hua Chu, Wen-Lan Wu, I-Mei Lin, Yu-Kai Chang, Yuh-Jen Lin, , and Pin-Chen Yang. Effects of yoga on heart rate variability and depressive symptoms in women: a randomized controlled trial. J Altern Complement Med 23(4): 310. (2017) https://doi.org/10.1089/acm.2016.0135
69. Borovikova LV, Ivanova S, Zhang M, Yang H, Botchkina GI, Watkins LR, et al. Vagus nerve stimulation attenuates the systemic inflammatory’ response to endotoxin. Nature. 2000;405:458–62. https://doi.org/10.1038/35013070.
70. Villemure C, Ceko M, Cotton VA, Bushnell MC. Neuroprotective effects of yoga practice: age-, experience-, and frequency-dependent plasticity. Front Hum Neurosci. 2015;9:281. https://doi.org/10.3389/fnhum.2015.00281.
71. Knobben S. A meta-analysis of the effectiveness of yoga on mental health; taking on a dual perspective reflecting the medical and positive perspective of mental health. Thesis of Master of Science in Psychology. University of Twente, Netherlands. 2013.
72. Psychosis and Schizophrenia in Adults. The NICE guideline on treatment and management. Updated Edition 2014. National Collaborating Centre for Mental Health.
73. Chu P, Gotink RA, Yeh GY, Goldie SJ, Hunink MGM. The effectiveness of yoga in modifying risk factors for cardiovascular disease and metabolic syndrome: a systematic review and meta-analysis of randomized controlled trials. Eur J Prev Cardiol. 2016;23(3):291–307. https://doi.org/10.1177/2047487314562741.
74. Cramer H, Haller H, Steckhan N, Michalsen A, Dobos G. Effects of yoga on cardiovascular disease risk factors: a systematic review and meta-analysis. Int J Cardiol. 2014;173(2):170–83.
75. Dorairaj Prabhakaran DM, et al. Effectiveness of a Yoga based cardiac rehabilitation (Yoga CaRe) program: a multi-center randomised controlled trial of patients with acute myocardial infarction from India. AHA 2018.
76. Hartley L, Dyakova M, Holmes J, Clarke A, Lee MS, Ernst E, Rees K. Yoga for the primary prevention of cardiovascular disease. Cochrane Database Syst Rev. 2014;5:CD010072.

Part III

Imaging and Laboratory Techniques

12 Next-Generation Techniques for Validating Yoga Effect on the Cardiovascular System

Kochhar Kanwal Preet, Yadav Raj Kumar, Sunil, and Shweta Sharma

12.1 Introduction

Yoga, an ancient discipline is a holistic intervention between mind and body aimed at physical, mental, emotional, and spiritual well-being. The following chapter gives an overview of the next-generation techniques for the scientific validation of yoga.

12.1.1 Types of Yoga

- *Restorative:* soothing and relaxing, a nap on the couch with as few as five poses in one class. This is ideal for injury or stress rehab.
- *Ananda Yoga:* Proper alignment, stretching, and controlled breathing are used to promote the flexibility needed to sit in the Lotus position.
- *Power Yoga:* These asanas include non-traditional yoga poses like push-ups and handstands without pause. This produces sweat and builds power, endurance, and flexibility which give more aerobic benefits instead of any other style of Yoga.

12.1.2 Benefits of Yoga

- Relaxes the body and helps to improve musculoskeletal fitness.
- It combines breathing techniques with poses that reduce stress:
- Promotes flexibility, blood flow, and mental focus.
- It enhances mental flexibility, information recall (Table 12.1)

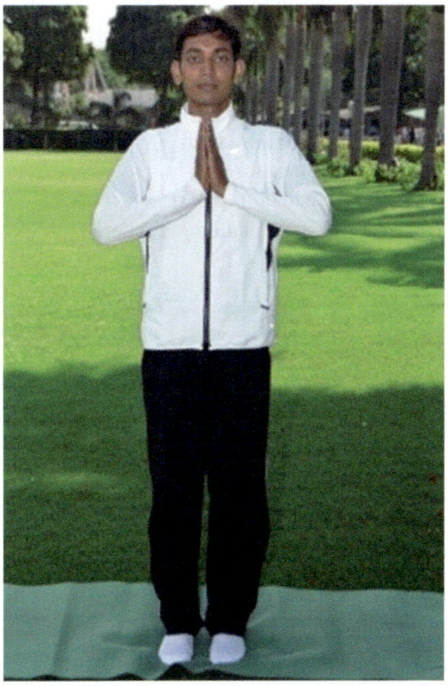

Department of Physiology, AIIMS

K. K. Preet (✉) · Y. Raj Kumar · Sunil · S. Sharma
Department of Physiology, All India Institute of Medical Sciences, New Delhi, India

I. Basu-Ray, D. Mehta (eds.), *The Principles and Practice of Yoga in Cardiovascular Medicine*,
https://doi.org/10.1007/978-981-16-6913-2_12

Table 12.1 Various breathing techniques in yoga with their physiological effects

Type of breathing practice	Manoeuvre	Known principle physiological effects
Slow breathing techniques		
Anulom-Vilom (Alternate breathing)	Inhalation with left then exhale with right nostril and continue	Cardiovascular and autonomic effects
Right nostril breathing	Breathing with right nostril while left nostril is closed	Excitatory effect, increased metabolism
Left Nostril Breathing	Breathing with left nostril while right nostril is closed	Relaxing effect, decreased metabolism, activates brain
Slow Bhastrika	Slow and deep exhalation, use both nostrils	Autonomic effects
Fast breathing techniques		
Kapalbhati	Fast and forceful exhalation followed by passive inhalation (use both nostrils)	Increased circulation to brain, cognitive excitation, respiratory effects
Bhramari	Exhalation with humming sound (use both nostrils)	Increased circulation to brain, cognitive excitation
Shitali	Inhalation through mouth with folded tongue (use both nostrils for exhalation)	Respiratory effects
Bhastrika (Fast & Mukha)	Fast exhalation	Altered circulation to brain, cognitive excitation, respiratory effects

12.1.3 Yoga and Cardiovascular Diseases

Exercise of high levels has been found to play a major role in preventing obesity, diabetes, and cardiovascular diseases. Evidence suggests that regular practice of yoga and meditation leads to an improvement in cardiovascular metabolic status [1, 2] and lipid peroxidation. In an Indian study, retardation of coronary atherosclerosis was evaluated by adopting a yoga-based lifestyle. The group practicing yoga showed a significant reduction in the number of angina episodes per week with improved exercise capacity and a decrease in body weight. The yoga group also showed a greater reduction in serum total cholesterol, LDL cholesterol, and triglyceride levels as compared to the control group [3]. Even the intervention of short-term yoga-based comprehensive lifestyle led to a significant reduction in body mass index (BMI), blood pressure (BP), and blood glucose [4, 5]. A recent study also suggested that psychological well-being, improved nutrition behaviors, and weight loss may foster by adopting a yoga-based, residential weight loss program [6, 7].

Another study showed that yoga postures such as *suryanamaskar* resulted in improved cardiorespiratory fitness [8]. In a previous study in young hypertensive and pre-hypertensive patients, it was observed that there was a significant reduction in BP (SBP/DBP: 2.0/2.6 mm Hg) following yoga [9]. Overall, yoga can modulate the progression of the inflammation of blood vessels at various steps of pathogenesis, thus counteracting the progression of CVD. Furthermore, yoga has been found to be beneficial when included in primary and secondary prevention strategies [10], as physical activity (exercises) has been found to have favorable effects not only on CVD risk factors but also on symptoms of CVD, functional capacity, and physiology of the person and the quality of life [11–13].

12.1.4 Mindfulness-Based Stress Reduction

Meditation is a physiological state of reduced metabolic activity and it is different from sleep which reduces physical and mental relaxation enhancing psychological and physiological balance and emotional stability. Mindfulness-based stress reduction (MBSR) is a type of meditation wherein breath is used as an object of awareness. Meditation has been reported to improve quality of life in patients suffering from diabetes mellitus, cardiovascular diseases, and other chronic conditions [14, 15].

12.1.5 Obesity and Yoga

Obesity is the one of biggest health challenges of the twenty-first century, not only because of its high prevalence among developed and developing countries but the large number of diseases for which obesity is the independent risk factor as well. Almost all systems of the body are affected by obesity and the main factors responsible for obesity are sedentary lifestyle, decreased physical activity, and unhealthy lifestyle including consumption of high energy-dense food, empty calories, high fat, high salt, and high sugar. Though the genetic mutations have been reported as a monogenic cause of obesity, it is now well known that obesity is basically polygenic in origin, in which environmental factors play a very important role. Among environmental factors, visual cues are one of the important environmental factors which are present everywhere and could affect feeding behavior. "High attention-grabbing property" of High energy-dense fatty foods gives more hedonic value to fatty foods in leading to hyperphagia and weight gain. Food-related visual cues are universally present everywhere which affects feeding behavior. Castellanos et al. (2009) have shown high energy-dense food images affects the visual attention bias in obese individuals so any intervention that can reduce attention bias toward food in obese subjects can play an important role in weight reduction program [16]. Both short-term and long-term Yoga-based lifestyle intervention has been shown by many studies as effective measures to reduce significant weight in overweight/obese individuals.

12.1.6 "Transitions in Modern Nutrition Practices: Paradigms Lost and Regained"

In virtually all populations, consumption of higher fat diets and decreased physical activity has been accompanied by the benefits of modernization. These changes in the pattern of diet and physical activity levels, combined with increasing longevity, have resulted in dramatic increases in the prevalence of type 2 diabetes mellitus in both developed and underdeveloped countries. However, the prevalence of various degrees of glucose intolerance like type 2 diabetes mellitus, impaired glucose tolerance (IGT), and impaired fasting glucose (IFG), varies considerably between populations.

12.1.7 The Obesity Epidemic

Lifestyle diseases including diabetes, hypertension, hyperlipidemia, obesity, and autonomic instability are the new pandemic of a modern lifestyle. Obesity is a global health problem, usually associated with an erratic lifestyle with a risk factor for many chronic diseases and also has serious implications for health-related quality of life (HRQOL). HRQOL is a cumulative outcome of poor health and has adverse social and emotional effects. Obesity has a commutative effect on poor HRQOL if it coexists with chronic diseases, compromised work life, and poor self-image. Therefore, it is useful to develop and promote a lifestyle intervention program that is not only effective in a short duration but also cost-effective and has good adherence as long-term lifestyle interventions have a poor adherence due to delayed benefits and high costs.

In the fight against diabetes and obesity, a much-improved knowledge about the pathophysiological and neurobehavioral mechanisms underlying these diseases is needed not only to prevent risky behaviors and to diagnose and treat the patients but also to develop new therapies which are safer and adjustable to each patient. As noted by Schmidt and Campbell (2013), [17, 18], treatment of eating disorders cannot remain "brainless," and the same principle applies to obesity when we consider the growing amount of literature highlighting the behavioral and brain changes/plasticity induced by obesity [19], effective bariatric surgery [20, 21], and neuromodulatory interventions [18, 22, 23] in animal models and human subjects.

12.1.8 Biochemical Studies as Tools for Assessment of Yoga and Meditation

Various studies pertaining to the analysis of biochemical markers for the effects of yoga and meditation have been carried out in the Integrated Health Clinic, AIIMS.

In a 2012 intervention study by Yadav et al. [24] with a cohort size of 86, improvement in the level of endorphins and cortisol and consequently a reduced level of stress was observed after the intervention of yoga-based lifestyle for 2 weeks. Similarly, Sarvottam et al. (2012) [5] showed a reduction in vascular inflammation through a significant improvement in parameters such as body weight, BMI, LDL, adiponectin, and IL-6 levels as a consequence of yoga-based lifestyle intervention. By keeping a track of the biochemical markers such as TC, LDL/HDL ratio, TG, FBS, IL-6, insulin, and insulin resistance (HOMA), well-marked change in diabetic risk factors was shown by Netam et al. (2015) [25] (Table 12.2).

12.1.9 Neuroimaging as Tool for Assessment of Effects of Yoga and Meditation

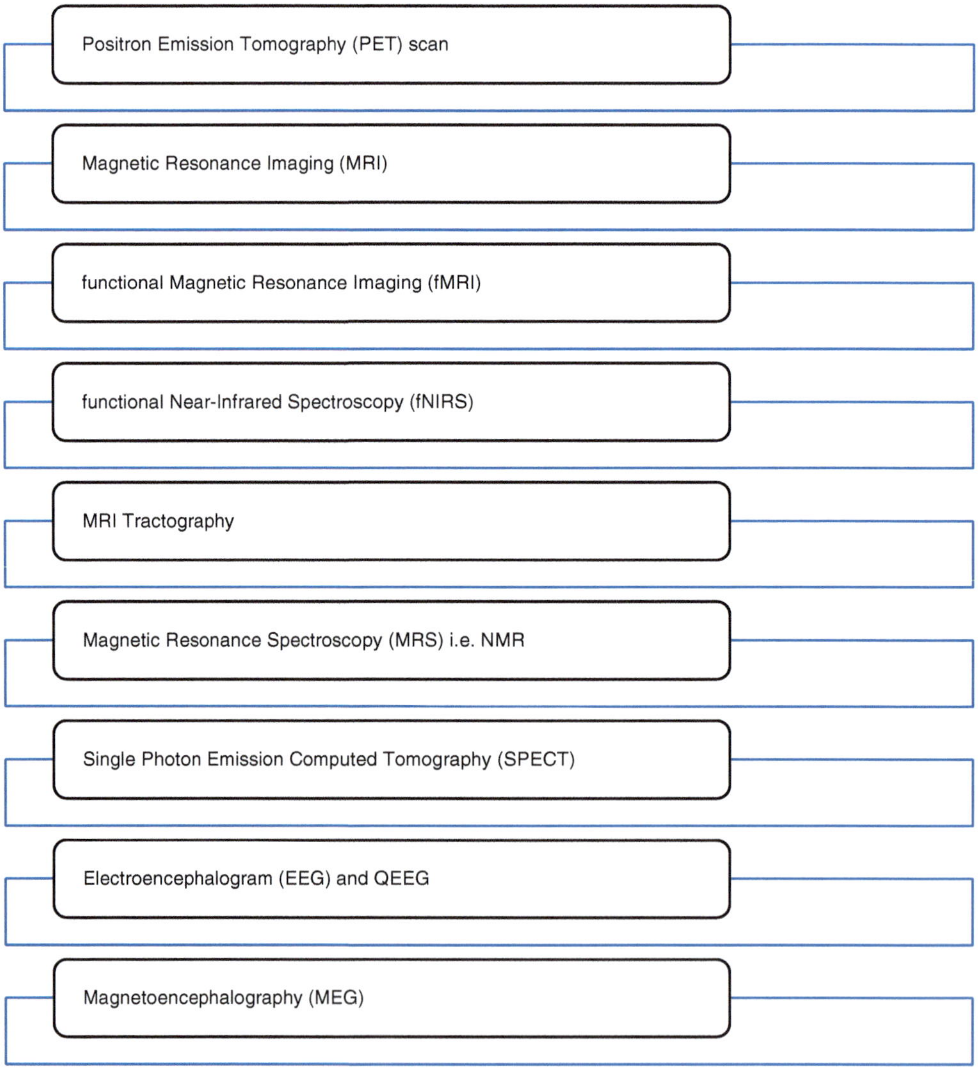

Table 12.2 Biochemical studies as tools for assessment of yoga and meditation

Author and study design	Material and methods	Result	Conclusion
Netam et al. (2015) Interventional study $n = 30$ overweight/ obsessed subjects [25]	Effect of 10 days yoga intervention on body weight, TC, LDL/HDL ratio, TG, FBS, *IL-6*, insulin, and insulin resistance (HOMA)	Significant change in diabetic risk factors	Short-term yoga-based lifestyle intervention reduces diabetic risk factors in overweight-obese subjects
Yadav et al. (2012) Interventional study $n = 86$ [24]	*Serum cortisol* and *endorphin* intervention: 2 week	Improvement in level of endorphin and cortisol after intervention	Yoga-based lifestyle intervention reduces stress
Sarvottam et al. (2012) Interventional study $n = 30$ [5]	Antropometic, lipid profile, FBS, *IL-6, adiponectin* & endothelin	Significant improvement in the parameter body weight, BMI, LDL, adiponectin & IL-6 levels.	Yoga-based lifestyle intervention can reduce vascular inflammation.

Cohen et al. (2009) used a PET scan to study cerebral blood flow before and after Yoga intervention and observed a significant increase in blood flow in different areas of frontal lobe after meditation [26].

Improvement in various cognitive functions by yoga, using EEG analysis, was reported by Magan et al., and Nagendra et al., through a comparison in the brain activity of long-term and short-term yoga groups; and yoga and non-yoga groups, respectively [24, 27].

The effects of yoga and meditation have also been analyzed by MRI in order to conclude improved emotional awareness response, increased gray matter concentration, and significantly lower pain sensitivity [28].

Another neuroimaging technique, fMRI, has been used widely to assess the activation of various areas of the brain after yogic and meditative interventions [29, 30] (Table 12.3).

12.1.10 Bereitschaftspotential as Tool for Assessment of Meditation

Bereitschaftspotential or Readiness potential/ Movement related cortical potentials couples EMG recording with motor cortex EEG. It is used to test motor planning, executive functions and also to test freewill induced movements vs movements in relation to sensory outputs, pre and post to intervention of meditation and yogic exercises.

12.1.11 Modern Methodologies and Techniques for Validating Benefits of Yoga and Traditional Indian Practices

1. Eye-tracking (module developed in our lab)
2. Non-invasive neuroimaging by fNIRS is a technique with better temporal resolution than MRI to identify brain areas activated in response to a stimulus (developed and standardized in our lab).
3. Wireless physiological monitoring of variables like heart rate, respiratory rate, skin temperature, blood flow, muscle tone, and electrodermal activity to establish an autonomic profile. (Developed and standardized in our lab.)
4. Body Composition Analyses and segmental fat versus lean body mass composition by Dexa/impedance analysis.

Table 12.3 Neuroimaging tools for assessment of yoga and meditation

Author & study design	Material & methods	Result	Conclusion
Magan et al. (2012) Interventional study $n = 34$ [24]	Comparing brain electrical activity among long-term and short-term meditators using EEG analysis	Long-term meditators involve larger and wider activation of brain areas	There is improvement in various cognitive functions by Yoga
Nagendra et al. (2015) Interventional study $n = 30$ [27]	EEG analysis in Yoga group and non-yoga group Intervention 5 months	Increase in $\alpha, \beta, and\ \delta$ EEG band powers significant reduction in θ and γ band powers.	
Cohen et al. (2009) Interventional study $n = 4$ [26]	PET scan for cerebral blood flow before and after yoga intervention.	Significantly increased blood flow in different areas of frontal lobe.	Brain experiences a "training effect" after meditation.
Holzel et al. Interventional study $n = 17$ [28]	Mindfulness-based stress reduction (MBSR) for 8 weeks	Gray matter concentration analyses by anatomical magnetic resonance imaging (MRI)	Increase gray matter concentration in posterior cingulated cortex, the temporal-parietal junction. Improves awareness emotional responding in meditators
Telles et al. $n = 26$ [29]	Random thinking, Non-meditative focused thinking, Meditative focusing, and effortless meditation or pure meditation	Functional magnetic resonance imaging (fMRI) Significant activation in the right middle temporal cortex, right inferior frontal cortex and left lateral orbital gyrus in meditators alone.	Activation of these Ares suggest that meditation is associated with sustained attention, memory, semantic Cognition & creativity.
Engstro et al. $n = 19$ [30]	On-off block-design: meditate(on) and Word (off) Each block for 2 min and a total of 8 blocks	Functional magnetic resonance imaging (fMRI) shows significant activation in the bilateral hippocampus	Hippocampus activity during meditation may be involved in memory consolidation

12.1.12 Functional Near-Infrared Spectroscopy (fNIRS)

fNIRS is an optical brain monitoring technology that is portable, safe, affordable, non-invasive and monitors changes in hemodynamic response within the cortex. It is based on the modified Beer–Lambert Law. It measures any change in the relative ratios of deoxygenated and oxygenated hemoglobin. The Optical window of this device is 700–900 nm [31].

The technique consists of fNIRS headband which is Flexible sensor pad with light sources and photodetectors (fixed source-detector separation of 2.5 cm) this configuration generates a total of 16 measurement locations (voxels) per wavelength as well as fNIRS system. The signals from the fNIRS sensor are sent to a Data Acquisition computer and via this, the fNIRS data is sent to the Protocol Computer where the signals are integrated (Fig. 12.1).

Unlike the other neuroimaging techniques, such as PET and fMRI, fNIRS neither require subjects to be in a supine position nor it strictly restricts the head movements, thus allowing to adopt a wide range of experimental tasks suitable for properly investigating eating disorders and food intake/stimuli. In addition, fNIRS uses a relatively low-cost instrumentation (with a sampling time in the order of the milliseconds and a spatial resolution of up to about 1 cm). On the other hand, although EEG is a useful electrophysiological technique, it has a very low spatial resolution making it difficult to precisely identify the activated areas of the brain.

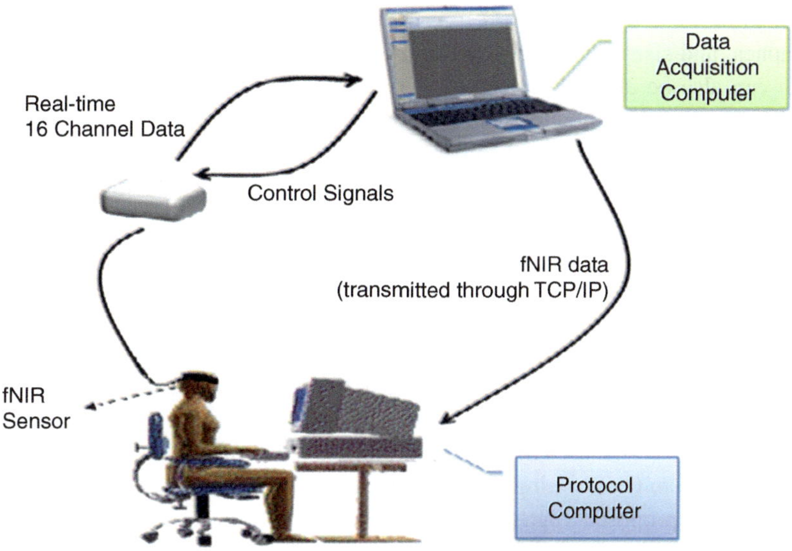

Fig. 12.1 fNIR system

fNIRS is a non-invasive vascular-based neuro-imaging technology that measures concentration changes of oxygenated-hemoglobin (O_2Hb) and deoxygenated-hemoglobin (HHb) in cortical microcirculation blood vessels. fNIRS relies on neurovascular coupling to infer changes in neural activity that is mirrored by changes in blood oxygenation in the region of the activated cortical area (i.e., the increase in O2Hb and the decrease in HHb). Unlike the BOLD signal of fMRI, which is gathered from the paramagnetic properties of HHb, the fNIRS signal is based on the changes in the intrinsic optical absorption of both HHb and O2Hb [32]. fNIRS systems vary in complexity from dual channels to "whole-head" arrays of several dozen channels. Data processing/analysis methods permit topographical assessment of real-time regional cortical hemodynamic changes.

fNIRS analysis is mainly done by time series method or time-domain method and it is virtually registered on brain surface to know the source of origin [31]. Bu et al. has shown a novel frequency domain approach for the analysis of fNIRS signal. Based on the previous studies, they divided the signal into five different frequency bands with known physiological significance [33]. These are:

(I) (0.6–2.0 Hz): Reflect the effects of cardiac activities
(II) (0.145–0.6 Hz): Reflect the effects of respiratory activities
(III) (0.052–0.145 Hz): Originate locally from intrinsic myogenic activity of smooth muscle cells in resistance vessels and this myogenic mechanism may be partly under autonomic control
(IV) (0.021–0.052 Hz): Closely regulated through tight neurovascular coupling and partial autonomic control
(V) (0.0095–0.021 Hz): Mainly the endothelial metabolic activity

It can be used to supplement the cognitive and behavioral assessment, inculcate advances in eliciting neurobiological and psychophysiological basis of psychiatry in general, and also to measure cortical oxygenation level [34].

12.1.13 Polysomnography as Tool for Assessment of Meditation

Polysomnography refers to a systematic process used to collect physiological parameters relevant to sleep. A polysomnogram (PSG) utilizes electroencephalogram (EEG), electrooculogram (EOG), electromyogram (EMG), electrocardiogram (ECG), and pulse oximetry, and airflow and respiratory effort, to evaluate for underlying causes of sleep disturbances. PSG is used for diagnosing sleep-related breathing disorders, which include obstructive sleep apnea (OSA), central sleep apnea, and sleep-related hypoventilation/hypoxia. It can also be utilized to evaluate for other sleep disorders, such as nocturnal seizures, narcolepsy, periodic limb movement disorder, and rapid eye movement sleep behavior disorder [35]. In the past decade, a number of observational studies have demonstrated an association between insomnia and incident cardiovascular disease morbidity and mortality, including hypertension, coronary heart disease, and heart failure [36]. A meta-analysis of cohort studies by Sofi et al. showed that 122,501 subjects free of baseline CVD disease with insomnia had a 45% increased risk of the development of or death from CVD during a 3- to 20-year follow-up [37]. A proposed yoga treatment and a follow-up with effects on sleeping cycles and parameters associated with sleep can be used to assess the risk of various cardiovascular diseases.

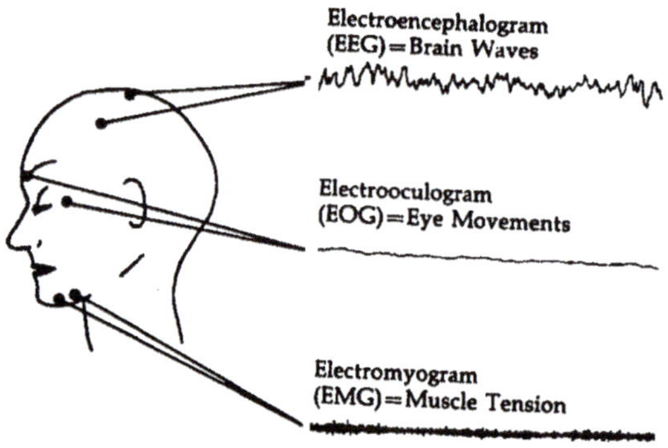

12.1.14 Eye Tracking as Tool for Assessment of Yoga

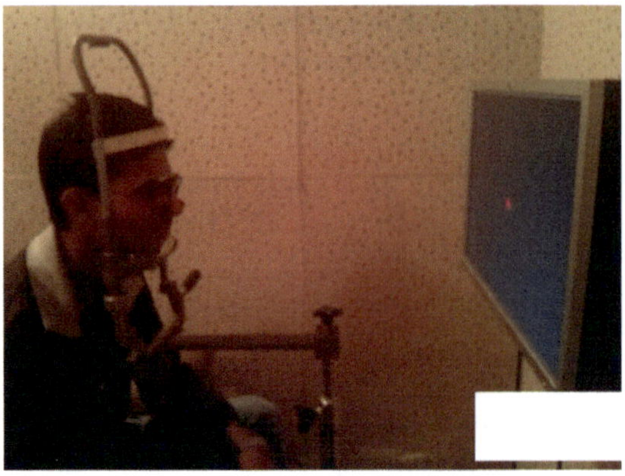

An eye tracker provides a complete eye movement evaluation environment including integrated stimulus presentation, simultaneous eye movement, and pupil diameter monitoring.

The ViewPointEyeTracker ® provides a basic and easy-to-use Data Analysis program. We can use this program to view and play back our data.

Each trail begins with a central fixation cross will for 1000 ms. Participant is instructed to fix his/her gaze on the fixation cross. The trial is followed by a pair of images, side by side, for 2000 ms. After the image pair, a visual probe, consisting of a pair of dots appears in the position of one of the preceding images. Although subjects would be aware that their eye movements are being tracked, they are instructed that their primary goal is to correctly identify the visual probe (Fig. 12.2).

12.1.15 Integrated Wireless Recording as a Tool for Assessment of Effects of Yoga

Some tests give the measure of sympathetic, some provide parasympathetic whereas some of them can be exploited for both as described below.

12.1.15.1 Deep Breathing Test (DBT)

Inspiration and expiration performed at a constant rate (one full cycle every 10 s) accentuate the normal respiratory sinus arrhythmia. Routine examination of this maneuver is performed at a rate of 6 breaths/min. The heart rate is continuously monitored and the difference between the maximum and minimum heart rate or the ratio of these two values is recorded. To quantify the test score the difference between maximal and minimal heart rate for each of the six cycles is determined and averaged to obtain the inspiratory–expiratory (I–E) difference in beats/min. This reflex is predominantly mediated by changes in parasympathetic (vagal) activity in humans. Both cardiac vagal inhibition and activation are tested.

1. Delta HR- difference between the maximal and minimal heart rate during inspiration and expiration, respectively, averaged for 6 cycles.

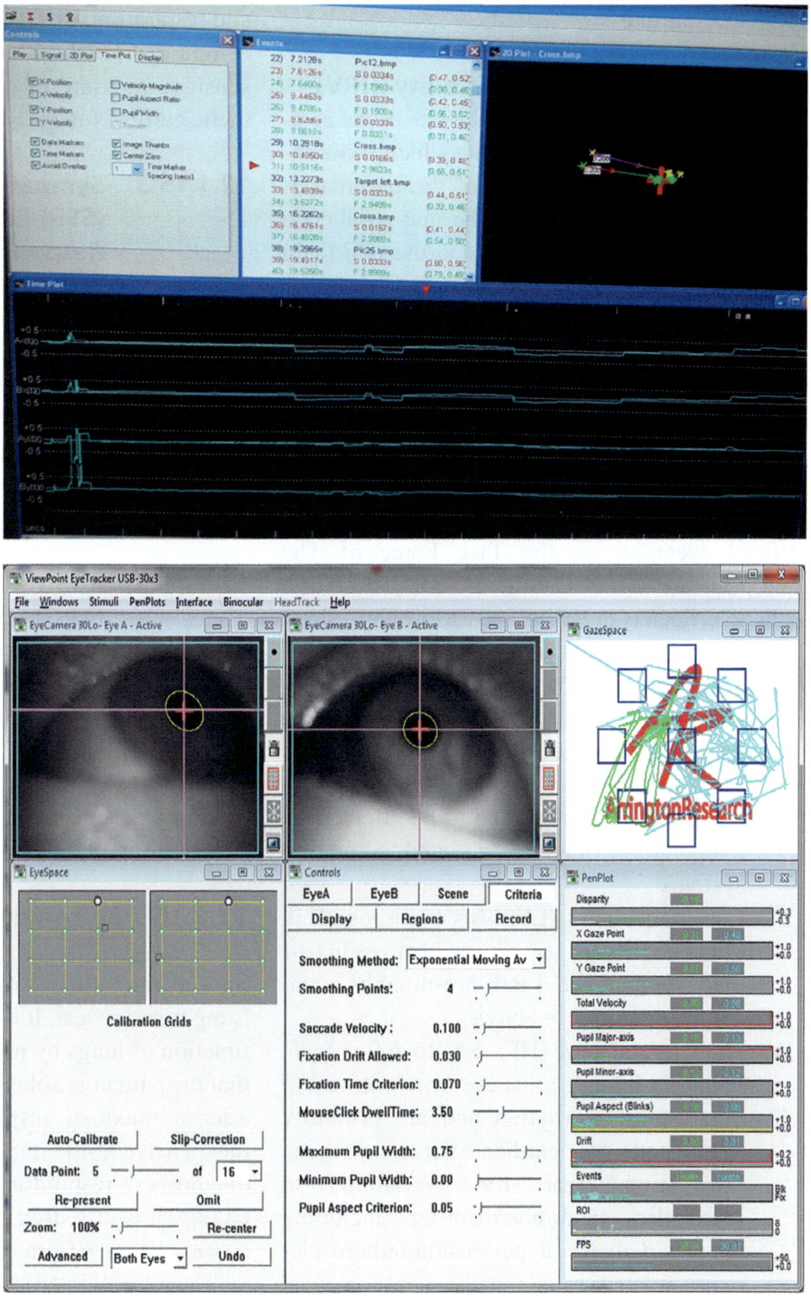

Fig. 12.2 Data Analyzing Windows

2. E:I ratio: ratio of the longest R–R interval and shortest R–R interval averaged over 6 cycles.

   Normal values:

   Delta HR –

- ≥15 bpm normal
- 11–14 bpm borderline
- ≤10 bpm abnormal

E: I ratio –

- $\geq$ 1.21 normal

12.1.15.2 Heart Rate Variability (HRV)

Heart rate variability (HRV) is the rate of the beat-to-beat variations of the heart rate which is dependent on the rate of discharge of the pacemaker, normally the sino-atrial node. The sino-atrial node in turn is influenced by activity in the two main divisions of autonomic nerves, which are controlled in a complex way by a variety of reflexes as well as by cortical factors [38]. There are three methods of HRV analysis (a) Time domain, (b) Frequency domain (c) Nonlinear Methods [39]. Frequency-domain method for this study has a consistent correlation between vagal or sympathetic activity. Frequency ranges are taken as defined according to the Task Force of The European Society of Cardiology and The North American Society of Pacing and Electrophysiology [39]. These frequencies are classified into:

(I) Ultra-low frequencies (ULF; >5-h cycle length) that include the circadian rhythm
(II) Very low frequencies (VLF; >25-s cycle length) that are supposed to be affected by temperature regulation and humoral systems
(III) Low frequencies (LF; >6-s cycle length in humans) that are sensitive to changes in cardiac sympathetic (and presumably parasympathetic) nerve activity
(IV) High frequencies (HF; 2.5- to 6.0-s cycle length in humans) that are synchronized to the respiratory rhythm and are primarily modulated by cardiac parasympathetic innervation. Heart Rate Variability in Metabolic syndrome/disorder including obesity, diabetes, hypertension, atherosclerosis, related to sympathovagal balance. Current research protocols are including neuromodulation, autonomic modulation and emotional and behavioral realignment.

Heart rate variability (HRV) can be used as a psychological and physiological stress indicator in the case of hypertension and other CVD and therefore can be used to monitor the impact of yoga. Research into heart rate variability (HRV) and respiration over the last century has led to the insight that HRV with deep breathing is a highly sensitive measure of cardiovagal or parasympathetic cardiac function [40].

12.1.15.3 Sympathetic Skin Response (SSR)/Electrodermal Response (EDA)/Galvanic Skin Response (GSR)

Sympathetic skin response (SSR) represents a potential generated in skin sweat glands; it originates by activation of the reflex arch with different kinds of stimuli. The potential of rapid habituation after repeated stimuli is formed by biphasic or triphasic slow wave activity with relatively stable latency and variable amplitude [41].

12.1.15.4 Photoplethysmography (PPG)

Photoplethysmography (PPG) is used to estimate the skin blood flow using infrared light. The PPG technology has been widely used for measuring oxygen saturation, cardiac output, blood pressure and assessing autonomic function, and also detecting peripheral vascular disease [42].

12.1.16 Spirometry

Spirometry is the most common and widely used Lung function test. It is a method of assessing the function of lungs by measuring the volume of air that the patient is able to expel out from the lungs after a maximal inspiration. This simple and inexpensive test is important in the detection and diagnosis of respiratory diseases like asthma and COPD. It is also used to differentiate obstructive airway diseases from restrictive diseases.

The general instructions given to subject are to sit straight, with his/her head erect, nose clip in place while holding the mouthpiece tightly between the lips. A number of dynamic and static lung volumes and capacities can be measured by spirometry. The main spirometry tests are Forced Vital Capacity (FVC) and Slow Vital Capacity (SVC). FVC is the volume of air exhaled by the subject as forcefully, as fast and completely as possible starting from full inspiration.

Predicted values are then calculated from age, size, weight, sex, and ethnic matched groups. The results of the test are then compared to the predicted values.

Main parameters which are measured are FEV1, FVC, and FEV1/FVC.

SVC is similar to FVC. It is the volume of air exhaled by the subject as slowly and maximally as possible starting from slow and maximal inspiration.

Once an acceptable test is performed it needs interpretation of flow–volume curves and volume–time graph.

12.1.17 Impulse Oscillometry

Impulse oscillometry is based on the forced oscillation technique (FOT) method which utilizes the application of external pressures to the respiratory system to measure respiratory impedance. Oscillating sound waves of single or multiple frequencies ranging between 5 and 35 Hz are generated by an external loudspeaker and delivered to the respiratory tract through the mouth. The impulses thus generated travel and superimposed upon the impulses from normal tidal breathing through the large and small airways. Impulses of higher frequencies (>20 Hz) travel shorter distances (usually up to the large airways), while impulses of lower frequencies (<15 Hz) travel deeper into the lung and reach the small airways including lung parenchyma. A transducer, working on the principle of change in pressure flow measures the inspiratory and expiratory flow and pressure, which are then separated from the breathing pattern by "signal filtering."

The procedure should be explained to the patient in a sitting position before starting. Tight seal between the mouthpiece and lips should be ensured to prevent any air leakage. The cheeks should be held firmly by the patient with his/her hands. The patient is then asked to perform normal breathing (tidal) in a relaxed state. The recording should be performed for at least 30–45 s. During this period, around 120–150 sound impulses are pushed into the lungs from which the mean reactance and resistance values are determined at a frequency ranging from 5 to 20 Hz.

A minimum of three tests should be performed and breathing segments containing artifacts should be discarded.

Therapies or adjunctive strategies like yoga used to treat respiratory diseases can also be evaluated by using spirometry and impulse oscillometry.

12.2 Conclusion

Today the era of biomarkers has become saturated and prone to many confounding variables but cyclic regulations and physiological waveforms are a more consistent and robust marker of an individual neurohormonal and psycho neuroimmune profile. The biochemical and electrophysiological markers, in combination with eye-tracking and wireless physiological monitoring, can be used to assess attention and autonomic variability which are important in the success of various medications and therapies, thus promising its benefit in bridging Physiology, Psychology, Psychiatry, Cardiology, Endocrinology, and integrated health. Contributions Concept protocol and equipment: Dr. KP Kochhar, Dr. Raj Kumar Yadav and Dr. Sunil.
Data search review and bibliography management: Riya Madan and Kushankur Pandit.
Protocols, support and graphics: Rinku Saini.
Secretarial Assistance Mrs. Prem Wati.

References

1. Vyas R, Dikshit N. Effect of meditation on respiratory system, cardiovascular system and lipid profile. Indian J Physiol Pharmacol. 2002;46:487–91.
2. Robergs R, Board Todd AR, Baker J, et al. Exercise and health impact of pranayama and yoga on lipid profile in normal healthy volunteers. Yoga Blood Lipid Profiles. J Exerc Physiol 2006;9.
3. Manchanda SC, Narang R, Reddy KS, Sachdeva U, Prabhakaran D, Dharmanand S, Rajani M, Bijlani R. Retardation of coronary atherosclerosis with yoga lifestyle intervention. J Assoc Physicians India. 2000;48:687–94.

4. Bijlani RL, Vempati RP, Yadav RK, Ray RB, Gupta V, Sharma R, Mehta N, Mahapatra SC. A brief but comprehensive lifestyle education program based on yoga reduces risk factors for cardiovascular disease and diabetes mellitus. J Altern Complement Med. 2005;11:267–74.
5. Sarvottam K, Yadav R, Mehta N, Pharmacol SM-IJP. Undefined effect of short term yoga on resting energy expenditure and lipid profile in overweight/obese subjects: a preliminary study. 2010.
6. Braun TD, Park CL, Conboy LA. Psychological well-being, health behaviors, and weight loss among participants in a residential, Kripalu yoga-based weight loss program. Int J Yoga Therapy. 2012;22:9–22.
7. Sarvottam K, Yadav RK. Obesity-related inflammation & cardiovascular disease: efficacy of a yoga-based lifestyle intervention. Indian J Med Res. 2014;139:822–34.
8. Mody BS. Acute effects of Surya Namaskar on the cardiovascular & metabolic system. J Bodyw Mov Ther. 2011;15:343–7.
9. Saptharishi LG, Soudarssanane MB, Thiruselvakumar D, Navasakthi D, Mathanraj S, Karthigeyan M, Sahai A. Community-based randomized controlled trial of non-pharmacological interventions in prevention and control of hypertension among young adults. Indian J Community Med. 2009;34:329–34.
10. Lavie CJ, Thomas RJ, Squires RW, Allison TG, Milani RV. Exercise training and cardiac rehabilitation in primary and secondary prevention of coronary heart disease. Mayo Clin Proc. 2009;84:373–83.
11. ACSM. ACSM's resource manual for guidelines for exercise testing and prescription. Philadelphia: Wolters Kluwer Health/Lippincott Williams & Wilkins; 2010.
12. Physical activity improves quality of life. https://atgprod.heart.org/HEARTORG/HealthyLiving/PhysicalActivity/Physical-activity-improves-quality-of-life_UCM_307977_Article.jsp. Accessed 13 Mar 2020.
13. Hartley L, Dyakova M, Holmes J, Clarke A, Lee MS, Ernst E, Rees K. Yoga for the primary prevention of cardiovascular disease. Cochrane Database Syst Rev. 2014; https://doi.org/10.1002/14651858.CD010072.pub2.
14. Young JDE, Taylor E. Meditation as a voluntary hypometabolic state of biological estivation. News Physiol Sci. 1998;13:149–53.
15. Keyworth C, Knopp J, Roughley K, Dickens C, Bold S, Coventry P. A mixed-methods pilot study of the acceptability and effectiveness of a brief meditation and mindfulness intervention for people with diabetes and coronary heart disease. Behav Med. 2014;40:53–64.
16. Castellanos EH, Charboneau E, Dietrich MS, Park S, Bradley BP, Mogg K, Cowan RL. Obese adults have visual attention bias for food cue images: evidence for altered reward system function. Int J Obes. 2009;33:1063–73.
17. Schmidt U, Campbell IC. Treatment of eating disorders cannot remain "brainless": the case for brain-directed treatments. Eur Eat Disord Rev. 2013;21:425–7.
18. Val-Laillet D, Aarts E, Weber B, Ferrari M, Quaresima V, Stoeckel LE, Alonso-Alonso M, Audette M, Malbert CH, Stice E. Neuroimaging and neuromodulation approaches to study eating behavior and prevent and treat eating disorders and obesity. NeuroImage Clin. 2015;8:1–31.
19. Burger KS, Berner LA. A functional neuroimaging review of obesity, appetitive hormones and ingestive behavior. Physiol Behav. 2014;136:121–7.
20. Geliebter A. Neuroimaging of gastric distension and gastric bypass surgery. Appetite. 1970;71:459–65.
21. Scholtz S, Miras AD, Chhina N, et al. Obese patients after gastric bypass surgery have lower brain-hedonic responses to food than after gastric banding. Gut. 2014;63:891–902.
22. McClelland J, Schmidt U, Campbell I, Bozhilova N. A systematic review of the effects of neuromodulation on eating behaviour: implications for brain directed treatments in eating disorders. J Eat Disord. 2013;1:O70.
23. Gorgulho AA, Pereira JLB, Krahl S, Lemaire JJ, De Salles A. Neuromodulation for eating disorders. Obesity and anorexia. Neurosurg Clin N Am. 2014;25:147–57.
24. Yadav RK, Magan D, Mehta N, Sharma R, Mahapatra SC. Efficacy of a short-term yoga-based lifestyle intervention in reducing stress and inflammation: preliminary results. J Altern Complement Med. 2012;18:662–7.
25. Yadav R, Khadgawat R, Sarvottam K, Yadav R, Netam R. Interleukin-6, vitamin D, and diabetes risk-factors modified by a short-term yoga-based lifestyle intervention in overweight/obese individuals. Indian J Med Res. 2015;141:775.
26. Cohen DL, Wintering N, Tolles V, Townsend RR, Farrar JT, Lou GM, Newberg AB. Cerebral blood flow effects of yoga training: preliminary evaluation of 4 cases. J Altern Complement Med. 2009;15:9–14.
27. Nagendra H, Kumar V, Mukherjee S. Cognitive behavior evaluation based on physiological parameters among young healthy subjects with yoga as intervention. Comput Math Methods Med. 2015;2015:821061.
28. Hölzel BK, Carmody J, Vangel M, Congleton C, Yerramsetti SM, Gard T, Lazar SW. Mindfulness practice leads to increases in regional brain gray matter density. Psychiatry Res Neuroimaging. 2011;191:36–43.
29. Nilkamal Singh ST. A fMRI study of stages of yoga meditation described in traditional texts. J Psychol Psychother. 2014; https://doi.org/10.4172/2161-0487.1000185.
30. Engström M, Pihlsgård J, Lundberg P, Söderfeldt B. Functional magnetic resonance imaging of hippocampal activation during silent mantra meditation. J Altern Complement Med. 2010;16:1253–8.

31. Izzetoglu M, Izzetoglu K, Bunce S, Ayaz H, Devaraj A, Onaral B, Pourrezaei K. Functional near-infrared neuroimaging. IEEE Trans Neural Syst Rehabil Eng. 2005;13:153–9.
32. Steinbrink J, Villringer A, Kempf F, Haux D, Boden S, Obrig H. Illuminating the BOLD signal: combined fMRI-fNIRS studies. Magn Reson Imaging. 2006;24:495–505.
33. Bu L, Li J, Li F, Liu H, Li Z. Wavelet coherence analysis of cerebral oxygenation signals measured by near-infrared spectroscopy in sailors: an exploratory, experimental study. BMJ Open. 2016;6:e013357.
34. Herold F, Wiegel P, Scholkmann F, Müller N. Applications of functional near-infrared spectroscopy (fNIRS) neuroimaging in exercise–cognition science: a systematic, methodology-focused review. J Clin Med. 2018;7:466.
35. Rundo JV, Downey R. Polysomnography. Handb Clin Neurol. 2019;160:381–92.
36. Javaheri S, Redline S. Insomnia and risk of cardiovascular disease. Chest. 2017;152:435–44.
37. Sofi F, Cesari F, Casini A, Macchi C, Abbate R, Gensini GF. Insomnia and risk of cardiovascular disease: a meta-analysis. Eur J Prev Cardiol. 2014;21:57–64.
38. Nussinovitch U, Katz U, Nussinovitch M, Nussinovitch N. Deep breath test for evaluation of autonomic nervous system dysfunction in familial dysautonomia. Isr Med Assoc J. 2009;11:615–8.
39. Malik M. Heart rate variability: standards of measurement, physiological interpretation, and clinical use. Circulation. 1996;93:1043–65.
40. Shields JW. Heart rate variability with deep breathing as a clinical test of cardiovagal function. Cleve Clin J Med. 2009;76:S37–40.
41. Kucera P, Goldenberg Z, Kurca E. Sympathetic skin response: review of the method and its clinical use. Bratisl Lek Listy. 2004;105:108–16.
42. Allen J. Photoplethysmography and its application in clinical physiological measurement. Physiol Meas. 2007;28(3):R1–R39. https://doi.org/10.1088/0967-3334/28/3/R01.

Yoga and Neuroimaging Current Status of Evidence

13

Sumana Venugopal, Venkataram Shivakumar, Bharath Holla, Shivarama Varambally, and B. N. Gangadhar

13.1 Introduction

Yoga is an ancient traditional practice existing over 5000 years which is a psycho-philosophical cultural method of lifestyle that reduces stress, induces relaxation and provides various health benefits. The word "Yoga" is derived from a sanskrit word "yuj" meaning "to join" which means the union of body, mind, and the soul. It aims for physical, mental, and spiritual well-being in a holistic way. Union also means uniting the individual consciousness with universal consciousness [1].

Yoga is becoming increasingly popular across the world as a lifestyle modification as well as a treatment approach. It includes various practices like yoga postures, breathing practices, meditation, relaxation techniques, guided imagery, etc., to improve physical and mental health [2]. Yoga has been widely advocated as one of the biopsychosocial models of treatment in various psychiatric disorders such as stress, depression, anxiety, psychosis, etc.

13.2 Emphasis on Mind-Body Link

Mind and body interact with each other constantly, even if we are aware of it or not. In fact, the ancient text "Yoga Vasishta" describes that most of the ailments of the body (vyadhi) originate through mental agitations (adhi).

The ancient texts like Bhagavad Gita, the Yoga *Sutras* of Patanjali, and Hathayoga talk about mind-body connection and how to improve the physical state through balanced mental health. To experience this mind-body connection, various limbs in Ashtanga yoga and Hatha yogic practices approach our body-mind integration through various practices. Thus, the mindfulness aspect of yoga has gained popularity in recent times.

There is early evidence that shows the association of yoga with increased body awareness and body responsiveness. Rani and Rao [3] found that participants who practiced yoga for 3 months reported greater awareness of bodily processes in comparison with a control group. Another study by Daubenmier [4] reported greater levels of body awareness and body responsiveness in yoga practitioners than participants taking exercise

S. Venugopal · V. Shivakumar · B. Holla (✉)
Department of Integrative Medicine, National Institute of Mental Health and Neurosciences (NIMHANS), Bengaluru, India
e-mail: hollabharath@nimhans.ac.in

S. Varambally
Department of Integrative Medicine, National Institute of Mental Health and Neurosciences (NIMHANS), Bengaluru, India

Department of Psychiatry, National Institute of Mental Health and Neurosciences (NIMHANS), Bengaluru, India

B. N. Gangadhar
Department of Psychiatry, National Institute of Mental Health and Neurosciences (NIMHANS), Bengaluru, India

I. Basu-Ray, D. Mehta (eds.), *The Principles and Practice of Yoga in Cardiovascular Medicine*,
https://doi.org/10.1007/978-981-16-6913-2_13

classes and the control group who did not practice yoga, aerobics, or any other mind-body practices. Numerous studies have suggested that yoga practice is associated with reduced stress and enhanced mood [5].

13.3 Role of Yoga in Brain Health and Disease

Yoga practices such as meditation, physical postures and breathing have drawn the attention of the medical community, and various studies have been undertaken for their possible beneficial effects on physical and mental health outcomes. Considering the positive impact of yoga on the body and mind, recent studies are emerging to explore the cognitive effects of yoga.

Previous research on yoga has shown the positive effects on depression, anxiety, bipolar disorder and many other psychiatric illnesses and age-related neurodegenerative diseases [6]. Practice of yoga has also been said to improve perceived cognition, improvement in spatial and verbal memory scores, working memory and attention-switching ability, cognitive performance in the domains of reaction time, improved scores in psychometric tests that included the letter cancelation test, trail making tests A and B, forward and reverse digit spans and auditory and visual reaction times for red light and green light, etc. in healthy individuals [7].

Yoga has also proved its effects for neurological rehabilitation purposes in building strength, flexibility, and coordination, promoting quality of life, as well as building self-esteem and so on. A few studies on yoga have also shown the positive effects of physical and psychological well-being in patients with brain injury. Improvement in strength, mobility, dexterity, and awareness of bodily sensations in the case of stroke patients, improved the quality-of-life of individuals with traumatic brain injury are few examples [8]. Currently, the interest has been piqued to assess the effect of yoga on brain structure, identify the regions of the brain involved and neural networks impacted by the short-term and long-term practice of yoga.

13.4 Aim of the Chapter

Yoga has been advocated as an add-on treatment approach in various neuropsychiatric disorders. However, the mechanistic effects of yoga on the brain are still elusive. Amongst the several techniques employed to understand the neurobiology of yoga, neuroimaging technique has been at the forefront. This chapter aims at summarizing the evidences from neuroimaging studies examining the neurobiological effects of yoga.

13.5 Mechanistic Insights to Yoga-Associated Health Benefits

There are different approaches to yoga which include spiritual, physiological, psycho-emotional, therapeutic, developmental purposes, etc. Yoga has been proved to be effective in health promotion and maintenance, and various studies have shown yoga's effects on psychological well-being and also coping with health challenges. Yoga, when practiced in a mindful manner, will have positive effects on strength, flexibility, stamina, improve balance and induces relaxation. To strengthen the statement, many studies have been conducted to show the mechanism of yoga by different measures [9].

Several studies over the last few years have made a sincere attempt at elucidating the potential mechanism underlying the effects of yoga. Amongst them, the most propounded mechanism of action is the downregulation of the hypothalamic–pituitary–adrenal axis and the sympathetic nervous system and subsequent increase in vagal tone. In fact, autonomic nervous system regulation involves various brain areas, including cortical areas to the brainstem and even the cerebellum, in which all of these structures act as brain networks suggesting a close link between yoga and brain [10]. To understand the critical link between yoga and its effects on the brain, researchers have used several neuroimaging techniques, which are briefly discussed below.

13.6 Brief Introduction to Neuroimaging

The brain is the body's most complex organ and requires various specialized techniques to observe the tissue inside the skull either directly or by indirect measures. In recent years there are a number of imaging techniques that are accepted as safe to be used in clinical settings and in research. Many imaging techniques are considered safe to be used in research studies. Some of them are magnetoencephalography (MEG), electroencephalography (EEG), positron emission tomography (PET), near-infrared spectroscopy (NIRS), and magnetic resonance imaging (MRI).

Our brain circuits produce electrical currents naturally, and this electrical activity can be captured as graphs using electroencephalography (EEG) by placing electrodes on the scalp. There are also magnetic fields formed around the electric current, which can be recorded by magnetoencephalography (MEG). Near-infrared spectroscopy (NIRS) also works with the same principle, only that it is an optical technique for measuring blood oxygenation in the brain. When electromagnetic waves in a near-infrared part of the spectrum with the wavelength of 700–900 nm are passed through the skull, the reflected attenuated waves by the hemoglobin are detected to provide an indirect measure of brain activity. In positron emission tomography (PET), a small amount of short-lived metabolically active radioactive substance is ingested, and the positron emitted by radioactive decay is detected by the scanner and measured to give 2 or 3-dimensional images. Magnetic Resonance Imaging (MRI) technique provides information about brain structure by using magnetic fields and radio waves in which the hydrogen atoms present in the brain are polarized under the strong magnetic field and emit radio-frequency signals to create two- or three-dimensional images. The most common MRI techniques used in the field of yoga research are functional MRI (fMRI), structural MRI (sMRI), magnetic resonance imaging (MRS) and diffusion tensor imaging (DTI).

13.7 Neuroimaging Evidence in Yoga

Yoga is known to bring changes in the mind and the body. But there is a lack of understanding of the underlying structural changes and functional mechanism associated with yoga. Recently there are a number of studies were conducted to examine the neurobiological correlation with yoga in the field of various psychiatric, neurological disorders and in healthy individuals. The majority of these studies have used functional neuroimaging techniques to understand the neural changes, and few of them are structural studies to show the long-term effects of yoga on the brain structure.

Neuroplasticity is one of the crucial features of the brain. Neuroplasticity is the ability of the nervous system to reorganize its structure, its functions and its connections in response to either internal or external stimulus like environment, learning, disease or stimulus through therapy at different levels of molecular to cellular to the system [11]. Many recent evidences have emerged to show the neuroplastic effect of various practices of yoga like postures, regulated breathing, meditation, and many other yogic techniques. These practices are noted to bring changes in the frontal cortex, hippocampus, anterior cingulate cortex, and insula [6].

Various studies are in progress to know the neuroplasticity induced by the practice of yoga. One of the studies examining changes in the brain of long-term Hatha Yoga and meditation practitioners reported a significant increase in gray matter volumes in them when compared with non-yoga practitioners [12]. There are also evidences that show the neuroprotective effect of meditation in increasing the cortical thickness. Lazer et al. found that there was an increased cortical thickness in the right anterior insula and right middle and superior frontal sulci in long-term meditation practitioners when compared to controls [13]. Pagnoni G and Cekic M assessed the changes in Gray matter volume in regular zen meditation practitioners and found that Meditators showed no age-related decline in the left putamen when compared with controls which are suggestive of neuroprotective effects of meditation on reducing the cognitive decline associated with normal aging [14]. Serum brain-derived neurotrophic factor (BDNF), which is considered to be the neuroprotective factor was found to be elevated after the practice of yogasanas and pranayama therapy for 3 months in adults with depression [15]. Based on the fact that BDNF is largely expressed in the hippocampus, Hariprasad et al. tested the possible effect of yoga on the hippocampus. Through magnetic resonance imaging, they found that practicing yoga for 6 months will lead to the increase in the volume of the bilateral hippocampus in elderly people concluding that Yoga can be a potential barrier to age-related neuro-senescence [16].

In a study, researchers compared the effect of meditation technique with usual care in Parkinson's disease patients to find an increase in gray matter density in the right amygdala, bilaterally in the hippocampus, left and right caudate nucleus, the left occipital lobe at the lingual gyrus and cuneus, the left thalamus, and bilaterally in the temporo-parietal junction indicating the neuroplastic effects of meditation [17].

There are a number of functional and structural studies conducted on long-term yoga to evaluate the neurobiological effects on healthy individuals. Many structural studies have shown the effect of yoga on brain structural changes after long-term practices. A study showed that long-term yoga and meditation led to changes like lower right amygdala volume and lower left hippocampus volume whereas another study reported greater left hippocampus gray matter volume in experienced yoga practitioners [18, 19]. Similarly, another study also reported an increase in gray matter volume after the practice of kundalini yoga [20].

Some of the studies report the slowing of age-related structural changes in the brain like gray matter volume differences in the left hemisphere (insula, frontal operculum, and orbitofrontal cortex), increases in hippocampal but not in occipital gray matter, and one functional study showed greater intra-network anteroposterior brain functional connectivity of the default mode network following long-term practice of yoga [16, 19, 21].

There are numerous functional studies done on long-term yoga practitioners, and few studies demonstrate the immediate effect. One study shows the deactivation in bilateral orbitofrontal, anterior cingulate, parahippocampal gyri, thalami, hippocampi., right amygdala following chanting of "OM" [22]. There are few studies on Sahaja yoga practice where they found the increase of activation in bilateral inferior frontal and temporal regions, and this activation reduced progressively deeper stages of meditation, and in another structural study, they found the increase in gray matter volume in meditators compared with non-meditators across the whole brain [23, 24].

Functional studies on yoga have shown the activation in the right prefrontal regions followed by meditation in long-term patanjali yoga practitioners, and in another study, slow breathing yoga practice induced the activation of dorsal pons, periaqueductal gray matter, cerebellum, hypothalamus, thalamus and lateral and anterior insular cortices [25, 26]. A study was conducted on yoga practitioners to observe the effect of yoga using structural, and diffusion tensor imaging techniques found that more insular gray matter in long-term practitioners correlated with more pain tolerance [27].

These real-time changes in the brain due to yoga using various neuroimaging techniques have provided deeper insights into the neural mechanism and its positive effects on our brain and mental well-being. Based on these evidences, we can use yoga in our clinical practice to treat various neuropsychiatric disorders.

Various studies on yoga have been conducted in the area of neurological disorders and have proved the neuroplasticity in many neurological disorders like epilepsy, stroke, Parkinson's disease, multiple sclerosis and so on. Studies have reported a reduction in seizure attacks following 6 months of yoga practice, as demonstrated using EEG changes [28]. Yoga also increases PNS activity [29]. An increase in GABA levels, PNS activity and reduction in stress levels can bring seizure control [30].

Many functional studies have been done on the psychiatric population and reports of significant improvement in certain brain regions after the practice of yoga. A recent fMRI study was conducted to see the effect of long-term yoga intervention on brain aging and related changes in mild cognitive impairment (MCI) individuals. It was found that there was increased connectivity between Default Mode Network and frontal medial cortex, right middle frontal cortex, posterior cingulate cortex, and left lateral occipital cortex of the brain, which correlates to the improvement in the verbal memory performance [31]. Similarly, there was a functional study conducted on the healthy elderly population to assess the effect of long-term yoga practice on the brain, which compared resting-state functional connectivity of the medial prefrontal cortex (MPFC) and posterior cingulate cortex-precuneus (PCC-Precuneus). Yoga practitioners showed a higher correlation between MPFC and the right angular gyrus (AGr), compared to the control and greater intra-network anteroposterior brain functional connectivity of the DMN, indicating healthier cognitive aging process [21]. Contrasting these results, a study was conducted to see the effect of yoga practice on MCI patients where they did not find any gray matter volume changes in dACC or hippocampus [20]. Recently a review was done to examine the underlying mechanisms of add-on yoga treatment on self-reflection through neuroimaging measures in schizophrenia patients. It stated that focused attention during the practice of yoga where a sustained posture, regulation in breathing and meditation techniques can facilitate brain mechanisms involving both low level autonomic, interoceptive networks and high-level cognitive networks resulting in better self-awareness [32].

FNIRS is a relatively newer technique of acquiring and analyzing the hemodynamic changes in the cortex. Only very few studies have been done using this technique in the field of yoga research. One fNIRS study was done to see the effect of kapalbhati on patients with schizophrenia in comparison to healthy individuals. Results of the study demonstrated a significant increase in bilateral prefrontal hemodynamic activity (increased HbO and total Hb) in healthy subjects, but a reduction in right prefrontal HbR compared to schizophrenia patients demonstrating hypo-responsiveness of prefrontal hemodynamics to Kapalbhati in schizophrenia [33].

There are few neuroimaging studies conducted to see the effect of yoga on depressive disorders. A functional study was conducted to see the effect of yoga meditation technique on major depressive disorder patients assessed through rs-fMRI scanning. After 2 weeks of intervention, patients showed a decrease in amplitude of low-frequency fluctuation values in the bilateral frontal pole and increased functional connectivity from the right dorsal medial prefrontal cortex (dmPFC) to the left dorsolateral prefrontal cortex (dlPFC) and the left lateral orbitofrontal cortex (OFC) indicating the regulation of the activities in prefrontal cortex correlating to modulation of brain activity in multiple emotion-processing systems [34]. In addition to functional and structural studies, very few spectroscopic studies have been done in yoga. One such study was done on subjects with a major depressive disorder to assess the thalamic GABA levels using MRS before and after yoga practice and found that there was a significant increase in GABA levels following 1 week of yoga which correlated with the mood improvement [35].

There are only a few neuroimaging studies conducted in the field yoga intervention for neurological disorders. A structural study was done to assess the effect of yoga meditation on Parkinson's disease patients using MRI scan. Increased gray matter density was found in the right *amygdala* and bilaterally in the hippocampus and in other neural networks indicating the important role of yoga in Parkinson's disease (16c). One early study has shown the effect of Sahaja yoga meditation practice on seizure control & EEG changes in patients of epilepsy. They found the shift in frequency from 0 to 8 Hz towards 8–20 Hz.of power spectral analysis of EEG and increase in the ratios of EEG powers in delta (D), theta (T), alpha (A), and beta (B) bands. There was also a decrease in the frequency of seizures after 3 months of practice and a further decrease after 6 months of Sahaja yoga practice [28].

13.8 Limitations

Although the current neuroimaging evidence shows the considerable effects of yoga on structural and functional changes in the brain, still there are many limitations regarding many aspects. First of all, none of these studies have taken into consideration the impact of lifestyle choices such as diet, recreational drugs, and physical exercise, which may act as the confounding factors. The second major limitation is the study design employed. Majority of these studies are lacking the rigorosity of randomized blinded sham-controlled study design. In addition, there is a lack of uniform yoga methodology in almost all the studies. Different schools of yoga have been used in different studies for a varied duration, making the comparison difficult. The third most important aspect is the sample size, which is very small in almost all the studies. Further, the majority of the studies are conducted in healthy individuals, especially long-term yoga practitioners. Results from these studies cannot be generalized to other healthy populations and diseased groups. Finally, there are also chances of publication bias which might have led to the smaller number of reported studies also, some of the studies fail to discuss negative results.

13.9 Future Directions

Preliminary evidence suggests the potential role of neuroimaging techniques in elucidating the mechanistic effects of yoga in neuropsychiatric disorders. Future directions are to use large sample sizes along with randomization. Also, more RTCs are to be conducted. Yoga intervention for the disease population to be carried out. Also, follow-up studies need to be carried out to determine the long-term effect of yoga.

13.10 Summary and Conclusion

As discussed above, current evidences suggest a significant effect of yoga on the brain as demonstrated by several neuroimaging studies. However, there is a need for uniform yoga practice with a robust study design encompassing multimodal imaging techniques to understand the neurobiological effects of yoga. Further, neuroimaging studies to understand the effects of yoga in neuropsychiatric disorders adopting rigorous study designs is the need of the hour.

References

1. Yardi N. Yoga for control of epilepsy. Seizure. 2001 Jan 1;10(1):7–12.
2. Basavaraddi IV. Yoga: its origin, history and development. Public diplomacy: in focus. 2015.
3. Jhansi Rani N, Krishna Rao PV. Body awareness and yoga training. Percept Mot Skills. 1994;79(3):1103–06. https://doi.org/10.2466/pms.1994.79.3.1103.
4. Daubenmier JJ. The relationship of yoga, body awareness, and body responsiveness to self-objectification and disordered eating. Psychol Women Q. 2005;29(2):207–19. https://doi.org/10.1111/j.1471-6402.2005.00183.x.
5. Impett EA, Daubenmier JJ, Hirschman AL. Minding the body: yoga, embodiment, and well-being. Sex Res Soc Policy. 2006 Dec 1;3(4):39–48.
6. Gothe NP, Khan I, Hayes J, Erlenbach E, Damoiseaux JS. Yoga effects on brain health: a systematic review of the current literature. Brain Plast. 2019;5:105–22.
7. Desai R, Tailor A, Bhatt T. Effects of yoga on brain waves and structural activation: a review. Complement Ther Clin Pract. 2015 May 1;21(2):112–8.
8. Donnelly KZ, Linnea K, Grant DA, Lichtenstein J. The feasibility and impact of a yoga pilot programme on the quality-of-life of adults with acquired brain injury. Brain Inj. 2017 Jan 28;31(2):208–14.
9. Herrick CM, Ainsworth AD. Invest in yourself: yoga as a self-care strategy. Nurs forum. 2000;35(2):32–6.
10. Macey PM, Ogren JA, Kumar R, Harper RM. Functional imaging of autonomic regulation: methods and key findings. Front Neurosci. 2016 Jan 26;9:513.
11. Cramer SC, Sur M, Dobkin BH, O'Brien C, Sanger TD, Trojanowski JQ, Rumsey JM, Hicks R, Cameron J, Chen D, Chen WG. Harnessing neuroplasticity for clinical applications. Brain. 2011 June 1;134(6):1591–609.
12. Froeliger B, Garland EL, McClernon FJ. Yoga meditation practitioners exhibit greater gray matter volume and fewer reported cognitive failures: results of a preliminary voxel-based morphometric analysis. Evid Based Complement Alternat Med. 2012;2012:821307.
13. Lazar SW, Kerr CE, Wasserman RH, Gray JR, Greve DN, Treadway MT, McGarvey M, Quinn BT, Dusek JA, Benson H, Rauch SL. Meditation experience is associated with increased cortical thickness. Neuroreport. 2005 Nov 28;16(17):1893.

14. Pagnoni G, Cekic M. Age effects on gray matter volume and attentional performance in Zen meditation. Neurobiol Aging. 2007 Oct 1;28(10):1623–7.
15. Naveen GH, Thirthalli J, Rao MG, Varambally S, Christopher R, Gangadhar BN. Positive therapeutic and neurotropic effects of yoga in depression: a comparative study. Indian J Psychiatry. 2013 Jul;55(Suppl 3):S400.
16. Hariprasad VR, Varambally S, Shivakumar V, Kalmady SV, Venkatasubramanian G, Gangadhar BN. Yoga increases the volume of the hippocampus in elderly subjects. Indian J Psychiatry. 2013 Jul;55(Suppl 3):S394.
17. Pickut BA, Van Hecke W, Kerckhofs E, Mariën P, Vanneste S, Cras P, Parizel PM. Mindfulness based intervention in Parkinson's disease leads to structural brain changes on MRI: a randomized controlled longitudinal trial. Clin Neurol Neurosurg. 2013 Dec 1;115(12):2419–25.
18. Gotink RA, Vernooij MW, Ikram MA, Niessen WJ, Krestin GP, Hofman A, Tiemeier H, Hunink MM. Meditation and yoga practice are associated with smaller right amygdala volume: the Rotterdam study. Brain Imaging Behav. 2018 Dec 1;12(6):1631–9.
19. Gothe NP, Hayes JM, Temali C, Damoiseaux JS. Differences in brain structure and function among yoga practitioners and controls. Front Integr Neurosci. 2018 Jun 22;12:26.
20. Yang H, Leaver AM, Siddarth P, Paholpak P, Ercoli L, St Cyr NM, Eyre HA, Narr KL, Khalsa DS, Lavretsky H. Neurochemical and neuroanatomical plasticity following memory training and yoga interventions in older adults with mild cognitive impairment. Front Aging Neurosci. 2016 Nov 21;8:277.
21. Santaella DF, Balardin JB, Afonso RF, Giorjiani GM, Sato JR, Amaro E Jr, Lazar S, Kozasa EH. Greater anteroposterior default mode network functional connectivity in long-term elderly yoga practitioners. Front Aging Neurosci. 2019;11:158.
22. Kalyani BG, Venkatasubramanian G, Arasappa R, Rao NP, Kalmady SV, Behere RV, Rao H, Vasudev MK, Gangadhar BN. Neurohemodynamic correlates of 'OM' chanting: a pilot functional magnetic resonance imaging study. Int J Yoga. 2011 Jan;4(1):3.
23. Hernández SE, Suero J, Rubia K, Gonzalez-Mora JL. Monitoring the neural activity of the state of mental silence while practicing Sahaja yoga meditation. J Altern Complement Med. 2015 Mar 1;21(3):175–9.
24. Hernández SE, Suero J, Barros A, González-Mora JL, Rubia K. Increased grey matter associated with long-term sahaja yoga meditation: a voxel-base-d morphometry study. PLoS One. 2016 Mar 3;11(3):e0150757.
25. Mishra SK, Khosa S, Singh S, Moheb N, Trikamji B. Changes in functional magnetic resonance imaging with yogic meditation: a pilot study. Ayu. 2017 Jul;38(3–4):108.
26. Critchley HD, Nicotra A, Chiesa PA, Nagai Y, Gray MA, Minati L, Bernardi L. Slow breathing and hypoxic challenge: cardiorespiratory consequences and their central neural substrates. PLoS One. 2015;10(5):e0127082.
27. Villemure C, Čeko M, Cotton VA, Bushnell MC. Insular cortex mediates increased pain tolerance in yoga practitioners. Cereb Cortex. 2014 Oct 1;24(10):2732–40.
28. Panjwani U, Selvamurthy W, Singh SH, Gupta HL, Thakur L, Rai UC. Effect of Sahaja yoga practice on seizure control & EEG changes in patients of epilepsy. Indian J Med Res. 1996 Mar;103:165–72.
29. Khattab K, Khattab AA, Ortak J, Richardt G, Bonnemeier H. Iyengar yoga increases cardiac parasympathetic nervous modulation among healthy yoga practitioners. Evid Based Complement Alternat Med. 2007;4(4):511–7.
30. Streeter CC, Gerbarg PL, Saper RB, Ciraulo DA, Brown RP. Effects of yoga on the autonomic nervous system, gamma-aminobutyric-acid, and allostasis in epilepsy, depression, and post-traumatic stress disorder. Med Hypotheses. 2012 May 1;78(5):571–9.
31. Eyre HA, Acevedo B, Yang H, Siddarth P, Van Dyk K, Ercoli L, Leaver AM, Cyr NS, Narr K, Baune BT, Khalsa DS. Changes in neural connectivity and memory following a yoga intervention for older adults: a pilot study. J Alzheimers Dis. 2016 Jan 1;52(2):673–84.
32. Rao N, Menon S. A heuristic model linking yoga philosophy and self-reflection to examine underlying mechanisms of add-on yoga treatment in schizophrenia. Int Rev Psychiatry. 2016 May 3;28(3):265–72.
33. Bhargav H, Raghuram N, HR N. Frontal hemodynamic responses to high frequency yoga breathing in schizophrenia: a functional near-infrared spectroscopy study. Front Psych. 2014 Mar 24;5:29.
34. Chen F, Lv X, Fang J, Yu S, Sui J, Fan L, Li T, Hong Y, Wang X, Wang W, Jiang T. The effect of body–mind relaxation meditation induction on major depressive disorder: a resting-state fMRI study. J Affect Disord. 2015 Sep 1;183:75–82.
35. Streeter CC, Gerbarg PL, Brown RP, Scott TM, Nielsen GH, Owen L, Sakai O, Sneider JT, Nyer MB, Silveri MM. Thalamic gamma aminobutyric acid level changes in major depressive disorder after a 12-week Iyengar yoga and coherent breathing intervention. J Altern Complement Med. 2020 Jan;26:190–7.

Part IV

Yoga for Various Cardiovascular Diseases

14 Yoga: A Holistic Approach for Cardiac Arrhythmia

Indranill Basu-Ray and Anindya Mukherjee

14.1 Introduction

Yoga has been speculated to exist since the 5000 BC, and it utilizes various postures and movements along with breathing methods to facilitate the physiology of various systems in the human body, which includes the autonomic nervous system (ANS), among others. The USA has seen a dramatic increase in the practice of yoga in the last decade and its clinical implications in the context of modern medicine have become an important subject for contemporary research [1]. ANS plays an important role in atrial arrhythmia generation and maintenance. Thus the unique interaction between cardiac ANS and yoga deserves further discussion and research.

14.2 Basics of Yoga

Yoga was believed to maintain a balance between mind, body, and soul. It has been broadly categorized into four major traditional types- Bhakti, Gnana (pronounced as ñana), Karma, and Kriya (with Hatha, Tantra, and Kundalini yoga subtypes) with various styles of practicing it (Table 14.1) [2]. According to Yoga, Ida (sympathetic) and Pingala (parasympathetic) "nadis" run along the spinal column crossing each other several times at strong energy centers known as chakras (spinal plexi) to finally join the Shushumna (central nervous system (CNS)) at the top. The wide variety of yoga practices that exist and has been studied do not demonstrate any superiority of any particular style [3].

14.3 Autonomic Function and Neurohormonal Modulation (Fig. 14.1)

Breathing exercises have been shown to increase heart rate variability (HRV) and improve the vago-sympathetic balance by modulating rate, depth, and pattern of respiration [4–7]. Yogic breathing acting via stretch receptors in the respiratory muscles relay vagal inputs to CNS to influence cognitive, emotional, behavioral, and somatic expressive outcomes [5, 6]. It also balances the parasympathetic system,

I. Basu-Ray (✉)
Memphis VA Medical Center, Memphis, TN, USA

The University of Memphis, Memphis, TN, USA

Department of Cardiology, All India Institute of Medical Sciences, Rishikesh, India
e-mail: indranill.basu-ray@va.gov; ibr@ibasuray.com

A. Mukherjee
Department of Cardiology, Nilratan Sircar Medical College, Kolkata, India

I. Basu-Ray, D. Mehta (eds.), *The Principles and Practice of Yoga in Cardiovascular Medicine*,
https://doi.org/10.1007/978-981-16-6913-2_14

gamma-aminobutyric acid (GABA) system and hypothalamo–pituitary–adrenal axis [4]. The "Om" chant reduces vagal tone, causes physiological relaxation and deactivation of the limbic system, while other yoga therapies reduce cortisol, CRP, and IL-6, thus attenuating endothelial and inflammatory disease processes [8–11]. Reduction of blood pressure and heart rate has been documented with yoga [12]. Please refer to Chap. 9 for detailed understanding of the effects of yoga in autonomic nervous system.

Table 14.1 Classification of Yoga

Types	Styles
Bhakti	Iyengar
Gnana	Vinyasa
Karma	Hot
Kriya	Ashtanga
	Sivananda
	Yin
	Restorative
	Anusara
	Prenatal
	Jivamukti
	Bikram

Cortisol, growth hormone (GH), thyroid-stimulating hormone (TSH) showed a reduction in levels with 4 months of meditation therapy which may contribute to reversing the chronic stress factors leading to disease [13]. Improvement of HRV, SDNNi, and rMSSD with yoga therapy has been documented in a randomized controlled trial [14]. A 50% reduction in premature ventricular contractions (PVC) and QT dispersion has been noted with deep breathing exercises [15]. Yoga therapy has also shown improvement in neurocardiogenic syncope management [16]. Reduction of malignant ventricular arrhythmias and sudden cardiac death has been documented with pranayama therapy by reduction of ventricular repolarization dispersion in patients with cardiac arrhythmias [17].

14.4 Cardiac Innervation

Heart receives a lateralized innervation with right-sided nerves innervating the right ventricle and left-sided nerves innervating the left ventri-

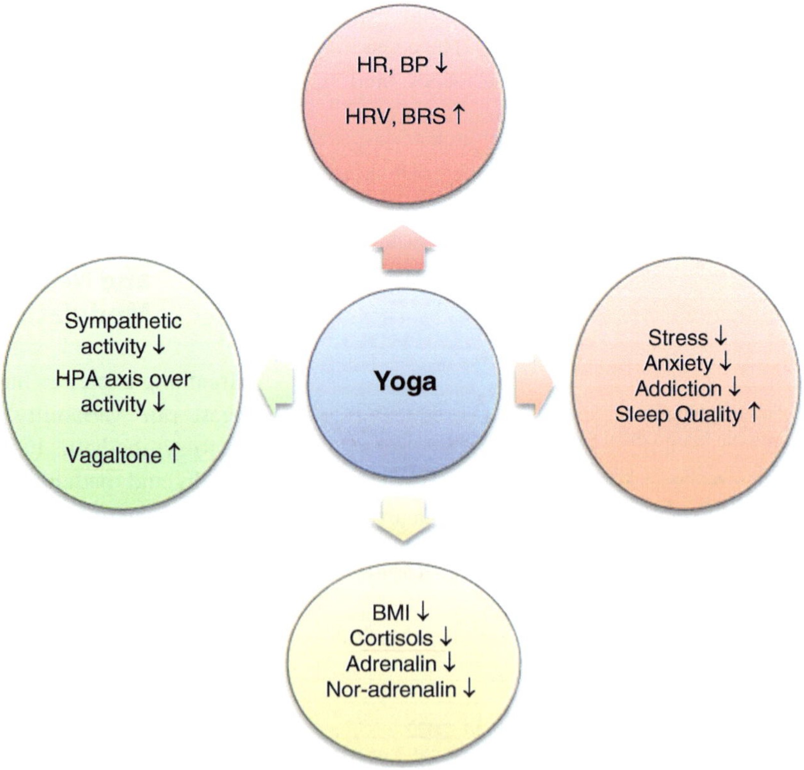

Fig. 14.1 Role of Yoga in primary prevention of cardiac arrhythmias. *BMI* body mass index; *BP* blood pressure; *BRS* breathing style; *HPA* hypothalamo-pituitary-adrenal; *HR* heart rate; *HRV* heart rate variability

cle. This results in asymmetrical stimulation of the heart in the pathological state leading to heterogenous repolarization, electrical instability, and re-entrant arrhythmias [18–20].

14.5 Psychiatry

Anxiety, depression, and other mental stress have been known to trigger cardiac arrhythmias such as atrial fibrillation (AF). Negative emotions increase the risk of AF by fivefold whereas a positive and happy mind reduces it [21–23]. There is no direct pathogenesis relating to emotional state and arrhythmias, but pathological consequences on neuroendocrine, immune, microcirculatory systems may result in cardiac arrhythmias [24–26]. Sympathetic system over activation leads to increased collagen production, extracellular matrix synthesis, increased TGF-β1, mononuclear infiltrate leading to atrial fibrosis, moreover, anxiety leads to activation of renin angiotensnsinaldosterone system (RAAS), leading to further atrial fibrosis and stretch [27–32]. AF also can be precipitated by activation of autonomic ganglia in pulmonary veins near their connection with the left atrium by emotional stress [33].

14.6 Autonomic Etiology of Dysrhythmias

14.6.1 Reflex Syncope

Neurocardiogenic syncope, situational syncope and carotid sinus hypersensitivity comprise reflex syncopes, of which the most common variety is neurocardiogenic associated with reduced blood volume, dehydration, and elevated sympathetic tone [34–38]. Conservative measures to control this consists of triggers like prolonged standing, dehydration, extreme temperatures, avoidance, handgrip, squat, leg-crossing (counterpressure maneuvers), adequate hydration, compression stockings, salt balance and tilt training [35, 36, 39–43]. More invasive procedures and potential medication use will then play their roles.

In 2015, Gunda et al. in their pilot study, documented the role of yoga in neurocardiogenic syncope [16]. Mean syncopes, mean of pre-syncopes and syncope functional questionnaire score (SFSQS) was significantly reduced in the yoga intervention arm ($p < 0.001$) Number of positive HUTT was also reduced in the yoga group. Yoga acts by accelerating blood volume return to the heart along with autonomic modulations [16]

14.6.2 Atrial Fibrillation (AF)

Premature atrial beats, increased sympathetic tone, increased β-adrenergic activation with vagal overcompensation in the milieu of the reduced refractory period and action potential duration give rise to AF [44–46]. These sudden variations in autonomic tone can also form the basis of other arrhythmias [47].

In 2013, The YOGA My Heart Study showed a significant reduction of symptomatic AF, asymptomatic AF and other symptomatic arrhythmias with yoga intervention [48]. Yoga not only demonstrated AF burden reduction but the reduction of baseline heart rate and blood pressure was also noted. The authors postulated increased baseline parasympathetic tone, reduction in ANS fluctuations as the cause behind limited atrial remodeling and thus reduced progression of AF [48].

14.6.3 Ventricular Arrhythmia

In the heart parasympathetic nervous system has a more focal localization and localized mainly in sino-atrial (SA) node, atrio-ventricular (AV) node and ganglionic plexi embedded in atrial fat pads. Thus increased parasympathetic tone decreases SA and AV nodal conduction but ventricular muscle being mainly innervated by sympathetic nerves is not much in control of the parasympathetic tone.

Myocardial infarction causes fibrosis and focal denervation in the ventricular musculature. This, along with surrounding tissue hypersensitivity, leads to variable tissue refractory period and generation of ventricular ectopy.

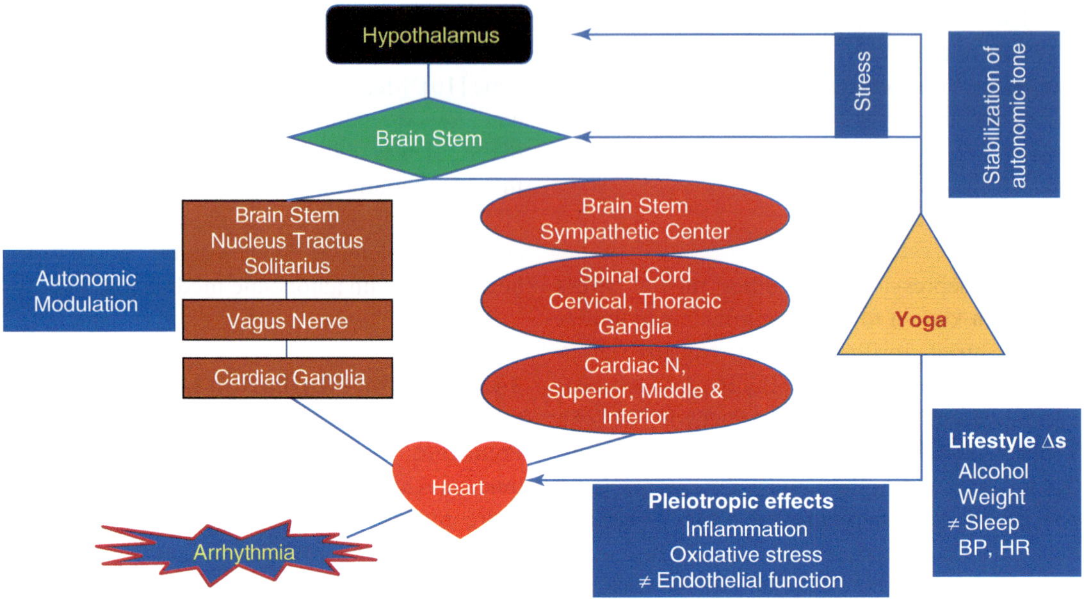

Fig. 14.2 Multipronged approach of yoga on human body and reduction of cardiac arrhythmias [47]

Table 14.2 Potential Yoga module for cardiac arrhythmias

Type of practices	Practice	Duration
Sukshmavyayam (loosening)	Standing: Loosening of fingers, wrist, elbow, shoulder, neck rotation, twisting synchronized with breathing Sitting: Loosening of toes, ankle, knees, and hip synchronized with breathing in sitting posture followed by quick relaxation technique (QRT)	10 min
Breathing practices	Hands in and out breathing, hands stretch breathing Ankle stretch breathing, Setubandhasana breathing Bhujangasana breathing, Tiger breathing followed by a quick relaxation technique	15 min
Asanas (Yoga postures)	Standing:Tadasana, ardhakatichakrasana, ardhachakrasana, trikonasana followed by QRT Sitting: Bhunamanasana, Paschuttasana, ardhamtsendrasana, janushirshasana followed by QRT Supine: setubandhasana, pavanamuktasana, anantpadmasana Prone: Bhuajangasana, makarasana, shalabhasana followed by DRT	20 min
Pranayama (Yoga breathing)	Complete yogic breathing, nadishudhi pranayama, Chandra anulom-vilom, bhramari pranayama,	10 min
Meditation	Om meditation, mindfulness meditation, chanting of A,U,M and OM	5 min

Nerve regeneration results in sympathetic hyperactivity among the denervated musculature, and this may further lead to ventricular arrhythmia (VA) and sudden cardiac death (SCD) [49–52]. VA management has found a new avenue focused on sympathetic modulation and related interventions [53].

Similarly, regular yoga practices help in parasympathetic stimulation, which is a useful adjunctive therapy. Three components of yoga viz. pranayama, asana, and dhyana modulate arrhythmia management with different mechanisms. Pranayama has the largest supportive evidence, and various breathing exercises and patterns modify ANS in various ways. Deep breathing results in stretch-induced inhibitory signaling, and there is a decrease in metabolic activity, suggesting parasympathetic augmentation. Also, stretch receptor activation above tidal volume reduces sympathetic tone in peripheral blood vessels through the Hering–Breuer reflex [54].

Overall, yoga plays a very important role in altering endothelial dysfunction, modulation of ANS and oxidative stress leading to a measurable reduction in arrhythmia and dysautonomia (Fig. 14.2).

14.7 Conclusion and Future Direction

Yoga is a very old complementary and alternative medicine (CAM) practice and has proven to be beneficial as an adjunct to modern medicine [47]. Yoga improves the HR and BP and reduces cardiac arrhythmia (CA) burden, likely by an increase in parasympathetic tone and reducing autonomic variations. Future studies are warranted to understand the different forms of yoga and their individual benefits in CA. Also, comparison with other forms of CAM needs further research. Studies regarding different arrhythmias and the effect of specific yoga interventions in them will shed light on the role of yoga in CA and cardiology practice overall.

A representative yoga module should be practiced under a trained yoga expert, and one can practice on his/her own once familiar with the practices (Table 14.2). We recommend the practice of complete yogic breathing and chanting of A, U, M and OM in shavasana during an episode of arrhythmia and palpitation while getting medical help.

References

1. Yoga Journal Releases 2012 Yoga in America Market study. Yoga J. 2012.
2. Patanjali CH. The yoga-sutra of Patanjali: a new translation with commentary (Shambhala classics) 2003: Shambhala; Shambhala Classics edition (April 1, 2003).
3. Cramer H, et al. Is one yoga style better than another? A systematic review of associations of yoga style and conclusions in randomized yoga trials. Complement Ther Med. 2016;25:178–87.
4. Streeter CC, et al. Effects of yoga on the autonomic nervous system, gammaaminobutyric-acid, and allostasis in epilepsy, depression, and post-traumatic stressdisorder. Med Hypotheses. 2012;78(5):571–9.
5. Brown RP, Gerbarg PL. Sudarshan Kriya yogic breathing in the treatmentof stress, anxiety, and depression. Part II – clinical applications and guidelines. JAltern Complement Med. 2005;11(4):711–7.
6. Brown RP, Gerbarg PL. Yoga breathing, meditation, and longevity. Ann N Y Acad Sci. 2009;1172:54–62.
7. Bernardi L, et al. Slow breathing reduces chemoreflex response to hypoxia andhypercapnia, and increases baroreflex sensitivity. J Hypertens. 2001;19(12):2221–9.
8. Saper RB, et al. Yoga for chronic low back pain in a predominantly minority population: a pilot randomized controlled trial. Altern Ther Health Med. 2009;15(6):18–27.
9. Telles S, Nagarathna R, Nagendra HR. Autonomic changes during "OM" meditation. Indian J Physiol Pharmacol. 1995;39(4):418–20.
10. Kiecolt-Glaser JK, et al. Stress, inflammation, and yoga practice. Psychosom Med. 2010;72(2):113–21.
11. Cheng TO. Effect of Tai Chi on endothelial function. Clin Cardiol. 2007;30(3):150.
12. Murugesan M, Taylor AG. Effect of yoga on the autonomic nervous system: clinical implications in the management of atrial fibrillation. 2017.
13. MacLean CR, et al. Effects of the transcendental meditation program on adaptive mechanisms: changes in hormone levels and responses to stress after 4 months of practice. Psychoneuroendocrinology. 1997;22(4):277–95.
14. Khattab K, et al. Iyengar yoga increases cardiac parasympathetic nervousmodulation among healthy yoga practitioners. Evid Based Complement Altern Med. 2007;4(4):511–7.
15. Yetkin E, et al. Beneficial effect of deep breathing on premature ventricular complexes: can it be related to the decrease in QT dispersion? Int J Cardiol. 2006;113(3):417–8.
16. Gunda S, et al. Role of yoga as an adjunctive therapy in patients with neurocardiogenic syncope: a pilot study. J Interv Card Electrophysiol. 2015;43(2):105–10.
17. Dabhade AM, et al. Effect of pranayama (breathing exercise) on arrhythmias in the human heart. Explore (NY). 2012;8(1):12–5.
18. Lane RD, Jennings JR. Hemispheric asymmetry, autonomic asymmetry, and the problem of sudden cardiac death. Denver: The MIT Press; 1995.
19. Taggart P. Brain-heart interactions and cardiac ventricular arrhythmias. Neth Heart J. 2013;21(2):78–81.
20. Fransson EI, et al. The association between job strain and atrial fibrillation: results from the Swedish WOLF study. Biomed Res Int. 2015;2015:371905.
21. Shusterman V, Lampert R. Role of stress in cardiac arrhythmias. J Atr Fibrillation. 2013;5(6):834.
22. Lampert R, et al. Triggering of symptomatic atrial fibrillation by negative emotion. J Am Coll Cardiol. 2014;64(14):1533–4.

23. Sterndorff B, Smith DF. Normal values for type A behaviour patterns in Danish men and women and in potential high-risk groups. Scand J Psychol. 1990;31(1):49–54.
24. Severino P, et al. Triggers for atrial fibrillation: the role of anxiety. Cardiol Res Pract. 2019;2019:1208505.
25. Pitsavos C, et al. Anxiety in relation to inflammation and coagulation markers, among healthy adults: the ATTICA study. Atherosclerosis. 2006;185(2):320–6.
26. Pasquini M, Berardelli I, Biondi M. Ethiopathogenesis of depressive disorders. Clin Pract Epidemiol Mental Health. 2014;10:166–71.
27. Nef HM, et al. Expression profiling of cardiac genes in Tako-Tsubocardiomyopathy: insight into a new cardiac entity. J Mol Cell Cardiol. 2008;44(2):395–404.
28. Alqaqa A. Anxiety and atrial fibrillation: an interesting bidirectional association. Curr Trend Cardiol. 2017;1(1):15–8.
29. Carney RM, Freedland KE, Veith RC. Depression, the autonomic nervous system, and coronary heart disease. Psychosom Med. 2005;67:S29–33.
30. Lefer DJ, Granger DN. Oxidative stress and cardiac disease. Am J Med. 2000;109(4):315–23.
31. Mlinarevic D, et al. Pathophysiological mechanisms of Takotsubo cardiomyopathy: a systematic review. Southeastern Eur Med J. 2017; https://doi.org/10.26332/seemedj.v1i1.31.
32. Szardien S, et al. Mechanisms of stress (Takotsubo) cardiomyopathy. Heart Fail Clin. 2013;9(2):197–205.
33. Mahida S, et al. Science linking pulmonary veins and atrial fibrillation. Arrhythmia Electrophysiol Rev. 2015;4(1):40–3.
34. Bartoletti A, et al. Hospital admission of patients referred to the emergency department for syncope: a single-hospital prospective study based on the application of the European Society of Cardiology Guidelines on syncope. Eur Heart J. 2006;27(1):83–8.
35. Sutton R. Reflex syncope: diagnosis and treatment. J Arrhythmia. 2017;33(6):545–52.
36. Sutton R, et al. Guidelines for the diagnosis and management of syncope (version 2009): the task force for the diagnosis and management of syncope of the European Society of Cardiology (ESC). Eur Heart J. 2009;30(21):2631–71.
37. Alboni P, Alboni M. Typical vasovagal syncope as a "defense mechanism" for the heart by contrasting sympathetic overactivity. Clin Auton Res. 2017;27(4):253–61.
38. da Silva RMFL. Syncope: epidemiology, etiology, and prognosis. Front Physiol. 2014;5:471.
39. Brignole M, et al. Isometric arm counter-pressure maneuvers to abort impending vasovagal syncope. J Am Coll Cardiol. 2002;40(11):2053–9.
40. Krediet CT, et al. Management of vasovagal syncope: controlling or aborting faints by leg crossing and muscle tensing. Circulation. 2002;106(13):1684–9.
41. Lee AKY, Krahn AD. Evaluation of syncope: focus on diagnosis and treatment of neurally mediated syncope. Expert Rev Cardiovasc Ther. 2016;14(6):725–36.
42. Shen W-K, et al. 2017 ACC/AHA/HRS guideline for the evaluation and Management of Patients with syncope: a report of the American College of Cardiology/American Heart Association task force on clinical practice guidelines and the Heart Rhythm Society. Circulation. 2017;136(5):e60–e122.
43. van Dijk N, et al. Effectiveness of physical counterpressure maneuvers in preventing vasovagal syncope: the physical counterpressure manoeuvres trial (PC-trial). J Am Coll Cardiol. 2006;48(8):1652–7.
44. Hoff HE, Geddes LA. Cholinergic factor in auricular fibrillation. J Appl Physiol. 1955;8(2):177–92.
45. Lewis T, Drury A, Bulger H. Observations upon atrial flutter and fibrillation. VI. Refractory period and rate of propagation in the auricle: their relation to block in the auricular walls and to flutter etc. Heart. 1921;8:84–134.
46. Xi Y, Cheng J. Dysfunction of the autonomic nervous system in atrial fibrillation. J Thorac Dis. 2015;7(2):193–8.
47. Akella K, Kanuri SH, Murtaza G, Rocca DGD, Kodwani N, Turagam MK, Shenthar J, Padmanabhan D, Basu Ray I, Natale A, Gopinathannair R, Lakkireddy D. Impact of yoga on cardiac autonomic function and arrhythmias. J Atr Fibrillation. 2020 Jun 30;13(1):2408. https://doi.org/10.4022/jafib.2408.
48. Lakkireddy D, et al. Effect of yoga on arrhythmia burden, anxiety, depression, and quality of life in paroxysmal atrial fibrillation: the YOGA My Heart Study. J Am Coll Cardiol. 2013;61(11):1177–82.
49. Vaseghi M, Shivkumar K. The role of the autonomic nervous system in sudden cardiac death. Prog Cardiovasc Dis. 2008;50(6):404–19.
50. Han J, Garciadejalon P, Moe GK. Adrenergic effects on ventricular vulnerability. Circ Res. 1964;14:516–24.
51. Shen MJ, et al. 40 - Neural activity and atrial tachyarrhythmias, in cardiac electrophysiology: from cell to bedside. In: Zipes DP, Jalife J, Stevenson WG, editors. Cardiac electrophysiology: from cell to bedside. 7th ed. Philadelphia, PA: Elsevier; 2018. p. 375–86.
52. Stavrakis S, et al. 44 - Role of the autonomic nervous system in atrial fibrillation. In: Zipes DP, Jalife J, Stevenson WG, editors. Cardiac electrophysiology: from cell to bedside. 7th ed. Philadelphia, PA: Elsevier; 2018. p. 419–25.
53. Bourke T, et al. Neuraxial modulation for refractory ventricular arrhythmias: value of thoracic epidural anesthesia and surgical left cardiac sympathetic denervation. Circulation. 2010;121(21):2255–62.
54. Nivethitha L, Mooventhan A, Manjunath NK. Effects of various Prānāyāma on cardiovascular and autonomic variables. Anc Sci Life. 2016;36(2):72–7.

Cardiometabolic Syndrome and Effects of Yoga

15

Sridip Chatterjee and Puneet Bhattacharya

15.1 Introduction

It is in evidence that being physically active is an important criterion for staying healthy. According to the American College of Sports Medicine (ACSM) and the Centers for Disease Control and Prevention, adults should be moderately physically active for at least 30 min on most—and preferably all—days of the week. Moderate physical activity is roughly that which uses approximately 150 kilocalories of energy per day, or 1000 kilocalories per week [1]. One can accomplish this by taking part in a less vigorous activity for a longer period or a more vigorous activity for a shorter period. The ACSM recommends exercising five days a week doing moderate activity, or three days a week for vigorous activity [2, 3]. It is amply clear that lack of following this recommendation stemming from a busy lifestyle is one of the most common causes of cardio-metabolic-syndrome (CMS). Changes in lifestyle from traditionally rustic to modern day urban living have led to stress and other mental aberrations including anxiety and depression. While acute stress is normal and can sometimes be beneficial, chronic stress is a harbinger of CMS. Experts agree that one best way to manage stress is through breathing and meditation protocols as seen in yoga that have been proven to relax the body and mind [4, 5]. The global burden of noncommunicable diseases (NCDs) is increasing alarmingly in adults. Two potential reasons for this include a deranged lifestyle associated with physical inactivity and stress. These are further augmented by an inappropriate diet. The global status report on Non-communicable Diseases (NCDs), published by World Health Organization in 2014, mentions that NCDs contribute 68% of all the deaths and are expected to increase gradually [6]. Physical inactivity is now identified as the fourth leading risk factor for global mortality. Scientific evidence indicates that physical inactivity levels are rising in many countries with major implications for the prevalence of non-communicable diseases (NCDs) and the general health of the population worldwide [7]. Cardiometabolic syndrome is thus emerging as a new form of NCDs and the leading cause of death in the world [8].

Scientific evidence indicates that the risk of coronary heart disease, myocardial infarction, stroke, peripheral vascular diseases, cerebrovascular arterial disease are the results of CMS [9]. The increasing prevalence of cardiometabolic syndrome is a serious health crisis worldwide that needs urgent attention. Physical inactivity, sedentary behavior, fat rich diet, mental stress, lack of sleep, and habitual dependency (smoking, alcoholism, tobacco use) are the lifestyle-related modifiable key factors that initiate CMS [10].

S. Chatterjee (✉) · P. Bhattacharya
Department of Physical Education, Jadavpur University, Kolkata, West Bengal, India
e-mail: sridipchatterjee.ped@jadavpuruniversity.ac.in; puneetbhattacharya.ped@jadavpuruniversity.in

I. Basu-Ray, D. Mehta (eds.), *The Principles and Practice of Yoga in Cardiovascular Medicine*,
https://doi.org/10.1007/978-981-16-6913-2_15

Clinically insulin resistance in skeletal muscles, adipose tissue, and liver plays a central role in the development of cardiometabolic syndrome.

15.2 Cardiometabolic Syndrome or Diseases

The phenomenon of cardiometabolic syndrome (CMS) is both complex and heterogeneous [11, 12]. The concept of insulin resistance syndrome or metabolic syndrome or syndrome X has been reported since the late 1980s. Early epidemiological and clinical studies held from the 1930s to 1950s clearly indicate that certain cardiovascular and metabolic risk factors tend to cluster together [13], finally give birth to a disease entity known as "cardiometabolic syndrome." Clinical observation conducted by Himsworth in the early 1930s brought out the occurrence of two types of diabetes mellitus. The first one caused due to insulin deficiency called the insulin sensitive type and the other due to dearth of some unidentified factors which insen-sitize the body to insulin called insulin insensitive type or insulin resistant as it was later known as. These pioneer thought-provoking research findings open a new window to answer the many unsolved hypotheses related to diabetes mellitus [14]. After 40 years of Himsworth's original observation, the National Diabetes Data Group in the USA came to the same conclusion [15]. Now it is finally established that there are two distinct types of diabetes mellitus, i.e., insulin-dependent diabetes mellitus (IDDM) and non-insulin-dependent diabetes mellitus (NIDDM). Gerald M. Reaven could be considered as the father of "Insulin Resistance" concept. In 1988, the famous Banting lecture was delivered by Dr. Reaven [16]. This is annually organized by the American Diabetes Association in the memory of Frederick Banting, a Canadian medical scientist who jointly won the Nobel Prize [17] in the area of Physiology/Medicine for the discovery of insulin and its therapeutic application. Therefore, Dr. Reaven was the first man who coined the term "Metabolic Syndrome or Syndrome X" [18]. On the basis of his extensive research experience, he proposed that insulin resistance is a single common phenomenon associated with the development of many other correlated symptoms or diseases in the human body. He hypothesized that it was a central feature in the development of coronary heart disease and type 2 diabetes mellitus, mainly through target tissue resistance to insulin action. From then till today many definitions, different guidelines have been proposed by some leading research organizations around the world, such as the World Health Organization (WHO) [19], the European Group for the study of Insulin Resistance (EGIR) [20], the National Cholesterol Education Program Adult Treatment Panel III (NCEP:ATPIII) [21], the American Association of Clinical Endocrinology (AACE) [22], the International Diabetes Federation (IDF) [23], and the American Heart Association/National Heart, Lung, and Blood Institute (AHA/NHLBI) [24], have attempted to incorporate all the different parameters used to define MetS (Table 15.1). However, all these organizations indicate some common correlated pathophysiological entities, including elevated fasting plasma glucose, dyslipidemia, obesity (visceral adiposity), insulin resistance, and hypertension.

As the time progressed it was evident that CMS led to increased prevalence of cardiovascular diseases and type II diabetes- the twin global epidemic [26, 27].

15.3 Etiology of Cardiometabolic Syndrome or Diseases and Yoga

The causative factors of cardiometabolic syndrome as reported in scientific literature are vastly diverse and widely cover many aspects of human health. Although extensive research has been carried out in recent decades on metabolic syndrome and diseases, the exact underlying etiology is still not completely understood. Many contributory factors and mechanisms have been proposed which include lifestyle factors as well as a wide variety of correlated pathophysiological conditions. In brief, two lines of research work on the etiological factors have been identified so far which are: Lifestyle related and

Table 15.1 Reported diagnostic criteria of metabolic syndrome

1.	**World Health Organization (WHO) Criteria**: The first attempt was made in 1998 by the WHO, which proposed that MetS may be defined by the presence of any one of Insulin resistance or impaired fasting glucose, type 2 diabetes mellitus (DM) or impaired fasting glucose (IFG) (>100 mg/dl) or impaired glucose tolerance (IGT), plus two of the following: • Abdominal obesity (waist-to-hip ratio > 0.90 in men or > 0.85 in women, or body mass index (BMI) > 30 kg/m^2. • Triglycerides 150 mg/dl or greater, and/or high-density lipoprotein (HDL)-cholesterol < 40 mg/dl in men and <50 mg/dl in women. • Blood pressure (BP) 140/90 mmHg or greater. • Microalbuminuria (urinary albumin secretion rate 20 μg/min or greater, or albumin-to-creatinine ratio 30 mg/g or greater) [19].
2.	**European Group for the Study of Insulin Resistance criteria**: Insulin resistance defined as insulin levels > 75th percentile of non-diabetic patients, plus two of the following: • Waist circumference 94 cm or greater in men, 80 cm or greater in women. • Triglycerides 150 mg/dl or greater and/or HDL cholesterol < 39 mg/dl in men or women. • BP 140/90 mmHg or greater or taking antihypertensive drugs. • Fasting glucose 110 mg/dl or greater [20].
3.	**National Cholesterol Education Program Adult Treatment Panel III (NCEP:ATPIII) criteria**: Any three or more of the following: • Waist circumference > 102 cm in men, > 88 cm in women. • Triglycerides 150 mg/dl or greater. • HDL cholesterol < 40 mg/dl in men and < 50 mg/dl in women. • BP 130/85 mmHg or greater. • Fasting glucose 110 mg/dl* or greater. * In 2003, the American Diabetes Association (ADA) changed the criteria for IFG tolerance from 110 mg/dl to 100 mg/dl [21].
4.	**American Association of Clinical Endocrinology criteria**: IGT plus two or more of the following: • BMI 25 kg/m^2 or greater. • Triglycerides 150 mg/dl or greater and/or HDL cholesterol < 40 mg/dl in men and <50 mg/dl in women. • BP 130/85 mmHg or greater [22].
5.	**International Diabetes Federation (IDF) criteria**: Central obesity (defined as waist circumference but can be assumed if BMI > 30 kg/m^2) with ethnicity-specific values,* plus two of the following: • Triglycerides 150 mg/dl or greater. • HDL cholesterol < 40 mg/dl in men and < 50 mg/dl in women. • BP 130/85 mmHg or greater. • Fasting glucose 100 mg/dl or greater. *To meet the criteria, waist circumference must be: for Europeans, >94 cm in men and >80 cm in women; and for South Asians, Chinese, and Japanese, >90 cm in men and >80 cm in women. For ethnic South and Central Americans, South Asian data are used, and for sub-Saharan Africans and Eastern Mediterranean and Middle East (Arab) populations, European data are used [23].
6.	**American Heart Association/National Heart, Lung, and Blood Institute (AHA/NHLBI) criteria**: Any three of the following: • Waist circumference 102 cm or greater in men, 88 cm or greater in women. • Triglycerides 150 mg/dl or greater. • HDL cholesterol < 40 mg/dl in men and < 50 mg/dl in women. • BP 130/85 mmHg or greater. • Fasting glucose 100 mg/dl or greater [24].
7.	**Consensus definition (incorporating IDF and AHA/NHLBI definitions)**: Any three of the following: • Elevated waist circumference (according to population and country-specific definitions). • Triglycerides 150 mg/dl or greater. • HDL cholesterol < 40 mg/dl in men and < 50 mg/dl in women. • BP 130/85 mmHg or greater. • Fasting glucose 100 mg/dl or greater [25].

Pathophysiological risk factors. In the following sections we explore these possible reported risk factors of CMS across the world and the prospective role of yoga for its prevention [9, 13, 24, 25, 28].

Lifestyle Related Risk Factors These are the primary risk factors for cardiometabolic syndrome. Yoga is purported to offer a holistic lifestyle model particularly that helps to inculcate good, healthy habits and foster positive attitude toward the philosophy of life, in turn modifying these lifestyle related risk factors of CMS [29, 30].

Physical Inactivity WHO report (2008) on the level of physical inactivity indicates that around 31% (men 28% and female 34%) of adults aged 15 years and above were insufficiently active globally. It is estimated that approximately 3.2 million deaths each year are due to insufficient physical activity [31, 32]. The principle reason for this is believed to be a sedentary lifestyle [1, 2, 6, 7]. Regular habit of yoga practice could be an economic, nonpharmacological, and noninvasive approach to fight against this inactivity epidemic worldwide as it includes doing physical activity like surya namaskar and other 'asanas'.

Sedentary Behavior Sedentary behavior is any type of working behavior characterized by energy expenditure $\leq$ 1.5 metabolic equivalents. Following a sedentary lifestyle pattern, such as persistent low levels of physical activity, watching TV, using computers sitting in cars and overeating, leads to positive energy balance, which is one of the major causes of metabolic dysfunction [33]. Positive energy balance leads to accumulation of body fat in the adipose tissue, overtime leading to insulin resistance [34]. Prolonged low level of physical activity causes chronic subclinical inflammation which is associated with cardiometabolic syndrome [35]. It is estimated that only 20% of the population is sufficiently physically active [36]. Cross-sectional and prospective observational studies reported that adults engaged in sedentary behavior for at least 8-10 hours per day in their waking hours [37] is a risk factor for the development of T2DM and CVD. Regular yoga practice not only negates but also helps assimilation of over nutrition. The yogic lifestyle also propagates appropriate eating including a plant based diet, low animal fat, lots of fibers all of which help both reduce truncal obesity and decrease insulin resistance.

Sleep Sleep is a basic requirement to maintain an optimal health status of the individual. It is important to regulate many physiological functions, including neurobehavioral performance [38], metabolism [39], appetite regulation [40], immune function [41], and hormone regulation [42]. It is reported that each healthy adult should have to sleep for 7 h per night [43]. However, 45 % of adults are not able to meet this requirement [39, 44]. A group of epidemiological and experimental studies reported that lack of sleep is directly associated with the adverse metabolic traits and cardiometabolic diseases [40, 45]. In a randomized study it was found that yoga practices for a period of 6 months improved different aspects of sleep (decreased time to fall asleep and increased total hours of sleep time) in a geriatric population [46]. Self-rated sleep quality was improved after cyclic meditation [47]. In a recent randomized control trial, it was reported that overall sleep and sleep quality improved significantly after 6 and 12 weeks of yoga practice (surya namaskar, asana, pranayama, and yoga nidra) and 6 weeks of aerobic exercise in type 2 diabetic women. It was interesting however to note that the yoga practicing group showed better improvement after 12 weeks compared to aerobic exercise group [48].

Wrong Food Selection and Unhealthy Dietary Pattern Wrong food selection and unhealthy dietary pattern play an important role in the development of cardiometabolic diseases, like diabetes mellitus, obesity, and cardiovascular diseases. Prolonged consumption of high-caloric ultra-processed food with high fat percentage cluster with sedentary behavior ultimately increase the excess accumulation of adipose tissue in the body. Unhealthy eating habits like low intake of antioxidant rich foods (green leafy vegetables and fruits), high intake of junk foods, and sodium-containing foods are important causative factors of metabolic syndrome. Excess intake of calories and less physical activity are responsible for high waist to hip ratio (Men >40 inches or >102 cm and Women >35 inches or >88 cm) [33, 49, 50]. The basic principle of diet from the yogic perspective is to eat small quantities of high-quality food, which promotes life force in a body without producing many metabolic toxins [51]. Overall, three types of food and diet pattern are described in yoga, *Sattvic* (pure and balanced diet), *Rajasic* (overnutrition and stimulating diet), and *Tamasic* (old stale food which induced laziness and sleep). According to the tradition of yoga *sattvic* food has the best health benefits, including consumption of freshly cooked food, low consumption of fried food and an overwhelming proportion of vegetables and fruits. [52]. Yoga has been known to modify over eating behavior leading to chronic obesity [53]. An experimental study actually concluded that 12 weeks of *hatha yoga* practice reduces compulsive eating (binge eating), lengthens meal times, and improves food quality [53, 54].

Mental Stress

Stress is also an important contributory factor for the development of CMS [55]. Oxidative stress accelerates the process of unnecessary cell damage. Oxidative damage implies an imbalance of production and inactivation of reactive oxygen species (ROS), which leads to cellular dysfunctions. ROS plays a distinct role as a causative agent of atherosclerosis, diabetes, hypertension, aging, Alzheimer's disease, kidney disease, and even certain forms of cancer [56–58]. Aberrant mental conditions including anxiety and depression both of which are both prevented or ameliorated by yoga and stress are the primary cause of many somatic abnormalities evidenced in CMS [59, 60]. In the 1970s, Dr. Herbert Benson at Harvard Medical School proposed that all mind–body techniques, including biofeedback, meditation, progressive muscle relaxation, autogenic training, tai chi, chi gong, yoga, and other such techniques, elicit a common physiologic response that Benson termed as relaxation response [61, 62]. Relaxation response not only reduce stress but negate the pathophysiological changes like release of dangerous chemicals including IL-6, TNF-alpha and such other players that accentuate atherosclerosis by initiating and sustaining inflammation in blood vessels. A substantial experimental and clinical research suggests that yoga not only decreases stress but also alters the accompanying inflammatory responses [63, 64].

Habitual Dependency A meta-analysis on cohort studies suggested that smoking may increase the CMS risk by 26%. Release of various neurotransmitters like catecholamines, vasopressin, corticotrophin-releasing hormone, adrenocorticotrophic hormone, growth hormone, etc. is stimulated by nicotine in smokers. Inflammatory biomarker levels like C-reactive protein, certain lipids like low-density lipoprotein and triglycerides, increase in smokers, mainly due to augmented release of free fatty acids triggered by very low lipoprotein activity [65, 66]. A meta-analysis of five studies indicates that people with alcohol use disorders (AUDs) have shown greater prevalence of cardiometabolic diseases [67]. Kuppili et al. in a narrative review of 16 studies reported the beneficial effects of short-term yoga practice in reducing the substance use disorder including nicotine dependency, alcohol use disorders, opioids use disorders, and cocaine use disorders [68].

Insulin Resistance Insulin resistance (IR) is an abnormal physiological condition associated with the metabolic process, where the insulin hormone becomes less effective or resistant at lowering blood sugars which directly increase the blood glucose levels outside the normal range and cause adverse health effects [13, 16]. Though multifactorial it is believed to be the predominant cause of Type II DM. An increase in blood glucose upon feeding stimulates pancreatic β-cells to release insulin into the circulation for carbohydrate metabolism. In insulin resistance, muscle, fat, and liver cells do not respond properly to insulin and thus glucose cannot easily be metabolized. As a result, the pancreatic β-cell needs to secrete more insulin to enable glucose to enter into the cells and undergo metabolism. The beta cells in the pancreas try to keep up with this increased demand for insulin by producing more and more. As long as the beta cells are able to produce enough insulin to overcome the insulin resistance, blood glucose levels stay in the normal range. However the increased presence of Insulin called Hyperinsulinemia accentuates many adverse reactions. Type II Diabetes is a condition of hyperinsulinemia where unless one approaches the last stages of the disease enough Insulin is found in the blood but it is ineffective leading to hyperglycemia [18, 25]. This pathophysiology of Insulin resistance is accentuated by physical inactivity and inappropriate diet leading to obesity which actually increases insulin resistance creating a vicious cycle of worsening disease states leading to a systemic disease pattern that affects almost every organ in the body. A detailed pathophysiologic consequence of this insulin resistant state is beyond the scope of this chapter but it finally leads to disease as varied as kidney failure to retinal damage and blindness and propensity to develop malignant coronary artery disease and cerebrovascular disorders [69]. Chapter 16 details the role of yoga in prevention and management of Diabetes.

Free Fatty Acid (FFA) Free fatty acid is the by-product of fat metabolism. Dysfunction in free fatty acid metabolism is also a key contributory factor related to the pathogenesis of hyperglycemia and dyslipidemia associated with the CMS much of which is driven by hyperinsulinemia [70]. Excess amount of FFAs released from the adipose tissue into the plasma and elevated FFAs concentration can impair the ability of insulin to stimulate glucose uptake and suppress hepatic glucose production. This excess FFAs finally delivered to the liver can increase hepatic VLDL (very low-density lipoprotein) triglyceride production and plasma triglyceride concentrations. Insulin is the major regulator of basal adipose tissue lipolytic activity. This critical cellular mechanism states that insulin resistance is the direct result of too many free fatty acids (FFAs) that have been released into the bloodstream by masses of excessive intra-abdominal fat cells. It appears that, in our muscles, FFAs interfere with insulin metabolism by putting an extra phosphorous molecule through the substances called insulin receptor substrate 1 and 2 (IRS1 IRS2). When IRS1 and IRS2 are phosphorylated, it can't bind insulin to a muscle cell's membrane and the cell is then insulin resistant and it can't get enough glucose to supply the energy it needs. High blood sugar levels are due, for the most part, to the inability of muscle cells to take in glucose. FFAs also go to the liver and, by interfering with insulin metabolism there, cause that organ to spew too much glucose into the blood, again raising blood glucose levels. In the pancreas, FFAs cause the β-cells (the ones that secrete insulin) to over-secrete. So, all together, a person's blood sugar and insulin levels will climb. In people who have type 2 diabetes, high serum levels of FFAs seem to account for 50% of their insulin resistance [69, 71, 72].

15.4 Central Obesity or Visceral Obesity or Abdominal Obesity

Central obesity, also known as android or visceral obesity is a feature of excess fat deposition in paraintestinal and omental areas of the abdomen. Visceral adipose tissue refers to excess fat stored around the internal organs and has been suggested as an independent risk factor for the CMS. It is a key contributory risk factor for impaired glucose tolerance, hyperinsulinemia, dyslipidemia, type 2 diabetes, hypertension, coagulation abnormalities, and CVD [12, 13, 73]. Though visceral obesity is a pathology of its own kind with observable adverse effects a general discussion on obesity and the role of yoga is described in Chap. 17.

15.5 Dyslipidemia or Abnormal Lipid Profile and Apolipoproteins

Dyslipidemia refers to abnormal levels of fat content in the blood. It is characterized by high levels of total cholesterol (above 200 mg/dl), triglycerides (above 150 mg/dl), low-density lipoprotein (LDL, above 100 mg/dl) cholesterol, very low-density lipoprotein (VLDL, above 30 mg/

dl), and low level of high-density lipoprotein (HDL, men below 40 mg/dl and women 50 mg/dl) cholesterol in the blood. Clinical evidence suggests that high levels of total cholesterol, LDL cholesterol, and VLDL cholesterol can build up fat deposition inside the walls of arteries, overtime this plaque narrowing the lumen of the arteries, producing atherosclerosis and leads to cardiovascular diseases. A more common mechanism is deposition of fat in the arterial walls causing inflammation and rupture of plaques leading to arterial obstruction due to collected debris. Both of this mechanism leads to myocardial infarction. A similar sequence of events lead to infarction in the brain leading to stroke and cerebrovascular disease. Low levels of HDL cholesterol with high levels of triglycerides are also associated with abnormal fat deposition inside the walls of arteries. However, high levels of HDL cholesterol actually protect our heart by helping to remove excess buildup of LDL cholesterol inside the arteries [70, 71, 74]. Apolipoproteins (apo) are the specialized group of proteins that helps to maintain lipid homeostasis by transporting cholesterol and lipids between cells. There are several types of apolipoproteins found in humans: Apolipoprotein A, B, C, D, E, F, G, and H. Some of them (apoA, apoB, and apoC) play a major role in lipid metabolism. For example, apoA makes up about 90% of the proteins in HDL. So, if there is a deficiency in apoA, it leads to a deficiency in HDL. Furthermore, increased levels of apoA5 lead to higher triglycerides levels while apoA1 works combined with apoE to reduce triglyceride levels. Apolipoprotein B (apoB) is the biggest among the lipoproteins found in LDL and VLDL. Increased level of apoB in the blood is a direct predictor of higher LDL VLDL concentration in the blood which is also a risk marker of coronary artery disease. In recent times apoA to apoB ratios are measured as an indicator of ischemic stroke, while apoC and apoA levels indicate a risk of coronary heart disease [75]. Yogic lifestyle including dietary modfication, exercise informed by yoga postures and decreasing stress has salutary effects on Hyperlipidemia. Chapter 18 outlines the role yoga plays in these disorders.

15.6 Atherosclerosis

Atherosclerosis is a condition that happens when lumen of the arteries becomes narrow and harder due to buildup of plaque around the artery wall. This actually disrupts the normal blood flow inside the body and subsequently increases the risk of complications, such as heart attack and stroke. CMS remains the most potent factor for atherosclerosis and its effects including myocardial infarction and cerebrovascular disease. Thus appropriate amelioration of this cluster of abnormalities provides primodial, primary as well as secondary prevention of these ailments. A large number of research has underlined the role yoga plays in curtailing CMS thus enhancing protection against these diseases [69, 70, 76]. Chapter 19 outlines the role yoga plays in primary and secondary coronary artery disease that is caused by atherosclerosis of the coronary arteries. Chapter 20 describes the role of yoga in strokes.

15.7 Dysfunctions Related to Systemic Metabolism

Systemic metabolism refers to efficient functioning of the multiple organ system within the body which works together to maintain a healthy state of metabolic homeostasis. Any kind of dysfunction in these systemic pathways is responsible for the development of metabolic imbalance in the body. The CNS is actively involved in the control of peripheral metabolism. A closed loop well communicating pathway exists that includes hypothalamic and other brain centers and peripheral tissues including the nerves in the gastrointestinal system to ensure a well balanced feedback loop for efficient functioning. It has become clear that different situations including addictions involved aberrations in the brain circuits that propels inappropriate behavior. Furthermore emotional imbalance particularly stress, can act on these pathways to disrupt the close feedback loop described above to create multiple pathologies. One important pathway in brain regulation of metabolism is the melanocortin system in the accurate nucleus of the hypothalamus. In this region, orexigenic neuropeptide Y/agouti-related peptide (NPY/AGRP) and anorexigenic pro-opiomelanocortin (POMC) neurons control glucose metabolism, expenditure of energy, and food intake behavior. AgRP is co-expressed with NPY and acts to increase appetite and decrease metabolism and energy expenditure. It is one of the most potent and long-lasting of appetite stimulators. Accumulated evidences sustain the notion that depression and other pathological mental states can activate such pathways to increase food intake despite the presence of overnutrition to lead to obesity. Other brain regions such as the amygdala and hippocampus that have strong role to play in emotions have neurons directed towards this system lending credence to the hypothesis that mood and mental states influence food intake. Hypothalamus with its sub-regions within the brain regulates food intake. The metabolic tissues (liver, intestine, adipose, and muscle) in the periphery send feedback signals to the hypothalamic circuit thus exerting metabolic control in healthy states. This normal feedback loop gets disrupted in CMS. In the peripheral system the tissues such as the liver, adipose, muscle, and intestine play major roles in energy intake and utilization. Exercise has been shown to affect whole-body metabolism through NPY/AGPR and POMC neurons of the hypothalamus. However, the exact inter-organ mechanism is still being uncovered [77, 78]. Yoga plays a dominant role possibly at multiple levels by modulating diet, exercise and attenuating mental diseases including anxiety, stress and depression. Chapter 11 underlines the role of mind and cardiovascular disease whereas Chaps. 9, 10 highlights the effects of stress.

15.8 Metabolic Dysfunction Induced by Liver

There are two distinct pathways through which hypothalamus controls liver metabolism, by stimulating the autonomic nerves and by releasing hormone from the pituitary gland. The hypothalamus regulates liver functions by neural and neuroendocrine connections. Under the influence of hypothalamus liver plays essential roles in glucose and lipid metabolism. Thereby, any disturbance in the metabolic function of the liver leads to abnormal metabolic health. The accumulation of excess lipids in the liver is associated with obesity and CVD and is an early indicator of insulin resistance. Hepatokines are the liver-derived hormones playing an important role in pathogenesis of CMS. Several hepatokines (hepassocin, angiopoietin-like 4, selenoprotein P, fibroblast growth factor 21, etc.) have been reported, as the link between accumulation of lipids in the liver and glucose intolerance and insulin resistance. These liver secreted hepatokines are likely to be predictive biomarkers for the metabolic disorders as we get a better understanding of their role and mechanism of action in the near future [79]. A large number of yogic postures are known to stretch the liver and the pancreas to improve their function. Dietary prudence associated with yogic lifestyle decreases carbohydrate and fat load in diet. Thus Pranayam and other yogic breathing techniques enhance parasympathetic drive. While the role of autonomic nerves in obesity is still a matter of debate there is some evidence that in obesity sympathetic activity is increased but its effectiveness is impaired. Yoga is thus known to play its role at multiple junctures to annul these metabolic aberrations. More research are underway to delineate their the exact cellular mechanism.

15.9 Metabolic Dysfunction Induced by Adipose Tissue

Considerable evidence has accumulated that adipose tissue plays a vital role in glucose and fat metabolism. White adipose tissue (WAT) is the major source of obesity and the site of inflammation, in turn, leads to insulin resistance and metabolic dysfunction. Several hormones produced by the adipose tissue have important effects on whole-body metabolism. Adipokines are specific type of hormones linked to obesity, diabetes, inflammation, atherosclerosis, and liver disease [69, 76]. Leptin is a peptide-based hormone and also a widely researched adipokine produces by the fat cells in adipose tissue and enterocytes in the small intestine that helps to regulate energy balance, suppressing food intake, increasing fatty acid oxidation via activation of 5'-AMP-activated protein kinase, thereby it maintains our healthy body weight. Leptin has been considered an anti-obesity hormone which sends feedback signals to the hypothalamus to inhibit food intake and decrease weight. Low leptin levels influence overfeeding and suppress energy expenditure, inhibit thyroid and reproductive hormones secretion and immune function. Adiponectin is a protein-based hormone and adipokine secreted by the mature adipocytes. Its physiological functions include regulation of glucose levels as well as fatty acid breakdown, reduction of inflammation and atherogenesis. Recent data indicate that serum levels of adiponectin decrease with obesity and are positively associated with insulin sensitivity [73]. On the basis of available evidence, it is safe to conclude that prevalence of increased adiposity is strongly associated with with metabolic dysfunction [80, 81]. Yoga has been known through multiple studies to increase adiponectin levels. See Chap. 17 to understand the role of yoga in obesity.

15.10 Metabolic Dysfunction Induced by Muscle Tissue

In normal physiological conditions the state of hyperglycemia initiates insulin secretion and glucose uptake in skeletal muscle, whereas this normal function is impaired in the state of insulin resistance which is a common feature of type 2 diabetes mellitus and obesity. Hypothalamus controls the glucose uptake in skeletal muscle via the sympathetic nervous system and probably through insulin dependent pathways. Insulin resistance disrupts this feedback mechanism which leads to metabolic complications [82, 83]. Muscles are important players in metabolic syndrome and forms a close knit entity with liver, fast store and the brain to control and regular metabolism. Many myokines are secreted during muscle contractions which increase energy expenditure, decrease inflammation, and have neuroprotective effects. In addition, myokines have autocrine, paracrine, and endocrine effects to maintain whole-body metabolism. Interleukin-6 (IL-6) is a well-recognized myokine secreted during muscular activity, producing effects on liver, adipose, and endocrine tissues. It also activates hepatic production and glucose during exercise. Individuals with metabolic abnormalities and obesity showed elevated levels of IL-6, thus possibly resistance to IL-6 signaling pathways. Evidence suggests that IL-6 concentration increases lipolysis in skeletal muscles, adipose tissues, and stimulates fatty acid oxidation in humans. Several studies reported a potential link between IL-6 and dyslipidemia. Multiple studies have shown that yoga reduced IL 6. Though the significance of which is uncertain. Emerging evidence also suggests that IL-6 deficiency results in cardiac lipotoxicity by deleterious effects on intracellular lipid accumulation and thus, generation of toxic lipid metabolites, leads to cardiac dysfunction, though the molecular mechanism of IL-6 in cardiac fatty acid metabolism is still under investigation [84]. In the same token it is also important to understand that high levels of IL 6 is also toxic to the body as it is an inflammatory marker that initiates rogue inflammation in the vascular system and other circuits including in COVID afflictions. Thus it is ostensible that body requires a well adjusted balance in production and destruction of IL 6 to maintain homeostasis. Myostatin is another important cytokine which negatively regulates muscle growth by preventing hyperplasia and hypertrophy. A lower level of serum myostatin is associated with the development of CMS, and central obesity, high triglycerides, and low HDL cholesterol levels. Emerging research trends indicate that myostatin may be used as a biomarker for metabolic disorders, higher levels of serum myostatin favorable metabolic profiles [78, 85].

15.11 Gastrointestinal and Endocrine Factors

Insulin and glucagon together regulate glucose homeostasis in the blood. In normal physiological response insulin helps cells to utilize blood glucose and store excess glucose in the form of glycogen for later use. In a condition when blood glucose level falls, during fasting and physical exercise, the hormone glucagon is secreted by the alpha cells of the pancreas. Glucagon then helps to convert stored glycogen into glucose in skeletal muscle and liver cells through a metabolic process called glycogenolysis. Glucagon stimulates liver to absorb amino acids from the blood and converts them into glucose through gluconeogenesis. Glucagon also stimulates adipose cells to release fatty acids into the blood and counteracts dyslipidemia. These glucagon mediated actions of rising blood glucose levels inhibit further glucagon release from the alpha cells through a negative feedback mechanism [70, 78]. The basal metabolic rate is controlled by the two thyroid hormones, thyroxine (T_3) and triiodothyronine (T_4) under the influence of thyroid stimulating hormone (TSH) release from anterior pituitary. T_3 and T_4 affect almost every cell in the body and bind to receptors on the mitochondria resulting in increased release of energy from the ATP. Scientific evidence indicates that overweight, obesity, type 2 diabetes mellitus, and dyslipidemia are directly associated with the insulin resistance, impaired synthesis of glucagon, hypothyroidism, and hyperthyroidism [86, 87]. Ghrelin, a peptide hormone secreted from the gastric mucosa in the stomach which stimulates appetite and growth hormone release, plays an important role in the metabolic process by acting on the CNS, food intake, modulating taste sensation, energy metabolism, and consequently fat mass. It is reported that ghrelin also acts to modulate thermogenesis in brown adipose tissue and lipid utilization in white adipose tissue. Ghrelin receptors are mostly found in the brain but also are found in the pancreas. The circulating level of ghrelin in the peripheral tissue is maintained by the balance among its secretion, degradation, and clearance rates. Ghrelin stimulates the brain which further influences our appetite, slows metabolism, and declines the body's natural ability to burn fat, thus increased fat deposition in the abdominal area. Serotonin, a neurotransmitter, is also secreted by the intestinal mucosa and has effects on glucose metabolism in the pancreas, liver, and adipose. It helps to have a normal bowel function and also reduces appetite when individual's stomach is full [88]. Serotonin levels increase in the brain with yoga and meditation practice. It is yet unclear as to the relation between release of serotonin in the brain and its level in the gut. Yoga may by some unknown mechanism provide satiety by increasing serotonin's availability in the gut.

15.12 Oxidative Stress

A large body of current evidence in biology and medicine postulates that oxidative stress is an important factor that contributes to the development of several disorders and diseases in the human body [56]. Oxidative stress generally occurs when there is an imbalance of free radicals and antioxidants in the body, which overtime leads to cell, tissue, and organ damage. Reactive oxygen species (ROS), reactive nitrogen species (RNS), and reactive chlorine species (RCS) are the terms collectively representing free radicals and other non-radicals' reactive derivatives. ROS, RNS, and RCS are the chemical by-product of basal metabolic functions [57]. These reactive species can be of two types: free radicals and non-radical derivatives. Among the reactive species some molecules are containing one or more unpaired electrons, thus known as free radicals, whereas some reactive species do not contain any unpaired electron, known as non-radicals. Antioxidants are the substances that neutralize these highly reactive free radicals by donating an electron. Generally free radicals are produced during natural physiological process can be either helpful or harmful for the body. Excessive production of free radicals or poor availability of natural antioxidants may lead to oxidative stress. Overproduction of ROS is associated with metabolic dysfunction and inflammatory signaling. Elevated inflammatory signaling combined with metabolic dysfunction is associated with the chronic diseases such as atherosclerosis, diabetes, obesity, and stroke [56–58].

15.13 Inflammatory Markers

A growing body of evidence emerges in recent times exploring that obesity, metabolic syndrome, type 2 diabetes mellitus, and cardiovascular diseases are linked to chronic inflammation in the body. C-reactive protein (CRP) is one such biomarker produced by the liver and a mediator of inflammation in the body. High level of CRP is a risk factor associated with CMS [89]. Increased levels of inflammatory markers (CRP, TNF-α, IL-1, and IL-6) have been linked with insulin resistance and multiple molecular mechanisms [78]. Yoga has been credited to decrease all these inflammatory markers.

15.14 Scientific Exposition of Yoga and Cardiometabolic Diseases

Cardiometabolic disease involves a cluster of conditions that alter fat and glucose metabolism, cause abdominal and ectopic fat deposition, develop insulin resistance, cause hypertension, and if unattended lead to cardiovascular diseases [69]. This section highlights the cascade of cardiometabolic syndrome factors acquired with drastic lifestyle changes overtime. The biochemical traits which are recognized as risk factors in terms of inherent and genetic markers have been excluded.

15.15 Yogic Concept of Disease

The Vasistha Samhita, an ancient hatha yogic text descriptively classifies diseases into two kinds, diseases caused by the mind known as *Adhija Vyadhi* (stress born psychosomatic or somatopsychic) and those by physical means called *Anadhija Vyadhi* (non-stress born) [90, 91]. Disease can manifest in either body or mind. The diseases that initiate in the mental level and then travel into the somatic (body) level are known as psychosomatic in nature, while other diseases that are born in the body and then travel into the mind are called somatopsychic. In essence yoga truly believes that all diseases have a mind and a body component. Even so called physical diseases based on western medicine according to yoga philosophy can have a mental component that either initiates or sustains the pathophysiology. Yoga as a therapy is essentially a mind–body medicine concept [92]. This section attempts to provide experimental proof of the role of yoga in CMS. A brief introduction to Vedic philosophy is also attempted to understand the nuances of yoga therapy.

Figure 15.1 describes the interaction between the various symptoms of cardiometabolic syndrome with the different phases of the human body and their correlation with the five different layers of existence as described in the *Taittiriya Upanishad* through *Pancha Kosha* theory. This theory is based on the five different layers of existence which have a counter impact on each other (*Annamaya*—physical body, *Pranamaya*—vital energy or pranic body, *Manomaya*—mental body, and *Vijnanamaya*—intellect or psychic body, and *Anandamaya Kosha*—super-conscious or blissful body) [93, 94]. Cardiometabolic syndrome is considered as a stress-induced disease disrupting the psycho-neuro-endocrine-immune system of the body. Yoga based on this philosophy acts at both mental and physical level to annul the pathophysiology of CMS [95]. *Ashtanga Yoga* (eight-fold path) of Rishi Patanjali explains various practical yogic techniques like *Bahiranga* (external) practices such as *yama, niyama, asana,* and *pranayama* help to build physical health while *antaranga* (internal) practices of pratyahara, *dharana, dhyana,* and *Samadhi* work on promoting mental health [96].

15.16 Obesity and Yoga

"Obesity" refers to an excessively high amount of body fat or adipose tissue accumulation resulting from energy intake that exceeds energy expenditure. This energy imbalance results from improper, inappropriate eating; consumption of large number of calories [97] associated with physical inactivity in association with stressful but sedentary lifestyles [98]. Both overweight (BMI of 25 kg/m) and obesity (BMI >30 kg/m ^{2}) are major epidemical risk factors in the occurrence of metabolic syndrome. Obesity is associated with over stimulation of the hypothalamic-pituitary-adrenal (HPA) axis [99] due to chronic stress [100] and metabolic abnormalities [101–103]. Obesity is associated with adipocyte hypertrophy, hyperplasia and inflammation. It is an independent predictor of cardiovascular disease, and mortality [104, 105].

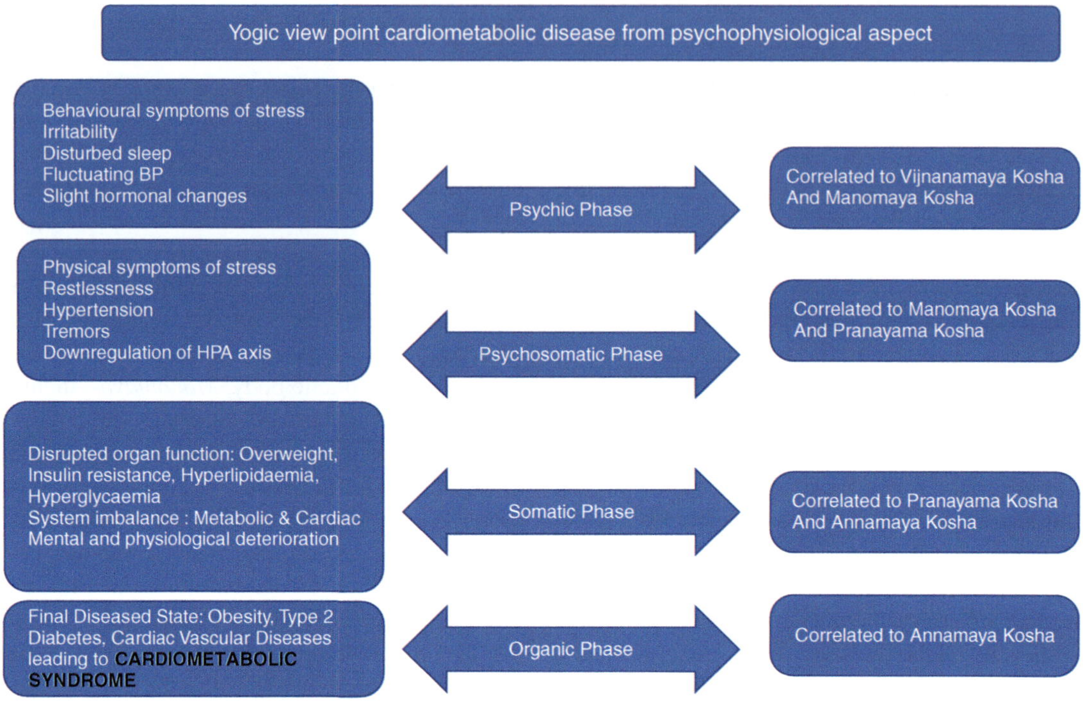

Fig. 15.1 Interrelation between yoga, cardiometabolic symptomatology, and Pancha Kosha Viveka Theory

Yogic physiological understanding on obesity is unlike western medicine that rotates more around the inappropriate mental states like anxiety, depression and stress fomenting pathophysiological changes that cause physical changes in the long run producing diseases and its manifestations. The Vedic philosophy of which yoga is a part considers the human body to be an integration of the mind, body, and soul. The Pancha Kosha theory as expressed above is a construct that has been available for thousands of years. While multiple layers of the human body part of this construct is not scientifically proven but the fact that many of these abnormalities are driven by inappropriate mental states including stress has been uncovered in the last one decade. Based on this thought and idea, obesity is considered a stress-induced disease-causing disturbance in the *Prana*—energy metabolism of the body. Thus stress in the mind—the so-called Manomaya kosha (mental layer) results in abnormalities at the Annayama—body [106–108].

Multiple clinical trials have substantiated that yoga induces relaxation and relieves stress but there is also attendant lowering of cortisol, [109] and other bad players including the cytokines [110]. Indirect benefit is seen due to lifestyle changes in both Diabetes and Hypertension [111]. We provide a few examples [112] here but they are dealt with more comprehensively in Chaps. 16 and 23.

There are numerous randomized controlled trials which show the reduction in body weight in obese urban population [113, 114].

Trials involving both short and long-term yoga practice have shown benefit albeit to different extent. Two studies collected data from various yoga camps which seemed encouraging, the first one where short-term yogic interventions of six days and five hours of practice with diet control showed decrease in BMI (1.6%), waist to hip ratio, fat free mass, total cholesterol (7.7%), high-density lipoprotein, cholesterol (8.7%), fasting serum leptin (44.2%), and an increase in postural stability and hand grip strength [115]. Another study in which 428 volunteers were assessed for seven days three hours daily the practice included breathing practices of pranayama (*bhastrika, kapalbhati, bahya,* and *anulom vilom*), meditation (*udgith*, OM recitation, and *pranav*) along with yoga postures. The volunteers attended the camps for 7 days (3 hours daily) during which they practiced the various breathing practices of *pranayam* (*bhastrika, kapalbhati, bahya,* and *anulom vilom*), meditation (*udgith,* OM recitation, and *pranav*), and undertook yoga postures. 65% had diabetes mellitus, 81 % had hypertension, 65% had hyperlipidemia, and 41% were obese and 21% had all four conditions. Post intervention results showed 56% patients lost weight, 38% hypertensive patients showed normal blood pressure recordings, 65% had decreased cholesterol among those who had hyperlipidemia [116]. Practice of yoga in the form of asanas, pranayama, and meditation for six months or more has shown better basal metabolic index, waist circumference and waist hip ratio. They have also been shown to curtail depression, and anxiety, thus a complete mind and body makeover [117].

Considerable evidence has accumulated that point to the effectiveness of yoga through the downregulation on the overactive hypothalamic-pituitary-adrenal axis (HPA) axis and the sympathetic adrenal medullary response to stress [118]. These leads to upregulation of anti-inflammatory markers like adiponectin.

A study by Lee et al, 2012 on sixteen post-menopausal women with more than 36% body fat who were assigned yogic training for sixteen weeks results showed significant decrease in body weight, percent body fat, lean body mass, body mass index, waist circumference, visceral fat area. On the other hand, adiponectin was significantly increased while blood pressure and cholesterol reduced significantly [119]. Another study by Supriya et al. 2017 on 52 patients with high BP and obesity were treated with one year of three hours a day yoga intervention the adiponectin levels in the yoga group increased by 20.1% [120].

On the other hand, leptin which is correlated to obesity, insulin resistance, and type 2 diabetes, showed significant reduction with regular yogic practice. Hatha Yoga exercise intervention on 26 obese women after 16 weeks of training showed significant reduction in serum leptin levels. This and other studies confirm that yoga induced correction of hormonal and cytokine aberrations in obesity [121]. In another study by Dilliraj et al, 2019 on obese adolescent students between 17 and 19 years of age who were given to perform a four-week suryanamaskar. The participants registered a decrease in serum leptin levels and BMI [122]. A study by Nikam et. al. concluded that practicing a group of five pranayama (*bhastrika pranayama, kapalbhati pranayama, bahya pranayama, anulom-vilom pranayama, and bhramari pranayama*) for a period of eight weeks significantly reduced the levels of lipid peroxidation and increased the activity of antioxidant enzymes [123]. Another study showed interesting but mixed results; effects of six weeks of high intensity yoga in healthy students did not significantly improve cardiovascular fitness but apolipoprotein A1 and adiponectin levels improved significantly compared to baseline. Findings suggest that yoga may have positive effects on blood lipids and an anti-inflammatory effect [124].

Similar results are note in other hormones that oppose the pathophysiological milieu in obesity. A study conducted on 79 centrally obese subjects suffering from metabolic syndrome of 58 ± 8 years of age a one-year yogic protocol showed significant increase in total circulating ghrelin and (control: −26%; yoga: +13%) decrease in obestatin hormones (control: +24%; yoga: −29%) [123] (Fig. 15.2).

15.17 Type 2 Diabetes and Yoga

A major growing epidemic among lifestyle related cardiometabolic risk diseases is type 2 diabetes. It is a common lifestyle disorder accompanied by an absolute or relative insulin resistance. This leads to hyperglycemia and also several cardiovascular difficulties if not treated and curbed. According to the International Diabetes Federation in 2017 there were an approximate 425 million people with diabetes, this figure projected to increase to 629 million by 2045 [125]. The causative risk factors of this disorder are quite related to obesity as all these are rooted under the cluster of metabolic diseases, thus physical inactivity, unhealthy eating habits, and psychological stress increase the severity of this disease, in fact lack of physical activity increases the risk of diabetes 3 times and risk of coronary disease 2.4 times [126].

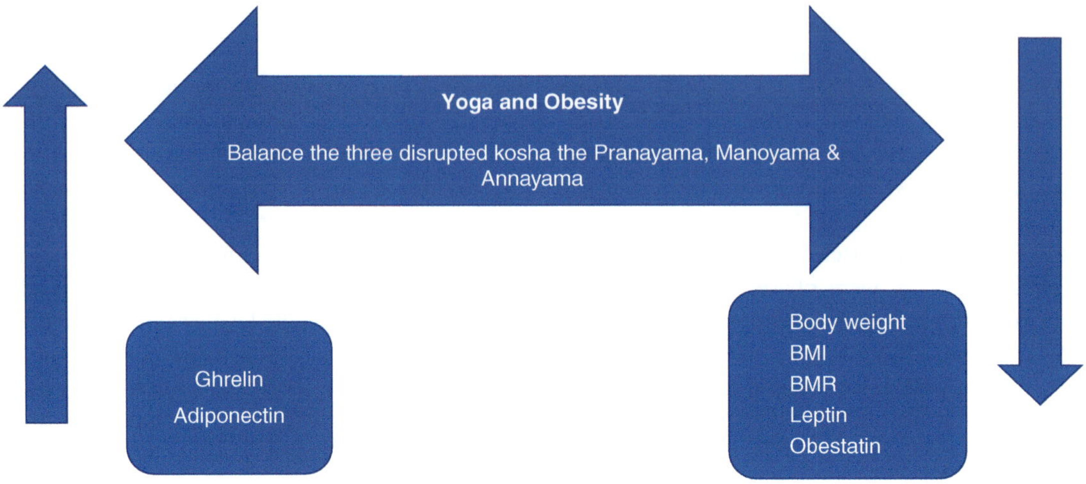

Fig. 15.2 Impact of yoga on obesity

Yoga creates an awareness of the body and mind, extensive research has shown biochemical, enzymatic, neurobiological, cellular, and genetic parameters to change positively with yogic practice. Yogic practice is based on a strict philosophy; it follows a code of conduct, a strict yogic diet, along with its various components which include cleansing process (*kriya*), postures (*asana*), controlled breathing (*pranayama*), meditation, relaxation, and chanting mantras [127, 128]. Diabetes mellitus however comes with a cluster of supplementary symptoms such as obesity, being physically unfit and having restricted joint mobility. While many of these problem circumvent from performing conventional physical activity [129]. It is different with yoga which is a more gentle for of exercise appropriate for all ages including elderly and those with mobility problems but equally effective [130].

There are enumerable research studies that shows yoga practice to be associated with better glycemic control. Effectiveness of mindfulness yoga on eating and exercise has shown positive impact on gestational diabetes [131], community based yogic interventions have proved to reduce oxidative stress [132], weight reduction [133], and lipid profile maintenance [134, 135].

Three months of yoga practice by 29 prediabetic patients resulted in significant decline in malondialdehyde ($p < 0.001$), relative to the control group, and a significant improvement in BMI, waist circumference, systolic blood pressure, and fasting glucose levels [136]. Another study measuring similar parameters but performed on 123 patients showed reduction in BMI, glycemic control, and malondialdehyde and increase in glutathione and vitamin C [137]. Pooled evidence of several studies confirms yoga's effectiveness in glycemic control and producing favorable lipid profiles [138–141] (Fig. 15.3).

Stress is ameliorated by the neurobiological benefits of *kriyas, jathis,* relaxation, and pranayama which also activates parasympathetic. Yoga is also known to improve heart rate variability responses measured by standard tests like the hand grip test and deep breathing test [142]. Yogic practices enhance vagal dominance through baroreflexes, muscle contraction, and breathing patterns. However, further researches on these are necessary [143]. Figure 15.3 illustrates the same.

In the second mechanism, yoga acts by downregulation of the HPA axis by reducing cortisol and catecholamines. It reduces perceived stress and HPA axis activation, thereby improving overall metabolic and psychological profiles, increasing insulin sensitivity, and improving glucose tolerance and lipid metabolism [144].

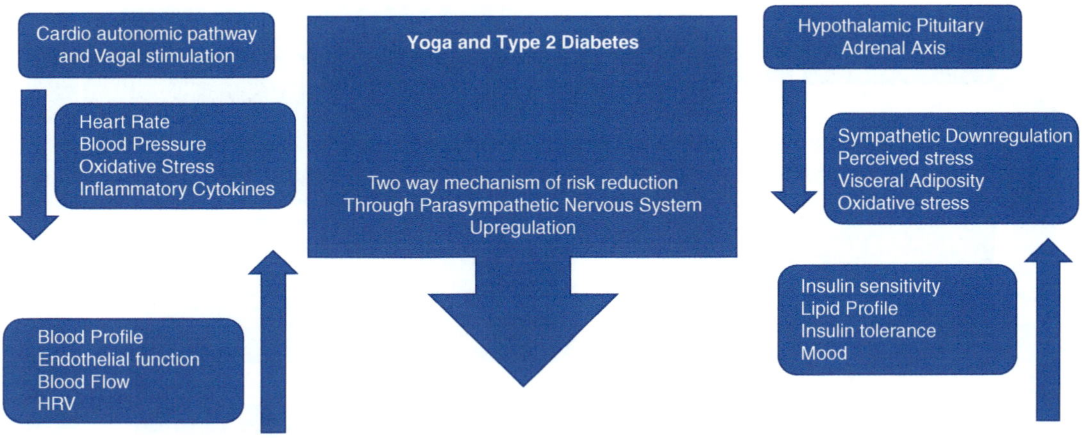

Fig. 15.3 Functional mind body mechanism in type two diabetics with practice of yoga

15.18 Cardiovascular Disease and Yoga

Cardiovascular diseases are a group of disorders associated with the heart and blood vessels, which include coronary heart disease, cerebrovascular disease and peripheral arterial disease. According to the WHO fact sheet 2017, CVDs are the number one cause of death globally [145]. Non-communicable diseases including coronary artery disease contribute to approximately 67% of global mortality and CVD is the number one cause of death and disability in the world [146, 147]. Yoga has been found to play a salutary role in both primary and secondary prevention of coronary artery disease (CAD). Chapter 19 details the current research on yoga and CAD.

15.19 Organokines and Yoga

Last few decades have discovered multiple bioactive molecules and their role in activating and inactivating the pathophysiological state of CMS. It is apparent that some of these are actually either activated or inactivated by Yogic practice. However more extensive studies are mandated to have a better understanding on the role and dose of yoga needed to curb the epidemic of non communicable diseases particularly CAD [148]. A few examples currently in evidence are elaborated below (Fig. 15.4).

15.19.1 Adipokines

It is important to understand the interaction of multiple chemokines and their activity in the pathophysiology of CMS to appreciate yoga's role. Obesity fosters secretion of adipokines from the adipose tissue. Adipose tissue dysfunction with decreased adipokine secretion produces obesity with metabolic, inflammatory, and cardiovascular complication [149, 150]. Adipokines such as leptin, adiponectin, tumor necrosis factor α (TNF-α), retinol binding protein 4 (RBP4), adipocyte fatty acid binding protein (A-FABP), resistin, vaspin, apelin, chemerin, omentin, and C1q/TNF-related proteins (CTRPs) are the main players involved in the spectrum of obesity-associated disorders [151, 152]. Detailed role of these entities are beyond the scope of this chapter but extensive date exists about their role in creation of the pathophysiological milieu in CMS [152–154].

In a study by Supriya et al. [120], revealed significant causing decrease in leptin, chemerin and increase in adiponectin concentrations in middle aged to 57+ 9 years metabolic syndrome affected male population with one year yoga training [155]. Even shorter interventions as low as fifteen days on an obese populations 36 = 11.2 years have shown decrease in BMI, waist circumference, hip circumference, lean mass, body water, and total cholesterol. The yoga group increased serum leptin ($p < 0.01$) and decreased LDL cholesterol ($p < 0.05$) [156]. Another short-term ten-day

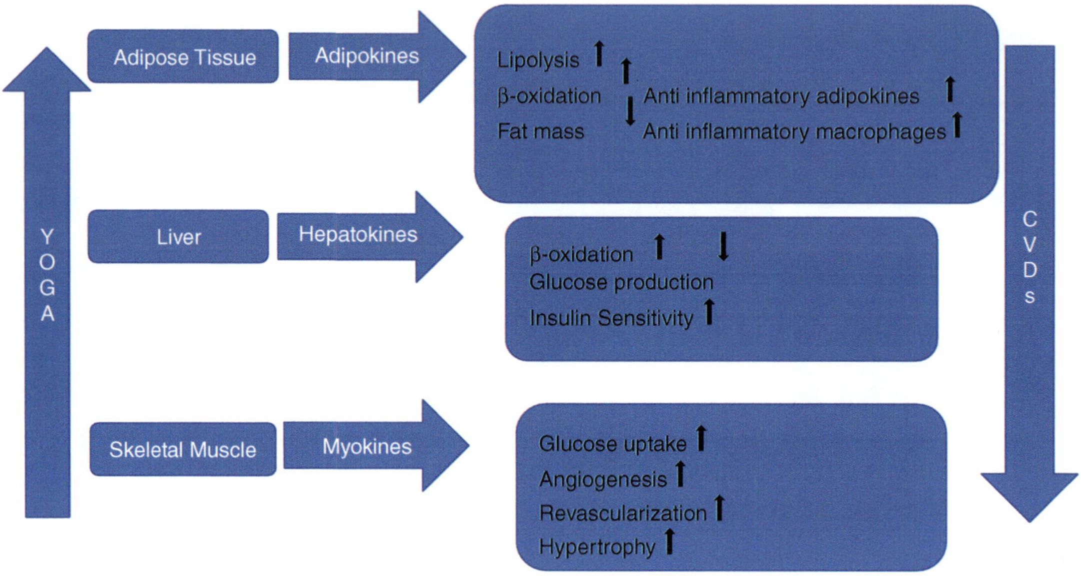

Fig. 15.4 Role of yoga on organokines to reduce cardiometabolic disorder

intervention of yoga asana and pranayama on 51 obese men measured primary positive outcome of significant weight loss, and the secondary outcome measures were clinical and laboratory correlates of CVD risk. This study concluded that yoga significantly reduced levels of interleukin-6 (IL-6) while adiponectin increased significantly, however endothelin-1 (ET-1) remained unchanged [157]. Endothelin it may be remembered is a vasoactive compound that increases vascular constriction and may play pathological roles in multiple conditions including hypertension and heart failure. These studies show that yoga practice begins to reflect instantaneous positive results which become more pronounced with passage of time and regular practice over the years.

15.19.2 Myokines

Myokines are proteins released from the skeletal muscle, mediated through physical exercise which affects skeletal muscle expression and the circulating myokine levels, such as IL-6, IL-15, angiopoietin-like 4, myostatin, and irisin [158]. IL-6 is one of the first myokines and it stimulates monocyte tissue factor production, provokes platelet hyperactivity, fibrinogen biosynthesis, enhances microparticle formation and erythrocyte aggregability. It suppresses proinflammatory cytokines and enhances anti-inflammatory mediators and antioxidants. However it level is increased in obesity and type II Diabetes indicating resistance to its action at the receptor or post receptor translation level. It is also true that many of the functions described in mice may not hold true for human. This remains an active research area where the exact role played by these new discovered molecules is far from clear [159]. Low-load resistance exercise like yoga also plays an advantageous role in thrombogenesis by reducing inflammatory processes and potentiating fibrinolytic features helping in reducing the risk of CVDs [160].

15.19.3 Hepatokines

Fetuin-A is a hepatokine that increases proinflammatory signaling and is increased during obesity, metabolic syndrome, and type 2 diabetes correlated with hepatic steatosis [161]. It increases the risk of myocardial infarctions and cardiac complexities [162, 163]. Yoga is known to increase the elaboration of Adiponectin which is reported to reduce hepatic Fetuin-A [164]. Another hepatokine is Selenoprotein P is positively correlated with insulin resistance, inflammation, and carotid thickness [165] in type 2 diabetic population and obese. However it has negative crosstalk with adiponectin, thus yoga can help improve adiponectin levels and reduce the secretions of selenoprotein P. Similary multiple hepatic enzymes have been discovered which is either increased or decreased with yoga but their exact function is unknown and thus their clinical significance is presently undetermined [166, 167].

15.20 Cardiovascular Diseases and Yoga Therapy

Research in the last decade has proved through multiple clinical trials the role of yoga in correcting the pathophysiological aberration and or symptomatology in various diseases [168].

15.20.1 Cardiac Autonomic Dysfunction

Autonomic dysfunction as elucidated by Heart Rate Variability (HRV) has been the hallmark of many cardiovascular disorders including heart failure and sudden cardiac death. In a systematic review of 59 studies with over 2358 patients; it was concluded that yoga increased HRV [143]. Brachial arterial reactivity improved after six weeks of yoga in a pilot study on patients with coronary artery disease [169]. Yoga has been shown to improve baroreflex sensitivity [170] and HRV [171].

15.20.2 Cardiac Arrhythmia

Lakkireddy et al. analyzed a three-month yogic program effect on 52 patients suffering with paroxysmal atrial fibrillation, anxiety and depression, and high blood pressure. Within the span of three months the numbers of symptomatic to asymptomatic atrial fibrillation episodes were significantly reduced, while BP, HR, anxiety, and depression scores were improved toward positive healthier outcomes [172]. Another study showed improved mental health scores in paroxysmal atrial fibrillation patients after twelve-week yoga intervention [173].

15.20.3 Coronary Artery Disease

Atherosclerosis manifested by fat accumulation in the blood vessel wall and vascular inflammation is the major cause of heart attacks and coronary deaths.

Secondary prevention for patients suffering from CAD includes lifestyle modifications to reduce risk of recurrent heart attack. Yoga has shown a strong correlation with decreasing risk factors for CAD. A study by Pal et al. performed randomized trial on 170 patients with CAD with yogic intervention for six months, there was significant reduction in blood pressure, HR, total cholesterol, triglycerides, LDL lipoproteins [174]. Cramer et al. showed similar but small benefit in angina scores [175]. Innes et al. [176] pooled 70 studies from 1970 to the year 2004 showing the improvement of insulin resistance, metabolic dysfunctions, and cardiovascular disease by reducing the activation of the sympathoadrenal system and HPA axis activity [144]. It is clearly evident that yoga while decreasing oxidative stress, vascular inflammation along with risk factor reduction is a strong management strategy along with modern medication to mitigate the fast increase in the CAD epidemic [177–179].

Ornish et al. [180], Manchanda et al. [181], and Yogendra et al. [182] led prospective, randomized and controlled trials on angiographically verified coronary artery disease patients with yoga intervention. All the studies showed regression in coronary lesions and enhancement in myocardial perfusions. Manchanda et al. also reported improvement in severe coronary artery symptomatic status and risk factor prolife. On the contrary to a life time change even short-term lifestyle changes and stress coping programs were seen to favor metabolic effects and reduce cardiometabolic risk elements [30].

It is beyond any doubt that comorbid mental condition like depression increase mortality in myocardial infarction. A meta-analytical study covering 3500 participants concluded that a three to six months yogic intervention improves anxiety and depression, these produce positive emotions which have a protective mediation against CAD [183]. Thus yoga remains one strategy that bring relief to both mental aberrations and the concomitant heart disease.

Manchanda et al. showed through multiple trials the role of yoga in primodial, primary and secondary prevention of CAD. Chapter 19 highlights those studies [181, 184]. Three controlled studies on advanced atherosclerotic coronary heart disease patients demonstrated that the practice of yoga and meditation with diet restrictions helped regression of coronary obstructions than in the experimental group [185–187].

15.20.4 Hypertension and Yoga

Several data and studies with controlled and uncontrolled show the effectiveness of yoga in treatment of hypertension [188–192]. In one randomized trial, yogic training as an antihypertensive therapy over an eleven-week period was found to be extremely effective [179]. A meta-analysis with nine RCTs pooled data on yoga and biofeedback have shown benefit in hypertension [193]. Although the reduction in blood pressure by yoga and meditation is modest, this could significantly decrease the risk of CVD, because it has been estimated that reducing systolic blood pressure by 3 mmHg in general population has the potential to reduce stroke mortality by 8 % and coronary heart disease (CHD) by 5% [194, 195]. The possible mechanism of reduction of blood pressure is considered to be reduced sympathetic activity and restoration of baroreceptor sensitivity by yoga [196]. Combined yoga practice for a period of six months significantly reduces basal metabolic rate in healthy adults which may be due to reduced psychophysiological arousal that is induced by stress and other mental aberrations all of which increase cardiovascular morbidity and mortality [197].

15.21 Cancer and Yoga

There has been evidence that poorly controlled metabolic syndromes like diabetes can promote oncogenesis or atleast help in proliferation of existing cancer cells thus aiding metastasis. It is thus unclear whether this is due to the disease itself or other factors. However better control of diabetes using lifestyle changes can certainly aid in decreasing such risk [198, 199]. Yoga independently plays a significant role in prevention of chemotherapy induced adverse effects and in multiple other pathways in oncogenesis and onco-proliferation which is beyond the topic of this chapter.

Quenching and decreased production of oxygen radicals also play an important role both in the process of metabolic aberrations and cancer pathophysiology [200].

15.22 Prophylactic Role of Yoga for Better Cardiometabolic Health

Research in the last few decades has completely modified our understanding of non communicable diseases. It has become apparent that psychosomatic illness as defined by modern medicine is very limited in its outlook. On the contrary a large of metabolic syndromes that is the largest causes of mortality and morbidity in the world including cardiovascular disease have a distinct underlying mental component that gives birth to and sustains the pathophysiology resulting in hypertension, diabetes mellitus Type II, stroke and coronary artery disease. Yoga by its essential philosophy derived from ancient Indian medical tradition called Ayurveda is the original so called "Mind-Body" medicine that correctly defines certain illness based on its psycho-physiological basis but also spells therapy accordingly. The failure of western medicine to quell these non-communicable disease pandemic have spurred research in to yoga and its effect [90, 94]. This new orientation in modern medicine have evoked an understanding of the role of stress a mental aberration and its physiological correlate which is essentially a chronic inflammatory reaction that lead to heart diseases and diabetes.

The concept of positive health was first introduced by Charaka. Charaka is widely considered one of the fathers of the ancient Indian medical system called Ayurveda. He is also the compiler of "Charaka Samhita" a foundation text of Ayurveda. According to Charaka body, mind, and soul, these three entities of human being are like a tripod; the human is sustained by their combination, they constitute the substratum for everything [204]. Mind–Body medicine is thus an inherent foundational concept in ayurveda. Yoga which is a part and parcel of ayurvedic therapeutics focuses on lifestyle changes, breathing techniques and mind control measures that not only bring physical diseases to culmination but also roots out the psychological causes like stress [92, 97, 205].

The ancient thinkers of India never regarded man as a mere biological entity, rather conglomerate being; where mind and body energy play a role to keep one healthy [97, 205]. In recent times psychology also accepted this basic aspect to recognize the correlation between the body and mind interaction as a whole [129, 205]. Peoples' lifestyle has undergone drastic changes in modern times, adversely affecting their health and happiness in many ways. Yoga is proving to be a boon in coping with the stresses and disorders caused by undesirable lifestyle changes [94]. The recognition of the mind–body relationship by the scientific medical community, Yoga has increasingly become a part of modern medicine [30, 64]. Mind, when it is disturbed, may make the body prone to psychophysiological disturbance (vikshepa) leading to incoordination between various organs thus lowering the efficiency of the body. According to Yoga mind has a very significant role to play not only in psychosomatic diseases, but also in every other form of disease, including the acute ones [90].

Traditional Yoga holds mental and bodily processes as mutually interdependent phenomena. From the Yogic view, the mind, the body, and consciousness are not held as separate entities. Therefore, structure and function of the human body is believed to be dictated by the effect of the mind at both psychological level and physical level (releasing neurotransmitters and hormones which act at the physical level) and conscious energy called "Prana". Prana is considered both an energy as well as a means of consciousness that pervades the mind-body complex to enable it to work in perfection. Thus any disruption in this mind-body-prana complex leads to a disease. Thus in Ayurveda the therapy is also directed towards all these three parameters. While the mind-body angle has got accepted in modern medicine giving credence to yoga as a viable complementary to actually treat diseases, the "consciousness-prana-energy" correlates is still be validated based on western medicine's reductionist principles. The practice of yoga thus assimilates three different levels. It invokes fitness in the body through physical postures called asanas. It balances the energy or prana through different breathing techniques cumulatively called "pranayama". It controls the mind and its vagaries through techniques like dharana (mindfulness) and dhyana (meditation). The yoga scriptures goes a step further and brings in the ability to change "consciousness" by attaining the so called "samadhi" [92, 97, 206]. The practice of *kriya, surya namaskara, and asana* (physical level), *pranayama* (psychophysiological level), and *meditation* (psycho-neurological level) integrates and harmonies mind and body to provide an ideal cardiometabolic health. A brief understanding of these different techniques is described below.

***Yamas* (Social Discipline) and *Niyamas* (Personal Discipline)** Yama and Niyama are initial two limbs of Yoga known as attitude forming yoga practices. Yamas' are certain rules of self-disciplines to train and regulate one's behavioral attitude toward social problems. Certainly, a particular positive attitude can be expressed as discipline, which then influences to modulate right behavior. Patanjali's yoga sutra mentions five different yamas, that is, behavior patterns or relationships between the individual and the outside world. Thus the yamas are the moral virtues or ethical code of conducts, for a normal healthy living. Niyamas are the rules or personal code of conducts prescribed for personal observation. Like the five yamas, the niyamas are not exercises or action to be simply studied. They are a set if behavioral and attitudinal correlates that every human being needs to follow to ensure a healthy and happy existence at both mental and physical level. The main objective of these vows is to eliminate all mental and emotional disturbances and help the aspirant to achieve metal stability which is believed to be a basic necessity for a disease free physical existence [90, 205, 207].

Yogic Kriyas Schools of Hatha Yoga begin with the practice of Kriyas or cleaning processes, usually classified into six divisions which consist of many subsections. These are Neti (nasal cleansing), Kapalbhati (force rapid breathing to ventilate and cleanse air passages), Dhauti (stomach wash), Basti (colon flushing), Nauli (manipulations of abdominal muscles to increase peristalsis), and Trataka (cleansing of the eye through steady gazing). They bring in control over the autonomic nervous system. The aim of the hatha yoga and therefore of the shatkarmas is to create harmony between the two major pranic flows, ida and pingala for attaining physical and mental balance. These ancient techniques are also used to balance the three doshas or humors in the body kapha (mucus) pitta (bile) and vata (wind). According to Ayurveda and hatha yoga, an imbalance of the doshas will result in illness. The nervous, digestive, respiratory, and excretory systems are very important to maintain our homeostasis so that the individual is able to maintain proper health and this is taken care of by these cleansing processes. Detailed understanding of the concepts of ayurveda is beyond the scope of this book. Readers are referred to other specialized writings [109, 110].

Suryanamaskar Surya Namaskara, or salutation to the sun, is an important yogic exercise which has been handed down from the sages of Vedic times. Surya Namaskara contains asana, pranayama, and meditational techniques all incorporated within the practice [208]. Sinha et al. [209] measured the energy cost and cardiovascular changes in healthy male volunteers during the practice of surya namaskara. They reported total energy cost throughout the practice of surya namaskar was 13.91 Kcal and at an average of 3.79 Kcal/min. During surya namaskara practice highest heart rate was recorded 101.6 ± 13.5 H/m. It is said that surya namaskar seemed to be ideal as an aerobic exercise as it involves both static stretching and slow dynamic component of exercise with optimal stress on the cardiorespiratory system [209]. Bhutkar et al. [210] studied the effect of surya namaskara on cardiorespiratory fitness. They found after 6 months of surya namaskara training, pulse rate, blood pressure reduced significantly and endurance measures by 40 mm endurance test increased significantly in both the male and female groups [210].

Asana Asanas are psycho-physical practices to culture the body and mind for further higher practices of yoga like *pranayama, pratyahara, dhyana,* etc. Patanjali's yoga sutra defines asana as that which is comfortable and easy, as well as firm. These are certain special pattern of postures that increase energy expenditure, improve long-term cardiorespiratory fitness (VO_2 max), oxidative capacity of skeletal muscles [211] and stabilize the mind and body [90]. They aim at establishing proper rhythm in the neuromuscular tonic impulses and improving the general tone of the muscles. The psycho-physiological advantages of asana are based on the following five principles [109, 110].

1. The use of gravity: The inverted postures such as the handstand, shoulder stand, and the reverse posture take advantage of gravity to increase the flow of blood to the desired part of the body.
2. Organ Massage: Different types of asana postures have a squeezing action on a specific organ or gland, resulting in the stimulation of that part of the body.
3. Stretching of the muscles, joints, and ligaments promotes the nerve conduction velocity, flexibility of the muscle, joint range of the motion, muscular endurance and strength, energy level, etc.

4. Deep breathing during yoga posture increases the oxygen supply to the target organ or gland, thereby enhancing the effect of asana.
5. Concentration as well as breathing slowly and deeply, we also focus our attention on the target organ or gland. This brings the mind into play, and greatly increases the circulation and energy supply to the organ or gland [90, 109, 110, 129, 212].

Pranayama Pranayama essentially is a voluntary control on the breathing process that is said to bring control over a wildly racing mind. Aberrant thoughts and emotions bring about physical damage secondary to elaboration of multiple cytokines and sympathetic over activity. Practice of pranayama quietens the mind and help control damaging emotions. Generally, it involves the manipulation of respiration beyond its normal limit, stretching it, speeding it up, and slowing it down in order to experience the full range of respiration on both gross and subtle levels. Traditional yogic texts claim that regular practice of pranayama has a direct effect on all the vital systems of the body. It has been reported that the state of arousal, attention, mental task, emotional disturbance, and behavioral pattern greatly influence our breathing pattern. During pranayama the different phases of breathing, puraka (inhalation), kumbhaka (holding), and rechaka (exhalation) are consciously made slow, deeper, and rhythmic to endow with calmness, quietness, tranquility, hemispheric balance, autonomic balance, psychosomatic balance, psychophysiological relaxation, and sense of well-being to the mind [90, 207, 213]. In physiological point of view pranayama are of two types: hypoventilation and hyperventilation. For example, *bhastrika* and *kapalbhati* may be considered as hyperventilatory type of pranayama. The rapid and deep breathing increases the alveolar ventilation, respiratory rate, heart rate, blood pressure, oxygen consumption, body temperature, and metabolic rate. While the hypoventilating techniques are generally tranquilizing pranayama (*anulom vilom, ujjayi, sheetali, sheetkari,* etc.) and their effect is just opposite to hyperventilation. It slightly increases the carbon dioxide levels (CO_2), reduces cardiorespiratory parameters, metabolic rate and frequency of brain waves. By the practice of kumbhaka, a controlled phase of holding the breath, more time is available for the exchange of gases between the blood and air which is beneficial for releasing CO_2 from active cells and put forth a positive physiological effect on cardiorespiratory parameters [95]. Scientific exposition on pranayama or yogic breathing elicits a positive effect on neurocognitive, neuroendocrine, cardiorespiratory, and biochemical efficiency in both the physiologic and clinical setups [170, 213, 214].

Bandha (Bind or Lock) and Mudra (Gesture) Mudra and Bandha are special features of hatha yoga generally practiced with the combination of asana and pranayama. Bandhas are included during the practice of pranayama particularly during the kumbhaka phase. Both mudra and bandha are essentially a voluntary contraction of a particular neuromuscular junction or sphincters of the body [94, 95].

Dharana (Concentration) and Dhyana (Contemplation) Multiple processes are detailed in yoga philosophy that leads to deep meditation (Dhyana) which based on the philosophy leads to higher levels of consciousness (samadhi). These processes include keeping the mind off unwanted thoughts-Pratyahara. Concentration and Mindfulness-Dharana and Meditation-Dhyana. Researches in the last few decades have shown multiple benefits of meditation. Regular practice of meditation reduced metabolic rate, heart rate, oxygen consumption, and increases carbon dioxide output. Calmness of mind is achieved with control over damaging emotions including anxiety, stress and depression. Mind is less distracted and swayed by external events and therefore calmer and worriless. Meditator will be able to solve day-to-day problems better and have more success in whatever activity undertaken [215]. Several studies have shown that meditation has positive effect on brain function and structure. Some early studies reported that meditation practice was associated with a decrease in oxygen consumption; reduced breath rate, heart rate, blood lactate, maintained blood pressure and an increase in slow alpha and occasional theta waves. Evidence shows that mindfulness meditation can increase both cortical thickness and gray matter, particularly in areas controlling emotional regulation and executive functioning. Meditation also improves the function of neurotransmitters (BDNF, GABA, melatonin, serotonin, etc.) and reduces the oxidative stress and over inflammation in the body. Meditation is believed to gradually diminish sympathetic dominance, resulting in a better balance in autonomic nervous system and hypothalamo-pituitary-adrenal axis [96]. It also brings about a hypometabolic state [97]. By modifying the state of tension and anxiety, mediation reduces stress induced sympathetic over reactivity [96, 99, 100]. Thus, a decrease in sympathetic response and ability to overcome stress can be a possible reason for the restoration of cardiometabolic health.

15.23 Conclusion

Now it may be concluded that integrated or separate approach of yoga techniques (*Yamas* and *Niyams, Yogic Diet, Kriya, Suryanamaskar, Asana, Pranayama, Bandha, Mudra, Dharana* and *Dhyana*) can improve quality of life, reduce the risk indices of cardiometabolic syndrome, and successfully prevent and manage cardiometabolic diseases, however research demands more in-depth study (clinical and therapeutic) for strong support. We hope that this evidence-based traditional-scientific approach will unfold some fundamental concept and set a direction for future research.

References

1. World Health Organization. WHO global recommendations on physical activity for health. Geneva: World Health Organization; 2010.
2. Riebe D, Franklin BA, Thompson PD, Garber CE, Whitfield GP, Magal M, Pescatello LS. Updating ACSM's recommendations for exercise preparticipation health screening. Medicine & Science in Sports & Exercise. Copyright 2015 by the American College of Sports Medicine.
3. 2018 Physical Activity Guidelines Advisory Committee. 2018 Physical Activity Guidelines Advisory Committee scientific report [Internet] [cited 2019 Apr 29]. Rockville MD. U.S. Department of Health and Human Services; 2018. Available from https://health.gov/paguidelines/second-edition/report/.
4. Cotman CW, Berchtold NC, Christie LA. Exercise builds brain heakey roles of growth factor cascades and inflammation. Trends Neurosci. 2007;30(9): 464–72.
5. Dishman RK, O'Connor PJ. Lessons in exercise neurobiology: the case of endorphins. Mental Health Phys Activity. 2009;2(1):4–9.
6. WHO. Noncommunicable diseases progress monitor, vol. 46. Geneva: World Health Organization; 2017.
7. WHO. Global status report on noncommunicable diseases: "Attaining the nine global noncommunicable disease targets; a shared responsibility.". World Health Organization, Geneva, Switzerland; 2014.
8. Baygi F, Herttua K, Jensen OC, Djalalinia S, Ghorabi AM, Asayesh H, Qorbani M. Global prevalence of cardiometabolic risk factors in the military population: a systematic review and meta-analysis. BMC Endocrine Disorders. 2020;20:8.
9. Einarson TR, Acs A, Ludwig C, Pantom UH. Prevalence of cardiovascular disease in type 2 diabetes: a systematic literature review of scientific evidence from across the world in 2007–2017. Cardiovasc Diabetol. 2018;17:83.
10. Hajar R. Risk factors for coronary artery disease: historical perspectives. Heart Views. 2017 Jul–Sep;18(3):109–14.
11. Gundu HR. Cardiometabolic diseases: a global perspective. J Cardiol Cardiovasc Ther. 2018;12(2):555834.
12. Gallagher EJ, LeRoith D, Karnieli E. The metabolic syndrome—from insulin resistance to obesity and diabetes. Endocrinol Metab Clin N Am. 2008;37:559–79.
13. Kraemer FB, Ginsberg HN, Reaven GM. Demonstration of the central role of insulin resistance in type 2 diabetes and cardiovascular disease. Diabetes Care. 2014 May;37(5):1178–81.
14. Himsworth H. Diabetes Mellitus: a differentiation into insulin-sensitive and insulin-insensitive types. Lancet. 1936;1:127–30.
15. National Diabetes Data Group. Report of the expert committee on glucosylated hemoglobin. Dibets Care. 1984;7:602–6.
16. Reaven GM. Banting lecture 1988. Role of insulin resistance in human disease. Diabetes. 1988;37:1595–607.
17. Vecchio I, Tornali C, Bragazzi NL, Martini M. The discovery of insulin: an important milestone in the history of medicine. Front Endocrinol (Lausanne). 2018 Oct 23;9:613.
18. Unwin N. The metabolic syndrome. J R Soc Med. 2006 Sep;99(9):457–62.
19. Alberti KG, Zimmet PZ. Definition, diagnosis and classification of diabetes mellitus and its complications. Part 1: diagnosis and classification of diabetes

mellitus provisional report of a WHO consultation. Diabet Med. 1998;15:539–53.
20. Balkau B, Charles MA. Comment on the provisional report from the WHO consultation. European Group for the Study of Insulin Resistance (EGIR). Diabet Med. 1999;16:442–3.
21. Expert Panel on Detection, Evaluation, and Treatment of High Blood Cholesterol in Adults. Executive Summary of the Third Report of The National Cholesterol Education Program (NCEP) Expert Panel on Detection, Evaluation, And Treatment of High Blood Cholesterol in Adults (Adult Treatment Panel III). JAMA. 2001;285:2486–97.
22. Einhorn D, Reaven GM, Cobin RH, Ford E, Ganda OP, Handelsman Y, Hellman R, Jellinger PS, Kendall D, Krauss RM, Neufeld ND, Petak SM, Rodbard HW, Seibel JA, Smith DA, Wilson PW. American College of Endocrinology position statement on the insulin resistance syndrome. Endocr Pract. 2003;9:237–52.
23. Alberti KG, Zimmet P, Shaw J. The metabolic syndrome: a new worldwide definition. Lancet. 2005;366:1059–62.
24. Grundy SM, Brewer HB Jr, Cleeman JI, Smith SC Jr, Lenfant C. Definition of metabolic syndrome: report of the National Heart, Lung, and Blood Institute/American Heart Association conference on scientific issues related to definition. Arterioscler Thromb Vasc Biol. 2004;24:e13–8.
25. Kassi E, Pervanidou P, Kaltsas G, Chrousos G. Metabolic syndrome: definitions and controversies. BMC Medicine. 2011;9:48.
26. Alberti KG, Eckel RH, Grundy SM, Zimmet PZ, Cleeman JI, Donato KA, Fruchart JC, James WP, Loria CM, Smith SC Jr, et al. Harmonizing the metabolic syndrome: a joint interim statement of the International Diabetes Federation Task Force on Epidemiology and Prevention; National Heart, Lung, and Blood Institute; American Heart Association; World Heart Federation; International Atherosclerosis Society; and International Association for the Study of Obesity. Circulation. 2009;120:1640–5.
27. Chatterjee A, Harris SB, Leiter LA, Fitchett DH, Teoh H, Bhattacharyya. Managing cardiometabolic risk in primary care: Summary of the 2011 consensus statement. Can Family Phys. 2012;58:389–93.
28. Eriksson J, Taimela S, Koivisto VA. Exercise and metabolic syndrome. Diabetologia. 1997;40:125–35.
29. Bhavanani AB. Role of yoga in prevention and management of lifestyle disorders. Yoga Mimamsa. 2017;49:42–7.
30. Bijlani RL, Vempati RP, Yadav RK, Ray RB, Gupta V, Sharma R, et al. A brief but comprehensive lifestyle education program based on yoga reduces risk factors for cardiovascular disease and diabetes mellitus. J. Altern Complement Med. 2005;11:267–74.
31. Physical Activity Guidelines Advisory Committee Report, 2008. To the Secretary of Health and Human Services. Part A: executive summary. Nutr Rev. 2009;67:114–20.
32. Guthold R, Stevens GA, Riley LM, Bull FC. Worldwide trends in insufficient physical activity from 2001 to 2016: a pooled analysis of 358 population-based surveys with 1·9 million participants. Lancet Glob Health. 2018;6:e1077–86.
33. Vincent GE, Jay SM, Sargent C, Vandelanotte C, Ridgers ND, Ferguson SA. Improving cardiometabolic health with diet, physical activity, and breaking up sitting: what about sleep? Front Physiol. 2017 Nov 8;8:865.
34. Grundy SM, Brewer HB Jr, Cleeman JI, et al. Definition of metabolic syndrome: report of the National Heart, Lung, and Blood Institute/American Heart Association conference on scientific issues related to definition. Circulation. 2004;109: 433–8.
35. Lawlor DA, Ebrahim S, Davey SG. The metabolic syndrome and coronary heart disease in older women. Findings from the British Women's Heart and Health Study. Diabetic Med. 2004;21:906–13.
36. Ravikiran M, Bhansali A, Ravikumar P, Bhansali S, Dutta P, Thakur JS, et al. Prevalence and risk factors of metabolic syndrome among Asian Indians: a community survey. Diabetes Res Clin Pract. 2010;8:269–73.
37. Colley RC, Garriguet D, Janssen I, Craig CL, Clarke J, Tremblay MS. Physical activity of Canadian adults: accelerometer results from the 2007 to 2009 Canadian Health Measures Survey. Health Rep. 2011;22:7.
38. Killgore WD. Human sleep and cognition: basic research. In: Kerkhof GA, Van Dongen HPA, editors. Progress in brain research, vol. 185. New York: Elsevier Science; 2010. p. 105–29.
39. Copinschi G, Leproult R, Spiegel K. The important role of sleep in metabolism. Front Horm Res. 2014;42:59–72.
40. Knutson KL. Impact of sleep and sleep loss on glucose homeostasis and appetite regulation. Sleep Med Clin. 2007;2:187–97.
41. Besedovsky L, Lange T, Born J. Sleep and immune function. Pflügers Arch Eur J Physiol. 2012;463:121–37.
42. Steiger A. Sleep and endocrine regulation. Front Biosci. 2003;8:s358–76.
43. Watson N, Badr M, Belenky G, Bliwise D, Buxton O, Buysse D, et al. Recommended amount of sleep for a healthy adult: a joint consensus statement of the American Academy of Sleep Medicine and Sleep Research Society. J Clin Sleep Med. 2015;38:843–4.
44. Centers for Disease Control Prevention. Unhealthy sleep-related behaviors 12 States, 2009. MMWR. 2011;60:233.
45. Schmid SM, Hallschmid M, Schultes B. The metabolic burden of sleep loss. Lancet Diabetes Endocrinol. 2015;3:52–62.

46. Manjunath NK, Telles S. Influence of yoga and Ayurveda on self-rated sleep in a geriatric population. Indian J Med Res. *2005*;121(5):683–90.
47. Patra S, Telles S. Positive impact of cyclic meditation on subsequent sleep. Med Sci Monit. 2009;15(7):CR375–81.
48. Ebrahimi M, Guilan-Nejad TN, Pordanjani AF. Effect of yoga and aerobics exercise on sleep quality in women with Type 2 diabetes: a randomized controlled trial. Sleep Sci. 2017 Apr–Jun;10(2):68–72.
49. Xu H, Li X, Hannah A, Kubena K, Guo S. Etiology of metabolic syndrome and dietary intervention. Int J Mol Sci. 2018 Dec 31;20(1):128.
50. Untangle food industry influences on health. Nat Med 2019;25:1629.
51. Swami D, Kokaje RS. Hatha pradipika of Svatmarama. 2nd ed. Lonavla, Pune, India: Kaivalyadhama, S.M.Y.M. Samiti; 1998.
52. Ramos-Jiménez A, Wall-Medrano A, Corona-Hernández RI, Hernández-Torres RP. Yoga, bioenergetics and eating behaviors: A conceptual review. Int J Yoga. 2015 Jul-Dec;8(2):89–95.
53. McIver S, McGartland M, O'Halloran P. Overeating is not about the food: women describe their experience of a yoga treatment program for binge eating. Qual Health Res. 2009;19:1234.
54. Carei TR, Fyfe-Johnson AL, Breuner CC, Brown MA. Randomized controlled clinical trial of yoga in the treatment of eating disorders. J Adolesc Health. 2010;46:346–51.
55. Jhon W, Newcomer MD. Metabolic syndrome and mental illness. Am J Manag Care. 2017;13:S170–7.
56. Li R, Jia Z, Trush MA. Defining ROS in biology and medicine. React Oxyg Species (Apex). 2016;1(1):9–21.
57. Forrester SJ, Kikuchi DS, Hernandes MS, Xu Q. Griendling. Reactive oxygen species in metabolic and inflammatory signaling. Circ Res. 2018;122(6):877–902.
58. Simioni C, Zauli G, Martelli AM, Vitale M, Sacchetti G, Gonelli A, Neri LM. Oxidative stress: role of physical exercise and antioxidant nutraceuticals in adulthood and aging. Oncotarget. 2018;9(24):17181–98.
59. Krikwood K, Rampes H, Tuffery V, Richardson J, Pilkington K. Yoga for anxiety: a systematic review of the research. Br J Sports Med. 2005;39:884–91.
60. Mehta P, Sharma M. Yoga as a therapy for clinical depression. Complement Health Pract Rev. 2010;15(3):156–70.
61. Wallace RK, Benson H, Wilson AF. A wakeful hypometabolic physiologic state. Am J Physiol. 1971;221:795–9.
62. Benson H, Beary JF, Carol MP. The relaxation response. Psychiatry. 1974;37:37–46.
63. Riley KE, Park CL. How does yoga reduce stress? A systematic review of mechanisms of change and guide to future inquiry. Health Psychol Rev. 2015;9(3):379–96.
64. Telles S, Singh N, Gupta RK, Balkrishna A. A selective review of dharana and dhyana in healthy participants. J Ayurveda Integr Med. 2016;7(4):255–60.
65. Dunn SL, Siu W, Freund J, Boutcher SH. The effect of a lifestyle intervention on metabolic health in young women. Diabetes Metab Syndr Obes. 2014 Sep 19;7:437–44.
66. Ki NK, Lee HK, Cho JH, Kim SC, Kim NS. Factors affecting metabolic syndrome by lifestyle. J Phys Ther Sci. 2016;28(1):38–45.
67. Vancampfort D, Hallgren M, Mugisha J, Hert MD, Probst M, Monsieur D, Stubbs B. The Prevalence of metabolic syndrome in alcohol use disorders: a systematic review and meta-analysis. Alcohol Alcohol. 2016;51(5):515–21.
68. Kuppili PP, Parmar A, Gupta A, Balhara YPS. Role of yoga in management of substance-use disorders: a narrative review. J Neurosci Rural Pract. 2018 Jan–Mar;9(1):117–22.
69. Kirk EP, Klein S. Pathogenesis and pathophysiology of the cardiometabolic syndrome. J Clin Hypertens (Greenwich). 2009;11(12):761–5.
70. Castro JP, El-Atat FA, McFarlane SI, Aneja A, Sowers JR. Cardiometabolic syndrome: pathophysiology and treatment. Curr Hypertens Rep. 2003;5(5):393–401.
71. Blaton V. How is metabolic syndrome related to the dyslipidemia? EJIFCC. 2007 Feb;18(1):15–22.
72. Ebbert JO, Jensen MD. Fat depots, free fatty acids, and dyslipidemia. Nutrients. 2013 Feb;5(2):498–508.
73. Gadde KM, Martin CK, Berthoud HR, Heymsfield SB. Obesity: pathophysiology and management. J Am Coll Cardiol. 2018;71(1):69–84.
74. Ruotolo G, Howard BV. Dyslipidemia of the metabolic syndrome. Curr Cardiol Rep. 2002 Nov;4(6):494–500.
75. Shapiro MD, Fazio S. Apolipoprotein B-containing lipoproteins and atherosclerotic cardiovascular disease. F1000Res. 2017 Feb 13;6:134.
76. Carson JS, Lichtenstein AH, Anderson CA, Appel LJ, Kris-Etherton PM, Meyer KA, Petersen K, Polonsky T, Horn LV. Dietary cholesterol and cardiovascular risk: a science advisory from the American Heart Association. Circulation. 2020;141:e39–53.
77. Sperling LS, Mechanick JI, Neeland IJ, et al. The Cardio Metabolic Health Alliance: working toward a new care model for metabolic syndrome. J Am Coll Cardiol. 2015;66(9):1050–67.
78. Priest C, Tontonoz P. Inter-organ cross-talk in metabolic syndrome. Nat Metab. 2019;1:1177–88.
79. Kim JH. Increased serum angiopoietin-like 6 ahead of metabolic syndrome in a prospective cohort study. Diabetes Metab J. 2019;43:521–9.
80. Berger A. Resistin: a new hormone that links obesity with type 2 diabetes. BMJ. 2001 Jan 27;322(7280):193.
81. Steppan CM, Bailey ST, Bhat S, Brown EJ, Banerjee RR, Wright CW, Patel HR, Ahima RS, Lazar

MA. The hormone resistin links obesity to diabetes. Nature. 2001;409(6818):307–12.
82. Han C, Rice MW, Cai D. Neuroinflammatory and autonomic mechanisms in diabetes and hypertension. Am J Physiol Endocrinol Metab. 2016 Jul 1;311(1):E32–41.
83. Münzberg H, Qualls-Creekmore E, Berthoud HR, Morrison CD, Yu S. Neural control of energy expenditure. Handb Exp Pharmacol. 2016;233:173–94.
84. Xu Y, Zhang Y, Ye J. IL-6: a potential role in cardiac metabolic homeostasis. Int J Mol Sci. 2018 Aug 21;19(9):2474.
85. Huang Z, Chen X, Chen D. Myostatin: a novel insight into its role in metabolism, signal pathways, and expression regulation. Cell Signal. 2011 Sep;23(9):1441–6.
86. Longhi S, Radetti G. Thyroid function and obesity. J Clin Res Pediatr Endocrinol. 2013;5(Suppl 1):40–4.
87. Sanyal D, Raychaudhuri M. Hypothyroidism and obesity: an intriguing link. Indian J Endocrinol Metab. 2016 Jul–Aug;20(4):554–7.
88. Ibrahim Abdalla MM. Ghrelin - physiological functions and regulation. Eur Endocrinol. 2015 Aug;11(2):90–5.
89. Ndumele CE, Pradhan AD, Ridker PM. Interrelationships between inflammation, C-reactive protein, and insulin resistance. J Cardiometab Syndr. 2006;1(3):190–6.
90. Kuvalayananda S, Vinekar SL. Yogic therapy basic principles and methods. Twari OP, Kaivalyadhama, Lonavla, India; 2019 (reprinted).
91. Nagarathna R, Nagendra HR. Yoga for hypertension and heart diseases. 2002 (reprinted). Bangalore, India: Vivekananda Yoga Research Foundation, Swami Vivekananda Yoga Prakashana.
92. Bhavanani AB. Yoga: The original mind body medicine. 2012. https://www.researchgate.net/publication/237077700
93. Bhavanani AB. Yoga is not an intervention but may yogopathy is. J Yoga. 2012;5(20):157–8.
94. Nagarathna R, Nagendra HR. Integrated approach of yoga therapy for positive health. Bangalore, India: Swami Vivekananda Yoga Prakashana; 2006.
95. Saraswati SM. Prana Pranayama Prana Vidya. Munger, Bihar, India: Yoga Publication Trust; 2002.
96. Rosmand R, Dallman MF, Bjorntorn P. Stress related cortisol secretion in men: relationships with abdominal obesity and endocrine, metabolic and hemodynamic abnormalities. Clin Endocrinol Metab. 1998;83(6):1853–9.
97. Bhavanani AB. Yogic perspectives of mental health. Ann SBV. 2014;3(1):47–52.
98. Mumukshananda S. Meditation and its preparation. Kolkata, India: The Ramakrishna Mission Institute of Culture; 2000.
99. Bjorntorp P. Neuroendocrine factors in obesity. J Endocrinol. 1997;155:193–5.
100. Björntorp P. The regulation of adipose tissue distribution in humans. Int J Obes Relat Metab Disord. 1996;20:291–302.
101. Kyrios M, Moore SM, Hackworth N, Buzwell SA, Crafti N, Critchley C, et al. The influence of depression and anxiety on outcomes after an intervention for prediabetes. Med J Aust. 2009;190:S81–5.
102. Dhananjai S, Sadashiv TS, Kumar R. Effect of a yoga practice in the management of risk factors associated with obesity: a pilot study. ISRJ. 2011;1:1–4.
103. Sohl SJ, Wallston KA, Watkins K, Birdee GS. Yoga for risk reduction of metabolic syndrome: patient reported outcomes from a randomized controlled pilot study. Evid Based Complement Alterat Med. 2016;2016:3094589.
104. Teychenne M, Ball K, Salmon J. Associations between physical activity and depressive symptoms in women. Int J Behav Nutr Phys Act. 2008; 5:27.
105. Dunn AL, Trivedi MH, Kampert JB, Clark CG, Chambliss HO. Exercise treatment for depression: efficacy and dose response. Am J Prev Med. 2005;28:1–8.
106. WHO Expert Consultation. Appropriate body mass index for Asian populations and its implications for policy and intervention strategies. Lancet. 2004;363:157–63.
107. Bray GA. Medical consequences of obesity. J Clin Endocrinol Metab. 2004;89:2583–9.
108. Taittiriyopanisad SS. Ch. 2: 1-6. Chennai: Shree Ramakrishna Publication; 2008. p. 88–134.
109. Hatha S. Yoga Pradipika of Svatmarama. Adyar: Adyar Library and Research Centre; 1994.
110. Digambarji S, Gharote ML. Gherenda Samhita. Lonavla: SMYM Samiti; 1978.
111. Parshad O. Role of yoga in stress management. West Indian Med J. 2004;53(3):191–4.
112. Yadav RK, Magan D, Mehta N, Sharma R, Mahapatra SC. Efficacy of a short term yoga based lifestyle intervention in reducing stress and inflammation: preliminary results. J Altern Complement Med. 2012;18:662–7.
113. Cozzolino D, Sasso FC, Cataldo D, Gruosso D, Giammarco A, Cavalli A, et al. Acute pressor and hormonal effects of beta-endorphin at high doses in healthy and hypertensive subjects: role of opioid receptor agonism. J Clin Endocrinol Metab. 2005;90:5167–74.
114. Rathi SS, Raghuaram N, Tekur P, Joshi RR, Ramarao NH. Development and validation of integrated yoga module for obesity in adolescents. Int J Yoga. 2018;11(3):231–8.
115. Rshikesan PB, Subramanyam P, Nidhi R. Yoga practice for reducing the male obesity and weight related psychological difficulties: a randomized controlled trail. J Clin Diagn Res. 2016;10:22–8.
116. Cramer H, Thoms MS, Anheyer D, Lauche R, Dobos G. Yoga in women with abdominal obesity: a randomised control trial. Dtsch Arztebl Int. 2016;30(113):654–2.
117. Telles S, Naveen VK, Balkrishna A, Kumar S. Short term health impact of yoga and diet change program on obesity. Med Sci Monit. 2010;16(1):CR35–40.

118. Gokal R, Shilliton L, Maharaj SR. Positive impact of yoga and pranayama on obesity, hypertension, blood sugar and cholesterol: a pilot assessment. J Alter Complemet Med. 2007;13(10):1056–7.
119. Dhananjai S, Sadashiv TS, Dutt K, Kumar R. Reducing psychological distress and obesity through yoga practice. Int J Yoga. 2013;6(1):66–70.
120. Ross A, Thomas S. The health benefits of yoga and exercise: a review of comparison studies. J Alter Complement Med. 2010;16(1):3–12.
121. Lee JA, Kim JW, Kim Y. Effects of yoga exercise on serum adiponectin and metabolic syndrome factors in obese postmenopausal women. Menopause. 2012;19(3):296–301.
122. Supriya R, et al. Yoga decreases anti-inflamatory adipokine in metabolic syndrome, high BP. Scand J Med Sci Sports. 2017;28(3):1130–8.
123. Lee JA, Kim D. Effects of Hatha yoga exercise on serum leptin and metabolic syndrome factors in menopause obese middle-aged women. Journal of life scence. 2010;20(7):1100–6.
124. Dilliraj G, Shanthi B, Kalai Selvi VS. Effects of yoga on "leptin-the satiety hormone" in the fight against the global threat-"obesity". Scholars Acad J Biosci. 2019; https://doi.org/10.21276/sajb.2019.7.2.5.
125. Yu AP, Ugwu FN, Tam BT, Lee PH, Lai CW, CSC W, Lam WW, Sheridan S, Sui PM. One year of Yoga training alters Ghrelin Axis in centrally obese adults with metabolic syndrome. Front Phsiol. 2018;9:1321.
126. Papp ME, Lindfors P, Nygren-Bonnier M, Gullstrand L, Wandell PE. Effects of high-intensity hatha yoga on cardiovascular fitness, adipocytokines and apolipoproteins in healthy students: a randomized controlled study. J Altern Complement Med. 2016;22(1):81–7.
127. International Diabetes Federation, Chapter 3, The global picture. In: IDF Diabetes Atlas. 8th ed. Brussels: International Diabetes Federation; 2017. p. 40–59.
128. Thangasami SR, Chandani AL, Thangasami S. Emphasis of yoga in the management of diabetes. J Diabetes Metab. 2015;6:613.
129. Khalsa SB. Yoga as a therapeutic intervention: a bibliometric analysis of published research studies. Indian J Physiol Pharmacol. 2004;48:269–85.
130. Raveendran AV, Deshpande A, Joshi SR. Therapeutic role of yoga in type 2 diabetes. Endocrinol Metab (Seoul). 2018;33(3):307–17.
131. Ramachandran A, Snehalatha C, Mary S, Mukesh B, Bhaskar AD, Vijay V, Indian Diabetes Prevention Programme (IDPP). The Indian Diabetes Prevention Programme shows that lifestyle modification and metformin prevent type 2 diabetes in Asian Indian subjects with impaired glucose tolerance (IDPP-1). Diabetologia. 2006;49:289–97.
132. Sahay BK. Role of yoga in diabetes. J Assoc Physicians India. 2007;55:121–6.
133. Youngwanichsetha S, Phumdoung S, Ingkathawornwong T. The effects of mindfulness eating and yoga exercise on blood sugar levels of pregnant women with gestational diabetes mellitus. Appl Nurs Res. 2014;27(4):227–30.
134. Hegde SV, Adhikari P, Shetty S, Manjrekar P, D'Souza V. Effect of community-based yoga intervention on oxidative stress and glycemic parameters in prediabetes: a randomized controlled trial. Complement Ther Med. 2013;21:571–6.
135. Rioux JG, Ritenbaugh C. Narrative review of yoga intervention clinical trials including weight-related outcomes. Altern Ther Health Med. 2013;19: 32–46.
136. Shantakumari N, Sequeira S, El deeb R. Effects of a yoga intervention on lipid profiles of diabetes patients with dyslipidemia. Indian Heart J. 2013;65:127–31.
137. Hedge SV, Adhikari P, Shetty S, Manjrekar P, D'Souza V. Effect of community-based yoga intervention on oxidative stress and glycemic parameters in prediabetes: a randomized controlled trial. Complement Ther Med. 2013;21(6):571–6.
138. Hegde SV, Adhikari P, Kotian S, Pinto VJ, D'Souza S, D'Souza V. Effect of 3-month yoga on oxidative stress in type 2 diabetes with or without complications. Diabetes Care. 2011;34(10):2208–10.
139. Telles S, Naveen VK, Balkrishna A. Serum leptin, cholesterol and blood glucose levels in diabetics following a yoga and diet change program Comment to: Statins and beta-cell function Lei Qian, Lihong Xu, Yi Lin, Yongde Peng Med Sci Monit 2010;16:HY1-2. Med Sci Monit. 2010;16:LE4–5.
140. Amita S, Prabhakar S, Manoj I, Harminder S, Pavan T. Effect of yoga-nidra on blood glucose level in diabetic patients. Indian J Physiol Pharmacol. 2009;53:97–101.
141. Aljasir B, Bryson M, Al-Shehri B. Yoga practice for the management of Type II diabetes mellitus in adults: a systematic review. Evid Based Complement Alternat Med. 2010;7:399–408.
142. Singh S, Kyizom T, Singh KP, Tandon OP, Madhu SV. Influence of pranayamas and yoga-asanas on serum insulin, blood glucose and lipid profile in type 2 diabetes. Indian J Clin Biochem. 2008;23:365–8.
143. Cohen BE, Chang AA, Grady D, Kanaya AM. Restorative yoga in adults with metabolic syndrome: a randomized, controlled pilot trial. Metab Syndr Relat Disord. 2008;6:223–9.
144. Vinutha HT, Raghvendra BR, Manjumanth NK. Effect of integrated approach of yoga therapy on autonomic functions in patients with type 2 diabetes. Indian J Endocrinol Metab. 2015;19(5):653–7.
145. Tyagi A, Cohen M. Yoga and heart rate variability: a comprehensive review of the literature. Int J Yoga. 2016;9(2):97–113.
146. Innes KE, Vincent HK. The influence of yoga-based programs on risk profiles in adults with type 2 diabetes mellitus: a systematic review. Evid Based Complement Alternat Med. 2007;4:469–86.
147. Cardiovascular Diseases (CVDs) - World Health Organization www.who.int › Newsroom › Fact

sheets › Detail. https://www.who.int/news-room/fact-sheets/detail/cardiovascular-diseases-(cvds).
148. World Health Organization. Prioritizing a preventable epidemic. A primer for the media on non-communicable diseases; 2011. Available from http://www.wpro.who.int/noncommunicable_diseases/ncd_primer.pdf.
149. Daubenmier JJ, Weidner G, Sumner MD, Mendell N, Merritt-Worden T, Studley J, et al. The contribution of changes in diet, exercise, and stress management to changes in coronary risk in women and men in the multisite cardiac lifestyle intervention program. Ann Behav Med. 2007;33(1):57–68.
150. Sarvottam Kand Yadav RK. Obesity-related inflammation & cardiovascular disease: efficacy of a yoga-based lifestyle intervention. Indian J Med Res. 2014;139(6):822–34.
151. Kloting N, Bluher M. Adipocyte dysfunction, inflammation and metabolic syndrome. Rev Endocr Metab Disord. 2014;15:277–87.
152. Yoo HJ, Choi KM. Adipokines as a novel link between obesity and atherosclerosis. World J Diabetes. 2014;5:357–63.
153. Oh JY. Regional adiposity, adipokines, and insulin resistance in type 2 diabetes. Diabetes Metab J. 2012;36:412–4.
154. Fasshauer M, Bluher M. Adipokines in health and disease. Trends Pharmacol Sci. 2015;36:461–70.
155. Xu A, Vanhoutte PM. Adiponectin and adipocyte fatty acid binding protein in the pathogenesis of cardiovascular disease. Am J Physiol Heart Circ Physiol. 2012;302:H1231–40.
156. Kralisch S, Fasshauer M. Adipocyte fatty acid binding protein: a novel adipokine involved in the pathogenesis of metabolic and vascular disease? Diabetologia. 2013;56:10–21.
157. Supriya R, Yu AP, Lee PH, Lai CW, Cheng KK, Yau SY, Chan LW, Yung BY, Siu PM. Yoga training modulates adipokines in adults with high-normal blood pressure and metabolic syndrome. Scand J Med Sci Sports. 2018;28(3):1130–8.
158. Telles S, Sharma SK, Yadav SN, Balkrishna A. A comparative controlled trial comparing the effects of yoga and walking for overweight and obese adults. Med Sci Monit. 2014;20:894–904.
159. Sarvottam K, Magan D, Yadav RK, Mehta N, Mahapatra SC. Adiponectin, Interleukin-6, and cardiovascular disease risk factors are modified by a short-term yoga-based lifestyle intervention in overweight and obese men. J Altern Complement Med. 2013;19(5):397–402.
160. Catoire M, Kersten S. The search for exercise factors in humans. FASEB J. 2015;29:1615.
161. Eckardt K, Gorgens SW, Raschke S, Eckel J. Myokines in insulin resistance and type 2 diabetes. Diabetologia. 2014;57:1087–99.
162. Chen YW, Apostolakis S, Lip GYH. Exercise-induced changes in inflammatory processes: Implications for thrombogenesis in cardiovascular disease. Ann Med. 2014;46(7):439–55.
163. Iroz A, Couty JP, Postic C. Hepatokines: unlocking the multiorgan network in metabolic diseases. Diabetologia. 2015;58:1699–703.
164. Weikert C, Stefan N, Schulze MB, Pischon T, Berger K, Joost HG, et al. Plasma fetuin-a levels and the risk of myocardial infarction and ischemic stroke. Circulation. 2008;118:2555–62.
165. Ix JH, Wassel CL, Kanaya AM, Vittinghoff E, Johnson KC, Koster A, et al. Fetuin-A and incident diabetes mellitus in older persons. JAMA. 2008;300:182–8.
166. Choi KM, Han KA, Ahn HJ, Lee SY, Hwang SY, Kim BH, et al. The effects of caloric restriction on fetuin-A and cardiovascular risk factors in rats and humans: a randomized controlled trial. Clin Endocrinol (Oxf). 2013;79:356–63.
167. Yang SJ, Hwang SY, Choi HY, Yoo HJ, Seo JA, Kim SG, et al. Serum selenoprotein P levels in patients with type 2 diabetes and prediabetes: implications for insulin resistance, inflammation, and atherosclerosis. J Clin Endocrinol Metab. 2011;96: E1325–9.
168. Kharitonenkov A, Adams AC. Inventing new medicines: the FGF21 story. Mol Metab. 2013;3:221–9.
169. Gimeno RE, Moller DE. FGF21-based pharmacotherapy: potential utility for metabolic disorders. Trends Endocrinol Metab. 2014;25:303–11.
170. Stephens I. Medical yoga therapy. Children. 2017;4:12.
171. Sivasankaran S, Pollard-Quintner S, Sachdeva R, Pugeda J, Hoq SM, Zarich SW, et al. The effect of a six-week program of yoga and meditation on brachial artery reactivity: Do psychosocial interventions affect vascular tone? Clin Cardiol. 2006;29: 393–8.
172. Bernardi L, Porta C, Spicuzza L, Bellwon J, Spadacini G, Frey AW, et al. Slow breathing increases arterial baroreflex sensitivity in patients with chronic heart failure. Circulation. 2002;105:143–5.
173. Madanmohan, Bhavanani AB, Prakash ES, Kamath MG, Amudhan J. Effect of six weeks of savasana training on spectral measures of short-term heart rate variability in young healthy volunteers. Indian J Physiol Pharmacol. 2004;48:370–3.
174. Lakkireddy D, Atkins D, Pillarisetti J, et al. Effect of yoga on arrhythmia burden, anxiety, depression, and quality of life in paroxysmal atrial fibrillation: the YOGA My Heart Study. J Am Coll Cardiol. 2013;61(11):1177–82.
175. Wahlstrom M, Rydell Karlsson M, Medin J, Frykman V. Effects of yoga in patients with paroxysmal atrial fibrillation—a randomized controlled study. Eur J Cardiovasc Nurs. 2017;16:57–63.
176. Pal A, Srivastava N, Tiwari S, et al. Effect of yogic practices on lipid profile and body fat composition in patients of coronary artery disease. Complement Ther Med. 2011;19(3):122–7.
177. Cramer H, Lauche R, Haller H, Dobos G, Michalsen A. A systematic review of yoga for heart disease. Eur J Prev Cardiol. 2015;22(3):284–95.

178. Innes KE, Bourguignon C, Taylor AG. Risk indices associated with the insulin resistance syndrome, cardiovascular disease, and possible protection with Yoga: a systematic review. J Am Board Fam Pract. 2005;18:491–519.
179. Manna I. Effects of yoga training on body composition and oxidant-antioxidant status among healthy male. Int J Yoga. 2018;11(2):105–10.
180. Shore R, Foster C, Pein R, Seebach E. Comparison of blood pressure lowering interventions. J Cardiopulm Rehabil. 2002;22:361–3.
181. Murugesan R, Govindarajulu N, Bera TK. Effect of selected yogic practices on the management of hypertension. Indian J Physiol Pharmacol. 2000;44:207–10.
182. Nikam SV, Nikam PS, Suryakar AN, Badade ZG, Nikam K. Effect of pranayama practice on lipid peroxidation and antioxidants in coronary artery disease. Int J Biol Med Res. 2010;1(4):153–7.
183. Ornish D, Brown SE, Scherwitz LW, Billings JH, Armstrong WT, Ports TA, et al. Can lifestyle changes reverse coronary heart disease? The Lifestyle Heart Trial. Lancet. 1990;336:129–33.
184. Manchanda SC, Narang R, Reddy KS, Sachdeva U, Prabhakaran D, Dharmanand S, Rajani M, Bijlani R. Retardation of coronary atherosclerosis with yoga lifestyle intervention. J Assoc Phys India. 01 Jul 2000;48(7):687–94.
185. Yogendra J, Yogendra HJ, Ambardekar S, Lele RD, Shetty S, Dave M, et al. Beneficial effects of yoga lifestyle on reversibility of ischaemic heart disease: caring heart project of International Board of Yoga. J Assoc Physicians India. 2004;52:283–9.
186. Goyal M, Singh S, Sibinga EM, Gould NF, Rowland-Seymour A, Sharma R, et al. Meditation programs for psychological stress and well-being: a systematic review and meta-analysis. JAMA Intern Med. 2014;174:357–68.
187. Manchanda SC, Naranag R, Reddy KS, Sachdeva U, Prabhakaran D, Dharmanand S, et al. Reversal of coronary atherosclerosis by yoga lifestyle intervention. Front Cardiovasc Health. 2000;2000:535–47.
188. Eraballi A, Raghuram N, Ramarao NH, Pradhan B, Rao PV. Yoga based lifestyle program in improving quality of life after coronary artery bypass graft surgery: a randomised controlled trial. J Clin Diagnostic Res. 2018;12(3):5–9.
189. Schmidt T, Wijga A, Von Zur MA, Brabant G, Wagner TO. Changes in cardiovascular risk factors and hormones during a comprehensive residential three month kriya yoga training and vegetarian nutrition. Acta Physiol Scand Suppl. 1997;640:158–62.
190. Gupta SK, Sawhney RC, Rai L, Chavan VD, Dani S, et al. Regression of coronary atherosclerosis through healthy lifestyle in coronary artery disease patients–Mount Abu open heart trial. Indian Heart J. 2011;63:461–9.
191. Datey KK, Deshmukh SN, Dalvi CP, Vinekar SL. "Shavasan": a yogic exercise in the management of hypertension. Angiology. 1969;20(6):325–33.
192. Sundar S, Agrawal SK, Singh VP, Bhattacharya SK, Udupa KN, Vaish SK. Role of yoga in management of essential hypertension. Acta Cardiol. 1984;39(3):203–8.
193. Bagga OP, Gandhi A. A comparative study of the effect of Transcendental Meditation (TM) and Shavasana practice on cardiovascular system. Indian Heart J. 1983;35(1):39–45.
194. Parati G, Steptoe A. Stress reduction and blood pressure control in hypertension: a role for transcendental meditation? J Hypertens. 2004;22(11): 2057–60.
195. Rana Singh RK, Singh VK. Clinical evaluation of some yogic practices in the management of essential hypertension. Indian Med J. 2013;107(3):105.
196. Anderson JW, Liu C, Kryscio RJ. Blood pressure response to transcendental meditation: a meta-analysis. Am J Hypertens. 2008;21(3):310–6.
197. Stamler J, Rose G, Stamler R, Elliott P, Dyer A, Marmot M. INTERSALT study findings. Public health and medical care implications. Hypertension. 1989;14(5):570–7.
198. Appel LJ. Lifestyle modification as a means to prevent and treat high blood pressure. J Am Soc Nephrol. 2003;14(7 Suppl 2):S99–S102.
199. Selvamurthy W, Sridharan K, Ray US, Tiwary RS, Hegde KS, Radhakrishan U, et al. A new physiological approach to control essential hypertension. Indian J Physiol Pharmacol. 1998;42(2): 205–13.
200. Chaya MS, Kurpad AV, Nagendra HR, Nagarathna R. The effect of long term combined yoga practice on the basal metabolic rate of healthy adults. BMC Complement Altern Med. 2006;6:28.
201. Boroughs LK, DeBerardinis RJ. Metabolic pathways promoting cancer cell survival. Nat Cell Biol. 2015;17:351–9.
202. Ward PS, Patel J, Wise DR, Abdel-Wahab O, Bennett BD, Coller HA, et al. The common feature of leukemia-associated IDH1 and IDH 2 mutations is a neurotrophic enzyme activity converting alpha-ketoglutarate to 2-hydroxyglutarate. Cancer Cell. 2010;17:225–34.
203. Korniluk A, Koper O, Kemona H, Dymicka-Piekarska V. From inflammation to cancer. Ir J Med Sci. 2017;186(1):57–62.
204. Mondal S. Science of exercise: ancient Indian origin. J Assoc Phys india. 2013;61:560–2.
205. Bhogal RS. Yoga and mental health and beyond. Lonavla, India: Published by Twari OP, Kaivalyadhama; 2018.
206. Chatterjee S, Mondal S. Modern theories of aging and contribution of yoga in its prevention – a critical review. Yoga Mimamsa. 2009;41(1):34–7.
207. Gore MM. Anatomy and Physiology of Yogic Practices, 4th revised and enlarged edition, 2019 (reprinted). Delhi, India: New Age Books.
208. Saraswati SS. Surya Namaskara: a technique of solar vitalization. Munger, Bihar, India: Yoga Publication Trust; 2007.

209. Sinha B, Ray US, Pathak A, Selvamurthy W. Energy cost and cardiovascular changes during the practice of Surya Namaskar. Indian J Physiol and Pharmacol. 2004;48:184–90.
210. Bhutkar PM, Bhutkar MV, Taware GB, Doijad V, Doddamani BR. Effect of suryanamaskar practice on cardio-respiratory fitness parameters: a pilot study. Al Ameen J Med Sci. 2008;1(2):126–9.
211. Ray US, Pathak A, Tomer OS. Hatha yoga practices: energy expenditure, respiratory changes and intensity of exercise. Evid Based Complement Altern Med. 2011;2011:241294.
212. Coulter HD. Anatomy of Hatha Yoga. Delhi, India: Motilal Banarasidass Publishers Private Limited; 2001.
213. Maheshananda S, Kulkarni DD. Scientific exposition on pranayama: a review. Pali, Rajasthan, India: Chouhan GS, Arogyadhama; 2012.
214. Saoji AA, Raghavendra BR, Manjunath NK. Effects of yogic breath regulation: a narrative review of scientific evidence. J Ayurveda Integr Med. 2019;10:50–8.
215. Telles S, Gerberg P, Kozasa EH. Editorial: physiologic effects of mind and body practices. Biomed Res Int. 2015;2015:983068.

16 Role of Yoga in Prevention and Management of Type 2 Diabetes Mellitus (T2DM) and Its Complications

Kashinath Metri, R Nagaratna and Amit Singh

16.1 Introduction

Diabetes Mellitus metabolic disorder characterized by chronic hyperglycemia due to decreased production and/or utilization of insulin is a leading cause of morbidity and mortality worldwide [1]. Type 2 Diabetes Mellitus (T2DM) contributes to 90% of diabetes mellitus cases. The global prevalence of T2DM has risen in the last three decades. A recent survey of 540 data from 111 countries reported that around 415 million people aged 20–79 years have T2DM, and it was estimated to increase to 642 million (uncertainty interval: 521–829 million) by 2040. India and China are the top [2] countries with the maximum number of people with T2DM [3]. Around 7.6% of the Indian population has T2DM [4].

Long-standing T2DM leads to complications such as cardiovascular disease (CVD) and cerebrovascular disease apart from neuropathy, retinopathy, and nephropathy [5, 6].

Unhealthy lifestyle is an important factor contributing to the increasing prevalence of both T2DM. Sedentary job, unhealthy diet, unmanaged chronic psychological stress, improper sleeping habits are the major factors. Hence, lifestyle modification is emphasized in most chronic health conditions, including T2DM.

Yoga is a form of mind–body practice and has become a popular complementary therapy in most of the countries across the globe [7]. Yoga emphasizes a healthy lifestyle promoting moderation in diet, adequate physical activity, healthy behavior, and adequate sleep in addition to practice of physical postures, a set of breathing techniques, relaxation techniques, and meditation [8, 9].

16.2 Yoga and Blood Glucose Control in T2DM

Blood glucose control is the primary objective in T2DM management. Optimal blood glucose control decreases the risk of diabetic complications [10] and enhances the quality of life in T2DM [11, 12].

Yoga improves fasting and postprandial blood glucose level in T2DM [13–15]. A large number of RCT studies have shown that yoga is effective in reducing HbA1C levels in T2DM [16]. A meta-analysis study has concluded that yoga can

K. Metri (✉)
Department of Yoga, Central University of Rajasthan, Bandar Sindri, Ajmer, Rajasthan, India
e-mail: kashinath@curaj.ac.in

R. Nagaratna · A. Singh
Division of Yoga and life Science, Swami Vivekanand Yoga Anusandhan Samsthan (SVYASA University), Bangalore, India

I. Basu-Ray, D. Mehta (eds.), *The Principles and Practice of Yoga in Cardiovascular Medicine*,
https://doi.org/10.1007/978-981-16-6913-2_16

be a potential intervention to reduce blood glucose in T2DM [17]. In a multicentric study, 3 months of intense yoga intervention produced a significant decrease in fasting and postprandial blood glucose by 32.6% & 34.7% respectively, in patients with T2DM [18]. Yoga also helps in reducing anti-diabetic medication/insulin requirement [19] and delays the progression of the disease [20]. It reduces insulin resistance and improves insulin sensitivity in patients with T2DM [21–23]. Various yogic postures and *sukshmavyamas* increase glucose uptake and reduce insulin resistance [24, 25].

Yoga helps in reducing the following T2DM indices:

- Fasting blood glucose
- Postprandial blood glucose
- Glaciated hemoglobin
- Insulin resistant

16.3 Yoga as a Preventive Measure for T2DM

As mentioned earlier, an unhealthy lifestyle is considered to be an important cause for T2DM in addition to age and genetic predisposition. Yoga is also a lifestyle that promotes health and helps prevent modern lifestyle-related diseases including T2DM. An unhealthy lifestyle contributes to weight gain, Obesity, reduced insulin sensitivity, and elevated blood pressure; these are the major risk factors for T2DM. Yoga helps in weight management, it reduces BMI, waist circumference, and hip circumference. Obesity is the most important risk factor for T2DM. Numerous scientific studies on yoga have reported the efficacy of yoga in correcting several obesity indices such as BMI, waist–hip ratio, and abdominal obesity among subjects with obesity. Further, Various psychological factors such as chronic stress, depression, anxiety, etc. are the potential risk factor for T2DM.

Yoga is an effective intervention for stress management; meditation and pranayama are simple and effective measures to reduce the stress and stress effects, instantly. Yoga reduces depression and anxiety, and improves the mood and psychological well-being. [26] by regulating hypothalamic–pituitary–adrenal (HPA) axis and it also enhances mood enhancer serotonin and GABA (Gama Acetyl Butyric acid) in the brain.

A randomized controlled study on patients with pre-diabetic conditions demonstrated the reduction in BMI, waist circumference, hip circumference, oral glucose tolerance, blood glucose level, and blood pressure following 8 weeks of yoga intervention, suggesting the preventive potential of yoga for T2DM. In a study significant decrease in the blood glucose level was observed in both diabetic and non-diabetic participants following 6 months of the yoga intervention compared to the baseline, this study suggests that yoga not only helps in reducing blood glucose levels, it is also a potential preventive measure for T2DM [27]. Another randomized controlled study of subjects at high risk of T2DM showed that following 3 months of yoga practice, there was a decrease in insulin mean insulin level, lipid profile, systolic and diastolic blood pressure, and fasting blood glucose level [28].

Yoga helps in improving the following risk factors of T2DM in healthy and pre-diabetes conditions:

- Fasting and postprandial blood glucose
- Anthropometric indices—Body mass index, waist circumference, hip circumference, Glaciated hemoglobin
- Insulin resistant
- Improves insulin sensitivity
- OGTT
- Chronic stress, depression, and anxiety

16.4 Cardio-Protective Effects of Yoga in T2DM

Cardiovascular disease (CVD) has been a major cause of mortality in T2DM. The prevalence of CVD and its severity is higher among T2DM patients compared to the controls. Patients with T2DM have a 2 times greater risk of cardiac disease compared to non-diabetic people [29]. The most prominent cardiac risk factors such as hypertension, dyslipidemia, obesity, systemic inflammation, and atherosclerosis are highly prevalent in T2DM patients. Patients with T2DM have a 4 times greater risk of hypertension, two times greater risk of dyslipidemia, and two times greater risk of atherosclerosis compared to controls which makes them more prone to CVD. Hypertension is the most common, independent, and preventable risk factor for CVD. Yoga is an effective method to improve blood pressure, many studies have shown that yoga reduces blood pressure and medication score, and prevents cardiac risk in hypertension [30]. It reduces blood pressure among T2DM patients as well. Yoga improves CVD risk factor indices [31].

> Yoga helps in improving following cardiac risk factors in T2DM:
>
> Systolic and diastolic blood pressure
> Insulin resistance
> Blood cholesterol (improves HDL)
> BMI, waist circumference, hip circumference, and obesity
> Stress, depression, and anxiety

Yoga also corrects dyslipidemia in T2DM. A 3-month yoga intervention reduced triglycerides, low-density lipoprotein (LDL), and cholesterol with an increase in high-density lipoprotein (HDL) in patients with T2DM.

A randomized controlled trial on patients with T2DM showed a significant decrease in blood glucose (FBS, PPBS, and HbA1C) level, dyslipidemia and increase in HDL cholesterol following 9 months of yoga intervention [19].

Chronic hyperglycemia in T2DM is associated with endothelial dysfunction, eventually leading to atherosclerosis and CVD. Atherosclerosis has been an important and independent cause of CVD, it increases the risk of CVD by two folds. Dyslipidemia is the major contributor to atherogenesis in T2DM.

Yoga improves dyslipidemia (reduce triglycerides, LDL, HDL, total cholesterol, and increase HDL). In a randomized controlled study 3 months yoga interventions demonstrated the reduction in dyslipidemia in T2DM patients. Evidence from several RCTs suggests that yoga reduces atherosclerotic plaque.

Anthropometric measures such as BMI, waist circumference, hip circumference are associated with increased risk of CVD. Yoga reduces BMI, waist circumference, and hip circumference among T2DM patients [26].

Endothelial dysfunction in T2DM leads to atherosclerosis. There are studies that showed a regression in atherosclerosis following yoga practice in patients with coronary artery disease [31]. A study found improvement in carotid artery lumen diameter following yoga intervention among patients with carotid artery stenosis [32], which suggests the potential benefits of yoga in reducing the risk of stroke [33].

T2DM increases the risk of T2DM by four folds.

Yoga improves dyslipidemia, blood pressure, BMI, and waist circumference which are considered to be independent risk factors for CAD [34–36].

Yoga reduces blood pressure in hypertensive individuals. Several RCTs have documented the decrease in the systolic, diastolic, and mean arterial blood pressure following yoga in hypertension [17, 37, 38]. Studies have also reported a decrease in antihypertensive medication requirements following yoga practices. Their RCT studies documented the improvement in blood pressure after yoga intervention among T2DM patients suggestive of yoga as a potential intervention to reduce cardiac risk factors in T2DM [39].

16.5 Prevention of T2DM Complication Through Yoga

Diabetic neuropathy and diabetic nephropathy are the most common complications of T2DM. Scientific evidence on yoga has shown its potential protective effect for diabetic neuropathy. Optimal control of blood glucose level is associated with decreased incidences of diabetic neuropathy and diabetic nephropathy in T2DM.

Yoga help in improving blood glucose levels in T2DM; thus, it is effective in the prevention of diabetic neuropathy and it also improves nerve conduction velocity among patients with T2DM [40]. Yoga reduces blood pressure and blood glucose level in T2DM which are the most important cause of diabetic nephropathy. Yoga improves variability indices of chronic kidney disease.

16.6 Cognitive Enhancement in T2DM Through Yoga

The patients with T2DM often experience cognitive impairment and dementia. Eventually, T2DM leads to severe forms of memory loss, such as in Alzheimer's disease [41]. Many longitudinal studies have reported the increased risk of cognitive decline among T2DM compared to the normal population [42].

Yoga is known to have cognition-enhancing property [43].

In numerous studies, yoga practice produced improvement in various cognitive domains such as attention, processing speed, memory, selective attention, concentration, etc. [44, 45]. A study found improvement in memory and attention following 3 months of yoga practice in subjects with T2DM [46].

16.7 Yoga and Mental Health in T2DM

Psychological factors such as chronic stress and depression are considered to be the risk factors of T2DM. Patients with depressive disorder were found to have two times higher risk of T2DM compared to controls. Major stressful life events increase the chances of T2DM. Yoga is an effective intervention in the management of stress. Numerous studies on yoga have shown its beneficial effects on stress. Yoga reduces perceived stress and serum cortisol levels in T2DM and it also helps in improving stress coping mechanisms [47–49]. Yoga reduces anxiety and depression and enhances mood in T2DM patients [50, 51]. Yoga has been shown to improve various hormones such as serotonin, endorphin, GABA, dopamine, which are mood enhancers and stress busters.

Yoga improves psychological well-being in T2DM:

Reducing depression, anxiety, chronic stress
Improves mood and positive thinking
Enhances stress coping strategy
Improves serotonin, GABA, and dopamine level

16.8 Autonomic Dysfunction

T2DM is characterized by autonomic dysfunction with increased sympathetic activity and reduced parasympathetic tone [52]. Increased sympathetic activity in T2DM is associated with poor blood glucose control and increased risk of CVD and incident MI [53]. Yoga helps correct autonomic dysfunction, it reduces sympathetic activity by downregulating the HPA axis and promotes parasympathetic activity in T2DM thus, it helps to reduce CVD risk in T2DM [54, 55]. It also enhances cardiac autonomic function and helps in reducing cardiac risk in T2DM.

16.9 Mechanism of Action: Molecular and Genetic Studies

Scientific evidence from a large number of RCT have confirmed the beneficial effects of yoga in T2DM. Several studies have been carried to understand the mechanism of action of yoga, which is attributed to bringing the change in health assessment. Autonomic dysfunction has been a hallmark in the cause, manifestation, and maintenance of several chronic health conditions including T2DM. Autonomic dysfunction is characterized by decreased parasympathetic tone and overactivity of the sympathetic nervous system. Yoga reduces sympathetic activity through downregulation of hypothalamic–pituitary–adrenal axis; this brings down serum cortisol and inflammatory markers which are involved in the pathology of T2DM. Studies on yoga have shown improvement in cardiac autonomic function. Asana practice in yoga involves stretching of skeletal muscle, which is associated with increased inhibition response.

Pranayama—a yogic breathing practice is a vital component of yoga. *Pranayama* practice involves slow and deep conscious breathing; this kind of practice is associated with increased parasympathetic tone via stimulation of the *vagus* nerve through stretch receptors in the lung tissues. Yoga enhances serotonin level, dopamine level, and endorphins, which are associated with enhanced mood, resilience, and improved stress-coping mechanism.

References

1. UK Prospective Diabetes Study Group. Tight blood pressure control and risk of macrovascular and microvascular complications in type 2 diabetes: UKPDS 38. Br Med J. 1998;317(7160):703.
2. Ogurtsova K, da Rocha Fernandes JD, Huang Y, Linnenkamp U, Guariguata L, Cho NH, et al. IDF diabetes atlas: global estimates for the prevalence of diabetes for 2015 and 2040. Diabetes Res Clin Pract. 2017;128:40–50.
3. Anjana RM, Pradeepa R, Deepa M, Datta M, Sudha V, Unnikrishnan R, et al. Prevalence of diabetes and prediabetes (impaired fasting glucose and/or impaired glucose tolerance) in urban and rural India: phase I results of the Indian Council of Medical Research-INdia DIABetes (ICMR-INDIAB) study. Diabetologia. 2011;54(12):3022–7.
4. Geldsetzer P, Manne-Goehler J, Theilmann M, Davies JI, Awasthi A, Vollmer S, Jaacks LM, Bärnighausen T, Atun R. Diabetes and hypertension in india: a nationally representative study of 1.3 million adults. JAMA Intern Med. 2014;178(3):363–72.
5. Cosentino F, Assenza GE. Diabetes and inflammation. Herz. 2004;29:749–59.
6. American Diabetes Association. American Diabetes Association: clinical practice recommendations. Diabetes Care. 2004;27:S1–9.
7. Schure MB, Christopher J, Christopher S. Mind–body medicine and the art of self-care: teaching mindfulness to counseling students through yoga, meditation, and qigong. J Couns Dev. 2008;86(1):47–56.
8. Rao M, Metri KG, Raghuram N, Hongasandra NR. Effects of mind sound resonance technique (yogic relaxation) on psychological states, sleep quality, and cognitive functions in female teachers: a randomized, controlled trial. Adv Mind Body Med. 2017;31(1):4–9.
9. Naoroibam R, Metri KG, Bhargav H, Nagaratna R, Nagendra HR. Effect of integrated yoga (IY) on psychological states and CD4 counts of HIV-1 infected patients: a randomized controlled pilot study. Int J Yoga. 2016;9(1):57–61.
10. The Diabetes Control and Complications Trial Research Group. The effect of intensive treatment of diabetes on the development and progression of long-term complications in insulin-dependent diabetes mellitus. N Engl J Med. 1993;329:977–86.
11. American Diabetes Association. Quality of life in type 2 diabetic patients is affected by complications but not by intensive policies to improve blood glucose or blood pressure control (UKPDS 37). UK Prospective Diabetes Study Group. Diabetes Care. 1999;22(7):1125–36.
12. Nathan DM, Singer DE, Godine JE, Harrington CH, Perlmuter LC. Retinopathy in older type II diabetics association with glucose control. Diabetes. 1986;35(7):797–801.
13. Pardasany A, Shenoy S, Sandhu JS. Comparing the efficacy of tai chi chuan and hatha yoga in type 2 diabetes mellitus patients on parameters of blood glucose control and lipid metabolism. Indian J Physiother Occup Therapy. 2010;4(3):11–6.
14. Amita S, Prabhakar S, Manoj I, Harminder S, Pavan T. Effect of yoga-Nidra on blood glucose level in diabetic patients. Indian J Physiol Pharmacol. 2009;53(1):97–101.
15. Subramaniyan TG, Subramaniyan N, Chidambaram M. Brisk walking and yoga as adjuvant therapy in management of type 2 diabetes mellitus. Int J Stud Res. 2012;2(1):43–6.
16. Bindra M, Nair S, Darotiya S. Influence of pranayama and yoga-asanas on blood glucose, lipid profile and HbA1c in type 2 diabetes. Int J Pharm Bio Sci. 2013;4(1):169–72.
17. Innes KE, Vincent HK. The influence of yoga-based programs on risk profiles in adults with type 2 diabetes mellitus: a systematic review. Evid Based Complement Alternat Med. 2007;4(4):469–86.
18. Singh A, Tekur P, Nagaratna R, et al. Impact of yoga on blood glucose level among patients with type 2 diabetes mellitus: a multicentre controlled trial. J Stem Cells. 2018;13(1):50–5.
19. Nagarathna R, Usharani MR, Rao AR, Chaku R, Kulkarni R, Nagendra HR. Efficacy of yoga based life style modification program on medication score and lipid profile in type 2 diabetes: a random-

ized control study. Int J Diabetes Dev Countries. 2012;32(3):122–30.
20. Singh S, Kyizom T, Singh KP, Tandon OP, Madhu SV. Influence of pranayamas and yoga-asanas on serum insulin, blood glucose and lipid profile in type 2 diabetes. Indian J Clin Biochem. 2008 Oct;23(4):365–8.
21. Sahay BK. Role of yoga in diabetes. JAPI. 2007;55:121–6.
22. Singh S, Kyizom T, Singh KP, Tandon OP, Madhu SV. Influence of pranayamas and yoga-asanas on serum insulin, blood glucose and lipid profile in type 2 diabetes. Indian J Clin Biochem. 2008;23(4):365–8.
23. Jyotsna VP, Ambekar S, Joshi A, et al. Prospective randomized controlled intervention trial: comprehensive yogic 20 Journal of Diabetes Research breathing program improves cardiac autonomic functions and quality of life in diabetes. Indian J Endocrinol Metab. 2012;16(Suppl 2):S489–91.
24. Kim SD. Effects of yogic exercises on life stress and blood glucose levels in nursing students. J Phys Ther Sci. 2014;26(12):2003–6.
25. Innes KE, Bourguignon C, Taylor AG. Risk indices associated with the insulin resistance syndrome, cardiovascular disease, and possible protection with yoga: a systematic review. J Am Board Fam Pract. 2005 Nov 1;18(6):491–519.
26. Kosuri M, Sridhar GR. Yoga practice in diabetes improves physical and psychological outcomes. Metab Syndr Relat Disord. 2009;7(6):515–8.
27. Chimkode SM, Kumaran SD, Kanhere VV, Shivanna R. Effect of yoga on blood glucose levels in patients with type 2 diabetes mellitus. J Clin Diagn Res. 2015;9(4):CC01.
28. Yang K, Bernardo LM, Sereika SM, Conroy MB, Balk J, Burke LE. Utilization of a 3-month yoga program for adults at high risk for type 2 diabetes: a pilot study. Evid Based Complement Altern Med. 2011;2011:257891.
29. Turner RC, Millns H, Neil HAW, Stratton IM, Manley SE, Matthews DR, Holman RR. Risk factors for coronary artery disease in non-insulin dependent diabetes mellitus: United Kingdom Prospective Diabetes Study (UKPDS: 23). BMJ. 1998;316(7134): 823–8.
30. Sivasankaran S, Pollard-Quintner S, Sachdeva R, Pugeda J, Hoq SM, Zarich SW. The effect of a six-week program of yoga and meditation on brachial artery reactivity: do psychosocial interventions affect vascular tone? Clin Cardiol. 2006;29(9):393–8.
31. Manchanda SC, Narang R, Reddy KS, Sachdeva U, Prabhakaran D, Dharmanand S, Rajani M, Bijlani R. Retardation of coronary atherosclerosis with yoga lifestyle intervention. J Assoc Physicians India. 2000;48(7):687–94.
32. Manchanda SC, Mehrotra UC, Makhija A, Mohanty A, Dhawan S, Sawhney JPS. Reversal of early atherosclerosis in metabolic syndrome by yoga: a randomized controlled trial. J Yoga Phys Therapy. 2013;3(1):1.
33. Manchanda SC, Narang R, Reddy KS, Sachdeva U, Prabhakaran D, Dharmanand S, Rajani M, Bijlani R. Retardation of coronary atherosclerosis with yoga lifestyle intervention. J Assoc Physicians India. 2000 Jul;48(7):687–94.
34. Jain SC, Uppal A, Bhatnagar SOD, Talukdar B. A study of response patterns of non-insulin dependent diabetics to yoga therapy. Diabetes Res Clin Pract. 1993;19(1):69–74.
35. Shantakumari N, Sequeira S. Effects of a yoga intervention on lipid profiles of diabetes patients with dyslipidemia. Indian Heart J. 2013;65(2):127–31.
36. Khatri D, Mathur KC, Gahlot S, Jain S, Agrawal RP. Effects of yoga and meditation on clinical and biochemical parameters of metabolic syndrome. Diabetes Res Clin Pract. 2007;78(3):e9–e10.
37. Singh S, Malhotra V, Singh KP, Madhu SV, Tandon OP. Role of yoga in modifying certain cardiovascular functions in type 2 diabetic patients. JAPI. 2004;52:203–6.
38. Kumar K. Reversing hypertension through yogic intervention.
39. Bijlani RL, Vempati RP, Yadav RK, Ray RB, Gupta V, Sharma R, Mehta N, Mahapatra SC. A brief but comprehensive lifestyle education program based on yoga reduces risk factors for cardiovascular disease and diabetes mellitus. J Altern Complement Med. 2005;11(2):267–74.
40. Malhotra V, Singh S, Tandon OP, Madhu SV, Prasad A, Sharma SB. Effect of yoga asanas on nerve conduction in type 2 diabetes. Indian J Physiol Pharmacol. 2002;46(3):298–306.
41. Roberts RO, Geda YE, Knopman DS, Christianson TJ, Pankratz VS, Boeve BF, Vella A, Rocca WA, Petersen RC. Association of duration and severity of diabetes mellitus with mild cognitive impairment. Arch Neurol. 2008;65(8):1066–73.
42. Cukierman T, Gerstein HC, Williamson JD. Cognitive decline and dementia in diabetes—systematic overview of prospective observational studies. Diabetologia. 2005;48(12):2460–9.
43. Froeliger B, Garland EL, Modlin LA, McClernon FJ. Neurocognitive correlates of the effects of yoga meditation practice on emotion and cognition: a pilot study. Front Integr Neurosci. 2012;6:48.
44. Ross A, Thomas S. The health benefits of yoga and exercise: a review of comparison studies. J Altern Complement Med. 2010;16(1):3–12.
45. Oken BS, Zajdel D, Kishiyama S, Flegal K, Dehen C, Haas M, Kraemer DF, Lawrence J, Leyva J. Randomized, controlled, six-month trial of yoga in healthy seniors: effects on cognition and quality of life. Altern Therapies Health Med. 2006;12(1):40.
46. Rajani SN, Indla YR, Archana R, Rajesh P. Role of yoga on cardiac autonomic function tests and cognition in type 2 diabetes. Int J Res Ayurveda Pharm. 2015;6(6):764.
47. Kozasa EH, Santos RF, Rueda AD, Benedito-Silva AA, De MoraesOrnellas FL, Leite JR. Evaluation of Siddha Samadhi yoga for anxiety and depres-

sion symptoms: a preliminary study. Psychol Rep. 2008;103(1):271–4.
48. Woolery A, Myers H, Sternlieb B, Zeltzer L. A yoga intervention for young adults with elevated symptoms of depression. Altern Therap Health Med. 2004;10(2):60.
49. Agte VV, Tarwadi K. Sudarshan kriya yoga for treating type 2 diabetes: a preliminary study. Altern Complement Ther. 2004 Aug 1;10(4):220–2.
50. Khalsa SB, Hickey-Schultz L, Cohen D, Steiner N, Cope S. Evaluation of the mental health benefits of yoga in a secondary school: a preliminary randomized controlled trial. J Behav Health Serv Res. 2012 Jan 1;39(1):80–90.
51. Büssing A, Michalsen A, Khalsa SB, Telles S, Sherman KJ. Effects of yoga on mental and physical health: a short summary of reviews. Evid Based Complement Alternat Med. 2012;2012:165410.
52. Vinik AI, Ziegler D. Diabetic cardiovascular autonomic neuropathy. Circulation. 2007;115(3):387–97.
53. Pop-Busui R, Evans GW, Gerstein HC, Fonseca V, Fleg JL, Hoogwerf BJ, Genuth S, Grimm RH, Corson MA, Prineas R, ACCORD Study Group. Effects of cardiac autonomic dysfunction on mortality risk in the Action to Control Cardiovascular Risk in Diabetes (ACCORD) trial. Diabetes Care. 2010;33(7):1578–84.
54. Tyagi A, Cohen M. Yoga and heart rate variability: a comprehensive review of the literature. Int J Yoga. 2016 Jul;9(2):97.
55. Vempati RP, Telles S. Yoga-based guided relaxation reduces sympathetic activity judged from baseline levels. Psychol Rep. 2002 Apr;90(2):487–94.

Yoga and Obesity

17

Ravi Kant and Nisha Batra

Obesity is a common, misunderstood, and a highly underestimated medical condition. Many societies, especially the poorly educated ones, do not consider obesity as a disease, but as a sign of well-being or a high social status. When health care professionals also ignore the problem -it contributes to an improper disease management and may result in a ineffective public health strategies to combat the obesity epidemic. Obesity affects people of all age groups in both the developed and developing countries. It has led to an increased occurrence of many diseases including Type 2 diabetes mellitus (T2DM), Cardiovascular disorders, cerebrovascular accidents, Gall bladder disease, various malignancies leading to an impaired quality of life, and a considerable economic burden on the society due to increased health care costs and loss of productivity.

17.1 Definition of Obesity

Obesity is defined as a condition of excessive fat accumulation in the adipose tissue, leading to an impaired quality of life [1]. However, the amount of excess fat in absolute terms is not the single determinant of obesity-related complications; the fat distribution in the body—around the trunk (abdominal or central obesity) and/or peripherally all over the body (peripheral obesity) should also be considered in diagnosing obesity. In general, central body fat distribution is associated with increased morbidity and mortality in people when compared to those with a more peripheral distribution [2].

For practical purposes, obesity is defined in terms of the Body Mass Index (BMI) of the person. BMI is obtained by dividing the weight of a person (in kilograms) by his or her height (in meters squared). Alternatively, it can also be calculated by dividing the weight (in pounds) by height (in inches squared) and then multiplying the value by 704.

Weight status is classified as per BMI proposed by various national and international health organizations [3–6] (Table 17.1).

This classification is not absolute as the incidence of obesity-related complications including Type 2 Diabetes Mellitus and Cardiovascular disorders vary a lot among different ethnic groups, even at identical BMI values. The best example of this disparity has been observed in the study involving Pima Indians, Taiwanese, and Japanese Americans who have been seen to have a higher prevalence of obesity-related complications at the same BMI when compared to most European populations [7].

The other evidence of ethnicity based variation emerged when the high prevalence of T2DM and cardiac disorders was observed in the Asian

R. Kant (✉) · N. Batra
Division of Diabetes and Metabolism, AIIMS, Rishikesh, India

I. Basu-Ray, D. Mehta (eds.), *The Principles and Practice of Yoga in Cardiovascular Medicine*,
https://doi.org/10.1007/978-981-16-6913-2_17

Table 17.1 Weight classification as per BMI

Weight classification	BMI (kg/m²)	Risk of obesity-related complications
Underweight	<18.5	
Normal weight	18.5–24.9	
Overweight	25.0–29.9	Increased
Obesity class I	30.0–34.9	High
Class II	35.0–39.9	Very high
Extreme obesity—Class III	≥40	Extremely high

Table 17.2 BMI cut-off values for Asia-Pacific population according to the WHO

Underweight	<18.5 kg/m²
Normal	18.5–22.9
Overweight	23–24.9
Obese	≥25

population with an average BMI below 25 kg/m² which clearly does not fit in the criteria of Obesity as discussed above. Various other studies have also demonstrated the differential distribution of BMI, body fat percentage, and fat distribution across various populations. The Asian population, in particular, has a higher percentage of body fat even with normal BMI cut-offs. These factors led the WHO to conduct a review consultation meeting regarding BMI classification, and the recommended cut-offs were modified as per ethnic groups in 2002, summarized in Table 17.2 [8, 9].

17.1.1 Childhood Obesity

Age needs to be considered in addition to weight and height when defining overweight and obesity in children as shown in Table 17.3.

There is a curvilinear relationship between BMI and body fat mass percentage; however, an element of uncertainty can always be present. Some people can have a normal body fat mass even at an obese BMI value, and it can be easily explained by increased muscle mass, and vice versa is also true best explained by low muscle mass of person. To conclude, BMI is not a very sensitive criterion for defining obesity.

However, various studies have proven a direct relationship between BMI and all-cause mortality rate, and hence, guidelines were made as per BMI-based criteria despite a variable relationship between BMI and body fat mass. A Large Prospective Cohort study done in the US Adult population not only showed a statistically significant increased risk of mortality in the overweight and obese population as compared to those with reference BMI values but also demonstrated that association was stronger when reported before the age of 70 years [10].

17.1.2 Waist Circumference as a Parameter of Central Fat Distribution

As already discussed, patients with abdominal obesity (also called central adiposity, visceral, android, or male-type obesity) are at increased risk for various obesity-related diseases including Diabetes Mellitus, hypertension, dyslipidemia, cardiac disorders, and nonalcoholic fatty liver disease [11–15]. The abdominal obesity patients also have increased rates of mortality when compared to those with increased lower body fat mass (peripheral fat distribution), who might be protected from metabolic complications [16, 17].

Waist circumference, which is highly correlated with abdominal fat mass, is considered as a surrogate marker of central or abdominal obesity and has been found to be an independent predictor of various metabolic complications.

This relationship between waist circumference and metabolic outcomes is strongest for diabetes risk, and this association is an independent and even better predictor of diabetes than BMI [18]. Recommended waist circumference thresholds for increased cardiometabolic complications are 40 inches (102 cm) in men and 35 inches (88 cm) in women. However, these values might not be applicable to high-risk ethnic groups (Asian population), where a lower threshold

Table 17.3 Definitions for childhood obesity

Age	Overweight	Obesity
<5 year	Weight-for-height > 2 standard deviations above WHO Child Growth Standards median	>3 standard deviations above the WHO Child Growth Standards median.
5–19 years	BMI-for-age more than 1 standard deviation above the WHO Growth Reference median	More than 2 standard deviations above the WHO Growth Reference median.

value of ≥35 in (90 cm) in Asian males and ≥ 31 inches (80 cm) in Asian females are considered abnormal.

17.2 Epidemiology of Obesity

The prevalence of obesity has increased all over the world in the past 50 years, reaching pandemic levels. WHO global estimates done in 2016 showed that more than 1.9 billion adults (18 years and above) accounting for 39% of the total world population were overweight and over 0.65 billion adults, a total of 13% of the world's adult population were obese.

The same is true for childhood obesity which has markedly increased in the last two or three decades. In 2016, an estimated 41 million children under the age of 5 years were overweight or obese. Once considered a high-income country problem, overweight and obesity prevalence, on the contrary, is now increasing in low- and middle-income countries, particularly in the urban population of these countries. In Africa, the number of overweight children under the age of 5 years has increased by 50% since 2000. Nearly half of the global population of overweight or obese children under 5 years of age in 2016 belonged to Asian countries. The prevalence of overweight and obesity among children and adolescents aged 5–19 years has risen dramatically from just 4% in 1975 to over 18% in 2016. Obesity-related diseases in adults, for example, T2DM, dyslipidemia, gallbladder disease, hypertension, nonalcoholic steatohepatitis (NASH), sleep apnea, and orthopedic complications, are now increasingly being observed in children as well [19].

17.3 Pathogenesis of Obesity

Energy homeostasis is defined as the balance between energy intake and energy expenditure. It involves various complex molecular and physiologic processes with constant communication within and among multiple organs, especially adipose tissue, skeletal muscle, liver, pancreas, gastrointestinal tract, and the central nervous system as well. Energy homeostasis is regulated by the integration of various signals from peripheral organs and central coordination in the brain [20]. The hypothalamus acts as a cerebral center of foremost importance in which various anorexigenic as well as orexigenic signals converge [21].

17.3.1 Physiology of Energy Homeostasis

A balanced interaction exists between two sets of neurons within the arcuate nucleus of the hypothalamus. Neurons secreting agouti-related protein (AgRP) and neuropeptide Y (NPY), when activated exert an orexigenic effect promoting food intake, whereas activation of neurons secreting pro-opiomelanocortin (POMC) and cocaine- and amphetamine-regulated transcript (CART) leads to anorexigenic effect, hence reducing food intake. The NPY/AgRP neurons also inhibit POMC/ CART neurons through γ-aminobutyric acid (GABA). These orexigenic and anorexigenic signals from the NPY/AgRP and POMC/CART neurons are transmitted to various other brain nuclei, leading to alterations in food intake and energy expenditure. The endocannabinoid system is also involved in the regulation of food intake, particularly the cannabinoid 1 (CB1) receptors (encoded by CNR1) and their endogenous ligands, anandamide. Disrupted CB1 gene in mice leading to an absence of CB1 receptors causes hypophagia in mice [22]. Randomized controlled trials (RCTs) done in obese people also proved that CB1 receptor antagonist treatment in humans decreases body weight highlighting the role of the Cannabinoid system in food ingestion in humans [23, 24].

Major peripheral organs too are involved in the regulation of food intakes such as stomach, gut, pancreas, and adipose tissue [21]. The stomach and the duodenum secrete an orexigenic peptide named ghrelin, which gets increased prior to eating and levels decrease after eating. The satiety signals are also transmitted from the gut to the brain via vagal afferent fibers synapsing in the nucleus tractus solitaries (NTS) in the hindbrain. This NTS has a role in various gustatory, satiety, and visceral sensations. Insulin, which is secreted by the pancreas, also has an anorexigenic effect via acting on arcuate nucleus. Another anorexigenic peptide is PYY, which is mainly secreted by the gastrointestinal tract after food ingestion [25]. Glucagon-like peptide-1 (GLP-1), one of the important anorexigenic peptides, is derived from preproglucagon and is secreted by the proximal gastrointestinal tract in response to ingestion of food. [26]. Leptin, serving as an important satiety signal, is secreted by the adipose tissue (Fig. 17.1).

17.3.2 Energy Metabolism

Obesity is basically caused by excessive calories intake compared to total energy expenditure over a long period of time. Large increases in body fat mass result from even small, but long-term differences in energy intake and expenditure. Total daily energy expenditure (TEE) consists of resting energy expenditure (REE), energy expended by physical activity and the thermic effect of food (TEF). REE accounts for a major portion of TEE approximately around 70% while energy expanded by physical activity and the thermic effect of food constitute 20% and 10%, respectively. REE represents the total energy expended for normal cellular and organ function in postabsorptive resting conditions while Energy expended in physical activity includes the energy utilized in volitional activity like exercise, as well as nonvolitional activities, including spontaneous muscle contractions, maintaining posture, and fidgeting. The TEF represents the energy that is consumed in various physiological processes after ingestion of a meal like digestion, absorption, and sympathetic nervous system activation. Obese people usually got increased rates of REE when compared to lean people of the same height because of a greater lean and adipose tissue cell mass. Various studies done in obese and lean subjects matched for either fat mass or lean body mass show that obese people have a small but potentially important reduction (approx. 75 kcal/day) in the thermic effect of food (TEF). This reduction in TEF might be because

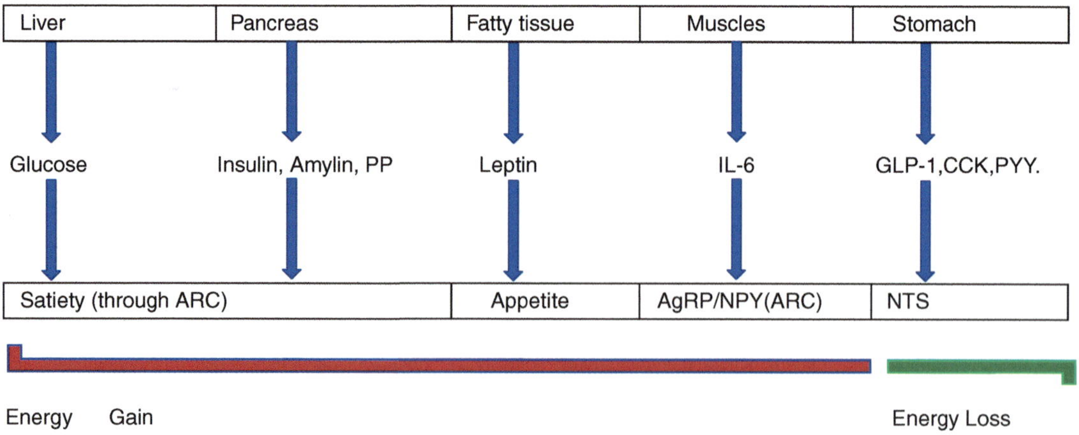

Fig. 17.1 Integration of peripheral metabolic signals and the central nervous system maintaining energy homeostasis

of insulin resistance or a blunted sympathetic nervous system activity which is frequently encountered in obesity.

Although extensive research has yet failed to reveal any significant defects in the energy metabolism in obese persons, the possibility of inherent abnormalities in energy metabolism contributing to the subsequent development of obesity still exists and this area is yet to be explored. One longitudinal study showed that daily TEE at 3 months of age was 21% lower in those infants who later became overweight as compared to those maintaining a normal weight in later years of age, [27] but a larger subsequent study did not confirm the findings of this study [28] The Baltimore Longitudinal Study on Aging followed 775 men for an average of 10 years and did not detect a relationship between initial REE and weight change [29]. However, this finding could be due to the fact that any currently available research technology is unable to detect small defects in energy metabolism which may be clinically relevant.

When energy intake exceeds energy expenditure, weight gain occurs, but the amount of weight gained varies among individuals. Genetic factors can influence the amount of weight gained with overfeeding. Data from a study that fed monozygotic twins an extra 1000 kcal/day for 84 days found that members of each twin pair gained similar amounts of weight thus supporting the involvement of genetic factors in the pathogenesis of obesity [30].

17.3.3 Genetics and Obesity

17.3.3.1 Monogenic Causes

Only a small percentage of obese people have a primary genetic cause for their obesity. Some single-gene mutations causing obesity have been identified such as leptin, leptin receptor, prohormone convertase 1, POMC, melanocortin 3 and 4 receptors, neurotrophin receptor TrkB (tyrosine receptor kinase B), and SIM1 (single-minded homolog 1).

Although rare, melanocortin 4 receptor (MC4R) mutations are the most commonly recognized monogenic cause of obesity [31].

As outlined above, the leptin-melanocortin pathway has an important role in food intake and energy balance. Leptin stimulates POMC neurons in the arcuate nucleus to produce a series of melanocortin peptides. The melanocortin α-MSH binds with high affinity to melanocortin 3 receptor (MC3R) and MC4R in the paraventricular nucleus [32, 33] which subsequently maintains a balance between energy intake and expenditure [34, 35]. Mutations in genes involved in the leptin-melanocortin tract have, to a greater or lesser extent, been associated with (childhood-onset) obesity. These mutations carry both dominant and recessive modes of inheritance, in contrast to the other monogenic causes, carrying only recessive modes of inheritance.

17.3.4 Syndromic Causes of Obesity

Obesity can also be part of a syndrome, where it is associated with various other congenital malformations, and/or intellectual deficits. Prader–Willi Syndrome, Bardet–Biedl syndrome, Carpenter syndrome, Cohen syndrome, and Alstrom syndrome are some of the known causes.

17.3.5 Polygenic Obesity

Obesity is likely to result from the interaction of many different gene–gene and gene–environment interactions. In contrast to the small number of single-gene mutations as rare causes of obesity, a large number of human genes have been identified that show variations in DNA sequences leading to obesity [36].

The use of the genome-wide association approach has identified over 80 loci with robust associations but usually with only modest contributions to overall genetic susceptibility to obesity or high BMI. It is a challenge to determine how these results fit into current models of the genetic architecture and pathophysiology of obesity, because no existing hypothesis explains all the data. The first major breakthrough in 2007 was the discovery of the fat mass and obesity-associated gene (FTO) as a potential obesity gene. Subsequently, other polygenic variants were identified after a large meta-analysis of genome-wide association studies (GWAS) for BMI. Domingue and co-workers showed that these genetic risk scores are positively correlated with BMI [37]. Notably, due to the small effect size of each single gene variant, most GWA studies are underpowered. Therefore, definite conclusions cannot be drawn from these studies. Hence, future research needs to focus on larger patient cohorts to further elucidate genetic variances in obesity-prone genes.

17.3.6 Epigenetics

Epigenetic programming in sperm cells, oocytes, and embryos plays an important role in the regulation of growth and metabolism. This can be seen in genetic obesity syndromes caused by imprinting defects, such as Prader–Willi and Temple syndrome. In both syndromes, imprinting disorders result in a phenotype characterized by short stature and neonatal feeding problems followed by hyperphagia and obesity. Exposure to environmental factors can also cause obesity through epigenetic mechanisms. This was first shown in the Dutch Hunger Winter study, where people prenatally exposed to famine during the second world war had significant epigenetic changes in the IGF2 gene compared to their unexposed siblings [38]. This area is still under-explored.

17.3.7 Environmental Factors and Obesity

A marked increase in the global prevalence of obesity has resulted largely from alterations in nongenetic factors which predominantly lead to increased energy intake and reduced physical activity. For example, more meals are now eaten outside rather than at home, there is greater availability of snack foods, serving sizes have become larger, and most importantly, the daily physical activity has now reduced because of our sedentary lifestyle and work activities. Church et al. [39] reported that energy expenditure related to occupation has drastically reduced in the last few decades, leading to a reduction in energy expenditure, hence contributing to increased mean body weight in the USA.

The dietary composition also has an important role as the prevalence of obesity has increased in direct proportionate to increased consumption of highly processed foods with higher levels of sugars and fats and a relatively low fiber diet. The Aborigines of northern Australia are a good example of showing the impact of changing lifestyles on metabolic complications. The weight and health status of this population has been compromised by exposure to a modern environment. Urbanized Aborigines are heavier than their hunter-gatherer kindred, who used to be very lean (BMI < 20.0 kg/m^2), and they have a high prevalence of T2DM and hypertriglyceridemia [40]. The traditional hunter-gatherer lifestyle of the Aborigines involved a low-fat, low-calorie diet of fish and plants with a high level of physical activity. In another study, short-term (7 weeks) re-exposure to the traditional lifestyle resulted in weight loss and significant improvements in glucose tolerance, fasting blood glucose, insulin, and triglyceride concentrations in urbanized Aborigines with T2DM and hypertriglyceridemia [41].

17.3.8 Stress and Obesity

Chronic social stress, often resulting due to poor interpersonal relationships, lack of self-esteem, job or unemployment stress is found to be significantly related to obesity and its associated illnesses. Chronic activation of the Sympathetic nervous system (SNS) and Hypothalamus-Pituitary-Adrenal axis (HPA) due to stress leads to an anabolic state which promotes fat storage within visceral depots, increases the risk of dyslipidemia, type 2 diabetes, cardiac disorders, and other facets of the metabolic syndrome. Stress also leads to weight gain and fat deposition via alterations in feeding behavior. Chronic stress leads to alteration in the pattern of food intake, dietary preferences may change, and modifies the rewarding properties of foods.

The stress response is critical for survival, as it helps a person to maintain energy homeostasis [42]. Stress, when acute, leads to activation of the sympathetic branch of the autonomic nervous system (ANS) followed by the hypothalamic–pituitary–adrenal (HPA) axis activation. ANS governs visceral functions including respiration, heart rate, maintenance of blood pressure, hormone release, and digestion. Sympathetic nervous system (SNS) activation leads to increased respiratory rate, blood pressure, and heart rate, and hence, activates catabolic pathways. The catecholamines bind to β-adrenergic receptors in adipose tissue and induce lipolysis via stimulation of hormone-sensitive lipase. This leads to the release of non-esterified fatty acids from adipocytes into the circulation. Glycogen gets hydrolyzed and gluconeogenesis is stimulated so that adequate glucose can be supplied to tissues requiring large amounts of energy, particularly, the brain, and skeletal and cardiac muscle [43].

Stress also leads to activation of the parvocellular cells of the paraventricular nucleus of the hypothalamus (PVN) leading to the release of corticotropin-releasing hormone (CRH) and arginine vasopressin into the hypothalamic–pituitary portal circulation, hence triggering the HPA axis. CRH leads to increased synthesis and release of adrenocorticotropic hormone (ACTH) from the anterior pituitary, which in return, acts on the adrenal cortex leading to the release of glucocorticoids from the zona fasciculata [44, 45]. Glucocorticoids stimulates lipolysis and gluconeogenesis and antagonizes the anabolic actions of insulin not only by inhibiting its release from pancreatic β cells, but also leading to insulin signaling defects, hence allowing glucose, fatty acids, and amino acids to be shunted to the tissues requiring them most.

In healthy individuals, this stress response, usually is short-lived. SNS activation is rapidly counterbalanced by the parasympathetic branch of the ANS and HPA response gets terminated via negative feedback loops. Indirect negative feedback from limbic structures such as the medial prefrontal cortex and hippocampus also plays an important role in terminating HPA axis response. This stress response, although, considered an integral part of survival and adaptation, becomes pathological when gets too prolonged. Chronic stress exposure leads to persistently elevated levels of basal catecholamines inducing downregulation or desensitization of adrenergic receptors in adipose tissue which, in turn, inhibits lipolysis and leads to insulin resistance.

Chronic activation of the HPA axis also leads to various metabolic complications. Many of the symptoms are similar to those of Cushing's syndrome, caused by hypercortisolism including the preferential adipose tissue accumulation in the abdominal area, hypertension, dyslipidemia, and insulin resistance [46–48].

In addition to the metabolic effects, stress also affects appetite and influences dietary preference. These effects are not always consistent—many people report that they tend to gain weight when they are stressed, whereas others report loss of appetite [49, 50]. Another important factor to consider is pre-existing weight as various studies have shown that patients who are overweight or at the upper limits of "normal" weight tend to gain weight more easily in response to stress than those who are of lower weight. Elevated insulin levels in heavier individuals may be responsible for this finding [51, 52]. Many people who increase food intake in response to stress report craving for foods high in fats and sugar. This "comfort food" effect is thought to activate brain reward systems and dampen stress responses. Imaging studies have revealed dysregulation of dopaminergic reward circuitry in these patients, the same as that found in drug addiction [50, 53]. Lack of sleep induced by stress may also be one of the factors responsible for obesity as it is known to disrupt the functioning of the ghrelin and leptin system leading to increased appetite and weight gain. The effect of stress in causing obesity is illustrated in Fig. 17.2.

17.4 Complications of Obesity

Obesity causes many serious medical complications impairing the quality of life and increasing the risk of premature death. These are enumerated in Table 17.4.

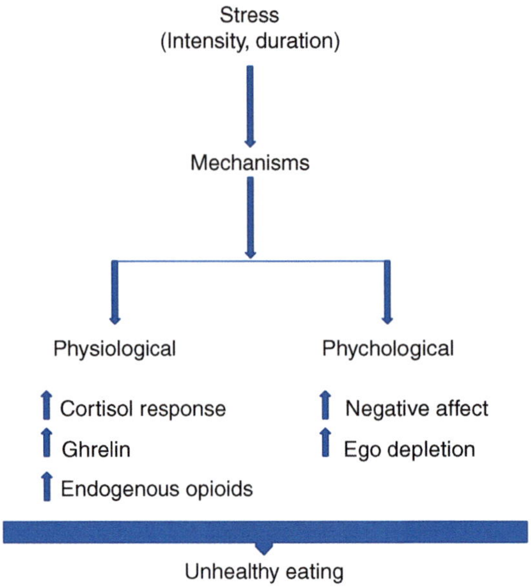

Fig. 17.2 Various mechanisms linking stress with obesity

Table 17.4 Complications of obesity

Metabolic and Endocrine diseases	
Type 2 diabetes mellitus	• The risk of diabetes is in linear association with BMI • Prevalence of diabetes in NHANES III was 13% in people with a BMI > 35 kg/m^2 when compared to 8% with a BMI of 30–34.9 kg/m^2 and only 2% in people with a BMI of 25.0–29.9 kg/m^2 [54]. • Insulin resistance is the main pathogenic mechanism.
Dyslipidemia	• Typical triad is hypertriglyceridemia, reduced HDL levels, and an increased fraction of small, dense LDL particles [55–57] • Strong association particularly in people with abdominal obesity [57] • Leads to an increased risk of cardiac diseases
Cardiovascular disease	
Hypertension	• Risk of hypertension in linear association with obesity • Framingham study showed 6.5–mm Hg increase in BP with every 10% increase in body weight [58].
Coronary heart disease	• Independent risk factor even after adjusting all other factors • More risk in those with (1) predominant central obesity and in those (2) who gained weight during young adolescence years • Risk begins to increase at a normal BMI cut-off value of 23.0 kg/m^2 in men and 22.0 kg/m^2 in women [59]
Cerebrovascular and thromboembolic disease	• Risk of ischemic stroke is approximately twice in obese as compared to lean persons • Risk of deep vein thrombosis and pulmonary embolism also increased especially in people with abdominal obesity
Pulmonary disease	
Restrictive lung disease	• Obesity decreases respiratory compliance, increasing the work of breathing, restricting ventilation, and limiting ventilation of lung bases.
Obesity-hypoventilation syndrome	• Partial pressure of carbon dioxide (PCO_2) is higher than 50 mm Hg • Decreased ventilatory responsiveness to hypercapnia or hypoxia (or both) and an inability of respiratory muscles to meet the increased ventilatory demand imposed by the mechanical effects of obesity • Pickwickian syndrome can occur
Obstructive sleep apnea	• Found in patients with BMI > 30.0 kg/m^2, excess of abdominal obesity, and increased neck girth (>17 inches in men, >16 inches in women) [60–62]
Cancers	• Overweight and obesity combined accounts for 14% of all cancer-related mortality in men and 20% in women [63] • Can lead to – GI malignancies: Liver, pancreas, stomach, esophagus, colon and rectum, and gallbladder – Renal cell carcinoma – Multiple myeloma, non-Hodgkin lymphoma – Prostate cancer in males – Ca uterus, cervix, ovary, and postmenopausal breast cancer in women [63]

(continued)

Table 17.4 (continued)

Gastrointestinal disease	
Gastroesophageal reflux disease	• Increased incidence of reflux symptoms in obese persons found in large epidemiologic studies [64, 65] and meta-analyses [66, 67]
Liver disease	• Spectrum of liver abnormalities known as nonalcoholic fatty liver disease (NAFLD), including steatosis and steatohepatitis • Prevalence of steatosis and steatohepatitis near 15% and 3%, respectively, in nonobese persons; 65% and 20% in persons with class I or II obesity; and 85% and 40% in extremely obese patients [68–71] • Surrogate marker of metabolic dysfunction in addition to BMI in obese people
Cholelithiasis	• The nurses' health study found the annual incidence of symptomatic gallstones 1% in women with a BMI > 30.0 kg/m2 and 2% in women with a BMI > 45.0 kg/m^2 [72] • Due to increased bile cholesterol supersaturation, enhanced cholesterol crystal nucleation, and decreased gallbladder contractility [73]
Pancreatitis	• Increased risk of GB stone induced pancreatitis • Higher morbidity and mortality
Others	• Increased risk of gout, osteoarthritis • Increased prevalence of cataracts • Infertility and birth defects increased

17.5 Management of Obesity

Various new pharmacotherapies are being developed for the management of obesity. Bariatric surgery has come up with a definite role and has been incorporated in the current guidelines with specific indications. But these therapies have some limitations including potential adverse effects, high cost, availability issues, and most importantly, lack of availability to the layperson. Hence, lifestyle and dietary intervention continue to remain the cornerstone of obesity management. Different types of physical exercises along with dietary modifications have been outlined in current guidelines for the management of Obesity.

Yoga, although an ancient science, having been in practice for thousands of years, has regained immense popularity in the last few years due to increasing stress, lifestyle changes, and a growing epidemic of obesity and related metabolic disorders.

17.6 Yoga: Basic Principles

The word yoga was originated from the Sanskrit word Yuj, which means to join or connect. This refers to connecting individual consciousness to universal consciousness. Yoga can also mean the process followed for managing one's mental states. Obesity is caused by an imbalance in energy intake and energy expenditure. A lack of mastery over the mind is increasingly seen as the source of many diseases including obesity, with reference to energy intake and energy expenditure [74, 75].

As per the ancient texts, *Ahara Vihara* and *Visranti* constitute the three sides of a conceptual triangle of harmonious human existence. *Ahara* denotes all the inputs to the body through various sense organs. *Vihara* represents the activities including yoga practices of Asana (body postures), Pranayama (breathing exercises), Suryanamaskara (Sun Salutation), etc. Visranti is the aspect of relaxation and sleep. Sleep quality is an important factor in the regulation of fat accumulation [76] and relaxation and awareness are essential in every yoga practice. The balance of all three sides of the triangle is the natural state of living. Yoga itself is defined as balance in all the activities [77]. Thus, with balance in Ahara Vihara Visranti, the bodily disorders can be effectively managed and a natural state of living can be embraced.

In Patanjali's Yoga Sutras, one of the foremost of Yogic texts, eight limbs are defined as follows. Yama (abstinences), niyama (observances), asana

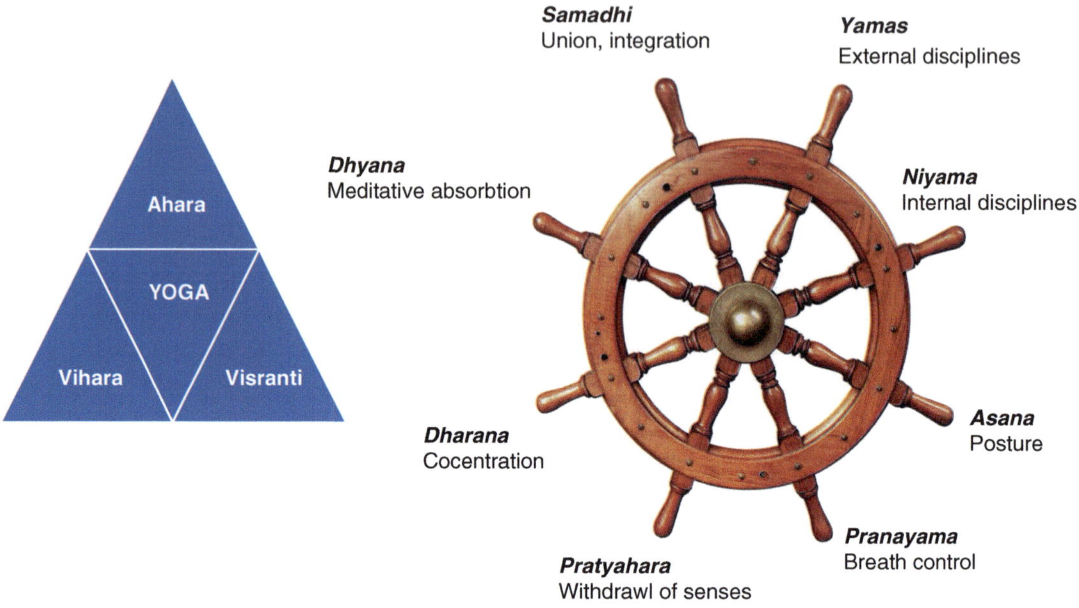

Fig. 17.3 Basic principles of Yoga as per ancient literature depicted as sides of triangle (**a**) and as eight limbs in Patanjali classification (**b**)

(postures), pranayama (breathing), pratyahara (withdrawal), dharana (concentration), dhyana (meditation), and samadhi (absorption) (Fig. 17.3).

17.7 Yoga: Role in Obesity

Various ancient yoga texts including *Hatha Yoga texts* have recognized obesity as a disorder and contain practices for managing obesity. The *Hathayogapradipika* explicitly mentions that symptoms of obesity can be reduced by yoga practices. Various asana (postures) and pranayama have been described specifically for managing obesity. Yoga - works on all dimensions of obesity including the physical, emotional, and mental aspects. Mechanisms by which yoga intervention can help with weight loss are enumerated in Table 17.5.

Table 17.5 Postulated Mechanisms by which Yoga helps in Obesity [78]

1. Energy expenditure during yoga sessions
2. Heightens mindfulness and reduce stress, reducing stress-induced overeating
3. Allows individuals to feel more connected to their bodies, leading to enhanced awareness of satiety and the discomfort of overeating
4. Maintains equilibrium between the sympathetic and parasympathetic wings of the autonomic nervous system leading to a dynamic state of health

A review of index medicus, covering the last few years does show significant literature on the effects of yoga on obesity. Holger Cramer et al. conducted a randomized controlled trial in young women with obesity and showed that an intensive yoga intervention lasting 12 weeks reduced participants' waist circumference, waist-hip ratio, body weight, BMI, and percentage of body fat and increased the percentage of muscle mass [79].

A Similar Randomized Controlled Trial conducted in Obese males by Rshikesan et al. showed remarkable improvement in anthropometric and psychological parameters including Weight, Percentage body fat, waist circumference [80].

Researchers from Hampton University in Virginia presented findings on the benefits of yoga and pranayama for teenagers at the American Heart Association's annual conference on Cardiovascular Disease Epidemiology and Prevention. Their study compared weight loss/gain in a group of overweight high school students practicing yoga for 12 weeks with those following daily routine. Students in the yoga group showed a 5.7% decrease in average body mass index and weight loss of six pounds, whereas students in the control showed a non-significant increase in average body mass index [81].

17.8 Yoga for Obesity

Various asana/pranayama have been designed specifically for the management of obesity. These are enumerated in Tables 17.6 and 17.7.

Table 17.6 Various asana with role in obesity

Asana	Technique	Special considerations
1. Wind relieving pose (Pawanmuktasana) (Fig. 17.4)	Practitioner lies upright on ground and raises the thighs up toward the abdominal muscles while holding knees tightly in hands.	• Strengthens abdominal muscles & reduces fat • Avoid uncontrolled hypertension, hernia, slipped disc, abdominal surgery, or testicular disorder
2. Cow face pose (Gomukhasana) (Fig. 17.5)	Practitioner kneels by crossing the legs and is made to raise arm of one side while the other arm reaches down behind the back, and hands clasped between the shoulder blades.	Causes release of endorphins inducing a feeling of relaxation within body and mind Contraindicated in patients with • Rotator cuff injury • Tennis elbow
3. Seated forward fold (Paschimottanasana) (Fig. 17.6)	Practitioner made to flex his hip joint while sitting on ground and bringing arms down to touch the feet.	• Contraindicated in asthma/ cardiac disorder • Avoid or do under supervision if spinal problem
4. Diamond pose (Vajrasana) (Fig. 17.7)	The practitioner sits on the heels with the calves beneath the thighs. Four finger gap kept between the kneecaps, and the first toe of both the feet touch each other and sit erect.	• Alters blood flow in the pelvic and abdominal region & strengthens the pelvic and lower back muscles • Avoid in case of osteoarthritis of the knee
5. Extended triangle pose (Utthita Trikonasana) (Fig. 17.8)	Practitioner widens legs right foot pivoted out to 90-degree angle and other kept inward. Exhaled, upper body turned in front of the right leg and right hand placed on floor beside the right foot. Left arm outstretched upwards and remains in this pose for 30 s.	• Increases core strength and stability, raises your consciousness • Avoid in case of back injury, giddiness or vertigo
6. Cobra pose (Bhujangasana) (Fig. 17.9)	Entered from a prone position. The palms are placed under the shoulders, pushing down until the hips lift slightly. The backs of the feet rest on the ground, the legs outstretched; the gaze is directed forwards, giving the preparatory pose.	• Strengthens deep muscles of back • Cardioprotective • Contraindicated in pregnancy & carpel tunnel syndrome
7. Plow pose (Halasana) (Fig. 17.10)	Pose entered from lowering back slightly for balance, and moving the legs over the head until the outstretched toes touch the ground and the arms may be stretched out on the ground away from the feet, giving the pose in the shape of a traditional plough.	• Strengthens neck, shoulder & abdominal muscles • Release of endorphins & alleviates stress • Avoid uncontrolled hypertension & cardiac illness
8. Peacock pose (Mayur asana)	In this asana, the body is raised like a horizontal stick holding the floor with both palms while the body is supported by the elbows.	• Tones up abdominal muscles • Considered an advanced asana • Avoid in uncontrolled hypertension, hernia
9. Mill churning pose (Chakki Chalanasana) (Fig. 17.11)	This posture mimics the movements of a hand-moved wheat grinder, common in the villages of India.	• Very effective in reducing abdominal obesity • Avoid in case of hernia, slipped disc or recent abdominal surgery

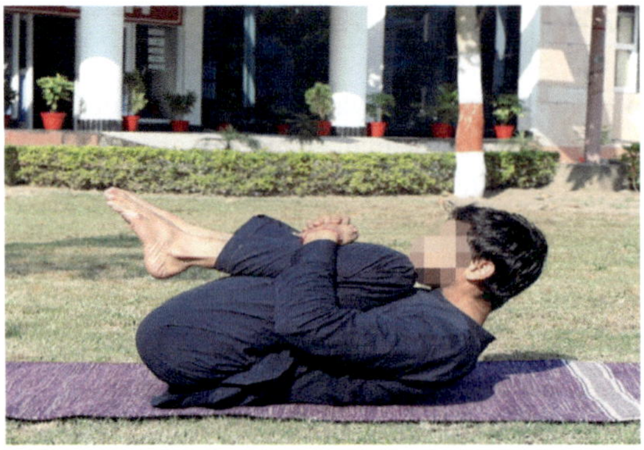

Fig. 17.4 Wind relieving pose (Pawanmuktasana)

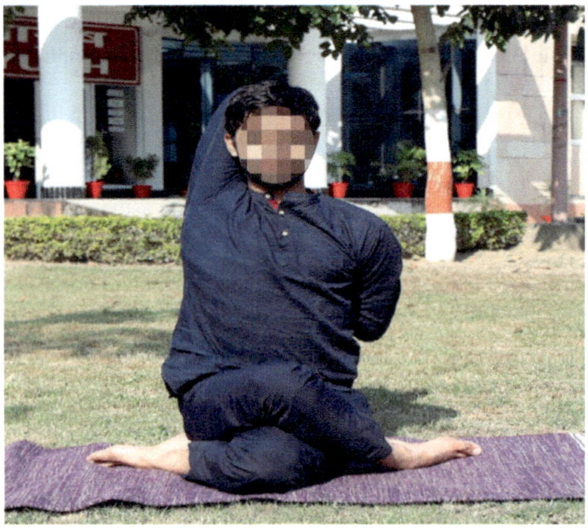

Fig. 17.5 Cow Face Pose (Gomukhasana)

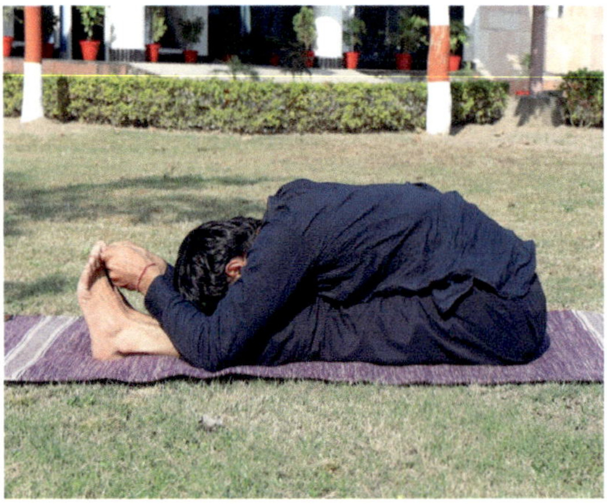

Fig. 17.6 Seated forward Fold (Paschimottanasana)

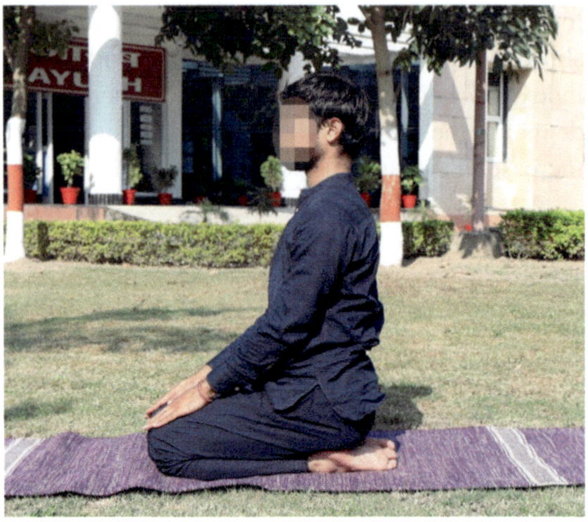

Fig. 17.7 Diamond Pose (Vajrasana)

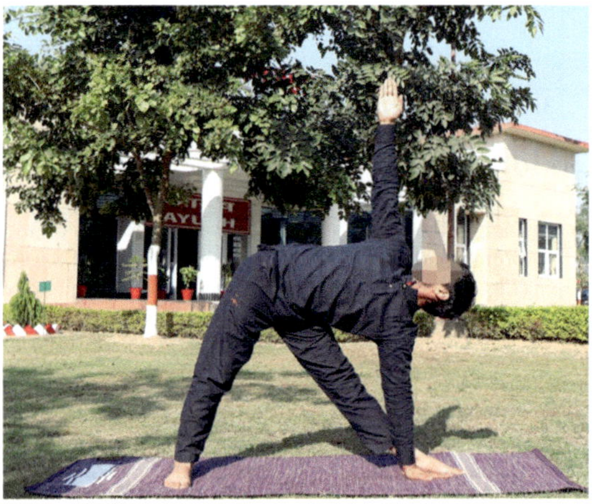

Fig. 17.8 Extended Triangle Pose (Utthita Trikonasana)

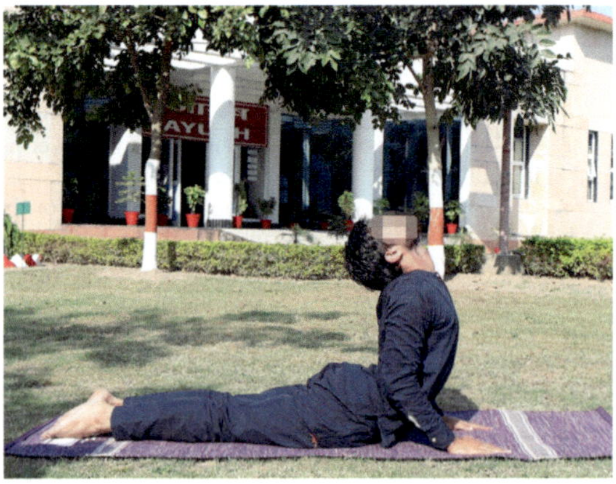

Fig. 17.9 Cobra Pose (Bhujangasana)

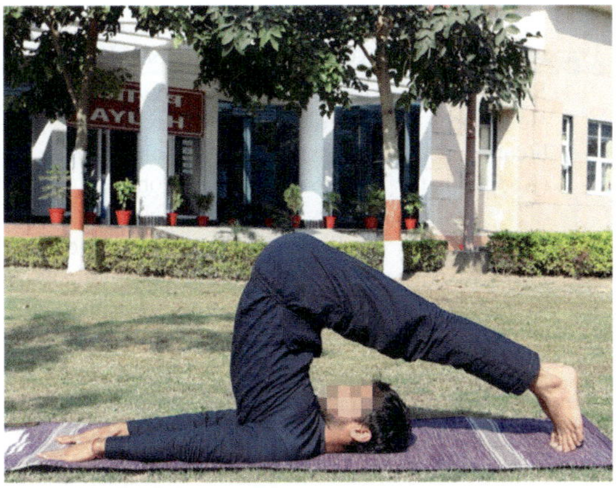

Fig. 17.10 Plow Pose (Halasana)

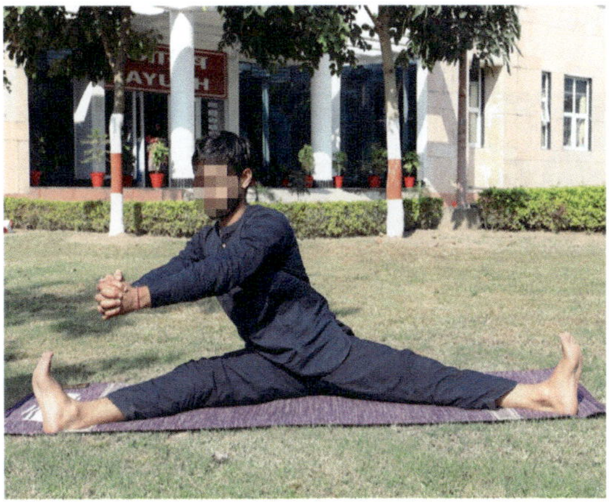

Fig. 17.11 Mill Churning Pose (Chakki Chalanasana)

Table 17.7 Various pranayama with role in obesity

Pranayama	Technique	Special considerations
1. Bee breathing technique (Bhramari) (Fig. 17.12)	Action of making a light humming sound during exhalation while practicing pranayama. Bhramari is a Sanskrit word derived from bhramar, which means "humming black bee." Practiced with a finger in each ear and remaining fingers over the eyes to reduce other auditory or visual stimulation and experience the relaxing effects of the sound.	• Good pranayama for hypertensive and patients with cardiac disease • One of the best relaxation exercises for mind • Decreases stress levels hence reducing craving for food
2. Alternate nostril breathing (Anulom Vilom pranayama) (Fig. 17.13)	Action of inhaling through one nostril, holding the breath in, then exhaling through the other nostril and reversing the sequence.	• Relaxes the mind • Improves concentration • Improves lung capacity

Pranayama	Technique	Special considerations
3. Breath of fire (Bhastrika) (Fig. 17.14)	Bhastrika basically means breathing like a bellows. Bellows is a device producing a strong current of air which was used to fan the fire in ancient days. Both inhalation and exhalation are forced in this exercise.	• Improves lung capacity • Alleviates stress • Contraindicated in hypertensive and unstable cardiac illness patients.
4. Skull cleansing breath (Kapalabhati)	Inhalation is normal while the exhalation is forceful. Done by pulling the belly inwards during exhalation forcing the diaphragm to move upwards	• Great way to reduce abdominal obesity • Needs to be done under the guidance of a qualified instructor • Contraindi-cated in hypertension, diabetic retinopathy

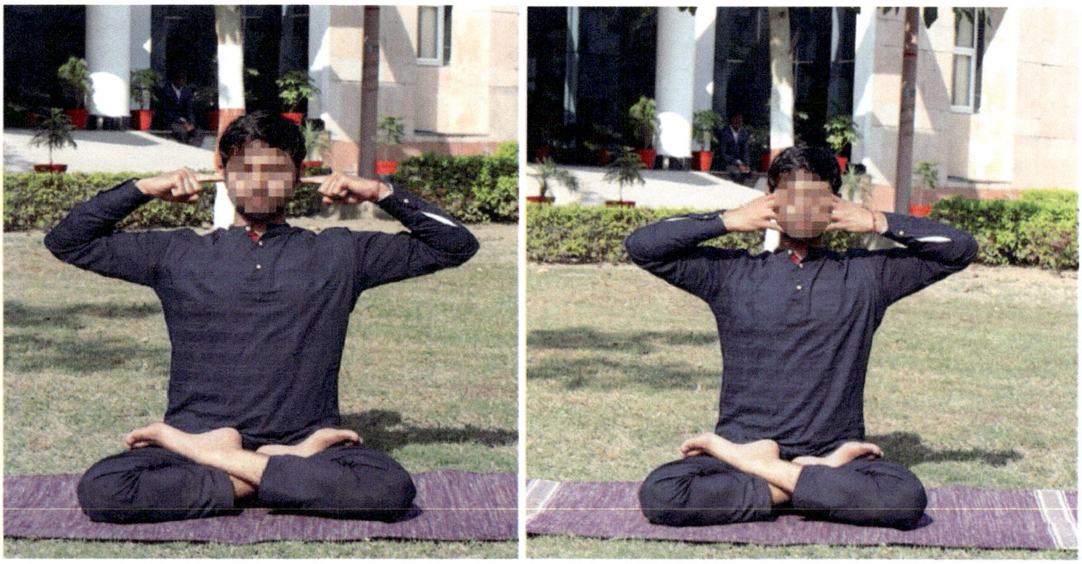

Fig. 17.12 Bee Breathing technique (Bhramari)

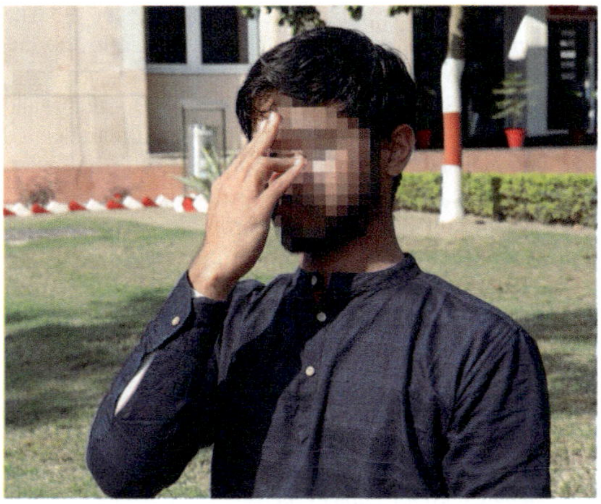

Fig. 17.13 Alternate Nostril Breathing (Anulom Vilom Pranayama)

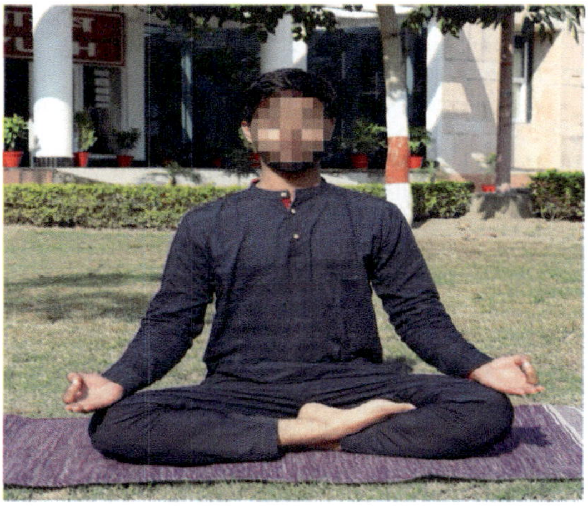

Fig. 17.14 Breath of Fire (Bhastrika)

17.9 Conclusion

Obesity is an often overlooked, chronic, complicated, and a serious disease. Yoga can be an effective component of a multi-faceted approach to combating obesity, along with dietary changes, moderate exercise, empowerment through education, and social support.

References

1. Garrow JS. Obesity and related diseases. London: Churchill Livingstone; 1988. p. 1–16.
2. Kissebah AH, Krakower GR. Regional adiposity and morbidity. Physiol Rev. 1994;74:761–811.
3. World Health Organization. Obesity: preventing and managing the global epidemic. Report of a WHO Consultation on Obesity. Geneva, Switzerland: WHO; 1998.
4. National Institutes of Health, National Heart, Lung and Blood Institute. Clinical guidelines on the identification, evaluation, and treatment of overweight and obesity in adults: the evidence report. Obes Res. 1998;6(Suppl 2):51S–209S.
5. U.S. Department of Health and Human Services. Nutrition and overweight. In: Healthy People 2010. Washington, DC: U.S. Government Printing Office; 2000.
6. U.S. Department of Agriculture and U.S. Department of Health and Human Services. Nutrition and Your Health: Dietary Guidelines for Americans.5th ed. Home and Garden Bulletin no. 232. Washington, DC: U.S. Government Printing Office; 2000.
7. Seidell JC, Kahn HS, Williamson DF, Lissner L, Valdez R. Report from a Centre for Disease Control and Prevention Workshop on use of adult anthropometry for public health and primary health care. Am J Clin Nutr. 2001;73:123–6.
8. WHO/IASO/IOTF. The Asia-Pacific perspective: redefining obesity and its treatment. Health Communications Australia: Melbourne. ISBN 0-9577082-1-1.2000.
9. James WPT, Chen C, Inoue S. Appropriate Asian body mass indices? Obesity Rev. 2002;3:139.
10. Patel AV, Hildebrand JS, Gapstur SM. Body Mass index and all-cause mortality in a large prospective Cohort of White and Black U.S. adults. PLoS One. 2014;9(10):e109153.
11. Janssen I, Katzmarzyk PT, Ross R. Waist circumference and not body mass index explains obesity-related health risk. Am J Clin Nutr. 2004;79:379.
12. Simpson JA, MacInnis RJ, Peeters A, et al. A comparison of adiposity measures as predictors of all-cause

mortality: the Melbourne Collaborative Cohort Study. Obesity (Silver Spring). 2007;15:994.
13. Koster A, Leitzmann MF, Schatzkin A, et al. Waist circumference and mortality. Am J Epidemiol. 2008;167:1465.
14. Jacobs EJ, Newton CC, Wang Y, et al. Waist circumference and all-cause mortality in a large US cohort. Arch Intern Med. 2010;170:1293.
15. Tsai AG, Wadden TA. In the clinic: obesity. Ann Intern Med. 2013;159:ITC3.
16. Snijder MB, Dekker JM, Visser M, et al. Trunk fat and leg fat have independent and opposite associations with fasting and postload glucose levels: the Hoorn study. Diabetes Care. 2004;27(2):372–7.
17. Jensen MD. Gender differences in regional fatty acid metabolism before and after meal ingestion. J Clin Invest. 1995;96:2297–303.
18. Wang Y, Rimm EB, Stampfer MJ, et al. Comparison of abdominal adiposity and overall obesity in predicting risk of type 2 diabetes among men. Am J Clin Nutr. 2005;81:555–63.
19. Barlow SE, Dietz WH. Obesity evaluation and treatment: Expert Committee recommendations. The Maternal and Child Health Bureau, Health Resources and Services Administration and the Department of Health and Human Services. Pediatrics.1998;102(3):E29.
20. Morton GJ, Cummings DE, Baskin DG, et al. Central nervous system control of food intake and body weight. Nature. 2006;443:289–95.
21. Badman MK, Flier JF. The gut and energy balance: visceral allies in the obesity wars. Science. 2005;307:1909–14.
22. Cota D, Marsicano G, Tschöp M, et al. The endogenous cannabinoid system affects energy balance via central orexigenic drive and peripheral lipogenesis. J Clin Invest. 2003;112:423–31.
23. Pi-Sunyer FX, Aronne LJ, Heshmati HM, et al. Effect of rimonabant, a cannabinoid-1 receptor blocker, on weight and cardiometabolic risk factors in overweight or obese patients—RIO-North America: a randomized controlled trial. JAMA. 2006;295:761–75.
24. Despres JP, Golay A, Sjostrom L. Effects of rimonabant on metabolic risk factors in overweight patients with dyslipidemia. Rimonabant in Obesity-Lipids Study Group. N Engl J Med. 2005;353:2121–34.
25. McGowan BM, Bloom SR. Peptide YY and appetite control. Curr Opin Pharmacol. 2004;4:583–8.
26. Deacon CF. Therapeutic strategies based on glucagon-like peptide 1. Diabetes. 2004;53:2181–9.
27. Roberts SB, Savage J, Coward WA, et al. Energy expenditure and intake from infants born to lean and overweight mothers. N Engl J Med. 1988;318:461–6.
28. Stunkard AJ, Berkowitz RI, Stallings VA, et al. Energy intake, not energy output, is a determinant of body size in infants. Am J Clin Nutr. 1999;69:524–30.
29. Seidell JC, Muller DC, Sorkin JD, et al. Fasting respiratory exchange ratio and resting metabolic rate as predictors of weight gain: the Baltimore longitudinal study on aging. Int J Obes Relat Metab Disord. 1992;16:667–74.
30. Bouchard C, Tremblay A, Despres JP, et al. The response to long term overfeeding in identical twins. N Engl J Med. 1990;322:1477–82.
31. Farooqi IS, Yeo GS, Keogh JM, et al. Dominant and recessive inheritance of morbid obesity associated with melanocortin 4 receptor deficiency. J Clin Invest. 2000;106:271–9.
32. Cone RD, et al. The melanocortin receptors: agonists, antagonists, and the hormonal control of pigmentation. Recent Prog Horm Res. 1996;51:287–317.
33. Farooqi IS, et al. Clinical spectrum of obesity and mutations in the melanocortin 4 receptor gene. N Engl J Med. 2003;348:1085–95.
34. Stutzmann F, et al. Prevalence of melanocortin-4 receptor deficiency in Europeans and their age-dependent penetrance in multigenerational pedigrees. Diabetes. 2008;57:2511–8.
35. Farooqi IS, et al. Dominant and recessive inheritance of morbid obesity associated with melanocortin 4 receptor deficiency. J Clin Invest. 2000;106:271–9.
36. Speliotes EK, Willer CJ, Berndt SI, et al. Association analyses of 249,796 individuals reveal 18 new loci associated with body mass index. Nat Genet. 2010;42:937–48.
37. Domingue BW, et al. Genetic and educational assortative mating among US adults. Proc Natl Acad Sci U S A. 2014;111:7996–8000.
38. Heijmans BT, et al. Persistent epigenetic differences associated with prenatal exposure to famine in humans. Proc Natl Acad Sci U S A. 2008;105:17046–9.
39. Church TS, Thomas DM, Tudor-Locke C, Katzmarzyk PT, Earnest CP, Rodarte RQ, Martin CK, Blair SN, Bouchard C. Trends over 5 decades in U.S. occupation related physical activity and their associations with obesity. PLoS One. 2011;6:e19657.
40. O'Dea K, White N, Sinclair A. An investigation of nutrition-related risk factors in an isolated aboriginal community in northern Australia: advantages of a traditionally-orientated life style. Med J Aust. 1988;148:177–80.
41. O'Dea K. Marked improvement in carbohydrate and lipid metabolism in diabetic Australian aborigines after temporary reversion to traditional lifestyle. Diabetes. 1984;33:596–603.
42. McEwen BS. Protective and damaging effects of stress mediators. N Engl J Med. 1998;338(3):171–9.
43. Lambert GW, Straznicky NE, Lambert EA, Dixon JB, Schlaich MP. Sympathetic nervous activation in obesity and the metabolic syndrome–causes, consequences and therapeutic implications. Pharmacol Ther. 2010;126(2):159–72.
44. de Kloet ER, Joels M, Holsboer F. Stress and the brain: from adaptation to disease. Nat Rev Neurosci. 2005;6(6):463–75.
45. Herman JP, Cullinan WE. Neurocircuitry of stress: central control of the hypothalamo-pituitaryadrenocortical axis. Trends Neurosci. 1997;20(2):78–84.
46. Rosmond R. Role of stress in the pathogenesis of the metabolic syndrome. Psychoneuroendocrinology. 2005;30(1):1–10.

47. Bjorntorp P. Do stress reactions cause abdominal obesity and comorbidities? Obes Rev. 2001;2(2):73–86.
48. Macfarlane DP, Forbes S, Walker BR. Glucocorticoids and fatty acid metabolism in humans: fuelling fat redistribution in the metabolic syndrome. J Endocrinol. 2008;197(2):189–204.
49. Pecoraro N, Reyes F, Gomez F, Bhargava A, Dallman MF. Chronic stress promotes palatable feeding, which reduces signs of stress: feedforward and feedback effects of chronic stress. Endocrinology. 2004;145(8):3754–62.
50. Adam TC, Epel ES. Stress, eating and the reward system. Physiol Behav. 2007;91(4):449–58.
51. Dallman MF. Stress-induced obesity and the emotional nervous system. Trends Endocrinol Metab. 2009;21(3):159–65.
52. Block JP, He Y, Zaslavsky AM, Ding L, Ayanian JZ. Psychosocial stress and change in weight among US adults. Am J Epidemiol. 2009;170(2):181–92.
53. Volkow ND, Wang GJ, Baler RD. Reward, dopamine and the control of food intake: implications for obesity. Trends Cogn Sci. 2011;15(1):37–46.
54. Cowie CC, Rust KF, Ford ES, et al. Full accounting of diabetes and pre-diabetes in the U.S. population in 1988-1994 and 2005-2006. Diabetes Care. 2009;32:287–94.
55. Reaven GM, Chen YDI, Jeppesen J, et al. Insulin resistance and hyperinsulinemia in individuals with small, dense, low density lipoprotein particles. J Clin Invest. 1993;92:141–6.
56. Terry RB, Wood PD, Haskell WL, et al. Regional adiposity pattern in relation to lipids, lipoprotein cholesterol, and lipoprotein subfraction mass in men. J Clin Endocrinol Metab. 1989;68:191–9.
57. Brown CD, Higgins M, Donato KA, et al. Body mass index and the prevalence of hypertension and dyslipidemia. Obes Res. 2000;8:605–19.
58. Kannel W, Brand N, Skinner J, et al. The relation of adiposity to blood pressure and development of hypertension. The Framingham Study. Ann Intern Med. 1967;67:48–59.
59. Stamler J, Wentworth D, Neaton JD. Is relationship between serum cholesterol and risk of premature death from coronary disease continuous or graded? Findings in primary screenees of the Multiple Risk Factor Intervention Trial (MRFIT). JAMA. 1986;256:2823–8.
60. Vgontzas AN, Tan TL, Bixler EO, et al. Sleep apnea and sleep disruption in obese patients. Arch Intern Med. 1994;154:1705–11.
61. Davies RJ, Stradling JR. The relationship between neck circumference, radiographic pharyngeal anatomy, and the obstructive sleep apnoea syndrome. Eur Respir J. 1990;3:509–14.
62. Katz I, Stradling J, Slutsky AS, et al. Do patients with obstructive sleep apnea have thick necks? Am Rev Respir Dis. 1990;141:1228–31.
63. Calle EE, Rodriguez C, Walker-Thurmond K, et al. Overweight, obesity and mortality from cancer in a prospectively studied cohort of U.S. adults. N Engl J Med. 2003;348:1625–38.
64. Romero Y, Cameron AJ, Locke GR III, et al. Familial aggregation of gastroesophageal reflux in patients with Barrett's esophagus and esophageal adenocarcinoma. Gastroenterology. 1997;113:1449–56.
65. Locke GR, Talley NJ, Fett SL, et al. Risk factors associated with symptoms of gastroesophageal reflux. Am J Med. 1999;106:642–9.
66. Corley DA, Kubo A. Body mass index and gastroesophageal reflux disease: a systematic review and meta-analysis. Am J Gastroenterol. 2006;101(11):2619–28.
67. Hampel H, Abraham N, El-Serag H. Meta-analysis: obesity and the risk for gastroesophageal reflux disease and its complications. Ann Intern Med. 2005:143–99.
68. Marcos A, Fisher RA, Ham JM, et al. Selection and outcome of living donors for adult to adult right lobe transplantation. Transplantation. 2000;69:2410–5.
69. Hilden M, Christoffersen P, Juhl E, et al. Liver histology in a "normal" population: examinations of 503 consecutive fatal traffic casualties. Scand J Gastroenterol. 1977;12:593–7.
70. Lee RG. Nonalcoholic steatohepatitis: a study of 49 patients. Hum Pathol. 1989;20:594–8.
71. Gholam PM, Kotler DP, Flancbaum LJ. Liver pathology in morbidly obese patients undergoing Roux-en-Y gastric bypass surgery. Obes Surg. 2002;12:49–51.
72. Stampfer MJ, Maclure KM, Colditz GA, et al. Risk of symptomatic gallstones in women. Am J Clin Nutr. 1992;55:652–8.
73. Hay DW, Carey MC. Pathophysiology and pathogenesis of cholesterol gallstone formation. Semin Liver Dis. 1990;10:159–70.
74. Rshikesan PB, Subramanya P. Effect of integrated approach of yoga therapy on male obesity and psychological parameters: a randomised controlled trial. J Clin Diagnostic Res. 2016;10(10):1–6.
75. Rshikesan PB, Subramanya P, Nidhi R. Yoga practice for reducing the male obesity and weight related psychological difficulties: a randomized controlled trial. J Clin Diagnostic Res. 2016;10(11):OC22–8.
76. Rshikesan PB, Subramanya P, Singh D. Sleep quality and body composition variations in obese male adults after 14 weeks of yoga intervention: a randomized controlled trial. Int J Yoga. 2017;10:128–37.
77. Nagaratna R, Nagendra HR. Yoga for obesity. 1st ed. Bengaluru: Swami Vivekananda Yoga Prakashana; 2014. p. 1–292.
78. Balayogi A. Yoga and modern medicine, possible meeting points. Pondicherry: ICYER; 2001.
79. Cramer H, Thoms MS, Anheyer D. Yoga in women with abdominal obesity—a randomized controlled trial. Dtsch Arztebl Int. 2016 Sep;113(39):645–52.
80. Rshikesan PB, Subramanya P, Nidhi R. Yoga practice for reducing the male obesity and weight related psychological difficulties: a randomized controlled trial. J Clin Diagn Res. 2016;10(11):OC22–8.
81. AHA Yoga & pranayama help overweight teens lose weight. 46th annual conference, poenix, CDC. March 2006; 2–5.

Yoga for Dyslipidemia

18

Jaideep Arya, Prashant Verma, Deepali Mathur,
Rahul Tyagi, Viraaj Pannu, and Akshay Anand

18.1 Background

Sedentary lifestyle and lack of physical activity are some of the possible reasons of Dyslipidemia [1]. Dyslipidemia is an epidemic in both developing as well as developed countries and is a major contributor to the formation of atherosclerosis. It is a well-established prevalent risk factor for stroke and coronary artery disease (CAD) [2, 3]. In a fast-developing country like India, problems of food, electricity, education, hospitals, and famine are soon vanishing. As a result, there is a reduced demand for physical work due to technological developments. Yet, the desire for perfect human health eludes the advancement of medicine. Hence, there is a need to achieve wellness which is bereft of non-communicable diseases.

J. Arya
Haryana Yog Aayog, Panchkula, Haryana, India

P. Verma
Interdisciplinary Centre for Swami Vivekananda Studies, Panjab University, Chandigarh, India

R. Tyagi · A. Anand (✉)
Neuroscience Research Lab, Department of Neurology, PGIMER, Chandigarh, India

D. Mathur
School of Biotechnology, KIIT University, Bhubaneshwar, Odisha, India

V. Pannu
Government Medical College and Hospital Sector 32, Chandigarh, India

Deteriorating lifestyle combined with poor environmental conditions require a holistic or "one health" approach, which is recently defined by WHO's as the sustainable goal for health administrators. Among various diseases, the scourge of dyslipidemia is growing among both developed and developing countries. High cholesterol levels is an insurmountable problem that has been projected by the pharmaceutical companies as untreatable without 'statins' and other cholesterol-lowering drugs. About 29.7 million people are believed to perish every year from raised cholesterol levels [4]. Studies reveal that dyslipidemia is fast affecting Indians. Recent studies suggest that 25%–30% of the Indian urban population and 15%–20% of rural Indians suffer from dyslipidemia. The prevalence is expectedly higher among high-income countries. Most commonly raised LDL, low HDL with increased triglyceride, defines dyslipidemia in the Indian sub-continent. In addition, elevated levels of apolipoprotein B, LDL, and total cholesterol correlate with coronary events [5]. Moreover, large number of dyslipidemia patients are found in the urban region than in rural region, which suggests that lifestyle changes are required to keep the respective marker levels in the normal range. Their results revealed that incorporation of exercise, yoga, aerobics, etc., in daily routine, regulated the lipid levels and avoiding the junk food may help in combating the very common and dreadful disease [5, 6]. Another cross-

I. Basu-Ray, D. Mehta (eds.), *The Principles and Practice of Yoga in Cardiovascular Medicine*,
https://doi.org/10.1007/978-981-16-6913-2_18

sectional study was proposed in all the 28 states of India and the first phase study was conducted in three different states and one union territory of India. The data was collected from both rural and urban parts of Tamil Nadu, Maharashtra, Jharkhand and Chandigarh. HDL, LDL, triglycerides and VLDL as well as socio-demographic details were collected.The results of the first phase showed that there was no significant difference between rural and urban populations. This study covered a population of 213 million people (≥ 20 years of age) using a stratified multistage sampling design. Among the four regions listed, lipid abnormalities (at least one) were found to be highest in Chandigarh (82.9%), followed by Jharkhand (80%), Maharashtra (77%) and Tamil Nadu (76.9%) [7].

According to previous reports, lipid levels in the bloodstream of the Asian population are perturbed to a greater extent than in non-Asian population [8, 9]. Furthermore, higher levels of triglycerides and lower levels of HDL cholesterol may serve as independent markers for the development of cardiovascular disease (CVD) [9–12]. Accumulating evidence indicates that there is a preponderance of low HDL cholesterol and less prevalence of high total cholesterol in Asian Indians than non-Asian Indians [13, 14]. Strikingly, South Asia lacks awareness about the consequences of dyslipidemia, and very few studies reported on its role on the burden of CVD, despite it is a well-established risk factor [13].

18.2 Dyslipidemia: An Overview, Stress and Disease Associated Mechanisms

Dyslipidemia is characterized by an altered lipid panel in the blood. These typically include (1) total cholesterol; (2) high-density lipoprotein cholesterol; (3) low-density lipoprotein (LDL) cholesterol; and (4) triglycerides (TG).

Dyslipidemia is also considered as a recognized risk factor for stroke and cardiovascular disorders [15]. Though in 40% to 60% of cases, the cause of dyslipidemia may be associated with any genetic alteration, but the lifestyle-related factors are critical in triggering the elevated lipid profile [16, 17]. A 4 year follow-up study conducted in the Japanese population concluded that smoking habits, increase in body mass index and snacking between meals is strongly associated with altered lipid profile. However, alcohol consumption and vegetarian diet were found to have anti-atherogenic effects on serum lipid profile [18]. An interesting study conducted in atherosclerosis-prone ApoE-null mice revealed that a combination of a high protein diet and exercise is beneficial in combating dyslipidemia [19]. This study also indicated an important role of diet and exercise even in a genetically predisposed model. Stress is another risk factor involved in inducing dyslipidemia [20].

18.2.1 Impact of Stress on Lipid Metabolism

There are a plethora of studies that have shown that stress triggers dyslipidemia. Stress which is nowadays an unavoidable problem, is caused as a result of excessive workload and a number of other reasons, and it plays an indispensable role in elevating blood cholesterol, triglyceride levels and LDL levels in the bloodstream of individuals [21, 22]. The harmful effect of stress is reported to disturb the lipid metabolism, which leads to the development and progression of a number of diseases, including stroke and cardiovascular diseases [23, 24].

18.2.2 Physiological Mechanisms

The heterogeneity of variation that occurs in metabolite levels due to stress is remarkable. Hormones such as glucocorticoids (cortisol) and catecholamines [neurotransmitters such as dopamine, epinephrine (adrenaline) and norepinephrine (nor-adrenaline)] are secreted in response to stressful conditions and are catabolic in nature. These neurotransmitters directly induce the release of free fatty acid and glycerol from adipose depots into the bloodstream [21]. Furthermore, they regulate the breakdown of glycogen, triglycerides, and proteins into simple molecules in order to yield energy [23]. Stress triggers the sympathetic nervous system and secrets catecholamines by corticotropin-releasing hormone (CRH), which in turn inhibits weight gain of the individual. It has been observed that acute stress quenches the appetite and curtails body weight gain in individuals. This might happen due to the stimulation of the hypothalamic–pituitary–adrenal axis region of the brain and secretion of CRH. On the contrary, chronic stress is linked with excessive food intake and eventually weight gain, which results in obesity [25, 26]. This happens due to the secretion of glucocorticoids and neuropeptide Y. Fifty percent of women who underwent sexual abuse during their childhood suffered from traumatic stress and gained a lot of weight with high concentrations of glucocorticoids in their urine [27]. Several studies describe the effect of stress on sleep which is linked with reduced leptin and increased ghrelin levels [28, 29]. Figure 18.1 illustrates the schematic representation of physiological mechanisms of dyslipidemia induced by stress.

Chronic stress also increases the appetite, reduces leptin levels, induces sleep loss and increases ghrelin levels [28, 29]. Furthermore, the presence of high amount of glucocorticoids in the bloodstream increases the fat of the viscera [30]. It is also suggested that chronic stress occurs due to a number of reasons which is also associ-

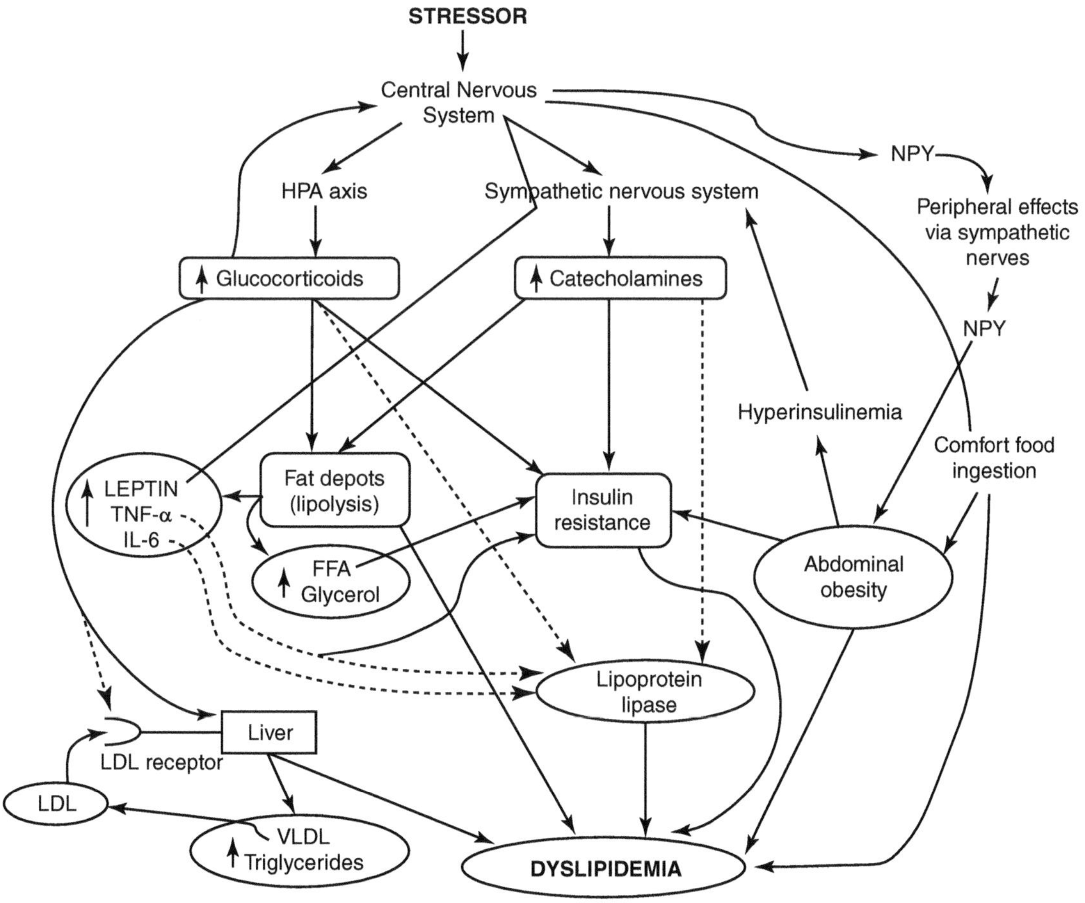

Fig. 18.1 Schematic representation of physiological mechanisms of dyslipidemia induced by stress. Hypothalamic–pituitary–adrenal axis (HPA), low-density lipoprotein (LDL), very low-density lipoprotein (VLDL), free fatty acids (FFA), neuropeptide Y (NPY), tumor necrosis factor (TNF-α), interleukin 6 (IL-6). Solid arrows show stimulatory effects; dashed arrows indicate inhibitory effects (Reproduced from Marcondes et al. 2012)

ated with high-calorie intake upregulates the expression of neuropeptide Y, a stress mediator. This eventually leads to hyperinsulinemia and hyperlipidemia [31, 32]. All these physiological mechanisms results from excessive eating due to chronic stress, which leads to obesity and subsequently alters the lipid levels causing dyslipidemia. Findings of Stoney et al. demonstrated that the rate by which exogenous fat is removed becomes minimum, and this occurs due to the occurrence of acute psychological stress in both healthy men and women [33]. Moreover, chronic psychological stress was found to elevate the cholesterol levels in the bloodstream of medical students [34]. Similar findings were observed by Yoo et al., 2011, suggesting increased cholesterol levels in the bloodstream of female law officers as compared to the general female population [35].

Patients undergoing depression and distress disorders were found to have a marked increase in cortisol concentrations which again might be caused due to stress conditions [36, 37]. Their lipid profile was abnormal with high triglycerides, LDL, total cholesterol and low HDL levels in their serum [36]. Berger et al. in 1980 reported that stress triggered by electric shock elevated the cholesterol levels in the plasma of animals [38]. Several lines of evidence indicate that stress changes the lipid levels in the bloodstream of rats. It was also observed about the elevated levels of LDL and very-low-density lipoprotein (VLDL), and reduced HDL levels when their mobility was restricted which could have triggered stress [39, 40]. It is known that the synthesis of triglycerides and VLDL in the liver is controlled by insulin. However, stress activates the sympathetic nervous system releasing catecholamines which in turn induces insulin resistance, eventually leading to uncontrolled triglyceride formation and VLDL production [21]. Thus, triglycerides present within VLDL particles are secreted in abundance by the liver into the bloodstream [41]. Moreover, apolipoprotein B (apo B) induced by cortisol is also secreted from the liver, which increases the concentration of VLDL in the blood [24]. VLDL particles then catabolize into LDL in the bloodstream.

The presence of an increased concentration of cortisol inhibits the hepatic LDL receptors, which impedes the LDL removal [21]. Xu et al. suggested that perilipin, a protein that plays an essential role in lipid metabolism, is phosphorylated by glucocorticoids and enhances the process of lipolysis of triglycerides into fatty acids and glycerol [42]. Furthermore, cortisol, norepinephrine and nor-adrenaline neurotransmitters suppress the activity of lipoprotein lipase resulting in reduced triglyceride removal from the bloodstream, decrease in HDL concentration, and increase in VLDL and LDL concentrations [21].

Additionally, proinflammatory cytokines, including tumor necrosis factor (TNF), interleukin 6 (IL-6), and leptin secreted from fatty cells, also play a crucial role in causing dyslipidemia. Evidence also indicate that TNF is indulged in the lysis of lipids in fat tissue and stimulates insulin resistance, IL-6 cytokine and leptin production [43]. IL-6 is involved in increasing the expression and activity of hydroxysteroid dehydrogenase 1 (11-HSD1). Both cytokines reduce lipoprotein lipase activity, which in turn increases the concentration of triglycerides in the bloodstream [41]. Hence, stress hormones (adrenaline, nor-adrenaline, and cortisol), insulin, adipose tissue metabolism, and cytokines play an indispensable role in causing dyslipidemia which is triggered by stress.

18.2.3 Cardiovascular Diseases

More than 25% of the world's population is suffering from the cardio-metabolic syndrome, including abnormal cholesterol levels. Arteries are affected by increased LDL and thus increase the risk of heart attack and coronary artery diseases (CAD) [44]. Table 18.1 illustrates different trials that support the role of yoga in dyslipidemia.

Most specifically, Yoga therapy helps to improve vascular as well as respiratory health in both pre- and post-diseased states. Health awareness through participation in health camps, semi-

Table 18.1 Table illustrating trials that support the role of yoga in dyslipidemia

Title	Journal	Date of publication	Authors	Study type	Sample size	Results/conclusion	Remarks
Effect of a Yoga Intervention on Lipid Profiles of Diabetes Patients with Dyslipidemia	Indian Heart Journal Vol. 65 Issue 2 (127–131)	March–April 2013	Nisha Shantakumari et al.	RCT	100	After a 3 month period the yoga + oral hypoglycemic intervention group showed a decrease in Total Cholesterol, LDL, and Triglycerides, while showing an increase in HDL as compared to the control group (oral hypoglycemics).	Dietary data was not recorded, thus nutrition was not matched amongst the two groups.
A Study on Effect of Yoga and Various Asanas on Obesity, Hypertension, and Dyslipidemia	International Journal of Basic and Applied Medical Sciences Vol. 2(1) (93–98)	January–April 2012	Vijay Tundwala et al.	RCT	150	After a 3 month period, the daily yoga intervention group showed a significant decrease in Body Mass Index, Waist-Hip Ratio, Systolic and Diastolic Blood Pressures, Total Cholesterol, LDL, VLDL, and Triglycerides with a significant increase in HDL levels as compared to the control group.	Dietary and lifestyle information was given to both the groups, however was not enforced in either. There are no remarks regarding the compliance of these groups to dietary and lifestyle advice or whether there was any significant variation in the compliance between these two groups in maintaining the dietary and lifestyle advice.

(continued)

Table 18.1 (continued)

Title	Journal	Date of publication	Authors	Study type	Sample size	Results/conclusion	Remarks
Importance of Yoga in Diabetes and Dyslipidemia	International Journal of Research in Medical Sciences Vol. 4(8)	August 2016	Riyaz Mohammed et al.	RCT	50	After 4 months, the yoga + oral hypoglycemic group showed no significant change in BMI, weight and HDL, significant reduction in Total Cholesterol, LDL, and Triglycerides, as compared to control (oral hypoglycemic only).	There was a significant rise in the bodyweight of the control group. This can be attributed to the use of sulphonylureas as the oral hypoglycemic agent.
Efficacy of a Validated Yoga Protocol on Dyslipidemia in Diabetic Patients: NMB-2017 India Trial	Medicines Vol. 6(4)	October 2019	Raghuram Nagarathna et al.	Stratified Cohort Study	17012	Those who met the selection criteria were taught the Diabetes Yoga Protocol (DYP) for 3 months. After the 3 month intervention, the significant conversion rates from abnormal to normal values were; 60.3% for Total Cholesterol, 73.7% for LDL, 63% for Triglycerides and 43.7% for HDL.	This study demonstrated a statistically significant positive co-relation between HbA1c and Total Cholesterol levels. Limitations include lack of appropriate control group, a large drop off rates, which may be ascribed to challenges in adopting the protocol or due to limitations in health conditions.

Title	Journal	Date of publication	Authors	Study type	Sample size	Results/conclusion	Remarks
Yoga and Meditation in Cardiovascular Disease	Clinical Research in Cardiology Vol. 103	January 2014	S.C Manchanda & Kaushal Madan	Review Article	N/A	This review article summarizes the studies relate to effects of yoga and meditation on a variety of cardiovascular diseases. The observations recorded include decrease in coronary heart disease in transcendental meditation practitioners by 48% over a 5 year period. Another study demonstrates yoga as helpful in the prevention of atrial fibrillation.	The authors conclude that the study has some major limitations: small sample sizes, inconsistencies in baselines, and methodologies adopted. Due to the cost-effective and safe nature of yoga/meditation, it can still be used for primary and secondary prevention of cardiovascular disease.
Risk Indices Associated with the Insulin Resistance Syndrome, Cardiovascular Disease, and Possible Protection with Yoga: A Systematic Review	The Journal of the American Board of Family Practice Vol. 8(6) (491–519)	November 2005	Kim E. Innes et al.	Meta-analysis	70 studies	The authors identified 70 eligible studies (1 observational, 26 uncontrolled, 21 Non-RCT, 22 RCTs). The authors observed from these studies the beneficial effects in several insulin resistance indices such as glucose tolerance, lipid profiles, blood pressure, oxidative stress, coagulation profiles, sympathetic activation as well as cardiovagal function.	The authors performed literature search using four computerized English and Indian Scientific databases. The search was restricted to studies from 1970 to 2004.

(continued)

Table 18.1 (continued)

Title	Journal	Date of publication	Authors	Study type	Sample size	Results/conclusion	Remarks
Yoga for the primary prevention of cardiovascular disease	Cochrane Systematic Review—Intervention	May 2014	Louise Hartley et al.	Meta-analysis	11 trials (800 participants)	Interventions ranged from 3 to 8 months duration. The results suggest the favorable effects on diastolic blood pressure, HDL, and triglycerides while showing uncertain effects on LDL.	The authors state that these results should be interpreted with caution, as the included studies were of short duration, small sample size and had risk of bias.
Obesity-related inflammation & cardiovascular disease: Efficacy of a yoga-based lifestyle intervention	Indian Journal of Medical Research Vol. 139(6)	June 2014	Kumar Sarvottam & Raj Kumar Yadav	Review	N/A	This review analyses the effect of yoga-based lifestyle intervention on the prevention and slowing down of the progression of cardiovascular as well as metabolic disorders. The mechanism postulated by the authors is attributed to the reduction in weight and stress, leading to a reduction in inflammation and inflammatory markers.	Authors have not compared the effect of other physical activities to a yoga-based lifestyle intervention. Creating ambiguity in the results analysis and comparison
Yoga—A promising technique to control cardiovascular disease	Indian Heart Journal Vol. 66(5) (487–489)	September 2014	S.C Manchanda	Review	N/A	This review suggests various studies conducted on the use of Yoga for both primary as well as secondary prevention of CVD. The evidence seen with the use of transcendental meditation for possibly reducing heart attacks, stroke, and deaths in CVD patients. The author also discusses studies that show a 48% risk reduction in all-cause mortality over a 5.4 year period.	The author discusses the various limitations in these studies, such as small sample sizes, absence of adequate controls and a lack of uniform methodologies.

Title	Journal	Date of publication	Authors	Study type	Sample size	Results/conclusion	Remarks
Effect of a multimodality natural medicine program on carotid atherosclerosis in older subjects: a pilot trial of Maharishi Vedic Medicine.	American Journal of Cardiology Vol. 89(8) (952–958)	April 2015	Fields JZ et al.	RCT	57	The subjects were divided into three groups. Practitioners of Maharishi Vedic Medicine(MVM), of modern medicine group and usual care(no care). The MVM group saw significant reductions in Intima-Media Thickness (a marker for atherosclerosis) compared to both the other groups (-0.15 ± -0.21, $n = 20$, $p = 0.004$)	The assessment of IMT was done by B-mode ultrasound of the Carotid artery. The mean age of the participants was 74 years.
Reversal of Early Atherosclerosis in Metabolic Syndrome by Yoga–A Randomized Controlled Trial	Journal of Yoga and Physical Therapy Vol. 3(1)	2013	S. C Manchanda et al.	RCT	100	At the end of 1 year, the yoga group showed a significant regression of Carotid intima-media thickness (0.842 ± 0.176 to 0.808 ± 0.204, $p < 0.001$) as compared to the control group. The author also found reductions in SBP, LDL, BMI, and Waist Circumference.	The various yogic exercises used were 1. Health Rejuvenating exercises 2. Breathing exercises 3. Asanas (Surya Namaskar etc) 4. Shav Asana 5. Preksha Dhyan
Adiponectin, Interleukin-6, and Cardiovascular Disease Risk Factors Are Modified by a Short-Term Yoga-Based Lifestyle Intervention in Overweight and Obese Men	The Journal of Alternative and Complementary Medicine Vol. 19(5)	May 2013	Kumar Sarvottam et al.	Non-Randomized Prospective study with pre and post design	51	A yoga protocol was initiated for 10 days in the men's group. Thirty subjects completed the study. The study showed significant reductions in IL-6(2.24 vs. 1.26 $p = 0.012$), adiponectin(4.95 vs. 6.26, $p = 0.014$). With no change in the Plasma ET-1 levels.	The findings in this study are suggestive of a 10 day short-term yoga protocol that can be useful in reducing the inflammatory and metabolic markers (reducing IL-6, increasing adiponectin) in overweight and obese groups.

nars, CHD awareness programs also prevent CHD progression. Thus the management platforms can be used to provide an evidence based approach to the general public. Some recent studies have shown that lonely, hopeless, helpless, and despondent CHD patients do worse as compared to those who feel at ease with their surroundings. However, randomized controlled studies depicting positive effects of yoga are meager.

18.2.4 Diabetes

Diabetes and dyslipidemia are co-morbid diseases. Dyslipidemia increases liver disorders resulting in poor digestion and increasing the glucose level in blood. Therefore, dyslipidemia may be an important risk factor for diabetes. It affects insulin secretion and leads to hyperglycemia. The co-morbidity of cardiovascular diseases with diabetes-induced dyslipidemia is high. Dyslipidemia along with Type-1 or Type-2 Diabetes has a high risk for CVD [45]. India is currently experiencing an epidemic of Type 2 diabetes mellitus (T2DM) and has the largest number of diabetic patients. It is often referred to as the Diabetes capital of the world. International Diabetes Federation (IDF) 2009 report reveals that the total number of diabetic subjects in India is 50.8 million.

Yoga provides a popular and simpler set of interventions for pre- and post-diseased conditions of Diabetics, not just because of its efficacy in the management, but also its strength in providing benefits to the practitioner, from mental and emotional distress, giving a sense of wellness. On the other hand, self-awareness potentially prevented the further progression of diabetes. Another study shows that Yoga can significantly reduce fasting blood glucose and a pre-prandial blood glucose level of Diabetics. A recent study was conducted with 4 men and 34 women of mild to moderate diabetes, in the age group of 30–60 years, which were selected from the outpatient clinic of G.T.B Hospital, Delhi. This study showed that Yoga significantly decreased VLDL, LDL, triglyceride, cholesterol, free fatty acids, serum lipase activity, and the fasting and pre-prandial blood glucose levels in diabetes after following proper yoga protocol.

Yoga has been established as an effective means to improve the overall health, especially in patients suffering from stress, hypertension, coronary atherosclerosis, heart failure, dyslipidemia, diabetes, anxiety, depression, and other similar conditions. This can also induce biochemical alterations that have a salutary effect of cardiac hemodynamics, blood lipids, fasting blood sugar, body mass, and stress. Like CKD, CHD, or ISD, stroke can be fully prevented by management. Katan et al. investigated the effect of yoga on the blood pressure and lipid profile of randomly selected individuals. His findings revealed a significant impact of 3 month yoga on these individuals by returning their blood pressure and lipid profile to the normal range [46]. These and other results need to be brought to the public discourse to heighten the awareness of Yoga by way of organizing such camps.

Rehabilitation therapy is a way that helps stroke survivors to refurbish skills that are forfeited when part of the brain experiences an ischemic insult. Although it it is an irreversible damage, rehabilitation can help the patients in improving functional neurological deficits. Physiotherapists and occupational therapists employ various techniques to enhance the physical strength, motor control and cognitive performance of stroke survivors and also assist them in managing their day-to-day activities.

Research has found that Yoga can remarkably lessen the risks and severity of permanent disability if incorporated along with treatment. Several lines of evidence indicate beneficial effects of yoga for people susceptible with an elevated risk of heart disease [47], anxiety or depression [48], cancer [49], and rheumatoid arthritis [50].

Yoga can also be utilized as self-administered practice in stroke recovery, as it can relieve the mind and body from stress [51]. Stroke survivors who perform Yoga regularly post-stroke may feel enhanced strength, improved flexibility, balance, and energy levels. Yoga is also found to be helpful in increasing the plasticity of the brain, a term called neuroplasticity [52]. Currently, it is well-known that within weeks of brain injury, there is new neuronal cells formation in the subventricular and sub-granular zone of dentate gyrus of the brain, which migrates to the damaged area and promote the regeneration process [53]. Whether these neurons are migratory or resident in local damaged areas of the brain is still unknown [54]. The brain has the potential to form new neural networks, connections/synapses, and reorganize itself. Studies have revealed that yoga practice can help to regenerate the damaged cells and adapt to damage caused by stroke. In addition, Yoga may act as an add-on therapy to stroke rehabilitation treatment and can greatly improve the damaged condition. Furthermore, quality of life can be improved, fear of losing control can be reduced, and patients can attain independence in their day-to-day activities with yoga practice post-stroke. Yoga mitigates motor control and increases the strength and perseverance of stroke survivors.

Lawrence et al. studied two randomized controlled trials and assessed the role of yoga in improving the quality of life and secondary outcome measures as a recovery of function for stroke survivors [55].

Studies pertaining the advantages of yoga in stroke care are still emerging [56, 57] Portz et al. investigated the after effects of Yoga and alterations in physical fitness of older patients with chronic stroke. Their findings revealed that it is crucial to adopt self-management interventions to provide safe physical activity [58].

18.3 Yoga: An Overview and Its Significance as a Therapeutic Module in Curing Diseases

Yoga is a healthy way of living that has origins in India [59–61] and was found thousands of years ago with the aim to attain prosperity and relieve suffering. It has now become prevalent and accepted all over the world [62–64]. "Yoga" arises from the Sanskrit root known as "yuj" [61, 65, 66], which means "to unite together" [66]. It is envisioned as a tree composed of "limbs" that solicits numerous practices such as common belief, physical postures, control of breath and senses, single-mindedness and meditation [64]

Yoga is the exercise of mind, body, and soul [61, 62, 67]. It is believed that yoga can facilitate the mental and spiritual health of an individual and is considered as one of the most vigorous drugless systems of treatment. The yoga protocol that can be practiced to cure dyslipidemia is given below:

Yoga Protocol Table 18.2

(A) **AYUSH International Day of Yoga Protocol 45 min**

(B) **Surya Namaskar (5times)- 5 min**

Figure 18.2 depicts the yoga protocol which can be used to treat dyslipidemia and other CVDs.

18.3.1 Mechanism of Action by Yoga

There are limited studies exploring cellular and molecular mechanisms governing the action of yoga therapy. Studies have shown the role of PPARδ (peroxisome proliferate activator receptor) agonists in activating lipid metabolism resulting in its actions on insulin sensitivity and adiposity [68]. PPARs regulate glucose, lipid, and lipoprotein metabolism in the cell. Preclinical evidences have shown the potential role of PPARs in reducing obesity-induced insulin

Table 18.2 Yoga protocol for dyslipidemia

S. No	Name of practice	Duration (min)
Yoga Protocol: Yoga for Dyslipidemia		
Part A: IDY protocol		
1	**Starting prayer**	2
2	***Sadalija/CalanaKryias*/Loosening practice** 1. Neck bending 2. Trunk movement 3. Knee movement	5
3	***Asanas*** (Postures) (1 min per Asana) **1. Standing position** *Tadasanas(*standing pose), *Trikonasana* (triangle pose), *Vrksasanas* (tree pose), *Padhhastasanas* (standing forward bend*) and ArdhaChakrasanas* (Halfmoon pose) **2. Supine position** *Setubandhasana* (Bridge pose), *Pavanamuktasana* (wind-relieving pose) *Savasana* (Corpse Pose) **3. Prone position** *Bhujangasana* (Cobra pose), *Salabhasanas* (Locust pose) *Vakraasanas*, (simple twist) **4. Sitting position** *Ardhaustrasana* (Half camel pose), *Sasankasanas* (Rabbit pose), *Badharasanas* (Gracious pose)	20
4	**Kapalbhati**	2
5	***Pranayama* (breathing practice)** (2 min per pranayam) Anuluma Viloma, Bhrammari, Sitali	6
6	***Dhyana* (meditation)**	8
7	***Sankalpa* (resolve)** I am completely healthy	1
8	***Santih Patha* (closing Prayer)**	1
	Time duration	45
Part B: *Surya Namaskar* (sun salutition)—5 repetitions		
	Pranamasana (Prayer pose), *Hastauttanasana* (Raised arms pose), *Hasta Padasana* (Hand to foot pose), *Ashwa Sanchalanasana* (Equestrian pose), *Dandasana* (Stick pose), *Ashtanga Namaskara* (Salute with eight parts), *Bhujangasana* (Cobra pose), *Parvatasana* (Mountain pose), *Ashwa Sanchalanasana* (Equestrian pose), *Hasta Padasana* (Hand to foot pose), *Hastauttanasana* (Raised Arms Pose), *Pranamasana* (Prayer pose)	5
	Total time duration	50

resistance and T2DM [69]. Studies report that Yoga therapy improves the lipid profile in subjects with Diabetes Mellitus by enhancing activities of hepatic lipase and pancreatic lipase [70, 71]. It has also been reported that Yoga creates a balance between the sympathetic and parasympathetic branches of CNS [72]. It also improves blood supply to various levels of cellular infrastructure. Insulin receptor expression has been found to be elevated due to improved blood supply to muscles resulting in enhanced glucose uptake by cells followed by a reduction in the blood sugar levels [73]. We argue that Asanas may modulate the cellular niche and enhance the accessibility of various enzymes, ultimately leading to reduction of LDL and TG. Figure 18.3 depicts the possible mechanism of reduction of cholesterol in the diabetic population.

18.3.2 Adverse Effects of Yoga

Similar to any kind of exercise if performed in an inaccurate way, Yoga too may lead to adverse effects. Recently, a 40 year lady suffered stroke due to rupture of one of the blood vessels in the neck while performing a tricky advanced yoga pose. Similarly, a 28 year old woman suffered a stroke while performing a "wheel" pose in 1973. Other cases with brain damage were reported in

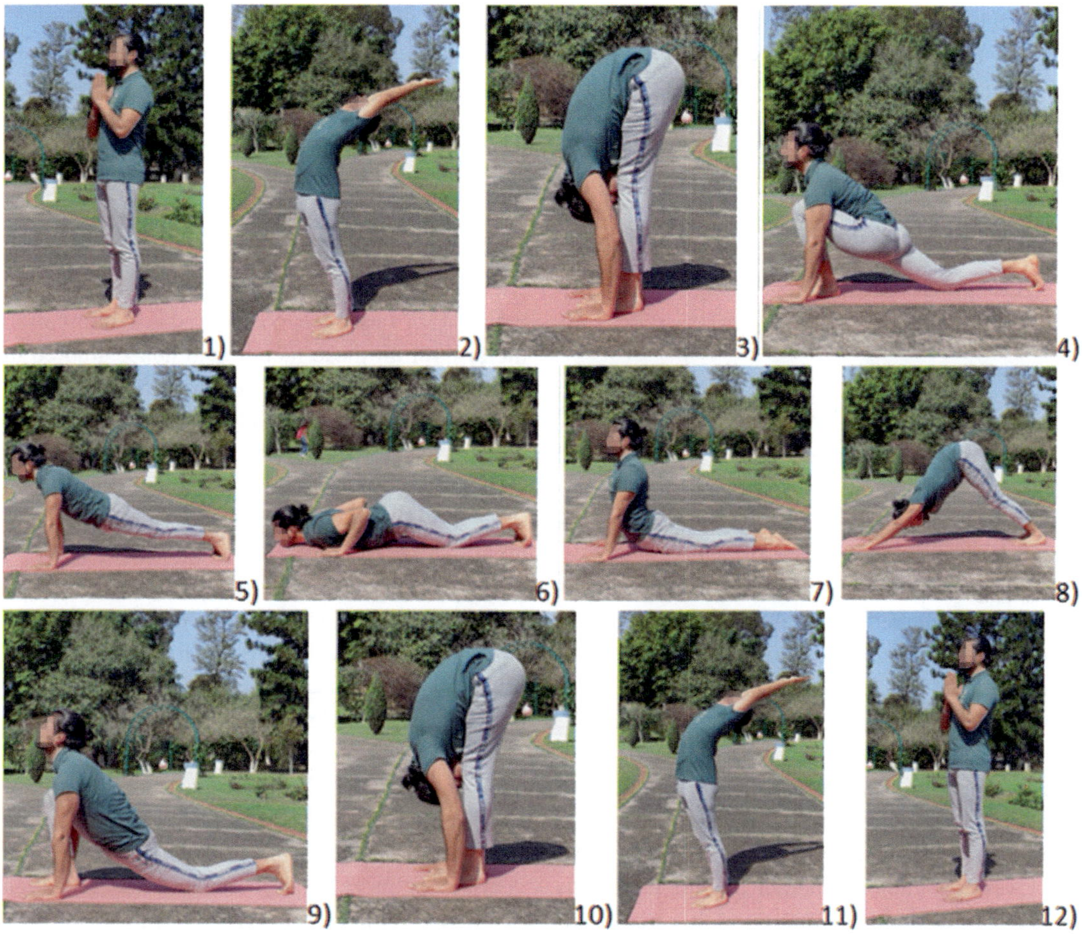

Fig. 18.2 Surya Namaskar Figure depicts the yoga protocol which can be used to treat dyslipidemia and several other CVDs. (**a**) Surya Namaskar (poses 1–12): 1: Pranamasana (Prayer pose), 2: Hastauttanasana (Raised arms pose), 3: Hasta Padasana (Hand to foot pose), 4: Ashwa Sanchalanasana (Equestrian pose), 5: Dandasana (Stick pose), 6: Ashtanga Namaskara (Salute with eight parts), 7: Bhujangasana (Cobra pose), 8: Parvatasana (Mountain pose), 9: Ashwa Sanchalanasana (Equestrian pose), 10: Hasta Padasana (Hand to foot pose), 11: Hastauttanasana (Raised Arms Pose), 12: Pranamasana (Prayer pose)

people performing tricky poses of yoga in 2009. Cramer et al. described adverse events of yoga that may occur if not performed safely. Hence utmost care must be taken while performing different poses of yoga, and advanced poses by beginners must be avoided.

18.3.3 Treatment of Dyslipidemia

(A) Drugs: Various approved drugs that are used to treat Dyslipidemia include:
   (a) 3-hydroxy-3methylglutaryl-coenzyme A (HMG–CoA) reductase inhibitors (the "statins")
   (b) The fibrates (gem fibrozi), clofibrate, and fenofibrate
   (c) Niacin/nicotinic acid
   (d) The bile acid-binding resin (colestipol) and cholestyramine
   (e) Statin [74]

(B) Exercise: These are very helpful for the prevention and treatment of dyslipidemia. There are certain exercises that can reduce the level of LDL and Triglycerides. These include (a) High Intensity Interval Training (HIIT): HIIT decreases the level of LDL, triglyceride and increase the level of HDL. This exercise is very useful in alleviating dyslipidemia. It improves insulin sensitivity and is beneficial to the heart [75]; (b) Cycling: Cycling is also known to reduce the risk factor for all CVD, decreasing LDL, important for regulation of BP. It has been shown that cycling reduces fat and improves BMI [76]; (c) Swimming: It is another useful exercise for human health. With regular swimming, it also reduces the risk of dyslipidemia, decreasing low-density lipoprotein [77]

18.3.4 Alternative Therapies and Dyslipidemia

Oxidative or nitrosative stress plays an indispensable role in the pathogenesis of ischemic stroke. Following ischemic insult, free radicals are accumulated in damaged tissue. A study measured the significantly elevated levels of malondialdehyde, a marker for oxidative stress in patients with acute ischemic stroke, as compared to controls. On the contrary, lutein which is an antioxidant, declined in them, suggesting the role of oxidative stress in stroke. These results indicate that oxidative stress is associated with ischemic stroke [78]. However, it is unclear whether oxidative stress is a result of ischemic injury or vice versa. Patil et al. investigated oxidative stress associated with stroke and the effect of yoga on stroke patients for a period of 3 months. They found a reduction in the malondialdehyde levels and an increase in antioxidant serum superoxide dismutase. According to this study, Yoga is useful in reducing the stress levels, one of the possible reasons for hypertension, especially in the elderly. Oxidative stress has been implicated as one of the underlying causes of hypertension. Yoga can reduce CVD's mortality and morbidity. Yoga is found to control the hypertension in the elderly [79]. Physical inactivity and stress are other reasons which cannot be ignored. Therefore, there are efforts to employ Yoga as a tool for integrative medicine for preventing CVDs. Yoga intervention has shown promising results in alleviating NCDs, especially CVDs. A study has reported that yoga has shown promising results in controlling blood pressure and lipid panel [80]. For promising and effective results, there is a need to develop and practice specific yoga protocols. A combination of stress therapy, dietary preferences and exercise may be beneficial in dyslipidemia. Yoga has been considered a combination therapy for all these factors and hence studied in the dyslipidemia management. Shantakumari et al. reported beneficial effects of 1 yoga protocol in Diabetes [70]. One of the largest studies conducted in India also reported a positive effect of Diabetes Yoga Protocol (DYP) in the management of Dyslipidemia [81].

The molecular mechanism governing the homeostasis of lipids through Yoga intervention has not yet been well studied. However, it is postulated that Yoga asanas enhance the niche in the liver and pancreas, resulting in the hepatic lipase and lipoprotein lipase level changes [82]. At the cellular level, enhanced oxygenation may have triggered an epigenetic shift followed by changes in the expression levels of molecules. Yoga intervention conducted in chronically stressed women resulted in reduced Methylation in the TNF gene [83]. Similarly, Yoga may be associated with balancing the lipid profile via homeostasis of expression of several metabolic biomarkers. More studies are required to validate the impact of yoga in human health.

There are a few Yoga protocols that are being validated through various studies. DYP (Diabetes Yoga Protocol) was performed in a study on Diabetes Patients associated with dyslipidemia. According to this study, dyslipidemia is also a risk factor for Diabetic patients resulting in cardiovascular complications. After DYP intervention, it is noted that there is a significant reduction in triglycerides and LDL and an increment in HDL levels. Therefore, Diabetes Yoga protocol

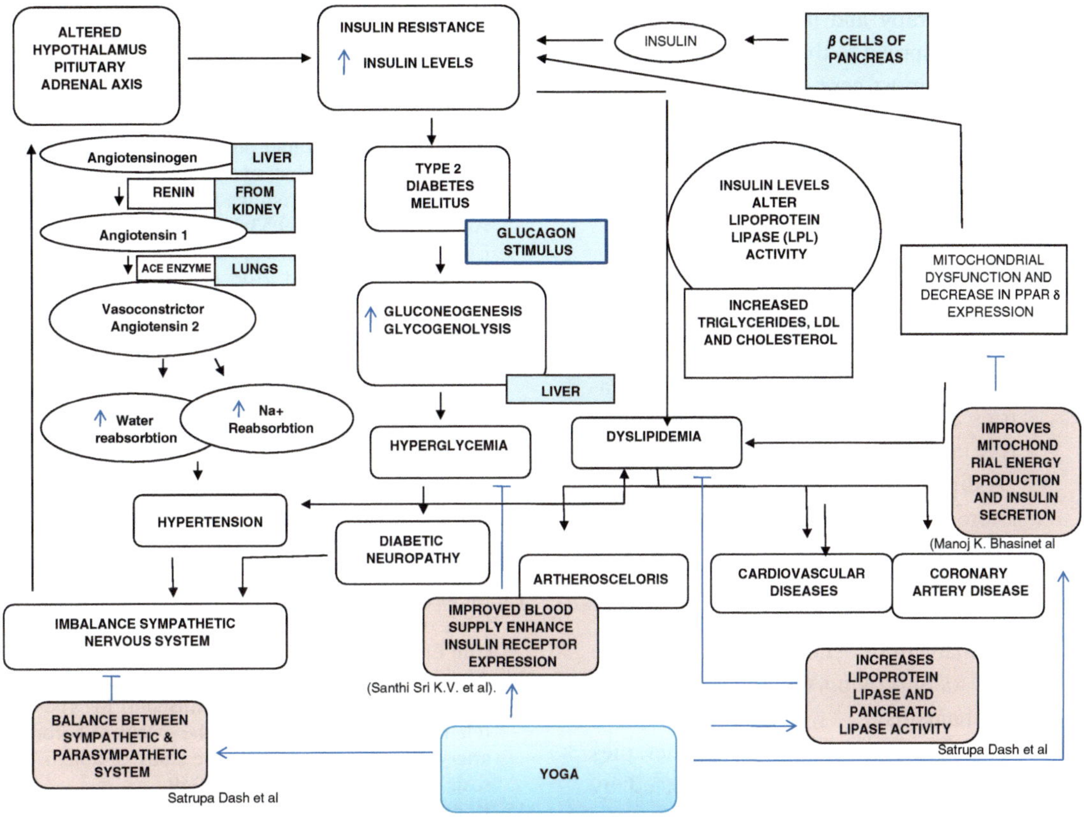

Fig. 18.3 Illustrates the possible mechanism of reduction of cholesterol in the diabetic population. Altered HPA axis may be crucial in developing metabolic disturbances resulting in hyperlipidemia in the diabetic population. YP may target balance between sympathetic and parasympathetic system, improving blood supply in hitherto inaccessible niches, improving lipase activity and improving mitochondrial efficiency

not only reduces T2DM but also benefits in cardiovascular diseases and their co-morbidity. One can adopt DYP as reliable medicine for Dyslipidemia and stroke studies [81].

18.4 Conclusion

In view of the tremendous health benefits of yoga therapy in reducing stress, hypertension and alleviating the development of chronic illnesses, it is advised that yoga practice must be incorporated by every individual in daily routine life in order to stay healthy and lead a stress and disease-free lifestyle. Several lines of evidence have emphasized the importance and effect of yoga as a tool for preventing cerebrovascular diseases, stroke, improving lipid profiles, lowering body mass index, diabetes mellitus, and other major illnesses. More studies of shorter or longer duration must be designed with a well-planned yoga protocol emphasizing on the role of yoga as an alternative therapy and the beneficial effects of yoga must be spread to the rural and urban areas. In addition, utmost care must be taken by yoga practitioners while performing advanced poses. Any inaccurate pose by an amateur may lead to adverse consequences.

Take-Home Message

- Dyslipidemia is an epidemic in both developing as well as developed countries and is a well-established prevalent risk factor of CVDs and ischemic stroke.
- Dyslipidemia is characterized by an altered lipid panel in the blood.
- Yoga is reported to have beneficial effects on prevention as well as management of CVDs and stroke
- Mechanism of beneficial effects may be due to improving cellular homeostatic mechanisms.
- Yoga along with alternative therapies may be investigated and suggested by clinicians.

References

1. Booth FW, Roberts CK, et al. Lack of exercise is a major cause of chronic diseases. Compr Physiol. 2012;2(2):1143–211. https://doi.org/10.1002/cphy.c110025.
2. Stone NJ, Robinson JG, Lichtenstein AH, Bairey Merz CN, Blum CB, Eckel RH, et al. ACC/AHA guideline on the treatment of blood cholesterol to reduce atherosclerotic cardiovascular risk in adults. Circulation. 2013;129(25 Suppl 2):S46–8. https://doi.org/10.1161/01.cir.0000437738.63853.7a.
3. Genest JG. Dyslipidemia and coronary artery disease. Can J Cardiol. 2000;16(Suppl A):3A–4A.
4. WHO website.www.who.int
5. Gupta R, Rao RS, Misra A, Sharma SK. Recent trends in epidemiology of dyslipidemias in India. Indian Heart J. 2017;69(3):382–92. https://doi.org/10.1016/j.ihj.2017.02.020.
6. Nagarathna R, Tyagi R, Kaur G, Vendan V, et al. Efficacy of a validated yoga protocol on dyslipidemia in diabetes patients: NMB-2017 India trial. Medicines (Basel). 2019;6(4):100.
7. Joshi SR, Anjana RM, Deepa M, et al. Prevalence of dyslipidemia in urban and rural India: the ICMR-INDIAB study. PLoS One. 2014;9(5):e96808. https://doi.org/10.1371/journal.pone.0096808.
8. Karthikeyan G, Teo KK, Islam S, McQueen MJ, Pais P, Wang X, et al. Lipid profile, plasma apolipoproteins, and risk of a first myocardial infarction among Asians: an analysis from the INTERHEART study. J Am Coll Cardiol. 2009;53:244–53.
9. Labreuche J, Touboul PJ, Amarenco P. Plasma triglyceride levels and risk of stroke and carotid atherosclerosis: a systematic review of the epidemiological studies. Atherosclerosis. 2009;203:331–45.
10. Amarenco P, Labreuche J, Touboul PJ. High-density lipoprotein-cholesterol and risk of stroke and carotid atherosclerosis: a systematic review. Atherosclerosis. 2008;196:489–96.
11. McBride PE. Triglycerides and risk for coronary heart disease. J Am Med Assoc. 2007;298:336–8.
12. Rizos E, Mikhailidis DP. Are high density lipoprotein and triglyceride levels relevant in stroke prevention? Cardiovasc Res. 2001;52:199–207.
13. McKeigue PM, Miller GJ, Marmot MG. Coronary heart disease in south Asians overseas: a review. J Clin Epidemiol. 1989;42:597–609.
14. Abdalamir M, Goyfman M, Chaus A, Dabbous F, Tamura L, Sandfort V, Brown A, Budoff M. The correlation of dyslipidemia with the extent of coronary artery disease in the multiethnic study of atherosclerosis. J Lipids. 2018;2018:5607349.
15. Kopin L, Lowenstein CJ. Dyslipidemia. Ann Intern Med. 2017;167(11):ITC81. https://doi.org/10.7326/aitc201712050.
16. Weiss LA, Pan L, Abney M, Ober C. The sex-specific genetic architecture of quantitative traits in humans. Nat Genet. 2006;38(2):218–22. https://doi.org/10.1038/ng1726.
17. García-Giustiniani D, Stein R. Genetics of dyslipidemia. Arq Bras Cardiol. 2016; https://doi.org/10.5935/abc.20160074.
18. Nakanishi N, Nakamura K, Suzuki K, Tatara K. Lifestyle and the development of dyslipidemia: a 4-year follow-up study of middle-aged Japanese male office workers. Environ Health Prev Med. 1999;4(3):140–5. https://doi.org/10.1007/bf02932270.
19. Cesar L, Suarez SV, Adi J, et al. An essential role for diet in exercise-mediated protection against dyslipidemia, inflammation and atherosclerosis in ApoE-/- mice. PLoS One. 2011;6(2):e17263. https://doi.org/10.1371/journal.pone.0017263.
20. Catalina-Romero C, Calvo E, Sánchez-Chaparro MA, et al. The relationship between job stress and dyslipidemia. Scand J Public Health. 2013;41(2):142–9. https://doi.org/10.1177/1403494812470400.
21. Stoney CM. Cholesterol and lipoproteins. In: Fink G, editor. Encyclopedia of stress. San Diego, CA: Elsevier; 2007. p. 478–83.
22. McCann BS, Warnick GR, Knopp RH. Changes in plasma lipids and dietary intake accompanying shifts

in perceived workload and stress. Psychosom Med. 1990;52(1):97–108.
23. Black PH, Garbutt LD. Stress, inflammation and cardiovascular disease. J Psychosom Res. 2002;52(1):1–23.
24. Brindley DN, McCann BS, Niaura R, Stoney CM, Suarez EC. Stress and lipoprotein metabolism: modulators and mechanisms. Metabolism. 1993;42(9):3–15.
25. Dallman MF, La Fleur SE, Pecoraro N, Gomez F, Houshyar H, Akana SF. Minireview: Glucocorticoids - food intake, abdominal obesity, and wealthy nations in 2004. Endocrinology. 2004;145(6):2633–8.
26. Nishitani N, Sakakibara H. Relationship of obesity to job stress and eating behavior in male Japanese workers. Int J Obesity. 2005;30(3):528–33.
27. Lemieux AM, Coe CL. Abuse-related posttraumatic stress disorders: evidence for chronic neuroendocrine activation in women. Psychosom Med. 1995;57(2):105–15.
28. Pejovic S, Vgontzas AN, Basta M, Tsaoussoglou M, Zoumakis E, Vgontzas A, Bixler EO, Chrousos GP. Leptin and hunger levels in young healthy adults after one night of sleep loss. J Sleep Res. 2010;19(4):552–8.
29. Spiegel K, Tasali E, Penev P, Van Cauter E. Brief communication: Sleep curtailment in healthy young men is associated with decreased leptin levels, elevated ghrelin levels, and increased hunger and appetite. Ann Intern Med. 2004;141(11):846–50. Björntorp & Rosmond, 1999
30. Björntorp P, Rosmond R. Hypothalamic origin of the metabolic syndrome X. Ann N Y Acad Sci. November 1999;892:297–307.
31. Bartolomucci A, Cabassi A, Govoni P, Ceresini G, Cero C, Berra D, Dadomo H, Franceschini P, Dell'Omo G, Parmigiani S, Palanza P. Metabolic consequences and vulnerability to diet-induced obesity in male mice under chronic social stress. PLoS One. January 2009;4(1):e4331.
32. Kuo LE, Czarnecka M, Kitlinska JB, Tilan JU, Kvetnanský R, Zukowska Z. Chronic stress, combined with a high-fat/high-sugar diet, shifts sympathetic signaling toward neuropeptide Y and leads to obesity and the metabolic syndrome. Ann N Y Acad Sci. December 2008;1148:232–7.
33. Stoney CM, West SG, Hughes JW, Lentino LM, Finney ML, Falko J, Bausserman L. Acute psychological stress reduces plasma triglyceride clearance. Psychophysiology. 2002;39(1):80–5.
34. O'Donnell L, O'Meara N, Owens D, Johnson A, Collins P, Tomkin G. Plasma catecholamines and lipoproteins in chronic psychological stress. J R Soc Med. 1987;80(6):339–42.
35. Yoo H, Franke WD. Stress and cardiovascular disease risk in female law enforcement officers. Int Arch Occup Environ Health. March 2011;84(3): 279–86.
36. Veen G, Giltay EJ, DeRijk RH, van Vliet IM, van Pelt J, Zitman FG. Salivary cortisol, serum lipids, and adiposity in patients with depressive and anxiety disorders. Metabolism. June 2009;58(6):821–7.
37. Vogelzangs N, Suthers K, Ferrucci L, Simonsick EM, Ble A, Schrager M, Bandinelli S, Lauretani F, Giannelli SV, Penninx BW. Hypercortisolemic depression is associated with the metabolic syndrome in late-life. Psychoneuroendocrinology. February 2007;32(2):151–9.
38. Berger DF, Starzec JJ, Mason EB, DeVito W. The effects of differential psychological stress on plasma cholesterol levels in rats. Psychosom Med. September 1980;42(5):481–92.
39. Bryant HU, Story JA, Yim GK. Assessment of endogenous opioid mediation in stress-induced hypercholesterolemia in the rat. Psychosom Med. November–December 1988;50(6):576–85.
40. Neves VJ, Moura MJCS, Tamascia ML, Ferreira R, Silva NS, Costa R, Montemor PL, Narvaes EAO, Bernardes CF, Novaes PD, Marcondes FK. Proatherosclerotic effects of chronic stress in male rats: altered phenylephrine sensitivity and nitric oxide synthase activity of aorta and circulating lipids. Stress. July 2009;12(4):320–7.
41. Black PH. The inflammatory response is an integral part of the stress response: Implications for atherosclerosis, insulin resistance, type II diabetes and metabolic syndrome X. Brain Behav Immunity. October 2003;17(5):350–64.
42. Xu XH, Shah PK, Faure E, Equils O, Thomas L, Fishbein MC, Luthringer D, Xu XP, Rajavashisth TB, Yano J, Kaul S, Arditi M. Toll-like receptor-4 is expressed by macrophages in murine and human lipid-rich atherosclerotic plaques and upregulated by oxidized LDL. Circulation. December 2001;104(25):3103–8.
43. Yudkin JS, Kumari M, Humphries SE, Mohamed-Ali V. Inflammation, obesity, stress and coronary heart disease: is interleukin-6 the link? Atherosclerosis. February 2000;148(2):209–14.
44. Zhang PY, Xu X, Li XC. Cardiovascular diseases: oxidative damage and antioxidant protection. Eur Rev Med Pharmacol Sci. 2014;18(20):3091–6.
45. Rašlová K. Diabetes and dyslipidemia: why are they so closely related? Vnitr Lek. 2016;62(11):908–11.
46. Katan M, Luft AA. Global burden of stroke. Semin Neurol. 2018;38:208–11. https://www.zora.uzh.ch/id/eprint/159894/
47. Cramer H, Lauche R, Haller H, Steckhan N, Michalsen A, Dobos G. Effects of yoga on cardiovascular disease risk factors: a systematic review and meta-analysis. Int J Cardiol. 2014;173(2):170–83.
48. Uebelacker LA, Epstein-Lubow G, Gaudiano BA, Tremont G, Battle CL, Miller IW. Hatha yoga for depression: a critical review of the evidence for efficacy, plausible mechanisms of action, and directions for future research. J Psychiatr Pract. 2010;16(1):22–33.
49. Bower JE, Woolery A, Sternlieb B, Garet D. Yoga for cancer patients and survivors. Cancer Control J. 2005;12(3):165–71.

50. Bosch PR, Traustadottir T, Howard P, Matt KS. Functional and physiological effects of yoga in women with rheumatoid arthritis: a pilot study. Altern Ther Health Med. 2009;15(4):24–31.
51. Lazaridou A, Phaethon P, Tzika AA. Yoga and mindfulness as therapeutic intervention for stroke rehabilitation: a systematic review. Evid Based Complement Altern Med. 2013;2013:357108.
52. Kress R. Research: increasing neuroplasticity with yoga. 2018.
53. Lindvall O, Kokaia Z. Neurogenesis following stroke affecting the adult brain. Cold Spring Harb Perspect Biol. 2015;7(11):a019034.
54. Nemirovich-Danchenko NM, Khodanovich MU. New neurons in the post-ischemic and injured brain: migrating or resident? Front Neurosci. 2019;13:588.
55. Lawrence M, Celestino Junior FT, Matozinho HH, Govan L, Booth J, Beecher J. Yoga for stroke rehabilitation. Cochrane Database Syst Rev Dec. 2017;8:12.
56. Thayabaranathan T, Andrew NE, Immink MA, et al. Determining the potential benefits of yoga in chronic stroke care: a systematic review and meta-analysis. Top Stroke Rehabil. 2017;24(4):279–87.
57. Harris A, Austin M, Blake TM, Bird ML. Perceived benefits and barriers to yoga participation after stroke: a focus group approach. Complement Ther Clin Pract. 2019;34:153–6.
58. Portz JD, Waddington E, Atler KE. Self-management and yoga for older adults with chronic stroke: a mixed-methods study of physical fitness and physical activity. Clin Gerontol. 2018;41(4):374–38.
59. DiBenedetto M, Innes KE, Taylor AG, Rodeheaver PF, Boxer JA, Wright HJ, et al. Effect of a gentle Iyengar yoga program on gait in the elderly: an exploratory study. Arch Phys Med Rehabil. 2005;86(9):1830–7.
60. Tran MD, Holly RG, Lashbrook J, Amsterdam EA. Effects of hatha yoga practice on the health-related aspects of physical fitness. Prev Cardiol. 2001;4(4):165–70.
61. Wahbeh H, Elsas SM, Oken BS. Mind-body interventions: applications in neurology. Neurology. 2008;70(24):2321–8.
62. Bower JE, Greendalee G, Crosswell AD, Garet D, Sternlieb B, Ganz PA, et al. Yoga reduces inflammatory signaling in fatigued breast cancer survivors: a randomized controlled trial. Psychoneuroendocrinology. 2014;43:20–9.
63. Fischer FH, Lewith G, Witt CM, Linde K, Ammon K, Cardini F, et al. High prevalence but limited evidence in complementary and alternative medicine: guidelines for future research. BMC Complement Altern Med. 2014;14:46.
64. Ross A, Thomas S. The health benefits of yoga and exercise: a review of comparison studies. J Altern Complement Med. 2010;16(1):3–12.
65. Garret R, Immink MA, Hillier S. Becoming connected: the lived experience of yoga participation after stroke. Disabil Rehabil. 2011;33(25–26):2404–15.
66. Taylor MJ. Yoga therapeutics: an ancient dynamic systems theory. Techniques Orthop. 2003;18(1):115–25.
67. Oken BS. Randomized, controlled, six-month trial of yoga in healthy seniors: effects on cognition and quality of life. Altern Ther Health Med. 2006;12(1):40–7.
68. Luquet S, Gaudel C, Holst D, Lopez-Soriano J, Jehl-Pietri C, Fredenrich A, Grimaldi PA. Roles of PPAR delta in lipid absorption and metabolism: a new target for the treatment of type 2 diabetes. Biochim Biophys Acta. 2005;1740(2):313–7.
69. Vázquez-Carrera M. Unraveling the effects of PPARβ/δ on insulin resistance and cardiovascular disease. Trends Endocrinol Metab. 2016;27(5):319–34.
70. Shantakumari N, Sequeira S, El Deeb R. Effects of a yoga intervention on lipid profiles of diabetes patients with dyslipidemia. Indian Heart J. 2013;65(2):127–31. https://doi.org/10.1016/j.ihj.2013.02.010.
71. Shradha B, Sisodia S. Diabetes, dyslipidemia, antioxidant and status of oxidative stress. Int J Res Ayurveda Pharm. 2010;1(1):33–42.
72. Udupa K, Sathyaprabha T. Influence of yoga on the autonomic nervous system. In: Based perspectives on the psychophysiology of yoga, vol. 67. New York: Springer; 2017.
73. Ansari RM. Kapalabhati pranayama: an answer to modern day polycystic ovarian syndrome and coexisting metabolic syndrome? Int J Yoga. 2016;9(2):163–7. https://doi.org/10.4103/0973-6131.183705.
74. American Diabetes Association, clinical practice recommendations 1999. Diabetes Care. 1999;22(Supp 1):S56–S59. www.diabetes.org.
75. Tian D, Meng J. Exercise for prevention and relief of cardiovascular disease: prognoses, mechanisms, and approaches. Oxidative Med Cell Longev. 2019;2019:1–11. https://doi.org/10.1155/2019/3756750.
76. Nordengen S, Andersen LB, Solbraa AK, Riiser A. Cycling and cardiovascular disease risk factors including body composition, blood lipids and cardiorespiratory fitness analysed as continuous variables: part 2—systematic review with meta-analysis. Br J Sports Med. 2019; https://doi.org/10.1136/bjsports-2018-099778.
77. Zheng F, Cai Y. Concurrent exercise improves insulin resistance and nonalcoholic fatty liver disease by upregulating PPAR-γ and genes involved in the beta-oxidation of fatty acids in ApoE-KO mice fed a high-fat diet. Lipids Health Dis. 2019;18(1) https://doi.org/10.1186/s12944-018-0933-z.
78. Polidori MC, Cherubini A, Stahl W, Senin U, Sies H, Mecocci P. Plasma carotenoid and malondialdehyde levels in ischemic stroke patients: relationship to early outcome. Free Radic Res. 2002;36(3):265–8. https://doi.org/10.1080/10715760290019273.
79. Patil SG. Effect of yoga on oxidative stress in elderly with grade-I hypertension: a randomized controlled study. J Clin Diagn Res. 2014; https://doi.org/10.7860/jcdr/2014/9498.4586.
80. Chu P, Gotink RA, Yeh GY, Goldie SJ, Hunink MM. The effectiveness of yoga in modifying risk factors for cardiovascular disease and meta-

bolic syndrome: a systematic review and meta-analysis of randomized controlled trials. Eur J Prev Cardiol. 2014;23(3):291–307. https://doi.org/10.1177/2047487314562741.

81. Nagarathna R, Tyagi R, Kaur G, Vendan V, et al. Efficacy of a validated yoga protocol on dyslipidemia in diabetes patients: NMB-2017 India trial. Medicines. 2019;6(4):100. https://doi.org/10.3390/medicines6040100.

82. Tziomalos K, Athyros V, et al. Dyslipidemia as a risk factor for ischemic stroke. Curr Top Med Chem. 2009;9(14):1291–7. https://doi.org/10.2174/156802609789869628.

83. Harkess KN, Ryan J, Delfabbro PH, Cohen-Woods S. Preliminary indications of the effect of a brief yoga intervention on markers of inflammation and DNA methylation in chronically stressed women. Transl Psychiatry. 2016;6(11):e965. https://doi.org/10.1038/tp.2016.234.

84. Song P, Zha M, Yang X, Xu Y, Wang H, Fang Z, et al. Socioeconomic and geographic variations in the prevalence, awareness, treatment and control of dyslipidemia in middle-aged and older Chinese. Atherosclerosis. 2019;282:57–66. https://doi.org/10.1016/j.atherosclerosis.2019.01.005.

19 Yoga for Primary and Secondary Prevention of Coronary Heart Disease

Subhash Chander Manchanda and Kushal Madan

19.1 Introduction

Despite tremendous advances in the prevention and treatment of cardiovascular disease, coronary heart disease (CHD) remains the leading cause of mortality and morbidity throughout the world, and its burden is increasing. According to the global burden of disease (GBD), deaths due to CHD have increased by 20% (7.3 million in 2007 to 8.93 million in 2017 [1]. Moreover, psychosocial stress, which is emerging as a strong risk factor for causation of CHD [2], has not been given adequate attention in the conventional preventive strategies. Hence, newer cost-effective strategies to prevent CHD and supplement the current treatment options are required. Yoga appears to be one such promising technique for the prevention of CHD. This chapter will review the current evidence regarding the role of yoga in the primary and secondary prevention of CHD.

19.2 What Is Yoga?

The word yoga comes from a Sanskrit word "YUG" which means to yoke or join together. It connotes joining the mind with the body or lower human nature to the higher [3]. Yoga is an ancient mind-body discipline that originated in India more than 5000 years earlier. It is an integrated system of self-culture which aims at the harmonious development of the body and the mind leading to physical well-being mental harmony culminating into positive thinking, happiness, and peace. The practice of yoga is becoming increasingly popular worldwide because of its health and stress-controlling benefits. Even United Nations has realized its importance and declared June 21 as the international day of yoga in 2015. Though there are several types of yoga the commonly practiced yoga consists of three components: (a) Stretching exercises or postures (Asanas), (b) Breathing techniques (Pranayams), (c) Concentration and thinking techniques (Meditation). Numerous scientific studies suggest that yoga is beneficial in chronic diseases including anxiety, depression, fatigue, low backache, arthritis, migraine, allergies, asthma, acid peptic disease, irritable bowel, diabetes mellitus, hypertension, cardiovascular disease etc. [4–7]. Yoga appears to be especially useful for primary and secondary prevention of CHD [8–11].

19.3 Yoga for Primary Prevention of CHD

Most of the major risk factors of coronary heart disease, viz. hypertension, diabetes mellitus, metabolic syndrome, obesity, psychosocial

S. C. Manchanda (✉) · K. Madan
Dharma Vira Heart Center, Sir Ganga Ram Hospital, New Delhi, India

I. Basu-Ray, D. Mehta (eds.), *The Principles and Practice of Yoga in Cardiovascular Medicine*,
https://doi.org/10.1007/978-981-16-6913-2_19

stress, dyslipidemia, and smoking, have been reported to be benefited by regular practice of yoga.

19.4 Hypertension

Hypertension (HTN) is a huge public health problem and is one of the major risk factors for CHD. According to GBD, hypertension contributed to 7.3 million deaths in 2017 [1]. Numerous randomized controlled studies and meta-analyses have demonstrated that both systolic (SBP) and diastolic blood pressure (DBP) are reduced in the majority of patients with mild or prehypertension [12–18]. The follow-up in these studies has varied from 6 to 48 weeks. Though the reduction in blood pressure is modest (SBP 5–10 mmHg & DBP 3–5 mmHg), this could significantly reduce the risk of CHD because it has been estimated that a reduction of SBP by 3 mmHg in the general population has the potential to decrease CHD mortality by 5% [19]. Though the reported studies have several limitations, including short follow-up, non-uniform methodologies and larger well-controlled long-term studies are needed, a scientific statement by American Heart Association has stated that transcendental meditation (TM) shows a modest decrease in blood pressure and have suggested that it is reasonable for all individuals with blood pressure more than 120/80 mmHg to consider TM as clinical adjunct method to lower blood pressure when clinically appropriate [20].

19.5 Diabetes Mellitus (DM), Metabolic Syndrome

DM is another major risk factor for CHD, and its incidence is increasing worldwide, especially in south Asian countries. According to GBD, DM was responsible for 1.37 million deaths in 2017. Yoga has been shown to be a simple therapeutic and preventive modality to lower blood sugar. A recent multicenter randomized study in 3366 patients with prediabetes demonstrated that new-onset diabetes could be prevented by 47% with yoga practice as compared to controls at 3 months follow-up [21]. Yoga intervention also resulted in A1c values returning to normal (less than 5.7%) in more subjects compared to control (52% vs. 39.9%). Several randomized control trials (RCTs) have been published to study the effect of yoga on DM for a period varying from 6 to 36 weeks [22–30]. These studies demonstrate that there is not only improvement in glucose tolerance but also in insulin resistance, central obesity, dyslipidemia, and blood pressure in these subjects. Some studies also suggest that yoga improves the autonomic functions and quality of life in DM patients [31]. Regular practice of yoga has also been shown to improve several components of metabolic syndrome like insulin resistance, body mass index, waist circumference, dyslipidemia, blood pressure, and A1c [32–36]. Yoga has also been reported to regress early atherosclerosis in metabolic syndrome as assessed by carotid intimal medial thickness in one study [36].

19.6 Obesity

Obesity, generalized as well as visceral both are independent risk factors for CHD, HTN, and DM. In low and middle-income countries, the prevalence of obesity is increasing. Global Burden of Disease has suggested that there may be approx. 1.4 billion people who are overweight. Visceral obesity has been considered to be a state of low-grade inflammation [37] which, if untreated, may later culminate in a chronic disorder. Several RCTs have demonstrated an improvement in body weight and or composition by yoga-based programs compared to control [38–41]. These studies have been performed in either healthy individuals or those with CVD risk factors such as HTN, type II DM and CHD. Yoga was associated with 1.5 to 13.5% decrease in body weight. By regular practice of yoga, it is shown that Central obesity is decreased in metabolic syndrome [36]. One study has shown a decrease in inflammatory markers of obesity after short-term yoga practice [37].

19.7 Smoking Cessation

Smoking and tobacco use are the most preventable causes of CHD and death. Quitting smoking decreases CHD, but it is a challenging task with poor success. Smoking cessation may be possible with yoga practices. A recent RCT has reported that a brief training of mindfulness meditation reduced smoking by 60% and also curbed craving in smokers. These changes were probably related to improved self-control as demonstrated by enhanced activity in the anterior cingulated and prefrontal cortex [42]. Recently two meta-analyses have suggested that yoga appears an effective complimentary therapy for smoking cessation [43, 44]. However, the studies have short follow-up and methodological limitations.

19.8 Psychosocial Stress

Psychosocial stress (especially depression, anxiety, and hostility) has emerged as a significant risk factor for hypertension, stroke, myocardial infarction, insulin resistance and cardiovascular mortality [45–47]. A large InterHeart study conducted in 52 countries suggested that psychosocial stress was an important risk factor for myocardial infarction (RR 2.67), almost as bad as smoking [2]. Recently American Heart Association has suggested that depression should be considered as a major risk factor like smoking, hypertension, diabetes, and obesity [48]. The exact mechanism by which stress causes heart disease is not clear, but it appears that this could be due to complex interaction of neuroendocrinal and autonomic nervous systems resulting in a change in behavior, inflammation, and other parameters (Fig. 19.1). Improvement in cardiovascular response and

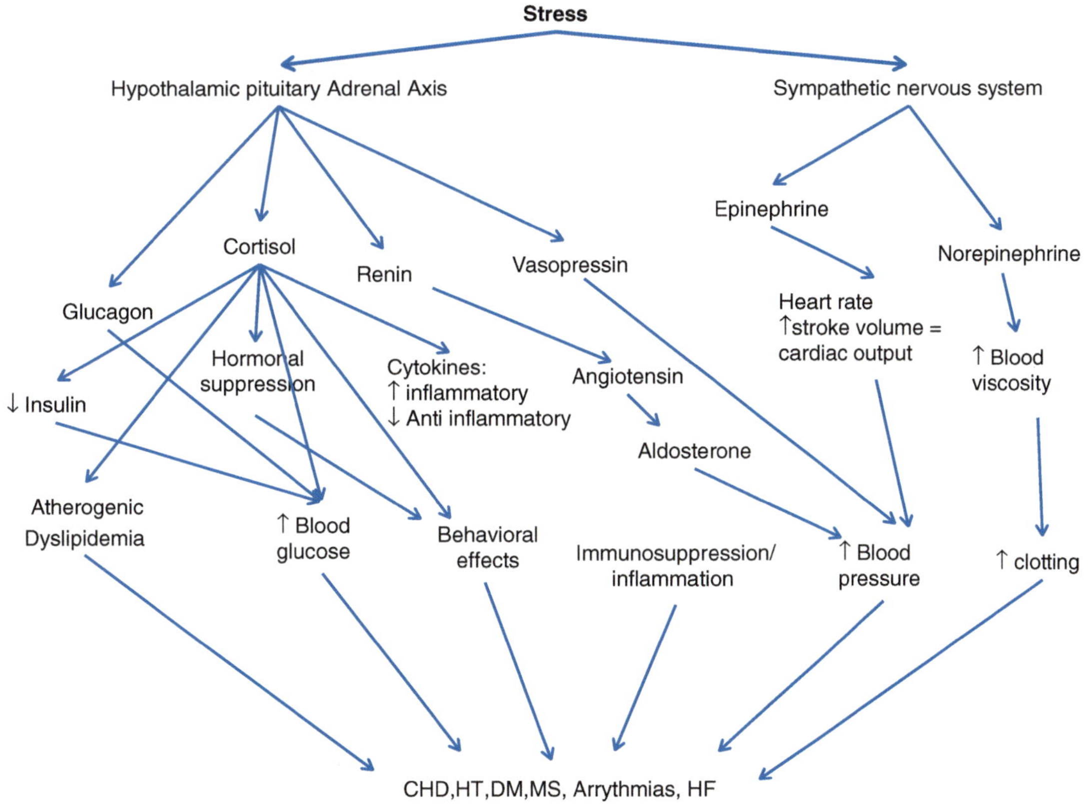

Fig. 19.1 Possible mechanism of stress-causing CVD

recovery from stress due to yoga has been demonstrated [49]. Several studies of yoga and meditation suggest that stress, anxiety, depression can be reduced significantly with regular practice [50–52]. One study suggests that yoga may be as useful as medicine to manage depression [53].

19.9 Dyslipidemia

Dyslipidemia is the leading risk factor for coronary heart disease and has been estimated to account for about 2.6 million deaths annually [1]. Several RCTs have shown significant improvement in lipid profiles by the practice of yoga for 6 weeks to 2 years in healthy subjects and in patients with HTN, DM, and CHD [41, 54–59]. A randomized trial has demonstrated a significant decrease in total cholesterol, triglycerides, LDLc and improvement in HDLc in diabetic patients with dyslipidemia [58]. A meta-analysis of 30 randomized control trials in 751 subjects demonstrated that LDL cholesterol decreased by 12 mg/dL as compared to controls [59]. However, many studies have utilized health education, diet control, and other therapies along with yoga. Hence, results have to be interpreted cautiously. It may be concluded that yoga may enhance the effect of the current drug regimen to lower lipids, and thereby the risk of CVD is reduced.

19.10 Inflammation, Oxidative Stress, and Procoagulant Status

Accumulating data suggest that inflammation contributes to the causation and progression of CHD [37, 60, 61]. Inflammatory mediators may prompt rupture of atherosclerotic plaque resulting in coronary thrombosis and acute ischemia. IL6, fibrinogen, C-reactive protein and TNF-alpha are the main inflammatory markers that have gained recognition, all of which have been considered as independent predictors of CHD. Adiponectin is cardioprotective important regulator of endothelial nitric oxide synthase and is also a key determinant of endothelial function. A yoga-based lifestyle intervention has been reported to reduce levels of IL6, IL18, CRP and TNF-alpha and thereby inflammation and increase in adiponectin in obese as well as normal-weight individuals [37].

Procoagulant changes due to oxidative stress have an important role in the development and progression of CHD, DM, and Metabolic Syndrome [62, 63]. In two uncontrolled studies in healthy adults, it was observed that 12–16 weeks of yogic practices resulted in a significant reduction in fibrinogen and increase in fibrinolytic activity [63, 64], suggesting that yoga may promote favorable changes in coagulation and fibrinogen system.

Several small studies [65–67] have demonstrated that yoga practices may reduce oxidative stress in both healthy population and chronic insulin-related disorders. Altered oxidative status is indicated by the increase in antioxidants and antioxidative enzymes and the reduction of free radicals.

19.11 Role of Yoga in Management of CVD Risk Score

Cardiovascular risk scores predict the possibility of occurring of CHD in the future. However, there are limited studies regarding the role of yoga on cardiovascular risk scores. One small short-term study has estimated the Framingham risk score (FRS) and 10 year cardiovascular disease risk reduction by yoga-based life style intervention [68]. In this study 386 subjects with low (0–1 CHD risk factors) to moderately high risk (10 year risk between 10% and 20% and 2 or more CHD risk factors) were given 2 weeks (2 h/day) practice of yoga. A significant reduction in FRS and estimated 10 year CVD risk was observed. Moreover, the reduction in FRS had a positive correlation with serum cholesterol and LDL. A decrease in BMI, SBP & DBP and Lipids was also reported. Another meditation-based intervention trial has also observed a 16% reduction in 10-year risk [69]. However, more trials with longer follow-up are needed to assess the role of yoga on CV risk scores.

19.12 Yoga for Secondary Prevention of CHD

Cardiac Rehabilitation Cardiac rehabilitation has been shown to be beneficial in the recovery process after myocardial infarction, coronary bypass surgery and coronary interventions but generally not followed. To further improve the quality of life and mortality, psychosocial intervention can be added to the rehabilitation program. Yoga practice leads to similar outcomes as cardiac rehabilitation like improved general well-being, better sleep and appetite, improved physical fitness, stress reduction, and lifestyle change [70]. A study utilizing yoga-based cardiac rehabilitation after coronary artery bypass surgery demonstrated a significant decrease in perceived stress, anxiety, depression, and negative effects [71]. The left ventricular ejection fraction was also reported to be improved with a reduction in blood glucose and decrease in LDL and increase in HDL. The largest multicenter randomized trial studying the effects of yoga-based cardiac rehabilitation after MI has been recently reported [72]. In this trial, 3859 patients with acute MI from 24 centers were randomized to yoga or enhanced standard care and followed for 22 months. It was observed that yoga improved the quality of life, self-rated health and early return to pre infarct activities. The major adverse cardiovascular events (MACE) (which included total mortality, non-fatal MI, stroke, and emergency cardiovascular hospitalization) were reduced from 7.4% to 6.4% but were not statistically significant. However, the patients who had high compliance with yoga practices showed a significant decrease in the MACE (RR 0.53, CI 0.39–0.83, $p < 0.003$). This landmark trial suggests that yoga could be a simple, safe, cost-effective technique of cardiac rehabilitation after myocardial infarction.

19.13 Regression of Atherosclerosis

Three controlled studies utilizing coronary angiography in advanced obstructive CHD demonstrated that yoga lifestyle (with low-fat vegetarian diet) caused retardation of progression and slight regression of coronary obstructions as compared to controls [38, 73, 74]. In addition, angina and exercise-induced ischemia were also significantly reduced in the yoga group. Although the regression of coronary atherosclerosis was minimal, it may translate into a very significant clinical benefit. One recent randomized control trial of TM has indeed reported that there was a 48% risk reduction of primary end point, which was composite of all-cause mortality, non-fatal MI and stroke over a period of 5.4 years in patients with CHD [75].

The presence of depression in patients after acute coronary syndrome, heart failure and bypass surgery increases mortality significantly [76]. As yoga can control depression, it may be extremely beneficial in these conditions. However, there is a paucity of studies in these conditions, and more studies are needed. A few studies suggest that yoga may be beneficial in controlling stress in patients with ICD implantation and may even reduce episodes of VF [77].

19.14 Cardiac Arrhythmias and Heart Failure

Cardiac arrhythmias and heart failure are serious complications of CHD. A few studies have reported that yoga may be useful to control premature ventricular ectopics and may also decrease atrial fibrillation (AF) burden in patients of paroxysmal AF [78, 79]. Yoga has also been reported to be useful in patients with heart failure, where it has been demonstrated to improve the peak oxygen consumption, left ventricular ejection fraction, improved biomarkers (NT Pro BNP, inflammatory markers) and quality of life [80, 81]. However, long-term studies are lacking.

Possible Mechanism of Action of Yoga in Heart Disease Precise mechanisms by which yoga may influence the heart are not entirely clear. It has been suggested that yoga affects the autonomic nervous system with an increase in the parasympathetic and under activity of the GABA system, which is the primary inhibitor of the neu-

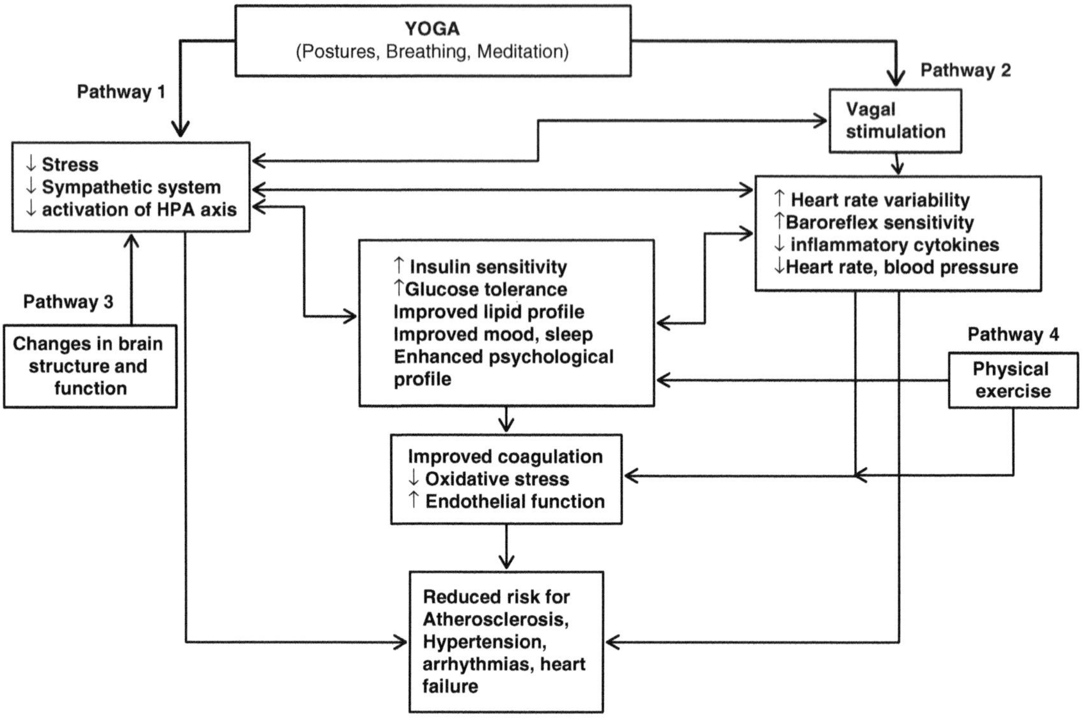

Fig. 19.2 Psychophysiology of yoga in heart disease—possible mechanisms (modified from Innes et al. [83])

rotransmitter system. This is achieved in part through stimulation of the vagus nerve and thereby may reduce allostatic load [82]. Innes et al. had postulated that yoga might reduce the risk of cardiovascular and metabolic disease through two interconnected pathways with the decrease in the activity of the hypothalamus–pituitary–adrenal axis (HPA axis) and decrease the activity of the sympathetic system [83]. Vagal stimulation during yoga also increases heart rate variability and baroreceptor sensitivity and decreases inflammatory cytokines, heart rate and blood pressure. Changes in brain structure, neurotransmitters, and physical exercise may also contribute to the beneficial effects of yoga in CHD (Fig. 19.2). These interactive pathways increase insulin sensitivity, improve lipid profiles and enhance psychological profile leading to decrease oxidative stress and ultimately conferring a protective effect against coronary heart disease, heart failure, hypertension, arrhythmias, and metabolic syndrome. Yoga has also been demonstrated to improve anxiety and depression, which also may be beneficial for the prevention of heart disease. Behavior changes like physical inactivity, insomnia, smoking, and excess alcohol may be corrected by yoga playing a further cardioprotective role.

19.15 Conclusion

Despite tremendous advances, CHD remains the leading cause of death and disability. Hence there is a need for additional strategies. Yoga, an ancient mind–body holistic lifestyle, appears to be a promising technique for primary and secondary prevention of CHD. Several RCTs suggest that yoga could help in controlling all the major risk factors for CHD, namely HTN, DM, insulin resistance, obesity, psychosocial stress, dyslipidemia, smoking, inflammation, and oxidative stress. The new onset of DM has been shown to be decreased by 47% by yoga practice. Yoga has also been shown to be extremely useful in secondary prevention of CHD, cardiac rehabilitation, arrhythmias, heart failure and may regress coronary atherosclerosis. Yoga appears to be a cost-effective, safe, and simple technique for cardiac rehabilitation after myocardial infarction. However, most reported studies have limitations like small sample size, short follow-up and poor methodologies. Hence, large well-controlled trials with clinical end points are needed. However, in view of existing knowledge and yoga being a cost-effective and simple technique without side effects, it appears appropriate to incorporate yoga for primary and secondary prevention of CHD where it can play a primary and/or complementary role.

References

1. GBD 2017 Causes of Death Collaborators. Global, regional, and national age-sex-specific mortality for 282 causes of death in 195 countries and territories, 1980–2017: A systematic analysis for the global burden of Disease Study 2017. Lancet. 2018 Nov 10;392(10159):1736–1788.
2. Yusuf S, Hawken S, Ounpuu S, Dans T, Avezum A, Lanas F, McQueen M, Budaj A, Pais P, Varigos J, Lisheng L, INTERHEART Study Investigators. Effect of potentially modifiable risk factors associated with myocardial infarction in 52 countries (the INTERHEART study): case-control study. Lancet. 2004 Sep 11–17;364(9438):937–52.
3. Ananda S. The complete book of yoga: harmony of body and mind. 1st ed. Delhi reprinted 2001: Orient; 1981.
4. Raub J. Psychophysiologic effects of hatha yoga on musculoskeletal and cardiopulmonary function: a literature review. J Altern Complement Med. 2002;8:797–812.
5. Meditation Practices for Health. State of the Research (2007) prepared for agency for Healthcare Research and Quantity; US Department of Health and Human Services. www.ahrg.gov
6. Büssing A, Michalsen A, Khalsa SB, Telles S, Sherman KJ. Effects of yoga on mental and physical health: a short summary of reviews. Evid Based Complement Alternat Med. 2012;2012:165410.
7. Taneja DK. Yoga and health. Indian J Community Med. 2014;39(2):68–72.
8. Manchanda SC, Madan K. Yoga and meditation in cardiovascular disease. Clin Res Cardiol. 2014 Sep;103(9):675–80.
9. Haider T, Sharma M, Branscum P. Yoga as an alternative and complimentary therapy for cardiovascular disease: a systematic review. J Evid Based Complement Altern Med. 2017 Apr;22(2):310–6.
10. Cramer H, Lauche R, Haller H, Steckhan N, Michalsen A, Dobos G. Effects of yoga on cardiovascular disease risk factors: a systematic review and meta-analysis. Int J Cardiol. 2014 May 1;173(2):170–83.
11. Levine GN, Lange RA, Bairey-Merz CN, Davidson RJ, Jamerson K, Mehta PK, Michos ED, Norris K, Ray IB, Saban KL, Shah T, Stein R, Smith SC, American Heart Association Council on Clinical Cardiology; Council on Cardiovascular and Stroke Nursing; and Council on Hypertension. Meditation and cardiovascular risk reduction: a scientific statement from the American Heart Association. J Am Heart Assoc. 2017 Sep 28;6(10):e002218.
12. Anderson JW, Liu C, Kryscio RJ. Blood pressure response to transcendental meditation: a meta-analysis. Am J Hypertens. 2008 Mar;21(3):310–6.
13. Yang K. A review of yoga programs for four leading risk factors of chronic diseases. Evid Based Complement Alternat Med. 2007 Dec;4(4):487–91.
14. Okonta NR. Does yoga therapy reduce blood pressure in patients with hypertension?: an integrative review. Holist Nurs Pract. 2012 May–Jun;26(3):137–41.
15. Hagins M, States R, Selfe T, Innes K. Effectiveness of yoga for hypertension: systematic review and meta-analysis. Evid Based Complement Alternat Med. 2013;2013:649836.
16. Wang J, Xiong X, Liu W. Yoga for essential hypertension: a systematic review. PLoS One. 2013 Oct 4;8(10):e76357.
17. Tyagi A, Cohen M. Yoga and hypertension: a systematic review. Altern Ther Health Med. 2014 Mar-Apr;20(2):32–59.
18. Posadzki P, Cramer H, Kuzdzal A, Lee MS, Ernst E. Yoga for hypertension: a systematic review of randomized clinical trials. Complement Ther Med. 2014 Jun;22(3):511–22.
19. Appel LJ. Lifestyle modification as a means to prevent and treat high blood pressure. J Am Soc Nephrol. 2003 Jul;14(7 Suppl 2):S99–S102.
20. Brook RD, Appel LJ, Rubenfire M, Ogedegbe G, Bisognano JD, Elliott WJ, Fuchs FD, Hughes JW, Lackland DT, Staffileno BA, Townsend RR, Rajagopalan S, American Heart Association Professional Education Committee of the Council for High Blood Pressure Research, Council on Cardiovascular and Stroke Nursing, Council on Epidemiology and Prevention, and Council on Nutrition, Physical Activity. Beyond medications and diet: alternative approaches to lowering blood pressure: a scientific statement from the American Heart Association. Hypertension. 2013 Jun;61(6):1360–83.
21. Nagarathna R, Ram V, Amit Singh R, Majumdar V, Patil S, Nagendra HR. Diabetes prevention through Yoga-based Lifestyle: a Pan-India randomized controlled trial. Diabetes. 2019 Jun;68(Suppl 1):129.
22. Khare K, Jain D. Effect of yoga on plasma glucose and serum fructosamine level in NIDDM. Yoga Mimamsa. 1999;33:1–9.
23. Agrawal R, Aradhana R, Hussain S, Beniwal R. Influence of yogic treatment on quality of life outcomes, glycaemic control and risk factors in

diabetes mellitus. Int J Diabetes Dev Countries. 2003;23:130–4.
24. Agte VV, Tarwadi K. Sudarshan Kriya yoga for treating type 2 diabetes: a preliminary study. Altern Compliment Therap. 2004;10(4):220–2.
25. Singh S, Kyizom T, Singh KP, Tandon OP, Madhu SV. Influence of pranayamas and yoga-asanas on serum insulin, blood glucose and lipid profile in type 2 diabetes. Indian J Clin Biochem. 2008;23(4):365–8.
26. Hegde SV, Adhikari P, Kotian S, Pinto VJ, D'Souza S, D'Souza V. Effect of 3-month yoga on oxidative stress in type 2 diabetes with or without complications: a controlled clinical trial. Diabetes Care. 2011 Oct;34(10):2208–10.
27. Nagarathna R, Usharani M, Rao A, Chaku R, Kulkarni R, Nagendra H. Efficacy of yoga based lifestyle modification program on medication score and lipid profile in type 2 diabetes – a randomized control study. Int J Diabetes Dev Countries. 2012;32(3):122–30.
28. Vaishali K, Kumar KV, Adhikari P, Unnikrishnan B. Effects of yoga-based program on glycosylated hemoglobin level serum lipid profile in community dwelling elderly subjects with chronic type 2 diabetes mellitus – a randomized controlled trial. Phys Occup Therapy Geriatrics. 2012;30(1):22–30.
29. Shantakumari N, Sequeira S, El Deeb R. Effects of a yoga intervention on lipid profiles of diabetes patients with dyslipidemia. Indian Heart J. 2013 Mar–Apr;65(2):127–31.
30. Jyotsna VP, Ambekar S, Joshi A, Dhawan A, Kumar N, Gupta N. Prospective randomized controlled intervention trial: Comprehensive yogic breathing program improves cardiac autonomic functions and quality of life in diabetes. Indian J Endocrinol Metab. 2012;2012(Suppl 2):S489–91.
31. Corey SM, Epel E, Schembri M, et al. Effect of restorative yoga vs stretching on diurnal cortisol dynamics and psychosocial outcomes in individuals with the metabolic syndrome: the PRYSMS randomized controlled trial. Psychoneuroendocrinology. 2014 Nov;49:260–71.
32. Kanaya AM, Araneta MR, Pawlowsky SB, et al. Restorative yoga and metabolic risk factors: the practicing restorative yoga vs. stretching for the metabolic syndrome (PRYSMS) randomized trial. J Diabetes Complicat. 2014 May–Jun;28(3):406–12.
33. Telles S, Sharma SK, Yadav A, et al. A comparative controlled trial comparing the effects of yoga and walking for overweight and obese adults. Med Sci Monit. 2014 May 31;20:894–904.
34. Schmidt T, Wijga A, Von Zur Mühlen A. Changes in cardiovascular risk factors and hormones during a comprehensive residential three month kriya yoga training and vegetarian nutrition. Acta Physiol Scand Suppl. 1997;640:158–62.
35. McCaffrey R, Ruknui P, Hatthakit U, et al. The effects of yoga on hypertensive persons in Thailand. Holist Nurs Pract. 2005 Jul–Aug;19(4):173–80.
36. Manchanda SC, Mehrotra UC, Makhija A, et al. Reversal of early atherosclerosis in metabolic syndrome by yoga: a randomized controlled trial. J Yoga Phys Ther. 2013;3:132. https://doi.org/10.4172/2157-7595.1000132.
37. Sarvottam K, Magan D, Yadav RK, Mehta N, Mahapatra SC. Adiponectin, interleukin-6, and cardiovascular disease risk factors are modified by a short-term yoga-based lifestyle intervention in overweight and obese men. J Altern Complement Med. 2013 May;19(5):397–402.
38. Manchanda S, Narang R, Reddy K, et al. Retardation of coronary atherosclerosis with yoga lifestyle intervention. J Assoc Phys India. 2000;48:687–94.
39. Udupa KN, Singh RH. The scientific basis of yoga. JAMA. 1972;220:1365.
40. Damodaran A, Malathi A, Patil N, et al. Therapeutic potential of yoga practices in modifying cardiovascular risk profile in middle aged men and women. J Assoc Phys India. 2002;50:633–40.
41. Mahajan A, Reddy K, Sachdeva U. Lipid profile of coronary risk subjects following yogic lifestyle intervention. Indian Heart J. 1999;51(1):37–40.
42. Tang YY, Tang R, Posner MI. Brief meditation training induces smoking reduction. Proc Natl Acad Sci U S A. 2013;110(34):13971–5.
43. Carim-Todd L, Mitchell SH, Oken BS. Mind-body practices: an alternative, drug-free treatment for smoking cessation? A systematic review of the literature. Drug Alcohol Depend. 2013 Oct 1;132(3):399–410.
44. Dai CL, Sharma M. Between inhale and exhale: yoga as an intervention in smoking cessation. J Evid Based Complementary Altern Med. 2014 Apr;19(2):144–9.
45. Kiecolt-Glaser JK, Mcguire L, Robles TF, Glaser R. Emotions, morbidity, and mortality: new perspectives from psychoneuroimmunology. Annu Rev Psychol. 2002;53:83–107.
46. Vitaliano PP, Scanlan JM, Zhang J, Savage MV, Hirsch IB, Siegler IC. A path model of chronic stress, the metabolic syndrome, and coronary heart disease. Psychosom Med. 2002;64:418–35.
47. Sharma M, Manchanda SC. Psychosocial risk factors and heart disease. J Prev Cardiol. 2011;2:57–65.
48. Lichtman JH, Froelicher ES, Blumenthal JA, et al. Depression as a risk factor for poor prognosis among patients with acute coronary syndrome: systematic review and recommendations: a scientific statement from the American Heart Association. Circulation. 2014 Mar 25;129(12):1350–69.
49. Mezzacappa ES, Kelsey RM, Katkin ES, et al. Vagal rebound and recovery from psychological stress. Psychosom Med. 2001;63:650–7.
50. Kirkwood G, Rampes H, Tuffrey V, Richardson J, Pilkington K. Yoga for anxiety: a systemic review of the research evidence. Br J Sports Med. 2005;39:884–91.
51. Pilkington K, Kirkwood G, Rampes H, Richardson J. Yoga for depression: the research evidence. J Affect Disord. 2005;89:13–24.
52. Shapiro D, Cook IA, Davydov DM, Ottaviani C, Leuchter AF, Abrams M. Yoga as a complementary treatment of depression: effects of traits and moods on

treatment outcome. Evid Based Complement Alternat Med. 2007;4:493–502.
53. Naveen GH, Thirthalli J, Rao MG, et al. Positive therapeutic and neurotropic effects of yoga in depression: a comparative study. Indian J Psychiatry. 2013 Jul;55(Suppl 3):S400–4.
54. Joseph S, Sridharan K, Patil S, et al. Study of some physiological and biochemical parameters in subjects undergoing yogic training. Indian J Med Res. 1981;74:120–4.
55. Patel C. Reduction of serum cholesterol and blood pressure in hypertensive patients by behaviour modification. J R Coll Gen Pract. 1976;26:211–5.
56. Naruka J, Mathur R, Mathur A. Effect of pranayamas practices on fasting blood glucose and serum cholesterol. Indian J Med Sci. 1986;40:149–52.
57. Mandape A, Bharshankar J, Phatak M. Effect of Raja yoga meditation on the lipid profile of healthy adults in Central India. J Med Sci Health. 2015;01:10–3.
58. Shantakumari N, Sequeira S, El Deeb R. Effects of a yoga intervention on lipid profiles of diabetes patients with dyslipidemia. Indian Heart J. 2013;65(2):127–31.
59. Jatuporn S, Sangwatanaroj S, Saengsiri AO, et al. Short-term effects of an intensive lifestyle modification program on lipid peroxidation and antioxidant systems in patients with coronary artery disease. Clin Hemorheol Microcirc. 2003;29(3–4):429–36.
60. Taube A, Schlich R, Sell H, Eckardt K, Eckel J. Inflammation and metabolic dysfunction: links to cardiovascular diseases. Am J Physiol Heart Circ Physiol. 2012 Jun 1;302(11):H2148–65.
61. Pullen PR, Nagamia SH, Mehta PK, Thompson WR, Benardot D, Hammoud R, Khan BV. Effects of yoga on inflammation and exercise capacity in patients with chronic heart failure. J Card Fail. 2008;14:407–13.
62. Ceriello A, Motz E. Is oxidative stress the pathogenic mechanism underlying insulin resistance, diabetes and cardiovascular disease? The common soil hypothesis revisited. Arterioscler Thromb Vasc Biol. 2004;24:816–23.
63. Chohan IS, Nayar HS, Thomas P, Geetha NS. Influence of yoga on blood coagulation. Thromb Hemost. 1984;51:196–7.
64. Schmidt T, Wijga A, Von Zur MA, et al. Changes in cardiovascular risk factors and hormones during a comprehensive residential three month kriya yoga training and vegetarian nutrition. Acta Physiol Scand Suppl. 1997;640:158–62.
65. Singh S, Malhotra V, Singh K, Sharma S. A preliminary report on the role of yoga asanas on oxidative stress in noninsulin dependent diabetes. Indian J Clin Biochem. 2001;16:216–20.
66. Bhattacharya S, Pandey U, Verma N. Improvement in oxidative status with yogic breathing in young healthy males. Indian J Physiol Pharmacol. 2002;46:349–54.
67. Sinha S, Singh SN, Monga YP, Ray US. Improvement of glutathione and total antioxidant status with yoga. J Altern Complement Med. 2007;13(10):1085–90.
68. Yadav R, Yadav RK, Sarvottam K, Netam R. Framingham risk score and estimated 10-year cardiovascular disease risk reduction by a short-term yoga-based LifeStyle intervention. J Altern Complement Med. 2017 Sep;23(9):730–7.
69. Edelman D, Oddone EZ, Liebowitz RS, et al. A multidimensional integrative medicine intervention to improve cardiovascular risk. J Gen Intern Med. 2006;21:728–34.
70. Telles S, Naveen KV. Yoga for rehabilitation: an overview. Indian J Med Sci. 1997 Apr;51(4):123–7.
71. Raghuram N, Parachuri VR, Swarnagowri MV, et al. Yoga based cardiac rehabilitation after coronary artery bypass surgery: one-year results on LVEF, lipid profile and psychological states: a randomized controlled study. Indian Heart J. 2014;66:490–502.
72. Prabhakaran D, Chandrasekaran AM, Singh K, Mohan B, Chattopadhyay K, Chadha DS, Negi PC, Bhat P, Sadananda KS, Ajay VS, Singh K, Praveen PA, Devarajan R, Kondal D, Soni D, Mallinson P, Manchanda SC, Madan K, Hughes AD, Chathurvedi N, Roberts I, Ebrahim S, Reddy KS, Tandon N, Pocock S, Roy A, Kinra S, Yoga-CaRe Trial Investigators. Yoga-based cardiac rehabilitation after acute myocardial infarction: a randomized trial. J Am Coll Cardiol. 2020 Apr 7;75(13):1551–61.
73. Ornish D, Brown SE, Scherwitz LW, Billings JH, Armstrong WT, Ports TA, McLanahan SM, Kirkeeide RL, Brand RJ, Gould KL. Can lifestyle changes reverse coronary heart disease? The Lifestyle Heart Trial. Lancet. 1990 Jul 21;336(8708):129–33.
74. Gupta SK, Sawhney RC, Rai L, et al. Regression of coronary atherosclerosis through healthy lifestyle in coronary artery disease patients–Mount Abu open heart trial. Indian Heart J. 2011;63:461–9.
75. Schneider RH, Grim CE, Rainforth MV, et al. Stress reduction in the secondary prevention of cardiovascular disease: randomized, controlled trial of transcendental meditation and health education in Blacks. Circ Cardiovasc Qual Outcomes. 2012;5:750–8.
76. Musselman DL, Evans DL, Nemeroff CB. The relationship of depression to cardiovascular disease: epidemiology, biology, and treatment. Arch Gen Psychiatry. 1998;55:580–92.
77. Toise SC, Sears SF, Schoenfeld MH, et al. Psychosocial and cardiac outcomes of yoga for ICD patients: a randomized clinical control trial. Pacing Clin Electrophysiol. 2014;37:48–62.
78. Prakash ES, Ravindra PN, Madanmohan AR, Balachander J. Effect of deep breathing at six breaths per minute on the frequency of premature ventricular complexes. Int J Cardiol. 2006 Aug 28;111(3):450–2.
79. Lakkireddy D, Atkins D, Pillarisetti J, Ryschon K, Bommana S, Drisko J, Vanga S, Dawn B. Effect of yoga on arrhythmia burden, anxiety, depression, and quality of life in paroxysmal atrial fibrillation: the YOGA my heart study. J Am Coll Cardiol. 2013;61(11):1177–82.
80. Gomes-Neto M, Rodrigues-Jr ES, Silva-Jr WM, Carvalho VO. Effects of yoga in patients with chronic heart failure: a meta-analysis. Arq Bras Cardiol. 2014 Nov;103(5):433–9.

81. Krishna BH, Pal P, Pal G, et al. A randomized controlled trial to study the effect of yoga therapy on cardiac function and N terminal Pro BNP in heart failure. Integr Med Insights. 2014;9:1–6.
82. Streeter CC, Gerbarg PL, Saper RB, Ciraulo DA, Brown RP. Effects of yoga on the autonomic nervous system, gamma-aminobutyric-acid, and allostasis in epilepsy, depression, and post-traumatic stress disorder. Med Hypotheses. 2012 May;78(5):571–9.
83. Innes KE, Bourguignon C, Taylor AG. Risk indices associated with the insulin resistance syndrome, cardiovascular disease, and possible protection with yoga: a systematic review. J Am Board Fam Pract. 2005 Nov–Dec;18(6):491–519.

Role of Yoga in Stroke Management: Current Evidence and Future Directions

20

Nishitha Jasti, Ashok Vardhan Reddy, Kishore Kumar Ramakrishna, Hemant Bhargav, and Girish Baburao Kulkarni

20.1 Introduction

Stroke is a preventable and treatable neurological emergency [1]. Stroke is defined by the World Health Organization as "Rapidly developing clinical signs of focal (or global) disturbance of cerebral function, lasting more than 24 h or leading to death, with no apparent cause other than that of vascular origin" [2].

In stroke, the damage to the brain parenchyma is either due to (1) Ischemia, in which the brain parenchyma is deprived of oxygen due to decreased blood supply, or (2) Haemorrhage, where there is rupture of the blood vessels. In the latter, there is extravasation of blood into the brain parenchyma and extravascular space, causing pressure effect on the surrounding parenchyma and may lead to disruption of various connections in the brain.

1. *Ischemia*: Ischemia can be caused by one of the three mechanisms: formation of the thrombus in the vessel narrowing its lumen (cerebral venous thrombosis or arterial thrombosis), dislodgement of the thrombus to a distant site (emboli) or reduction in the total perfusion due to cardiac pump failure, hypotension, hypovolemia, or any other cause.
2. *Hemorrhage*: It includes four subtypes: subarachnoid hemorrhage; intracerebral hemorrhage; subdural hemorrhage; and epidural hemorrhage. Subarachnoid hemorrhages often originate from bleeding due to aneurysms, arteriovenous malformations, bleeding diathesis or trauma. Intracerebral hemorrhage is most commonly due to uncontrolled hypertension. Other causes include the use of anticoagulants, drugs, trauma, vascular malformations and amyloid angiopathy. Subdural and epidural hemorrhages are typically caused by head trauma.

Over the last two decades, morbidity and mortality associated with stroke have changed due to the advances in acute ischemic stroke treatment through intravenous thrombolysis, endovascular thrombectomy and other surgical procedures. Despite these advances, the significant number of patients still sustain chronic consequences such as residual deficits, cognitive decline and psychological distress; they are also vulnerable to stroke recurrence. As per the Global Burden of Disease (GBD) study (2016), the lifetime risk of developing a stroke is 24.9% in those with age more than 25 years [3]. The adjusted prevalence rate of stroke is more in the

N. Jasti · K. K. Ramakrishna (✉) · H. Bhargav
Department of Integrative Medicine, National Institute of Mental Health and Neurosciences (NIMHANS), Bengaluru, India

A. V. Reddy · G. B. Kulkarni
Department of Neurology, National Institute of Mental Health and Neurosciences (NIMHANS), Bengaluru, India

I. Basu-Ray, D. Mehta (eds.), *The Principles and Practice of Yoga in Cardiovascular Medicine*,
https://doi.org/10.1007/978-981-16-6913-2_20

urban (334–424/100,000) than in the rural areas (84–262/100,000). These prevalence rates suggest the need for training manpower and promoting rehabilitation services for stroke-related morbidity across the globe. Ischemic stroke is the most common subtype of stroke, which contributes to 75–80% according to various studies [4]. In a study investigating the functional outcome in stroke survivors at the end of 28 days of stroke onset, it was found that 42.4% had mild disability, 43% had a moderate disability, and 14.6% were bedridden (Rankin score 5) [4]. The incidence of cerebral venous thrombosis (CVT) is less than 1% globally. However, it is more common in India, with higher incidence in females due to exposure to specific risk factors like postpartum state and hormonal supplementation. Incidence of Intra-cranial hemorrhage (ICH) ranges from 20% to 25% among all strokes. In comparison to patients with arterial stroke, CVT patients have better recovery and 60% recover completely. About 8% of the CVT patients report mortality [5].

20.2 Clinical Features

The symptoms at presentation depend on the etiological type of the stroke:Ischemic (IS) or hemorrhagic (HS). If symptoms improve within 24 h, it is Transient Ischemic Attack (TIA). Signs and symptoms depend on the artery involved or area of hemorrhage in IS and HS, respectively.

Symptoms of IS may include unilateral facial weakness, weakness of upper limb and/or lower limb, blurring of vision in one eye, language disturbances like difficulty to speak and understand, loss of consciousness, seizures, sensory loss on one side of the body, sudden-onset giddiness, imbalance, speech difficulties (dysarthria and anarthria), swallowing difficulties, deviation of the tongue to one side, excessive sleepiness and memory loss.

Patients with HS may present with sudden-onset severe headache followed by neurological deficit, loss of balance, incoordination, unilateral weakness of limbs, seizures, confusion, and drowsiness.

The most common symptoms of CVT include headache, vomiting, seizures, and hemiparesis. CVT involving the peripheral system usually presents with headaches, seizures, and focal motor weakness. When the deep venous system is involved, the symptoms are more severe, resulting in altered mental status and bilateral motor deficits. High mortality and morbidity are observed with the involvement of basal ganglia and thalamus [5].

20.3 Risk Factors

The risk factors for stroke can be divided into those which can be modified (modifiable) and those which cannot be modified (non-modifiable) (Refer Table 20.1). It is evident that modifiable risk factors are closely related to lifestyle, and lifestyle modification programs could be useful in reducing the risk of stroke.

20.4 Limitations of Conventional Management Care

Despite the advances in conventional management, stroke still continues to significantly contribute to the global burden in terms of mortality and morbidity. There seems to be very less awareness on stroke burden, warning signs, acute management services available, the prevention

Table 20.1 Risk factors of stroke

Modifiable risk factors	Non-modifiable risk factors
Cigarette smoking	Age > 65 years
Alcohol	Positive family history
Hypertension	African or South-Asian ethnicity
Diabetes Mellitus Type 2	Bleeding disorders
High cholesterol	High cholesterol due to genetic defects
Overweight	Head injury
Lack of exercises	
Improper diet	
Oral contraceptive pills	

strategies, effective rehabilitative therapies that can be availed [6]. Despite impressive emergency management, the conventional system of medicine faces some limitations such as limited resources, costly investigations and treatment procedures, limited trained professionals and rehabilitation personnel. It also majorly centralizes on illness-oriented approach rather than on the wellness-oriented approach, not directing much attention towards the holistic health promotion and preventive strategies in the currently healthy population.

20.5 Need for Holistic Interventions such as Yoga

The life of a patient changes markedly after stroke. They start to significantly depend on the caregivers for their daily needs due to the post-stroke disabilities. These disabilities make the patients susceptible to develop mental illnesses that may range from dysthymia to as serious as suicidal tendencies. This implicates the need for holistic therapies such as yoga-based lifestyle, which aim at improving quality of life on both physical and psychosocial domains. There is growing evidence indicating the potential use of yoga in improving an individual's functional status post-stroke. Moreover, many patients seek medical assistance in the form of certain herbal formulations, behavioural, and lifestyle recommendations to prevent stroke occurrence, recurrence and also its associated co-morbidities. This indicates the need to integrate the conventional and traditional systems of medicine to reduce the burden of stroke around the globe.

20.6 Introduction to Yoga Therapy and Rationale for Its Use in Stroke Management

National Health Interview survey has defined yoga as a combination of breathing exercises, physical postures, and meditation to calm the nervous system and balance body, mind, and spirit [7]. The practice of yoga includes Yama (social ethics), Niyama (individual code of conduct), Asana (physical postures), Pranayama (regulated breathing), Pratyahara (restraint of senses), Dharana (focussed awareness), Dhyana (defocussed awareness to the state of meditation) and Samadhi (state of self-absorption). These practices primarily focus on enhancing the stability of one's body, breath, and mind. Due to this ability, yoga has emerged as a potent therapeutic option to address psycho-somatic disorders. Yoga is a safe, adaptable, and cost-effective therapeutic option that empowers the subject to be self-reliant.

20.7 Understanding of Stroke from Yoga Perspective: The Concept of Five Layers of Existence

Yoga therapy (YT) is based on the principle of *Pancha koshas* that has been derived from *Taittriya Upanishad* [8]. This approach looks into an individual at five layers of existence, namely: physical layer (*Annamaya kosha*), layer of the life force (*Pranamaya kosha*), layer of mental processes (*Manomaya kosha*), layer of intellect (*Vijnanamaya kosha*), and layer of bliss (*Anandamaya kosha*).

According to the *Guna* theory from Yoga philosophy, stroke is a disorder that is most likely to occur in *rajas* (characterized by intense passion and relentless desires) or *tamas* (characterized by inertia and ignorance) predominant personalities [9]. *Rajasic* personalities tend to relentlessly work towards their high-set goals while ignoring the basic needs of their body and get overwhelmed with fear, anxiety, and an array of negative emotions in the due process of achieving so (*kama esa krodha esa rajo guna samudbhavah B.G 3.37*) [10]. This results in cycles of maladaptive thoughts and emotions that initiate turbulence in the *Manomaya kosha,* which graduates into *Pranamaya kosha*. This results in the haphazard functioning of *prana* (life force) at the level of *Pranamaya kosha. Prana* functions at various levels viz., *prana* (in head region) *udana* (thorax) *samana* (in gastrointestinal tract) *vyana*

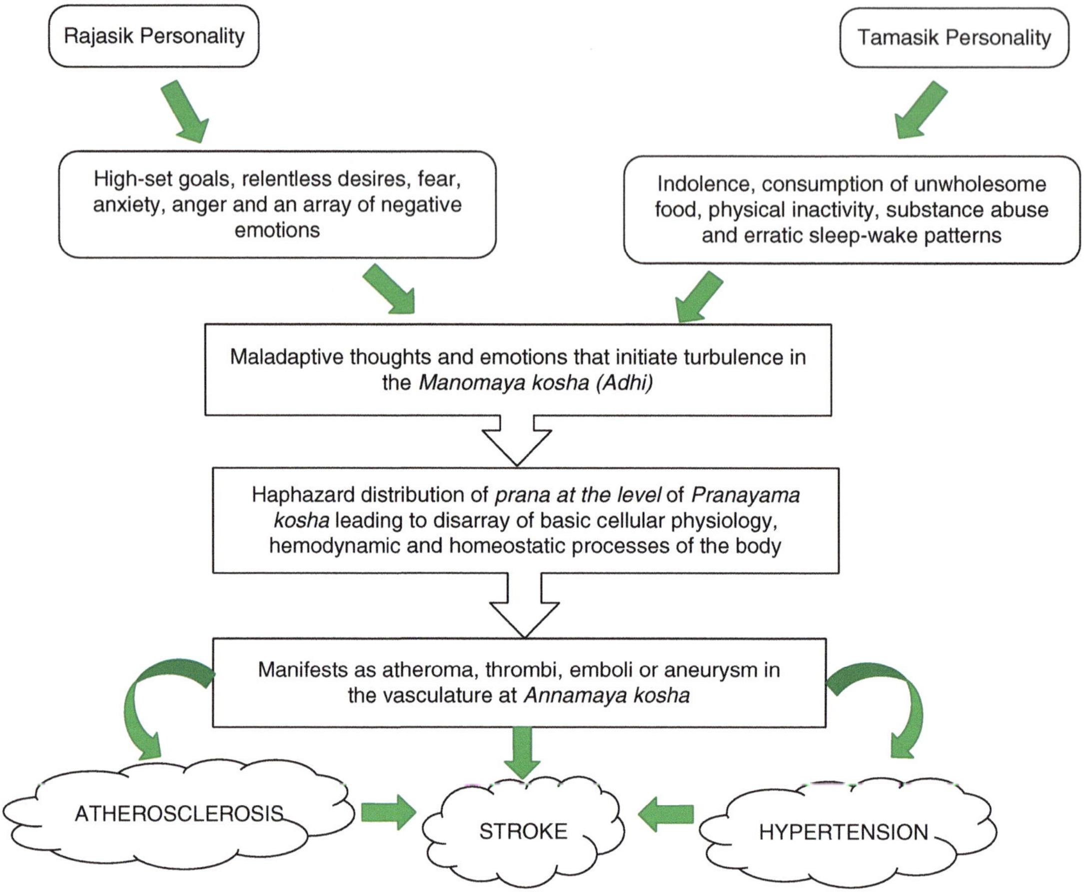

Fig. 20.1 Understanding Stroke from Yoga Perspective

(through the whole body) and *apana* (urogenital tract). According to the genetic imprints of an individual and the influence of his/her lifestyle, *prana* tends to accumulate in particular regions and becomes scanty elsewhere, manifesting as various symptoms. In stroke, *vyana* is greatly vitiated. This disturbance in the *Pranamaya kosha* results in a disarray of basic cellular physiology, hemodynamic, and homeostatic processes of the body (fat metabolism, regulation of blood pressure, etc.), leading to formation of atheroma, thrombi, emboli, or aneurysm in the vasculature at *Annamaya kosha*. This further manifests as various disorders such as hypertension, atherosclerosis, stroke, and so on. On the other hand, tamasic personalities are indolent and seem reluctant about their well-being due to inertia resulting in the consumption of unwholesome food, erratic food intake patterns, lack of physical activity, substance abuse and prolonged sleep duration. These wrong lifestyle patterns lower the resilience to cope with stress and renders *Manomaya kosha* to be very vulnerable to maladaptive thought patterns and emotions. Further, the turbulence in *Manomaya kosha* penetrates into *Annamaya kosha* via *Pranamaya kosha* as aforementioned (refer Fig. 20.1). Once such disturbances set in, the individual is likely to develop stroke or related risk factors like hypertension, diabetes, and coronary heart disease. After such disorders develop, the morbidity in the *Annamaya kosha* starts to intensify the turbulence in *Manomaya kosha* leading to elevated levels of psychological stress, depression, anxiety, and fear of death. This vicious cycle keeps functioning and negatively influences the prognosis of the disorder, highlighting the need for yoga therapy to address such disorders.

20.8 Yoga for Prevention of Stroke: Current Evidence

Modern lifestyle disorders such as hypertension, type 2 diabetes, dyslipidaemia, atherosclerosis, and latent conditions like oxidative stress and chronic psychological stress are potential risk factors that build the foundation for stroke occurrence and recurrence. Yoga has been demonstrated to be useful in significantly downplaying these risk factors and positively modulate one's health [11]. Chronic mental stress is the common trigger for Hypertension, Diabetes, Heart diseases and other lifestyle disorders. Yoga fosters better mental adaptability, efficiency, and resilience by increasing the levels of GABA (Gamma Amino Butyric Acid) and further modulating the neuroendocrine axis and cortisol levels [12, 13]. Several studies have been conducted to evaluate the short-term and long-term effects of yoga on Hypertension. A meta-analysis of nine randomized controlled trials (RCTs) has shown that Transcendental Meditation (TM) could reduce systolic blood pressure by 4.7 mmHg (CI 1.9–7.4) and diastolic blood pressure by 3.2 mmHg (CI 1.3–5.6), when compared to controls [14]. In an RCT, 11-week yoga therapy program was found to be equally effective as anti-Hypertensive drug therapy [15]. Specifically, the practice of *laghu shankhprakshalana* (systematic yogic purgation), *shavasana* (corpse yogic pose), *sukha pranayama* (6 breaths/min, with awareness), and TM have shown a consistent reduction in both systolic and diastolic blood pressures [14, 16–18]. Long-term beneficial effects of yoga at 8 weeks, 8 months and after 4 years were also assessed. There was persistence in reduction of both systolic and diastolic blood pressures in the treatment arm in contrast to the health education—control group across the timepoints [19]. Even though evidence suggests moderate reductions in blood pressure with yoga, it still translates into a significant reduction in the risk of CVD. It is estimated that a reduction in systolic blood pressure by 5 mmHg in a healthy population results in a fall of stroke mortality by 14% and coronary heart disease (CHD) by 9% [20]. Considering the dearth of evidence on the usefulness of yoga in the management of hypertension, AHA has classified TM, Yoga and other meditation techniques under second and third classes of recommendation for its implementation in clinical practice. Manchanda et al. have demonstrated the potential of yoga therapy in decelerating and reversing atherosclerotic processes that could prospectively result in cardiovascular or cerebrovascular accidents [21–23]. Carotid intimal-medial thickness (cIMT) was shown to reduce in patients with metabolic syndrome with 1 year of yoga practice [22]. Positive changes have been observed on coronary angiography and parameters like body mass index (BMI), waist circumference, LDL (low-density lipoprotein), triglycerides (tgy), angina and exertion induced ischemia have significantly reduced with the simultaneous increase in HDL (high-density lipoprotein) in advanced cases of atherosclerosis following the practice of yoga-based lifestyle [21, 22]. Appreciating the association of dyslipidaemia with coronary heart disease and ischemic stroke, many RCTs have been conducted to understand the role of yoga in dyslipidaemia. The results report that the total cholesterol has shown a variation of 5.8–25.2%, tgy by 22.0–28.5% and LDL-c by 12.8–26% across 6 weeks to 12 months in these studies [24–26]. Similar trend in lipid profile has been demonstrated in a population with type 2 diabetes also [24]. A metanalysis of 12 RCTs investigating effects of yoga in adults with type 2 diabetes showed significant reductions in glycosylated hemoglobin, fasting blood glucose, postprandial blood glucose, total cholesterol and LDL levels with an increase in the levels of HDL [27]. In addition to the above, oxidative stress worsens the scenario. Regular practice of yoga for about 3 months has been found to reduce the malondialdehyde levels (an indicator of oxidative stress) and increase the levels of glutathione, superoxide dismutase and vitamin-C (antioxidants) in patients with diabetes and hypertension [28–30]. From the above studies, evidence suggests a significant protective role of yoga towards the prevention of stroke and cardiovascular disorders.

20.9 Current Evidence: Yoga for Post-Stroke Rehabilitation

Stroke results in considerably severe physical and psychosocial distress leading to compromise on the quality of life and loss of independence of an individual [31]. Post-stroke hemiparesis, aphasia, headaches, falls, pain, and depression stand as major concerns, towards which yoga has a potential role to play. Bastille et al., studied the effect of yoga on balance, timed mobility and quality of life on the Berg Balance Scale (BBS), Timed Movement Battery [TMB] and Stroke Impact Scale [SIS], respectively in 4 cases of chronic post-stroke hemiparesis. 1.5-h yoga session twice weekly over 8 weeks, improved timed mobility in 3 cases and balance in 2 cases [32]. A prospective randomized controlled trial confirmed the results of the above study on post-stroke balance and fear of falling [33]. Further, another pilot study demonstrated substantial improvement in pain, range of motion at neck and hip, upper limb strength and 6-min walk scores in patients with chronic stroke with 8-week Yoga intervention [34]. Besides hemiparesis, aphasia is another physical symptom that is greatly distressing and seeks attention. 12 weeks of Kundalini yoga was shown to improve aphasia on Boston Aphasia Exam and fine motor coordination on O'Connor Tweezer Dexterity Timed Test in patients with stroke [35]. In the similar context, a case study that involved practice of Alternate nostril breathing (20 min/day for 17 weeks) and consumption of coconut oil (1 tablespoon a day) have translated into a significant improvement in anomic aphasia and paraphasia on Western Aphasia Battery-Revised (WAB-R) tool [36]. Uni-nostril yogic breathing alongside traditional speech therapy has been found beneficial in improving the affect and language abilities in stroke patients [37]. The long-term debilitating effects of stroke is very devastating for the patient making them vulnerable to mental illnesses. There is sufficient evidence demonstrating the potential of yoga in reducing anxiety and improving mood [28, 38]. The results of an RCT exploring the role of 6 week yoga program on post-stroke anxiety and depression displayed greater improvements in the depression on Geriatric Depression Scale (GDS15) and state trait anxiety on State Trait Anxiety Inventory (STAI) in the intervention group (yoga and exercise) than the control group (exercise) [29]. Another study exploring multiple array of symptoms in stroke patients has displayed improvement in quality of life associated with memory, perceived motor function and perceived recovery [30]. Garrett et al. and Portz et al. qualitatively studied the experiences of patients with stroke after 10-week yoga intervention. The participants reported greater sensitivity, calmness, acceptance, and connectedness to the present self and with others. Improvement was reported in perceived strength, range of motion, walking ability, endurance, gait speed, flexibility, and balance [39, 40]. These findings conform to the necessity of inclusion of yoga and meditation techniques into post-stroke rehabilitation programs.

20.10 General Guidelines to Adapt Yoga Therapy for Stroke Rehabilitation

Yoga therapy involves the practice of physical postures, controlled breathing techniques, mindfulness-based chanting practices, devotional sessions and yogic counseling sessions to enhance physical, cognitive, and psychosocial functioning. However, yoga for post-stroke individuals has to be greatly modified considering the general physical disabilities to improve compliance, feasibility, and self-reliance. Below-listed are few points to be considered while adapting the yoga module for post-stroke patients.

- The module should be brief, but should include all the components of YT.
- Instructions should be short and clear. Multiple short sessions should be conducted rather than one long session.

- Graduated yoga module: only easy to perform and very essential practices are introduced in the first week of therapy; gradually necessary practices are introduced in succession according to the performance of the patient. (see the module below)
- The sequence should be well planned. It will be wise not to change postures frequently from standing to sitting or lying abruptly.
- Involvement of whole body in each session. This will ensure proper circulation and will prevent bedsores and deep vein thrombosis due to inactivity.
- Avoid inversions in the module.
- Avoid postures that exert extreme pressure and sudden movements of the neck like *Sarvangasana* and *Halasana*.
- Avoid acute forward and backward bends in the module like *Ardhachakrasana, Padahasthasana, Chakrasana,* etc.
- Avoid balancing postures like *Vrikshasana, Garudasana*, etc.
- Avoid fast breathing practices like *Kapalbhati* and *Bhastrika* as it might lead to episodes of dizziness.
- Avoid the practices involving breath retention like *Kumbhakas* and *Bandhas* as they might be strenuous to the subject.
- Encourage repetitions of each practice in the first week. The short module can be repeated for three times interspaced with sufficient resting periods.
- The patient should be encouraged to memorize the yoga module in the correct sequence and be self-reliant.
- Inclusion of instructions on breath awareness.
- Inclusion of instructions to enhance their mindfulness during the practice.
- Inclusion of visualization techniques, especially when mobility is greatly compromised will aim at improving motor learning, planning, and coordination [41]. The patient should be encouraged to visualize the practice mentally if he/she is incapacitated to perform any specific practice.
- Inclusion of instructions sensitizing the subject about the sensory awareness.
- Acknowledge even the minute improvements and communicate to the patient.
- It is best to include a 15-min counseling session every day at the end of the yoga practice to encourage the patient and promote the practice of yoga through positive reinforcement.
- Use of support is strongly recommended during the initial phases of the practice. However, the effort has to be made to slowly discontinue the usage of support according to the functional improvement in the subject.
- Therapist/ caregiver should assist the passive range movements in severe cases.

20.11 Graduated Yoga Module for Stroke

Generally, a yoga module can be split into six components: loosening exercises, breathing techniques, *Asanas, Pranayama*, chanting, and guided meditation. Of the six components, substantial emphasis should be laid on the *Pranayama,* chanting, and guided meditation techniques as these practices target the deeper *koshas, i.e., Pranamaya* and *Manomaya koshas.* Moreover, these practices can be done even in a severe degree of immobility.

Considering the positive impacts of yoga therapy on overall well-being of patients with stroke, a graduated 4-week yoga protocol has been designed based on the available scientific evidence. This 4-week yoga training program might serve as an adjunct therapy for enhancing functional independence and recovery of patients in the post-stroke rehabilitation phase.

Details of the graduated yoga program for post-stroke rehabilitation are as follows:

1. *First week (to be practiced three times a day for the first week, once a day after week-1)*
   - Whole body joint loosening with mindfulness and breath synchronization: Feet, ankles, knees, hips, fingers, wrists, elbows, shoulders, and neck—10 rounds each while sitting in a chair. If these practices cannot be done actively, the therapist can administer passive joint movements.

2. *Second week (preparatory breathing practices in sitting + instant relaxation technique + first week practices)*

   - Preparatory breathing practices in sitting using chair support: Twisting, side bending, hand stretch breathing, hands in and out breathing with "*M-kara*" chanting—10 rounds of each practice.
   - Instant relaxation technique in the supine pose: Quick and sequential tightening of all body parts from toes to head followed by letting go and relaxation (2 rounds).

3. *Third week [asanas (physical postures)—first 5 rounds without holding the pose, sixth round hold the pose for 10 breaths + first and second week practices]*

   - Prone: *Bhujangasana* (cobra pose), *Ardha Shalabhasana* (half locust pose), *Makarasana* stretch (crocodile pose).
   - Supine: *Utthita Padasana* (alternate straight leg rising), *Ardha Pavanamuktasana kriya* (half-wind releasing pose), *Setubandhasana* (bridge pose), *Shavasana* (corpse pose).

4. *Fourth week [asanas (physical postures)—first 5 rounds without holding the pose, sixth round hold the pose for 10 breaths + first, second week and third week practices]*

   - Standing with wall support (holding for support if required): second week practices in standing position + *Padasanchalana* (alternate leg movements with breath synchronization). *Trikonasana* (triangle pose), *Ardha Kati Chakrasana* (half-waist pose).
   - Sitting with wall support: *Vakrasana* (sitting twisted pose), *Patangasana* (butterfly flapping 100 counts), *Ardhabaddhakonasana* (half butterfly pose), *Moola bandha* (anal lock).

5. *Pranayama practice (yogic controlled breath) in sitting meditative pose, as a regular common practice after physical postures from the first to fourth week*

   - *Nadishuddi Pranayama* (alternate nostril breathing)
   - *Bhramari* in *Shanmukhi Mudra* (humming bee breath)
   - *Nadanusandhana* (chanting of sounds—*AAA*, *UUU*, *MMM,* and *AUM* 9 rounds each, while being mindful and feeling the vibrations in the body)

6. *Relaxation in Shavasana (corpse pose) as a regular common practice after pranayama from the first to fourth week*

   - Deep abdominal breathing with prolonged exhalation in *Shavasana* (the duration of inhalation and exhalation for each respiratory cycle should be maintained at a 1:3 ratio, respectively).
   - Part by part relaxation of the body from head to toes.

Precautions to be Taken

– Do not encourage overdoing the practice. This might result in adversities like myalgia, fatigue, and cramps.
– Avoid frequent changes in starting posture through the course of the module. Changes in the posture should be assisted by a caregiver or therapist.
– Avoid strenuous practices in the first few weeks and gradually increase the complexity of the postures.
– Ensure empty bladder and bowel before yoga practice.
– Ensure light stomach conditions while practicing yoga.

20.12 Yoga and Ayurveda-Based Lifestyle Advices for Post-Stroke Care

Besides improvement in functional status of the patient, therapy also aims at regulating one's life-style to reduce the risk of recurrence of stroke and its associated co-morbidities. Table 20.2 provides Yoga and Ayurveda-based lifestyle advices that are to be followed Post-stroke. These recommendations can be classified under three major headings; *ahara* (dietary regimen), *vihara* (behavioral changes) and *vichara* (mental changes).

Table 20.2 Yoga and ayurveda-based lifestyle advices for stroke

Ahara (dietary regimen)	*Vihara* (behavioral changes)	*Vichara* (mental changes)
Do's		
– *Sattvik* food: fresh, sweet, juicy, and nourishing foods like fresh fruits, leaves and vegetables. Whole grains and cereals should be preferred. – Easily digestible, seasonal, and locally available foods should be preferred. – Include foods rich in vitamins, minerals, and antioxidants, especially Beta carotene, anthocyanins, flavonoids, and lycopene rich (e.g.; black grapes, papaya, tomatoes, black rice, cocoa) – Intake of sesame oil and moderate consumption of fat. – Warm milk is recommended. – The temperature of food being consumed should be warm – *Yuktahara*: moderate food consumption – *Mitahara*: the quantity of food taken should fill half of the stomach, liquids should fill another quarter, and the last quarter of the stomach is to be left free to ensure proper digestion.	– Physical activity involving whole body mobilization – Exposure to fresh air breeze – Sleeping on hard bed – Proper sleep-wake pattern – Warm water bath everyday – Regular evacuation of bowels – Gentle massage to the whole body with warm sesame oil every day. – Steam bath once a week after gentle massage – Lukewarm sesame oil enema at least once a week under supervision – Adherence to therapy recommendations – Mindfulness with each activity – Reading and imbibing traditional wisdom from prominent ancient scriptures like Bhagavad Gita, Bible, or Quran, etc.	– Attitude of surrender towards the higher principle of life – Being compassionate – Strong will and perseverance – Unshakeable faith – Enthusiasm and optimism – Feeling of connectedness to self and others – Contentment and peace – Introspection into one's own life and his spiritual growth – Ability to stay tranquil in the odds.
Do nots		
– Excess intake of food – Long-term fasting and starvation – Red meat – Cold and reheated food – Food items that have lost their natural oil. – Processed food – Excess salt and sodium intake – White sugar – Alcohol – Recreational Drugs	– Smoking – Daytime sleep – Excess comforts leading to compromise on minimal physical activity – Indolence – Avoid hot water for head bath – Staying awake late in the night – Overexertion – Exposure to extreme temperatures – Excess sensual indulgences of taste, touch, smell, vision, and sound. – Suppression of natural urges like hunger, thirst, urination, defecation, etc. – Avoid the company of vicious and pessimistic company	– Excess mentation – Irritability, anger, and hatred – Fear, specially the fear of death – Lust and relentless desires – Low mood and sadness – Helplessness and hopelessness – Procrastination – Dejection – Guilt feelings

20.13 Probable Mechanism of Action

The definite mechanisms of how yoga helps in post-stroke rehabilitation are not lucidly understood. In physical domain, it enhances microcirculation in the joints and facilitates restoration of proper tone in the muscle fibers resulting in improvement of strength, range of motion and gait with a reduction in stiffness [42, 43]. It further improves balance, coordination of fine and complex movements. These improvements empower the patient and improve their functional independence. Studies suggest that yoga regulates the HPA axis resulting in the reduction of cortisol levels. This enhances well-being through alleviation of stress, promotion of better neuro-endocrine-immune functioning and metabolic profile of an individual [12, 13]. There is extensive evidence on the efficacy of yoga in bringing balance in the functions of the autonomic nervous system. Its ability to maintain the vagal tone transcribes into better cardiovascular functioning, which reduces the risk of stroke, associated risk factors and co-morbidities [12]. There are a few studies that demonstrate the efficacy of yoga on significantly increasing the levels of brain-derived neurotrophic factor (a key-regulator of neuroplastic processes), which might play some role in the recovery of brain lesions, improve the functional status of the individual and offer further neuroprotection [44–47]. The improvement in mood and reduction in anxiety with the practice of yoga could be attributed to the upregulation of GABAergic (Gamma Amino Butyric Acid) activity in addition to the reduction in cortisol levels [48]. Further, yoga philosophy and meditative practices bring changes in the perception and behavior of an individual that allows them to accept their current shortcomings [39]. This enhances the confidence levels of an individual and empowers them to establish a proper bio-psychosocial domain with the external.

20.14 Limitations of Current Evidence in Yoga and Future Directions to Overcome the Limitations in Yoga Research in Stroke

There are many brief reports, case series and only two randomized control trials exploring the effects of yoga therapy on stroke in comparison to waitlist controls. Moreover, these trials study a very small sample because of which the results lack generalisability. Large multicentric trials are needed to study this area systematically with a subsequent period of follow-up. The current literature has very few comparable studies to perform a metanalysis, suggesting the need for a standard protocol for conducting further studies in terms of detailing all characteristics of the intervention, outcome measures and utility of standard tools of assessment, reporting compliance and adverse events of the intervention. Further, long-term effects have not been investigated, which could be explored in the forthcoming studies. Cochrane review of literature on stroke reveals a high risk of bias in performance, attrition outcomes, detection, and reporting [49]. On the basis of GRADE (Grading of Recommendations Assessment, Development, and Evaluation) criteria, the overall quality of the evidence available seems to fall between low and moderate [50].

20.15 Conclusion

The literature suggests Yoga-based lifestyle practices play a significant role in the prevention of stroke and post-stroke rehabilitation. This suggests a dire need for the integration of Yoga therapy with the current conventional medical systems to reduce morbidity and mortality due to stroke, its risk factors and co-morbidities.

References

1. National Collaborating Centre for Chronic Conditions (UK). Stroke: national clinical guideline for diagnosis and initial management of acute stroke and transient ischaemic attack (TIA). London: Royal College of Physicians; 2008.
2. Sacco RL, Kasner SE, Broderick JP, Caplan LR, Connors JJ, Culebras A, et al. An updated definition of stroke for the 21st century: a statement for healthcare professionals from the American Heart Association/American Stroke Association. Stroke. 2013;44(7):2064–89.
3. Gorelick PB. The global burden of stroke: persistent and disabling. Lancet Neurol. 2019;18(5):417–8.
4. Pandian JD, Sudhan P. Stroke epidemiology and stroke care services in India. J Stroke. 2013;15(3):128.
5. Ferro JM, Canhão P, Stam J, Bousser M-G, Barinagarrementeria F. Prognosis of cerebral vein and dural sinus thrombosis: results of the international study on cerebral vein and dural sinus thrombosis (ISCVT). Stroke. 2004;35(3):664–70.
6. Das S, Das SK. Knowledge, attitude and practice of stroke in India versus other developed and developing countries. Ann Indian Acad Neurol [Internet]. 2013 [cited 2020 Mar 25];16(4):488–93. Available from: https://www.ncbi.nlm.nih.gov/pmc/articles/PMC3841586/
7. Black LI, Clarke TC, Barnes PM, Stussman BJ, Nahin RL. Use of complementary health approaches among children aged 4–17 years in the United States: National Health Interview Survey, 2007–2012. Natl Health Stat Rep [Internet]. 2015 Feb 10 [cited 2020 Mar 26];(78):1–19. Available from: https://www.ncbi.nlm.nih.gov/pmc/articles/PMC4562218/
8. Chinmayananda S. Taittiriya Upanishad. Central Chinmaya Mission Trust; 2014.
9. Jasti N, Bhargav H, Metri K, Choudhary P. Theory of Trigunas and its relevance to mental health. J Relig Health.
10. Swarupananda S. Srimad Bhagavad Gita. Advaita Ashrama (A publication branch of Ramakrishna Math, Belur Math); 2016.
11. Mishra SK, Singh P, Bunch SJ, Zhang R. The therapeutic value of yoga in neurological disorders. Ann Indian Acad Neurol. 2012;15(4):247.
12. Streeter CC, Gerbarg PL, Saper RB, Ciraulo DA, Brown RP. Effects of yoga on the autonomic nervous system, gamma-aminobutyric-acid, and allostasis in epilepsy, depression, and post-traumatic stress disorder. Med Hypotheses. 2012;78(5):571–9.
13. Thirthalli J, Naveen GH, Rao MG, Varambally S, Christopher R, Gangadhar BN. Cortisol and antidepressant effects of yoga. Indian J Psychiatry. 2013;55(Suppl 3):S405.
14. Anderson JW, Liu C, Kryscio RJ. Blood pressure response to transcendental meditation: a meta-analysis. Am J Hypertens. 2008;21(3):310–6.
15. Murugesan R, Govindarajulu N, Bera TK. Effect of selected yogic practices on the management of hypertension. Indian J Physiol Pharmacol. 2000 Apr;44(2):207–10.
16. Bhavanani AB, Sanjay Z, Madanmohan. Immediate effect of sukha pranayama on cardiovascular variables in patients of hypertension. Int J Yoga Ther [Internet]. 2011 Oct 1 [cited 2020 Mar 17];21(1):73–6. Available from: https://iaytjournals.org/doi/abs/10.17761/ijyt.21.1.y007g51341634172
17. Mashyal P, Bhargav H, Raghuram N. Safety and usefulness of Laghu shankha prakshalana in patients with essential hypertension: a self controlled clinical study. J Ayurveda Integr Med [Internet]. 2014 [cited 2020 Mar 17];5(4):227–35. Available from: https://www.ncbi.nlm.nih.gov/pmc/articles/PMC4296435/
18. Santaella DF, Lorenzi-Filho G, Rodrigues MR, Tinucci T, Malinauskas AP, Mion-Júnior D, et al. Yoga relaxation (savasana) decreases cardiac sympathovagal balance in hypertensive patients. Medical Express [Internet]. 2014 Oct [cited 2020 Mar 17];1(5):233–8. Available from: http://www.scielo.br/scielo.php?script=sci_abstract&pid=S2358-04292014000500233&lng=en&nrm=iso&tlng=en
19. Patel C, Marmot MG, Terry DJ, Carruthers M, Hunt B, Patel M. Trial of relaxation in reducing coronary risk: four year follow up. BMJ [Internet]. 1985 Apr 13 [cited 2020 Mar 17];290(6475):1103–6. Available from: http://www.bmj.com/cgi/doi/10.1136/bmj.290.6475.1103
20. Stamler J, Rose G, Stamler R, Elliott P, Dyer A, Marmot M. INTERSALT study findings. Public health and medical care implications. Hypertension. 1989;14(5):570–7.
21. Manchanda SC, Narang R, Reddy KS, Sachdeva U, Prabhakaran D, Dharmanand S, et al. Reversal of coronary atherosclerosis by yoga lifestyle intervention. In: Dhalla NS, Chockalingam A, Berkowitz HI, Singal PK, editors. Frontiers in cardiovascular health [Internet]. Boston, MA: springer US; 2003 [cited 2020 Mar 3]. p. 535–47. (Progress in experimental cardiology). Available from: https://doi.org/10.1007/978-1-4615-0455-9_39.
22. Manchanda SC, Mehrotra UC, Makhija A, Mohanty A, Dhawan S, Sawhney JPS. Reversal of early atherosclerosis in metabolic syndrome by yoga-a randomized controlled trial. J Yoga Phys Ther. 2013;3(1):1.

23. Manchanda SC, Narang R, Reddy KS, Sachdeva U, Prabhakaran D, Dharmanand S, et al. Retardation of coronary atherosclerosis with yoga lifestyle intervention. J Assoc Physicians India. 2000;48(7):687–94.
24. Shantakumari N, Sequeira S, El Deeb R. Effects of a yoga intervention on lipid profiles of diabetes patients with dyslipidemia. Indian Heart J [Internet]. 2013 Mar 1 [cited 2020 Mar 17];65(2):127–31. Available from: http://www.sciencedirect.com/science/article/pii/S0019483213000369
25. Mohammed R, Banu A, Imran S, Jaiswal RK. Importance of yoga in diabetes and dyslipidemia. IJRMS. 2016; https://doi.org/10.18203/2320-6012.ijrms20162320.
26. Tundwala V, Gupta RP, Kumar S, Singh VB, Sandeep BR, Dayal P, et al. A study on effect of yoga and various asanas on obesity, hypertension and dyslipidemia. Int J Basic Appl Med Sci. 2012;2(1):93–8.
27. Cui J, Yan J-H, Yan L-M, Pan L, Le J-J, Guo Y-Z. Effects of yoga in adults with type 2 diabetes mellitus: A meta-analysis. J Diabetes Investig [Internet]. 2017 Mar [cited 2020 Mar 26];8(2):201. Available from: https://www.ncbi.nlm.nih.gov/pmc/articles/PMC5334310/
28. Cramer H, Lauche R, Anheyer D, Pilkington K, de Manincor M, Dobos G, et al. Yoga for anxiety: a systematic review and meta-analysis of randomized controlled trials. Depress Anxiety. 2018;35(9):830–43.
29. Chan W, Immink MA, Hillier S. Yoga and exercise for symptoms of depression and anxiety in people with poststroke disability: a randomized, controlled pilot trial. Altern Ther Health Med. 18:34–43.
30. Immink MA, Hillier S, Petkov J. Randomized controlled trial of yoga for chronic poststroke hemiparesis: motor function, mental health, and quality of life outcomes. Top Stroke Rehabil. 2014;21(3):256–71.
31. Warren N, Ayton D. Loneliness as social suffering: social participation, quality of life, and chronic stroke. In: World suffering and quality of life. New York: Springer; 2015. p. 159–70.
32. Bastille JV, Gill-Body KM. A yoga-based exercise program for people with chronic poststroke hemiparesis. Phys Ther. 2004;84(1):33–48.
33. Schmid AA, Van Puymbroeck M, Altenburger PA, Schalk NL, Dierks TA, Miller KK, et al. Poststroke balance improves with yoga: a pilot study. Stroke. 2012;43(9):2402–7.
34. Schmid AA, Miller KK, Van Puymbroeck M, DeBaun-Sprague E. Yoga leads to multiple physical improvements after stroke, a pilot study. Complement Ther Med. 2014;22(6):994–1000.
35. Lynton H, Kligler B, Shiflett S. Yoga in stroke rehabilitation: a systematic review and results of a pilot study. Top Stroke Rehabil. 2007;14(4):1–8.
36. Mohapatra B, Shisler Marshall R, Laures-Gore J. Yogic breathing and ayurveda in aphasia: a case study. Top Stroke Rehabil. 2014;21(3):272–80.
37. Marshall RS, Basilakos A, Williams T, Love-Myers K. Exploring the Benefits of Unilateral Nostril Breathing Practice Post-Stroke: Attention, Language, Spatial Abilities, Depression, and Anxiety. J Altern Complement Med [Internet]. 2013 Oct 11 [cited 2020 Mar 16];20(3):185–94. Available from: https://www.liebertpub.com/doi/abs/10.1089/acm.2013.0019
38. Cramer H, Lauche R, Langhorst J, Dobos G. Yoga for depression: a systematic review and meta-analysis. Depress Anxiety. 2013;30(11):1068–83.
39. Garrett R, Immink MA, Hillier S. Becoming connected: the lived experience of yoga participation after stroke. Disabil Rehabil. 2011;33(25–26):2404–15.
40. Portz JD, Waddington E, Atler KE, Van Puymbroeck M, Schmid AA. Self-management and yoga for older adults with chronic stroke: a mixed-methods study of physical fitness and physical activity. Clin Gerontol. 2018;41(4):374–81.
41. Nicholson VP, Keogh JW, Choy NLL. Can a single session of motor imagery promote motor learning of locomotion in older adults? A randomized controlled trial [Internet]. Clinical Interventions in Aging. 2018 [cited 2020 Mar 12]. Available from: https://www.dovepress.com/can-a-single-session-of-motor-imagery-promote-motor-learning-of-locomo-peer-reviewed-article-CIA
42. DiBenedetto M, Innes KE, Taylor AG, Rodeheaver PF, Boxer JA, Wright HJ, et al. Effect of a Gentle Iyengar Yoga program on gait in the elderly: an exploratory study. Arch Phys Med Rehabil [Internet]. 2005 Sep 1 [cited 2020 Mar 26];86(9):1830–7. Available from: http://www.sciencedirect.com/science/article/pii/S0003999305003175
43. Ebnezar JNP, Yogitha B. Effectiveness of yoga therapy with the therapeutic exercises on walking pain, tenderness, early morning stiffness and disability in osteoarthritis of the knee joint - a comparative study. J Yoga Phys Therapy. 2012;2:3.
44. Naveen GH, Thirthalli J, Rao MG, Varambally S, Christopher R, Gangadhar BN. Positive therapeutic and neurotropic effects of yoga in depression: a comparative study. Indian J Psychiatry. 2013;55(Suppl 3):S400.
45. Tolahunase MR, Sagar R, Faiq M, Dada R. Yoga- and meditation-based lifestyle intervention increases neuroplasticity and reduces severity of major depressive disorder: A randomized controlled trial. Restor Neurol Neurosci [Internet]. 2018 Jan 1 [cited 2020 Mar 26];36(3):423–42. Available from: https://content.iospress.com/articles/restorative-neurology-and-neuroscience/rnn170810
46. Naveen GH, Varambally S, Thirthalli J, Rao M, Christopher R, Gangadhar BN. Serum cortisol and BDNF in patients with major depression—effect of yoga. Int Rev Psychiatry [Internet]. 2016 May 3 [cited 2020 Mar 26];28(3):273–8. Available from: https://doi.org/10.1080/09540261.2016.1175419.

47. Hara Y. Brain plasticity and rehabilitation in stroke patients. J Nippon Med Sch Nippon Ika Daigaku Zasshi. 2015;82(1):4–13.
48. Streeter CC, Whitfield TH, Owen L, Rein T, Karri SK, Yakhkind A, et al. Effects of yoga versus walking on mood, anxiety, and brain GABA levels: a randomized controlled MRS study. J Altern Complement Med. 2010;16(11):1145–52.
49. Lawrence M, Junior FTC, Matozinho HH, Govan L, Booth J, Beecher J. Yoga for stroke rehabilitation. Cochrane Database Syst Rev [Internet]. 2017 [cited 2020 Mar 16];(12). Available from: https://www.cochranelibrary.com/cdsr/doi/10.1002/14651858.CD011483.pub2/full
50. Thayabaranathan T, Andrew NE, Immink MA, Hillier S, Stevens P, Stolwyk R, et al. Determining the potential benefits of yoga in chronic stroke care: a systematic review and meta-analysis. Top Stroke Rehabil. 2017;24(4):279–87.

Meditation and Yoga in the Treatment of Addictive Disorders

21

Debesh Mallik, Tyree Dingle, and Sarah Bowen

21.1 Introduction

Substance Use Disorder (SUD) has been defined as a chronic relapsing disorder of brain reward, motivation, memory, and related circuitry, with dysfunction in these circuits leading to biological, psychological, social, and spiritual manifestations [1, 2]. SUD is further often characterized by progressive substance use, difficulty abstaining from use despite harmful consequences, craving, problems with interpersonal relationships, emotional regulation, poor self-awareness, and exposure to trauma [1, 3]. Furthermore, the Diagnostic and Statistical Manual for Mental Health Disorders-V (DSM-V) describes additional criteria for a SUD to be excessive time spent in pursuing substances, poor task management, tolerance, and withdrawal [4].

21.2 Epidemiology

According to the United Nations Office on Drugs and Crime, approximately 29.5 million meet the criteria for SUD. In the USA alone, 19.5 million people meet criteria, yet only 4.2 million of those individuals have received any form of SUD treatment [5]. Additionally, in the United States, drug overdose has become the leading cause of accidental death [6, 7], and excessive alcohol use has led to an estimated 88,000 deaths [8]. Globally, men with alcohol use disorder (AUD) are at twice the risk of mortality than the general population, and women with AUD have a generally higher mortality rate than men with AUD [9]. Furthermore, in 2016 over 632,000 alcohol, tobacco, and drug-related deaths were reported, costing taxpayers more than 740 billion dollars [10–12]. A primary cause of these harms is the exceptionally high rates of relapse seen in SUD, with estimates anywhere from 40 to 60% of individuals who have undergone substance abuse treatment relapsing [13].

Given the prevalence of SUDs and the current rates of relapse, there is a great need for efficacious treatment modalities. A literature review by Dutra et al. (2008) found that among the most prominent behavioral treatments for SUD, the combination of contingency management and cognitive behavioral therapy yielded the greatest effect sizes, and cognitive behavioral therapy and relapse prevention alone yielded low-to-moderate effect sizes [14]. Relapse rates remain high, however, warranting further treatment innovation and research. In recent decades, evidence is emerging in support of the efficacy of mindfulness-based interventions (MBIs) for the treatment of SUDs [15–18].

Order of authorship reflects respective contributions.

D. Mallik (✉) · T. Dingle · S. Bowen
Pacific School of Graduate Psychology,
Pacific University, Hillsboro, OR, USA
e-mail: debeshmallik@pacificu.edu

I. Basu-Ray, D. Mehta (eds.), *The Principles and Practice of Yoga in Cardiovascular Medicine*,
https://doi.org/10.1007/978-981-16-6913-2_21

21.3 Pathophysiology

To better treat SUD, we must first understand its underlying mechanisms. One of the most empirically supported models of addiction is the self-medication hypothesis [19–24]. This hypothesis proposes that rather than using substances to seek euphoria, individuals are attempting to alleviate or escape distressing emotional states (see Fig. 21.1). While this may provide temporary relief from unpleasant states, prolonged substance use may lead to the development of SUD. SUD often brings further distressing states, which subsequently perpetuates the self-medication cycle.

Buddhist perspectives on addiction center on the notion that suffering is ubiquitous. However, as the self-medication hypothesis suggests, many individuals attempt to remove psychological pain, which often causes further pain and pathology. From this perspective, what may seem like the solution to suffering may actually be fundamentally causal [25]. To further explain, similar to the self-medication hypothesis, Buddhist philosophy posits that substance use is often an attempt to escape suffering; however, it is a "false refuge" as the effects of the substance are short-lived [26, 27]. The individual becomes attached to, or "craves," the substance for its ability to temporarily alleviate suffering. This craving causes individuals to lose contact with the present moment, as they place attention on the future cessation of suffering or upcoming substance-induced euphoria. From this perspective, addiction is a strong form of attachment to the false promise the substance brings, i.e., escape from suffering or onset of highly pleasant states [26–27].

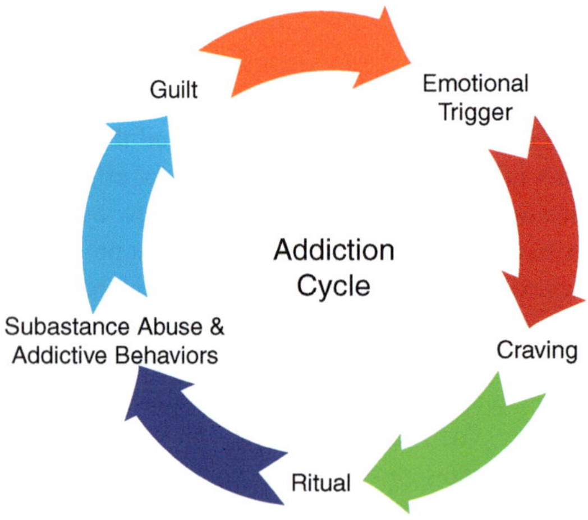

Fig. 21.1 The self-medication hypothesis. Substance use can lead to aversive emotional states that result in individuals seeking temporary relief through further substance use. This pattern of negative reinforcement often perpetuates further substance use

21.4 Treatment Options

21.4.1 Mindfulness

Mindfulness practices are thought to alleviate the suffering caused by attachments, e.g., attachment to substances, by directing and reorienting attention to the present moment, and cultivating awareness of how the mind behaves. Mindfulness practice is a specific form of meditation that relates back to Buddhist teachings. Vipassana, which is Pali for, "to see things as they really are," is one type of mindfulness meditation practice. The practice of Vipassana is based on developing *Sila*, or adhering to a moral code of conduct, strengthening *Samadhi*, or concentration practices in which one observes arising and passing sensations with non-judgment, and *Panna*, or the development of wisdom through these practices when an individual understands the fleeting and everchanging nature of reality [28]. Mindfulness-Based Interventions (MBIs) are heavily informed by Vipassana philosophy and practice. In current scientific literature, the term *mindfulness* is used to describe a state, trait, and practice. State mindfulness has been defined by Garland and Howard (2018) as, "a state of metacognitive awareness characterized by an attentive and nonjudgmental monitoring of moment-by-moment cognition, emotion, sensation, and perception without perseveration on thoughts of past and future" (p. 2) [29]. There are two primary forms of mindfulness practice. Concentration practices focus on a single specific object or sensation (the breath, bodily sensation, physical object, etc.) while noticing and letting go of distractions, while open monitoring practice involves holding a metacognitive view of the entire organism-environment field, in which the individual is aware of internal stimuli (thoughts, emotions) and external stimuli (perceptions), noticing the impermanence of both [21, 30]. Trait mindfulness is described as the ability an individual gains through mindful practice to become mindful in day-to-day living, resulting in decreased reactivity to internal emotional experiences [31]. Mindfulness meditation, according to a Buddhist model of addiction, may be a beneficial component to the treatment of addictive behaviors.

Current MBIs for addiction tend to follow the general 8-week group format that was set forth by Mindfulness-Based Stress Reduction (MBSR) [32] and Mindfulness-Based Cognitive Therapy (MBCT) [33]. Two of the most widely studied MBIs for addiction are Mindfulness-Based Relapse Prevention (MBRP) [34] and Mindfulness-Oriented Recovery Enhancement (MORE) [35]. These interventions follow a structured 8-week group format in which each session lasts for approximately 2 h. Sessions are led by a clinician, who guides individuals through various mindfulness practices such as mindful breathing, body scans, urge surfing, and mindful walking. Practices are often followed by a period of inquiry, or verbal exploration of the experience, and homework is assigned in the form of noticing triggers, cravings, and engaging in mindfulness practices outside of the group period [29, 34].

MBIs apply mindfulness meditation practice and skills as a way to teach individuals how to relate differently to internal experiences [36], by recognizing that they do not have to automatically react to their thoughts or urges [27], can foster distance between cravings and actions [26], and have the agency to choose valued behaviors in moments of distress. Through mindfulness practice, individuals can foster these skills, which may aid in breaking down the cyclical process of addiction. MBIs have been found to reduce key risk factors, such as negative affect [37–39], cravings [39–41], and psychiatric severity [37]. Studies also show reductions in substance use [14, 35], specifically, alcohol, opiate, nicotine, marijuana, and methamphetamine use [16], providing evidence that mindfulness training may be an advantageous component in the treatment of SUDs.

Though MBIs have demonstrated efficacy in treating SUD [16], the research as to why mindfulness is an effective treatment modality is still nascent. Still, some potential mechanisms of change have been explored and are shedding light on the means by which MBIs affect change. A literature review on MBIs for SUD by Priddy et al. (2018) found support in the scientific literature for the promotion of cognitive control, restructuring rewards, and decreasing stress reactivity as mechanisms of mindfulness in the treatment of SUD [42]. Another recent literature review by Garland and Howard (2018) describes restructuring of rewards, changes in executive functioning, dispositional mindfulness, stress reactivity, craving, cue-reactivity, and thought suppression as proposed mechanisms of MBIs [29]. These authors state that an emerging body of evidence points toward the restructuring reward hypothesis as a potential mechanism for MBIs in the treatment of addiction. The hypothesis posits that mindfulness may shift the salience of drug-related rewards back to natural (non-drug-related) rewards that were prominent before substance addiction began.

Further, the strengthening of self-control behaviors that often becomes dysregulated during substance abuse may also be a mechanism of mindfulness training [29]. The same review specifies that after undergoing an MBI, individuals had improved response inhibition, working memory, and decision-making. Increases in executive functions suggest that MBIs may help to increase personal agency over habitual responses that play a role in problematic substance use. Increased trait mindfulness may be another mechanism, as the review found that trait mindfulness strongly mediated the relationship between MBIs and craving.

In addition, there are other possible mechanisms of change found in the MBI literature on SUD treatment. Mindfulness practice may lessen problematic substance use by reducing stress reactivity, as indicated by heart rate variability (HRV), defined as the amount of time between each heartbeat. Evidence suggests that stress can worsen problematic substance use and that HRV is the body's way of recovering from stress. HRV in individuals with SUDs has been shown to increase after undergoing MBRP and/or MORE, leading researchers to hypothesize that through mindfulness practice, individuals can recover from stress at a faster rate. Decreased craving seen in MBI studies is supported in both lab-based and clinical research looking at the reduction in craving mediating outcomes of MBIs. The review states MBIs may address the role thought suppression plays in addiction by reducing the amount of thought suppression in individuals as it is known to amplify craving levels [29].

21.4.2 Alternative Mind–Body Practices for the Treatment of SUD

Although research on mindfulness-based approaches has received considerable attention for the treatment of SUD, there are various meditation techniques that may offer benefit to these populations. Numerous clinical trials have demonstrated the efficacy of MBIs in treating SUD [15, 29, 42]; however, one meta-analysis of nine randomized clinical trials (RCTs) concluded that MBRP had small effects on severe substance-related outcomes (withdrawal, craving, and negative consequences) [43]. Given the mixed results of MBIs for addictive behaviors, it may be necessary to explore alternative mind–body practices for the treatment of SUD. Meditation is a practice that originated over 5000 years ago [44] and is central to various cultural and religious traditions, some of which have influenced the practice and philosophy of mindfulness meditation. Several of these contemplative practices have been evaluated as clinical technologies for individuals with SUD and will be reviewed individually in the following sections.

21.4.3 Transcendental Meditation

Transcendental Meditation (TM) has gained notable popularity and visibility in the West since its first introduction to western culture in 1959 by Maharishi Yogesh [45]. TM is a seated practice done with the eyes closed for 20 min twice a day. A mantra is repeated for the duration of the practice to shift focus away from external stimuli and settle the mind inwardly [46]. Repetition of the mantra has been posited to lead to an increasingly quiet awareness, eventually leading to complete silence [46]. TM has been described as a simple and natural practice whereby a person experiences a state of restful alertness [47]. According to Maharishi's philosophy, the mind is hierarchically structured in layers that are progressively more subtle, abstract, and unified [48]. At the opposite spectrums of this continuum lie the "lower self" which only deals with the relative/changing aspects of existence, and the "higher self", which is the aspect of being that is unchanging, absolute, and completely integrated [48]. Maharishi's philosophy purports that the higher or transcendent self can be accessed through a deep practice of TM.

One of the earliest evaluations of TM for SUD, conducted by one of MBRP's progenitors in the late 1970s, found TM to be a useful practice for high-risk college student drinkers [49]. Since then, multiple investigations of TM for SUD have been carried out. A review and meta-analysis conducted by Alexander and colleagues (1994) included 19 studies evaluating TM for SUD. Authors found TM to have a medium effect size on both negative affect (e.g., depression, anger, hostility, anxiety), and positive affect (e.g., self-concept, well-being, self-esteem, internal locus of control) [48]. The meta-analysis also revealed a medium effect size for TM on alcohol use, and large effect size for cigarette use, cannabis use, and illicit drug use. Of note, the majority of subjects in the review were currently incarcerated and most effect sizes were only calculated for subjects in the TM or control conditions reporting substance use at pretest.

Although there was initially an abundance of trials on TM, in the 20 years since this meta-analysis was published, there have only been three further evaluations of TM for SUD. Of the three investigations, one RCT of TM compared to a waitlist control in a sample of university students found no between-group differences in smoking and illicit drug use but did find lower alcohol use among male but not female students in the TM condition [47]. The second study was a quasi-experimental study investigating the efficacy of integrating TM into SUD treatment [50]. This study found no significant differences between TM and TAU conditions overall but did find that those who were in the TM condition who practiced as recommended were less likely than the rest of the entire sample to return to drinking and exhibit heavy drinking post-discharge. Further, amount of TM practice was found to be inversely correlated with stress, craving, and alcohol use at follow-up. The third study, an RCT evaluating the effect of TM compared to biofeedback, neurotherapy, and TAU, found that TM and biofeedback groups reported significantly more days abstinent than other conditions, with TM emerging as the group with the highest rates of abstinence at 18-month follow up [51]. The review suggests that TM practice can help reduce substance use and its associated consequences by neutralizing accumulated stress and restoring psychophysiological balance, increasing serotonin, reducing cortisol, and stabilizing autonomic response during exposure to stressful stimuli [48]. With respect to impulsive behavior associated with SUDs, TM may reduce aggression, hostility, rule infractions, and recidivism in correctional populations and reduce impulsivity and aggression in non-correctional samples. In addition, TM has been found to reduce negative affect and bolster positive affect, thereby stabilizing emotions that characterize the affective sequelae of addiction.

Given the numerous trials exploring TM for SUD, TM shows promise as a contemplative practice for SUD recovery; however, it should be taken into consideration that the majority of these trials were conducted over 20 years ago, and have low methodological quality [52]. Further, the majority of this research has taken place in correctional settings; as such, future RCTs should investigate the efficacy of TM in SUD treatment settings, and should further explore mechanisms of change involved in TM practice.

21.5 Evidence for Yoga

While the meaning and practice of yoga have evolved, particularly in the West, the original Sanskrit definition of yoga translates into the union of the human being with the transcendent, or samadhi [53, 54]. Of note, samadhi from a Hindu perspective differs from how the Vipassana literature defines it. In the Hindu context, samadhi has been defined as one-pointed concentration leading to union with Divine Consciousness, or God, and the cessation of mental activity [55]. The philosophy of yoga outlined by the Hindu sage Patanjali in the second century BC is based on the eight limbs of Ashtanga Yoga, comprising the yamas (ethical disciplines), niyamas (individual observances), asana (posture), pranayama (breath control), pratyahara (withdrawal of senses), dharana (concentration), dhyana (meditation), and samadhi (self realization/enlightenment) [56]. Despite the fact that various forms of yoga exist and significant overlap exists across practices, the four main forms of yoga are: (1) hatha yoga—primarily involving the practice of physical techniques (e.g., asanas and pranayama) to attain purity, (2) raja yoga or the king of yogas involving meditation with the intention to reach samadhi, (3) jnana yoga—involving knowledge and wisdom, and (4) karma yoga—involving selfless action as a form of prayer. Of the forms of yoga, hatha yoga has emerged as the most commonly practiced form and has potential medical and clinical benefit. In addition, there have been several investigations of raja yoga for a variety of medical and clinical pathologies.

There has been an emerging interest in yoga as an adjunctive intervention for SUDs in the last decade. Nascent reviews have investigated the utility of hatha yoga for the treatment of SUDs

[57–60]. In the most recent review, 16 studies were examined, including 12 RCTs [58]. Although one RCT showed no effect relative to controls, overall findings suggest that hatha yoga shows promise as an adjunctive treatment modality for SUD, specifically involving tobacco, alcohol, opiates, cocaine, and barbiturates. Further, the review suggests that hatha yoga can be implemented in both outpatient and inpatient settings and can help reduce negative affective symptoms associated with SUD (e.g., low motivation, depression, stress, craving, and anxiety) while improving quality of life. Another recent study found that yoga can be delivered at medication-assisted treatment programs with high rates of adherence to at-home practice [61]. Further, the Veterans Health Administration recently compiled a research agenda to improve opioid safety, one of the committees findings was to improve access to non-opioid therapies such as yoga via telemedicine, especially for those who have difficulty accessing in-person treatment [62].

To date, only one study has explicitly investigated raja yoga meditation as an adjunctive treatment intervention for individuals with SUD [63]. Informed by the understanding that SUD may contain a spiritual deficiency, this quasi-experimental study asked participants in an outpatient SUD treatment center to concentrate on the point between their eyebrows, or third eye, for 20 min each session, focusing on their relationship with a higher power and chanting a mantra personally meaningful to them. Results showed that participants in the raja yoga meditation condition had a greater likelihood of maintaining abstinence compared to the relaxation and treatment-as-usual conditions. This study concluded that raja yoga could offer clinical benefit in preventing relapse in a partially buprenorphine-supported sample, and could be an alternative or additive spiritual supplemental practice to the 12-steps [63].

Despite the many advantages found in integrating yogic techniques into SUD treatment settings, results should be interpreted with caution. Most studies reviewed report favorable short-term outcomes; however, there remains a paucity of data on the long-term effects of yoga for individuals with SUD. Future studies should include long-term outcome data and rigorous study methodology to assess whether it is advisable to implement yoga as an adjunctive treatment modality for SUD.

Numerous theories and investigations of purported change mechanisms associated with yoga as a treatment for addictive behaviors have been explored in recent years. One way in which yoga may benefit individuals with SUD is that yoga is considered a holistic intervention that induces homeostasis that leads to long-term benefits in managing the reward deficiency syndrome that characterizes SUD [64]. SUD is often characterized by negative affect, and heightened arousal; relapse can function as a means to avoid aversive emotional content, or as a response to stressful cues [60]. In this context, a relapse often occurs when an individual is in an "automatic pilot" state indicative of mid-brain activation sometimes referred to as "fight or flight." Recent studies show that yoga can modulate the "fight or flight" stress response system involved in SUD. More specifically, yoga can return the autonomic nervous system to balance by downregulating the HPA axis when triggered by external or internal stimuli [65], and by decreasing stress via reducing levels of cortisol and ACTH [66]. In addition, detoxification from substances often involves increased heart rate and blood pressure; yoga could be helpful in ameliorating stress associated with substance detoxification by lowering heart rate and blood pressure [52, 67].

21.5.1 Qigong

The only other locatable literature on mind–body practices for treatment of SUD suggests that Qigong meditation may show promise as an adjunctive treatment intervention for individuals with SUD. *Qigong* (pronounced as *Chee Kung*), is an ancient Chinese health practice purported to have unique therapeutic benefits [68]. Qigong is a general term for complementary and alternative practices that integrate body, breath, and psychological adjustment into a cohesive whole through specific breathing practices [69]. Qigong is similar to hatha yoga in that it is an Eastern form of contemplative practice that utilizes breathing techniques and body movements, but differs in its culture of origin (i.e., China vs. India), and is comprised of movements that are generally slower and more gentle than hatha yoga movements. The meditative aspect of qigong typically involves a standing practice in which mantras are mentally repeated along with the integration of breath with body postures akin to Tai Chi. The highest form of qigong meditation involves sitting quietly without thinking, which differs from mindfulness practice in which a practitioner notices thoughts with curiosity and non-judgment. Of note, practices considered to be yoga, mindfulness, reiki, and transcendental meditation in the West are all considered qigong in China.

To date, there have been several investigations of qigong in the treatment of SUD in both China and the United States. One study conducted on 1403 individuals in residential SUD treatment in China found that individuals who underwent the combination of qigong practice with qi healing performed significantly better than TAU controls in smoking cessation [70]. Another study randomized detoxification-seeking heroin addicts to either qigong, medication, or a no-treatment control group. Results suggest that participants in the qigong group showed a more rapid reduction of withdrawal symptoms, and greater reductions in anxiety and substance use compared to treatment controls [71]. In a more recent study, participants in residential SUD treatment in the United States self-selected into either a qigong or stress management treatment for 4 weeks [72]. Both groups reported significant improvement in negative affect, but the qigong group reported a significantly higher treatment completion rate and greater reductions in craving than the stress management group. Furthermore, the study found that females in the qigong meditation group reported significantly greater reductions in anxiety and withdrawal symptoms than in the other group [72]. The most recent RCT of qigong meditation for SUD found qigong to be superior to a sham qigong control group in reducing cue-elicited craving and depression in a cocaine-dependent treatment sample [73].

Qigong literature suggests that the practice of qigong produces a strong "qifield" that may promote health benefits for individuals in recovery from SUD. However, there is a paucity of data on how specifically the *qifield* may aid in recovery from SUD. Perhaps due to limited empirical investigations of qigong meditation for addictive disorders, there is also a dearth of information on how this contemplative practice aids in the recovery process.

The results of these studies are preliminary and should be interpreted with caution. Several methodological weaknesses were found in these studies, such as self-selection, lack of structurally equivalent control groups, and lack of statistical analytic methods to rule out placebo effects [69]. Future studies should be conducted with greater methodological rigor and should investigate how qigong specifically aids in the recovery process of SUD.

21.5.2 Conclusion and Recommendations

Considering the body of evidence supporting meditation and yoga for the treatment of SUD, it seems apparent that these contemplative practices may not only be beneficial for individuals with addictive behaviors but may share some mechanisms of change. As SUD is characterized by mid-brain activation and fight-or-flight reactivity [74], it is beneficial to cultivate coping mechanisms that shift decision-making from "automatic pilot" to skillful responding with personal agency. The practice of mindfulness meditation, transcendental meditation, qigong, and yoga all seem to achieve this aim. The evidence base of MBIs for SUD has grown tremendously in recent years, but research on other contemplative practices such as yoga and qigong are still in their infancy. Moving forward, the development of structured protocols that integrate these practices into SUD treatment may be useful in combating this destructive epidemic. Further, as there remains a dearth of evidence for mechanisms underlying qigong meditation for SUD, future clinical trials should assess both efficacy and putative change agents of this practice in SUD treatment settings. In addition, the interaction between the cardiovascular system, stress, and substance use, and related consequences is becoming readily apparent. Future clinical trials on mind–body practices for SUD treatment should continue to track HRV data alongside other biomarkers of stress reactivity to clarify this relationship in order to better serve these populations. Further, researchers and agencies that treat addiction have suggested that SUD may contain spiritual components [75, 76]. As such, future investigations of contemplative practices that include the spiritual component of meditation, such as raja yoga meditation, may further broaden the utility of meditation practices for individuals in SUD recovery.

Considering the body of evidence for mind–body practices in the treatment of SUD, clinicians treating SUD should attempt to integrate efficacious interventions that include contemplative practices (e.g., Mindfulness-Based Interventions, Acceptance and Commitment Therapy, Dialectical Behavioral Therapy, Yoga) into their therapeutic repertoire. When working with clients, practitioners may encourage their client(s) to close their eyes, or lower their gaze, and gently gather their attention inward, noticing the physical sensations of the breath in their abdomen, and bring a gentle curiosity to noticing and labeling what thoughts, emotions, and sensations are arising at the moment. While using the sensations of breathing as an anchor to remain in contact with their body and direct experience. A simple exercise of this nature for as little as 5 min may help foster increased mindful awareness. Further, as other budding alternative contemplative practices in SUD treatment become held to higher scientific scrutiny, clients may be better served through the integration of practices such as qigong and transcendental meditation. The devastating epidemic of SUD continues to cause harm both in the USA and globally, and we may be better able to serve those that are suffering by learning from our wisdom traditions and integrating these practices into our clinical settings.

References

1. American Society of Addiction Medicine. Public policy statement: definition of addiction. 2011. August 15. https://www.asam.org/docs/default-source/public-policy-statements/1definition_of_addiction_long_4-11.pdf?sfvrsn=a8f64512_4
2. Koob GF, Volkow ND. Neurocircuitry of addiction. Neuropsychopharmacology. 2010;35(1):217–38.
3. Rehm J, Marmet S, Anderson P, et al. Defining substance use disorders: do we really need more than heavy use? Alcohol Alcohol. 2013;48(6):633–40.
4. American Psychiatric Assocaition. Diagnostic and statistical manual of mental disorders. 5th ed. Washington, DC: The Association; 2013.
5. SAMHSA. Reports and detailed tables from the 2017 national survey on drug use and health (NSDUH). 2017. https://www.samhsa.gov/data/nsduh/reports-detailed-tables-2017-NSDUH. Accessed 20 Feb 2019.
6. Madras BK. The surge of opioid use, addiction, and overdoses: responsibility and response of the US health care system. JAMA Psychiat. 2017;74(5):441–2.
7. Rudd RA, Seth P, David F, Scholl L. Increases in drug and opioid-involved overdose deaths—United States, 2010–2015. MMWR Morb Mortal Wkly Rep. 2016;65(50–51):1445–52. https://doi.org/10.15585/mmwr.mm655051e1.
8. Centers for Disease Control and Prevention. Fact sheets—alcohol use and your health. 2018. Retrieved from https://www.cdc.gov/alcohol/fact-sheets/alcohol-use.htm
9. Roerecke M, Rehm J. Alcohol use disorders and mortality: a systematic review and meta-analysis. Addiction. 2013;108(9):1562–78. https://doi.org/10.1111/add.12231.
10. CDC. Tobacco-related mortality. 2016. https://www.cdc.gov/tobacco/data_statistics/fact_sheets/health_effects/tobacco_related_mortality/index.htm. Accessed 27 Feb 2019.
11. NIAA. Alcohol facts and statistics. 2017. https://www.niaaa.nih.gov/alcohol-health/overview-alcohol-consumption/alcohol-facts-and-statistics. Accessed 27 Feb 2019.
12. NIDA. Overdose related deaths. 2017. https://www.drugabuse.gov/related-topics/trends-statistics/overdose-death-rates. Accessed 27 Feb 2019.
13. NIDA. Drugs, brains, and behavior: the science of addiction. 2018. https://d14rmgtrwzf5a.cloudfront.net/sites/default/files/soa.pdf. Accessed 20 Feb 2019.
14. Dutra L, Stathopoulou G, Basden SL, Leyro TM, Powers MB, Otto MW. A meta-analytic review of

psychosocial interventions for substance use disorders. Am J Psychiatry. 2008;165(2):179–87.
15. Bowen S, Witkiewitz K, Clifasefi SL, et al. Relative efficacy of mindfulness-based relapse prevention, standard relapse prevention, and treatment as usual for substance use disorders: a randomized clinical trial. JAMA Psychiat. 2014;71(5):547–56.
16. Chiesa A, Serretti A. Are mindfulness-based interventions effective for substance use disorders? A systematic review of the evidence. Subst Use Misuse. 2014;49(5):492–512.
17. Garland EL, Gaylord SA, Boettiger CA, Howard MO. Mindfulness training modifies cognitive, affective, and physiological mechanisms implicated in alcohol dependence: results of a randomized controlled pilot trial. J Psychoactive Drugs. 2010;42(2):177–92.
18. Zgierska A, Rabago D, Chawla N, Kushner K, Koehler R, Marlatt A. Mindfulness meditation for substance use disorders: a systematic review. Subst Abus. 2009;30(4):266–94.
19. Khantzian EJ. The self-medication hypothesis of addictive disorders: focus on heroin and cocaine dependence. Am J Psychiatry. 1985;142(11):1259–64.
20. Audrain-McGovern J, Rodriguez D, Epstein LH, Cuevas J, Rodgers K, Wileyto EP. Does delay discounting play an etiological role in smoking or is it a consequence of smoking? Drug Alcohol Depend. 2009;103(3):99–106.
21. Dworkin ER, Wanklyn S, Stasiewicz PR, Coffey SF. PTSD symptom presentation among people with alcohol and drug use disorders: comparisons by substance of abuse. Addict Behav. 2018;76:188–94.
22. Ertl V, Saile R, Neuner F, Catani C. Drinking to ease the burden: a cross-sectional study on trauma, alcohol abuse and psychopathology in a post-conflict context. BMC Psychiatry. 2016;16:202.
23. Garland EL, Pettus-Davis C, Howard MO. Self-medication among traumatized youth: structural equation modeling of pathways between trauma history, substance misuse, and psychological distress. J Behav Med. 2013;36(2):175–85.
24. Shadur JM, Hussong AM, Haroon M. Negative affect variability and adolescent self-medication: the role of the peer context. Drug Alcohol Rev. 2015;34(6):571–80.
25. Hayes SC. Buddhism and acceptance and commitment therapy. Cogn Behav Pract. 2002;9(1):58–66.
26. Groves P, Farmer R. Buddhism and addictions. Addict Res. 1994;2(2):183–94.
27. Marlatt GA. Buddhist philosophy and the treatment of addictive behavior. Cogn Behav Pract. 2002;9(1):44–9.
28. Krygier JR, Heathers JA, Shahrestani S, Abbott M, Gross JJ, Kemp AH. Mindfulness meditation, well-being, and heart rate variability: a preliminary investigation into the impact of intensive Vipassana meditation. Int J Psychophysiol. 2013;89(3):305–13.
29. Garland EL, Howard MO. Mindfulness-based treatment of addiction: current state of the field and envisioning the next wave of research. Addict Sci Clin Pract. 2018;13(1):14.
30. Vago DR, Silbersweig DA. Self-awareness, self-regulation, and self-transcendence (S-ART): a framework for understanding the neurobiological mechanisms of mindfulness. Front Hum Neurosci. 2012;6:296.
31. Baer RA, Smith GT, Hopkins J, Krietemeyer J, Toney L. Using self-report assessment methods to explore facets of mindfulness. Assessment. 2006;13(1):27–45.
32. Kabat-Zinn J. Full catastrophe living: using the wisdom of your body and mind to face stress, pain, and illness. New York: Delta Publishing; 1990.
33. Segal ZV, Williams JMG, Teasdale JD, Kabat-Zinn J. Mindfulness-based cognitive therapy for depression. New York: The Guilford Press; 2018.
34. Bowen S, Chawla N, Marlatt GA. Mindfulness-based relapse prevention for addictive behaviors: a clinician's guide. New York: Guilford Press; 2010.
35. Garland EL, National Association of Social Workers. Mindfulness-oriented recovery enhancement for addiction, stress, and pain. Washington, DC: NASW Press; 2013.
36. Witkiewitz K, Bowen S. Depression, craving and substance use following a randomized trial of mindfulness-based relapse prevention. J Consult Clin Psychol. 2010;78(3):362–74.
37. Glasner-Edwards S, Mooney LJ, Ang A, et al. Mindfulness based relapse prevention for stimulant dependent adults: a pilot randomized clinical trial. Mindfulness (NY). 2017;8(1):126–35.
38. Schroevers MJ, Brandsma R. Is learning mindfulness associated with improved affect after mindfulness-based cognitive therapy? Br J Psychol. 2010;101(Pt 1):95–107.
39. Zemestani M, Ottaviani C. Effectiveness of mindfulness-based relapse prevention for co-occurring substance use and depression disorders. Mindfulness. 2016;7(6):1347–55.
40. Witkiewitz K, Bowen S, Douglas H, Hsu SH. Mindfulness-based relapse prevention for substance craving. Addict Behav. 2013;38(2):1563–71.
41. Garland EL, Manusov EG, Froeliger B, Kelly A, Williams JM, Howard MO. Mindfulness-oriented recovery enhancement for chronic pain and prescription opioid misuse: results from an early-stage randomized controlled trial. J Consult Clin Psychol. 2014;82(3):448–59.
42. Priddy SE, Howard MO, Hanley AW, Riquino MR, Friberg-Felsted K, Garland EL. Mindfulness meditation in the treatment of substance use disorders and preventing future relapse: neurocognitive mechanisms and clinical implications. Subst Abus Rehabil. 2018;9:103–14.
43. Grant S, Colaiaco B, Motala A, et al. Mindfulness-based relapse prevention for substance use disorders: a systematic review and meta-analysis. J Addict Med. 2017;11(5):386–96.
44. Dakwar E, Levin FR. The emerging role of meditation in addressing psychiatric illness, with a focus

on substance use disorders. Harv Rev Psychiatry. 2009;17(4):254–67.
45. Yogi M. Thirty years around the world: 1957–1964. Stichting Drukkerij en Uitgeverij MVU; 1986.
46. Yogi M. Life supported by natural law. Washington, DC: Age of Enlightenment Press; 1986.
47. Haaga DAF, Grosswald S, Gaylord-King C, et al. Effects of the transcendental meditation program on substance use among university students. Cardiol Res Pract. 2011;2011:537101.
48. Alexander CN, Robinson P, Rainforth M. Treating and preventing alcohol, nicotine, and drug abuse through transcendental meditation. Alcohol Treat Q. 1994;11(1–2):13–87.
49. Marlatt GA, Marques JK. Meditation, self-control, and alcohol use. In: Stuart RB, editor. Behavioral self-management: strategies, techniques, and outcomes. New York: Brunner/Mazel; 1977. p. 117–53.
50. Gryczynski J, Schwartz RP, Fishman MJ, et al. Integration of Transcendental Meditation(R) (TM) into alcohol use disorder (AUD) treatment. J Subst Abus Treat. 2018;87:23–30.
51. Taub E, Steiner SS, Weingarten E, Walton KG. Effectiveness of broad spectrum approaches to relapse prevention in severe alcoholism: a long-term, randomized, controlled trial of Transcendental Meditation, EMG biofeedback and electronic neurotherapy. Alcohol Treat Q. 1994;11(1–2):187–220.
52. Ospina MB, Bond K, Karkhaneh M, et al. Meditation practices for health: state of the research. Evid Rep Technol Assess. 2007;155:1–263.
53. Sengupta P. Health impacts of yoga and pranayama: a state-of-the-art review. Int J Prev Med. 2012;3(7):444–58.
54. Yogananda P. The yoga of the Bhagavad Gita: an introduction to India's universal science of God-realization: selections from the writings of Paramahansa Yogananda. Los Angeles: Self-Realization Fellowship; 2007.
55. Fort AO. Vijñānabhikṣu on two forms of Samadhi. Hindu Studies. 2006;10(3):271–94.
56. Bonura KB. The psychological benefits of yoga practice for older adults: evidence and guidelines. Int J Yoga Therap. 2011;21:129–42.
57. Khanna S, Greeson JM. A narrative review of yoga and mindfulness as complementary therapies for addiction. Complement Ther Med. 2013;21(3):244–52.
58. Kuppili PP, Parmar A, Gupta A, Balhara YPS. Role of yoga in management of substance-use disorders: a narrative review. J Neurosci Rural Pract. 2018;9(1):117–22.
59. Posadzki P, Choi J, Lee MS, Ernst E. Yoga for addictions: a systematic review of randomised clinical trials. Focus Altern Complement Ther. 2014;19(1):1–8.
60. Sarkar S, Varshney M. Yoga and substance use disorders: a narrative review. Asian J Psychiatr. 2017;25:191–6.
61. Uebelacker LA, Van Noppen D, Tremont G, Bailey G, Abrantes A, Stein M. A pilot study assessing acceptability and feasibility of hatha yoga for chronic pain in people receiving opioid agonist therapy for opioid use disorder. J Subst Abus Treat. 2019;105:19–27.
62. Becker WC, Krebs EE, Edmond SN, et al. A research agenda for advancing strategies to improve opioid safety: findings from a VHA state of the art conference. J Gen Intern Med. 2020;35:978–82. https://doi.org/10.1007/s11606-020-06260-9.
63. Mallik D, Bowen S, Yang Y, Perkins R, Sandoz EK. Raja yoga meditation and medication-assisted treatment for relapse prevention: a pilot study. J Subst Abus Treat. 2019;96:58–64.
64. Miller D, Miller M, Blum K, Badgaiyan RD, Febo M. Addiction treatment in America: after money or aftercare? J Reward Defic Syndr. 2015;1(3):87–94.
65. Sengupta P, Krajewska-Kulak E. Is mind-body relaxation by yoga is effective to combat with lifestyle stress? Ann Med Health Sci Res. 2013;3(Suppl 1):S61–2.
66. Vedamurthachar A, Janakiramaiah N, Hegde JM, et al. Antidepressant efficacy and hormonal effects of Sudarshana Kriya Yoga (SKY) in alcohol dependent individuals. J Affect Disord. 2006;94(1–3):249–53.
67. Bharshankar JR, Mandape AD, Phatak MS, Bharshankar RN. Autonomic functions in Raja-yoga meditators. Indian J Physiol Pharmacol. 2015;59(4):396–401.
68. Jahnke R, Larkey L, Rogers C, Etnier J, Lin F. A comprehensive review of health benefits of qigong and tai chi. Ame J Health Promot. 2010;24(6):e1–e25.
69. Shinnick P. Qigong: where did it come from? Where does it fit in science? What are the advances? J Altern Complement Med (New York, NY). 2006;12(4):351–3.
70. Xu WY. Establishing *qigong* field to cease smoking. Zhineng Qigong Sci. 1996;11:38.
71. Li M, Chen K, Mo Z. Use of qigong therapy in the detoxification of heroin addicts. Altern Ther Health Med. 2002;8(1):50–9.
72. Chen KW, Comerford A, Shinnick P, Ziedonis DM. Introducing qigong meditation into residential addiction treatment: a pilot study where gender makes a difference. J Altern Complement Med. 2010;16(8):875–82.
73. Smelson D, Chen KW, Ziedonis D, et al. A pilot study of Qigong for reducing cocaine craving early in recovery. J Altern Complement Med (New York, NY). 2013;19(2):97–101.
74. Everitt BJ, Robbins TW. Neural systems of reinforcement for drug addiction: from actions to habits to compulsion. Nat Neurosci. 2005;8(11):1481–9.
75. Miller WR. Researching the spiritual dimensions of alcohol and other drug problems. Addiction. 1998;93(7):979–90.
76. ASAM. ASAM releases new definition of addiction. 2011. https://www.asam.org/docs/pressreleases/asam-definition-of-addiction-2011-08-15.pdf. Accessed 20 Feb 2019.

22 Yoga and Cardiovascular Disease Prevention in African Americans and Hispanics

Keith C. Norris and Bettina M. Beech

22.1 Introduction

Despite numerous advances in the prevention and treatment of cardiovascular disease (CVD) and CVD risk factors, CVD remains a leading cause of morbidity and mortality in the USA and globally [1]. The effective prevention and treatment of CVD often requires the combination of pharmacologic and non-pharmacologic approaches, typically directed at CVD risk factors [1, 2]. However, the prevention of CVD is more commonly grounded in non-pharmacologic approaches, especially primary prevention of key CVD risk factors such as hypertension, diabetes, obesity, hypercholesterolemia, inactivity, smoking, and stress [1–3]. The therapeutic lifestyle changes required as part of a comprehensive non-pharmacologic approach are particularly important since many of these CVD risk factors are behavioral and modifiable [1, 2]. Health care providers may use evidence-based tools for CVD prevention, for example, brief motivational interviewing or the 5A's (Ask, Advise, Assist, Assess, Arrange) to ask patients about diet and exercise patterns, their smoking status, provide lifestyle advice, and participate in local initiatives or services that may provide support services and promote healthy lifestyle change [4]. By contrast, health care providers may encourage the use of approaches considered alternative for addressing CVD in Western Allopathic medicine such as naturopathy, meditation, and yoga [5–7]. The identification and effective communication of key CVD risk-attributable behaviors (such as dietary intake, physical inactivity, excessive alcohol intake, smoking, and stress reduction), should engage and encourage patients to be proactive in the implementation of therapeutic lifestyle changes including the practice of yoga and meditation [1–3].

The term yoga is Sanskrit for "union" or "to yoke." All forms of yoga share common elements, including the use of controlled breathing (pranayama), physical postures (asanas), and meditative techniques (dhyana) to achieve well-being and mind–body union and balance [8]. Of the numerous schools of yoga, Hatha yoga is the most commonly practiced in the USA and since most elementary courses of Hatha yoga focus on physical exercises consisting of various postures and breathing techniques yoga is commonly viewed as an exercise with a series of poses [9].

K. C. Norris (✉)
Division of General Internal Medicine and Health Services Research, Department of Medicine, David Geffen School of Medicine, University of California, Los Angeles, CA, USA
e-mail: kcnorris@mednet.ucla.edu

B. M. Beech
Department of Health Systems and Population Health Science, College of Medicine, University of Houston, Houston, TX, USA

University of Houston Population Health, Jackson, MS, USA

I. Basu-Ray, D. Mehta (eds.), *The Principles and Practice of Yoga in Cardiovascular Medicine*,
https://doi.org/10.1007/978-981-16-6913-2_22

Yoga is considered to improve bodily functions through the manipulation of cardiovascular, respiratory, metabolic, and other control mechanisms [10]. Whereas asanas are generally understood, the central role that pranayamas and dhyana have in yoga are less well appreciated in the USA. Further, there is a more limited understanding that yoga is truly a holistic ancient Indian discipline designed to bring balance and health to the physical, mental, emotional, and spiritual dimensions of the individual [8, 9].

Yogic cognitive-behavioral practices are among the most widely used complementary approaches and have gained significant interest in recent years given the need to create high-value (cost-effective and high-quality) alternative solutions to today's health care challenges. Studies suggest that these yogic/meditative practices have significant positive effects on the mind–body system and thereby can increase wellness and support the healing process from disease [11]. The 2007 National Health Interview Survey found that yoga is one of the top 10 CAM health approaches used among U.S. adults, with an estimated 6% of adults having used yoga for health purposes in the previous 12 months [12]. By 2012 an estimated 9.5% of adults reported practicing yoga and by 2017 over 14% of adults reported practicing yoga, with yoga and meditation (also 14%) now exceeding the use of chiropractic care (10.3%) and are the two most common alternative medicine practices outside of nutritional supplements and [13]. It should be noted that in most instances intrinsic to yoga is a meditative component or dhyana [9]. Thus, the holistic vision of health and well-being within yoga is consistent with the traditional view of health in the USA and is an essential aspect of the lives of all human beings occupying a central place in the social construct of every community. In English, the word health is derived from the Anglo-Saxon root "hale," which means whole or holy [14, 15]. Health, in its ultimate sense, might be viewed as the physical expression of the totality of individuals, families, and communities, truly the re-establishment of wholeness. Thus, yogic cognitive-behavioral practices treat the mind, body, and spirit as inseparable and interdependent, establishing a communion between spirit and the science of medicine [16].

While the practice of yoga has been consistently increasing in the USA, its use is not evenly distributed across racial/ethnic groups with 17.1% non-Hispanic White adults reporting to practice yoga in 2017, nearly twice that of African American (9.3%) and Hispanic adults (8.0%) [13]. Given the persistent distrust by minorities of the U.S. health care system [17], it seems there might be an even higher level of use of a well-established, non-Western Allopathic approach to health such as yoga. Further, with the disproportionately high rates of CVD risk factors such as hypertension, diabetes, obesity, and physical inactivity and stress among African American and Hispanic individual [1, 2], the potential role of yoga as a high-value approach to primary and even secondary CVD prevention for African American and Hispanic communities seems substantial. While the underlying cellular mechanisms that explain these emerging clinical benefits are not well known, they appear to enhance gene expression in key inflammatory response and stress-related pathways as well as energy metabolism, mitochondrial function, insulin secretion, and telomere maintenance pathways [12, 18–21].

22.2 Yoga and the African American Community

African American individual, particularly women, have had a long history with the reliance on yoga for healing. Krishna Kaur, an African American female pioneer in the 1970s practiced a form of yoga that focused on awakening Kundalini energy through meditation, pranayama, chanting, and physical asana. Kaur studied yoga under Yogi Bhajan and postulated that yoga could provide and restore peace and amity to African American populations who have endured centuries of oppression, anguish, and injustice. Indeed many [22–27], but not all [28–30] studies have reported increased levels of blood pressure and CVD risk related to racial discrimination against the African American community.

22.3 Yoga Trials with African American Participants

A direct and positive relation between blood pressure and CV risk has been well-established and the primary prevention of elevated blood pressure provides an opportunity to interrupt and prevent the long-standing cycle of managing hypertension and its associated sequalae [1, 2]. The greatest long-term potential for avoiding hypertension is to utilize a range of prevention strategies such as yoga early in life [2]. Hatha Yoga is a moderately safe form of exercise that appears to be beneficial for the primary and secondary prevention of CVD, however, few clinical trials have directly investigated the effectiveness of yoga for the primary prevention of CVD among the African American community; the population group with arguably the highest prevalence of hypertension in the nation [31].

The Jackson Heart Study (JHS) is a multicenter investigation of predictors of CVD in 5301 African Americans residing in the Jackson, Mississippi metropolitan area, and the largest cardiovascular cohort study of African Americans adult ever conducted [32]. A fairly recent randomized, hybrid phase-in/crossover design ancillary trial to JHS was conducted to examine the effects of yoga practice on mitigating CVD risk factors among adults diagnosed with hypertension or pre-hypertension. Participants were randomized to one of five intervention conditions delivered over 24-weeks: high-frequency yoga, moderate-frequency yoga, low-frequency yoga, guided walking, and health education classes. At the post-intervention follow-up, there was a significant difference ($p = 0.007$) in the pooled yoga intervention retention (78.3%) compared with the guided walking condition (60%) and the education group (74.3%); however, there was no difference at the 48-week follow-up [33].

One feasibility/acceptability study was conducted to evaluate a novel, Internet-based cultural dance-modified yoga intervention designed for African American women. A convenience sample of 24 women (mean age 43.4 years) completed the 4-week intervention which consisted of seven, 10-min yogic dance training modules. Concepts from hatha yoga and the Chakra systems were integrated with movements from West African dance demonstrated by African American female models of varying body sizes and stretching levels to provide a range of role models [34]. The videos were rated as acceptable and enjoyable by participants, however, given the nature of this small feasibility study, blood pressure outcome data was not reported.

A randomized pilot study with 83 African American adults diagnosed with hypertension was conducted to examine the outcomes of an 8-week mindful meditation program compared to a social support control group [35]. An 11/4 mmHg decrease in systolic/diastolic blood pressure was observed in those randomized to the active intervention condition. At follow-up demonstrated a 22/17 mmHg difference in blood pressure between the two groups demonstrated an intervention effect. Relatively high participation at each data collection point (80%) and 100% data ascertainment was achieved in this trial, providing confidence in the study findings.

22.4 Yoga and the Hispanic Community

While the practice of yoga among Hispanics in the USA is slowly growing, the Observatory of Natural Therapies, based in Catalonia reported that among 2000 individuals interviewed between the ages of 16 and 65 that yoga was the most commonly used alternative therapy at 32.5%. [36]. Persons of Hispanic or Latino/a origin now represent the largest minority group in the U.S., making up 18% of the total population in 2018 [37]. The limitation of yoga participation in the U.S. Hispanic or Latino/a population may be due to a sense of limited accessibility and may explain why Spanish yoga classes are anticipated to be the next big trend in the yoga world [38]. This may open the door to yoga practices for health prevention and early intervention for an increasing portion of the U.S. Hispanic or Latino/a population. Similar to African Americans, Hispanics in the USA have been reported to have increased levels of blood pressure and CVD risk related to racial discrimination [26, 28]. Thus, stress reduction strategies like yoga may have particular benefits for Hispanics as part of a CVD prevention program.

22.5 Yoga Trials with Hispanic Participants

Park et al. reported a 95% adherence rate in 100 English-speaking or Spanish-speaking participants (40% Hispanic, 45% White, 15% Other) with attendance at 12 of the 16 chair yoga sessions for 75-year-old community-dwelling adults with lower-extremity osteoarthritis [39]. While not a CVD-related trial, it demonstrated a high level of adherence to yoga among Spanish-speaking Hispanic participants when presented in Spanish. A survey patients of 161 consecutive adult patients (mean age 61 years) in an inner-city cardiology clinic (59% female, 37% Black, 34% Hispanic) found 66.0% of Black and 51% of Hispanic compared to only 43% of White patients expressed an interest in learning meditation to reduce the impact of stress in their lives [40]. This suggests a high percentage of Black and Hispanic cardiac patients are interested in contemplative practices and might be willing to participate in yoga-based trials. A 2-year follow-up using qualitative interviews on 39 urban elementary school teachers and staff (44% White, 36% Black, and 15% Other) who participated in an onsite fitness facility with an integrative wellness program. The program included group exercise classes, yoga, mindfulness, and nutrition competitions and the authors found it improved several health-related outcomes including key CVD risk factors such as mood, motivation to eat healthily, and improved sleep health-related outcomes among [41].

In addition, a 10-week Your Own Greatness Affirmed (YOGA) program among 30 urban inner-city 4th–8th grade students (50% Black and 50% Hispanic) found yoga significantly improved students' stress, positive affect, and resilience [42].

There are few reported randomized controlled trials for yoga in Hispanic persons. For example, one study underway will recruit 126 Hispanics/Latinos aged ≥18 years into a positive psychological intervention (¡Alégrate!) that includes daily positive events, a positive reappraisal of stressful events, effective expression of gratitude, performing acts of kindness, and regular practice of mindfulness and meditation, among others or a wait-list control on blood pressure and inflammatory markers [43]. While it did not include yoga in the positive psychological intervention although its attributes resemble that of yoga and suggests an increase in interest in contemplative interventions in Hispanic or Latino/a individuals for CVD prevention.

22.6 Limitations to Yoga Trials and Cardiovascular Disease in African American and Hispanic Individuals

In general, racial and ethnic minorities in the U.S. are underrepresented in clinical trials [44]. A qualitative investigation on barriers to practicing yoga among 24 participants from a low-income, urban housing community (25% Black and 12.5% Hispanic) found a perception that yoga lacks physicality and weight loss benefits, fear of injury, lack of ability/self-efficacy to perform the practices, preference for other physical activities, and scheduling difficulties [45]. Fortunately, meta-analyses and systemic reviews indicate that yoga and meditative therapies are equally effective as conventional antidepressants in the treatment of depression and anxiety disorders [46–48], providing promise that yoga and meditation may have similar effects for primary and secondary CVD prevention. Out of 37 yoga-based randomized controlled trials (RCTs) in a systematic review and 32 in a linked meta-analysis both yoga and exercise controls showed a significant improvement for body weight (−2.3 kg), systolic blood pressure (−5.2 mmHg), low-density lipoprotein cholesterol (−12.1 mg/dl), and high-density lipoprotein cholesterol (3.2 mg/dl) compared to non-exercise controls [49]. There were no significant differences between yoga, exercise controls, and non-exercise controls in fasting blood glucose or glycosylated hemoglobin [49]. Finally, among 113 patients treated with antihypertensive drugs, stress reduction (consisting of rice diet, walks, yoga, relaxation, and stress management) was shown to be as effective for blood pressure control as a high fruit and vegetable/low salt diet (DASH diet) or exercise control group (consisting of DASH diet and walks), reinforcing the benefits of stress reduction strategies, although there were no African American or Hispanic participants [50].

22.7 Conclusion

In summary, unlike conventional Western allopathic medicine which often treats most individuals with the same cardiovascular symptoms with a similar treatment, complementary practices such as yoga introduce a more personalized and holistic approach recognizing that each individual is unique in space and time. Importantly, no single approach is ideal for all people. For instance, a widely used breathing program derived from yoga is Sudarshan Kriya [11, 51, 52], which uses specific rhythms of breathing to transform overpowering emotions to eliminate stress and restore peace of mind and thus support the various organs and systems within the body [53].

A combination of different approaches will often be needed to create a high-value and culturally acceptable individualized CVD prevention program. In general, due to mistrust African American and Hispanic individuals may be less likely to adhere optimally to Western Allopathic treatment recommendations [54, 55] and thus providing alternative approaches to CVD health that will complement traditional Western Allopathic practices is prudent. Practice recommendations should consider those that focus on CVD health prevention and emphasize diet, lifestyle, emotional well-being, and stress management [12, 56, 57] such as yoga which can facilitate stress reduction and self-healing, maximizing coherence and effectiveness of self-healing [58, 59]. Complementary and alternative practices such as meditation, yoga, and even prayer, which act, in part, through enhancement of the relaxation response, the counterpart of the stress response, are emerging as effective therapeutic interventions for stress disorders such as hypertension, CVD, and more [12, 20] and may have a particularly effective role in the primary and secondary prevention of CVD in African American and Hispanic individuals.

References

1. Virani SS, Alonso A, Benjamin EJ, Bittencourt MS, Callaway CW, Carson AP, et al. Heart disease and stroke statistics-2020 update: a report from the American Heart Association. Circulation. 2020;141(9):e139–596. https://doi.org/10.1161/cir.0000000000000757.
2. Whelton PK, Carey RM, Aronow WS, Casey DE Jr, Collins KJ, Dennison Himmelfarb C, et al. 2017 ACC/AHA/AAPA/ABC/ACPM/AGS/APhA/ASH/ASPC/NMA/PCNA Guideline for the prevention, detection, evaluation, and management of high blood pressure in adults: a report of the American College of Cardiology/American Heart Association Task Force on Clinical Practice Guidelines. Circulation. 2018;138(17):e484–594. https://doi.org/10.1161/cir.0000000000000596.
3. Levine GN, Lange RA, Bairey-Merz CN, Davidson RJ, Jamerson K, Mehta PK, et al. Meditation and cardiovascular risk reduction: a scientific statement from the American Heart Association. J Am Heart Assoc. 2017;6(10) https://doi.org/10.1161/jaha.117.002218.
4. National Guideline C. National Institute for health and care excellence: clinical guidelines. In: Hypertension in adults: diagnosis and management. London: National Institute for Health and Care Excellence (UK); 2019. Copyright (c) NICE 2019.
5. Mooventhan A, Nivethitha L. Role of yoga in the prevention and management of various cardiovascular diseases and their risk factors: a comprehensive scientific evidence-based review. Explore (NY). 2020; https://doi.org/10.1016/j.explore.2020.02.007.
6. Prasad K, Sharma V, Lackore K, Jenkins SM, Prasad A, Sood A. Use of complementary therapies in cardiovascular disease. Am J Cardiol. 2013;111(3):339–45. https://doi.org/10.1016/j.amjcard.2012.10.010.
7. Sirois FM, Jiang L, Upchurch DM. Use and disclosure of complementary health approaches in US adults with cardiovascular disease. Am J Cardiol. 2018;122(1):170–4. https://doi.org/10.1016/j.amjcard.2018.03.014.
8. Pascoe MC, Bauer IE. A systematic review of randomised control trials on the effects of yoga on stress measures and mood. J Psychiatr Res. 2015;68:270–82. https://doi.org/10.1016/j.jpsychires.2015.07.013.
9. Sengupta P. Health impacts of yoga and pranayama: a state-of-the-art review. Int J Prev Med. 2012;3(7):444.

10. Kuntsevich V, Bushell WC, Theise ND. Mechanisms of yogic practices in health, aging, and disease. Mt Sinai J Med. 2010;77(5):559–69. https://doi.org/10.1002/msj.20214.
11. Zope SA, Zope RA. Sudarshan kriya yoga: breathing for health. Int J Yoga. 2013;6(1):4–10. https://doi.org/10.4103/0973-6131.105935.
12. Barnes PM, Bloom B, Nahin RL. Complementary and alternative medicine use among adults and children: United States, 2007. Natl Health Stat Rep. 2008;(12):1–23.
13. Clarke TC, Barnes PM, Black LI, Stussman BJ, Nahin RL. Use of yoga, meditation, and chiropractors among U.S. adults aged 18 and over. NCHS Data Brief. 2018;(325):1–8.
14. Bohm D. Wholeness and the implicate order. London: Routledge; 2002.
15. Gove PB. Webster's third new international dictionary of the English language, unabridged, vol. 1. Springfield: Merriam-Webster; 1981.
16. Denner SS. The science of energy therapies and contemplative practice: a conceptual review and the application of zero balancing. Holist Nurs Pract. 2009;23(6):315–34. https://doi.org/10.1097/HNP.0b013e3181bf3784.
17. Sullivan LS. Trust, risk, and race in American medicine. Hast Cent Rep. 2020;50(1):18–26. https://doi.org/10.1002/hast.1080.
18. Bhasin MK, Dusek JA, Chang BH, Joseph MG, Denninger JW, Fricchione GL, et al. Relaxation response induces temporal transcriptome changes in energy metabolism, insulin secretion and inflammatory pathways. PLoS One. 2013;8(5):e62817. https://doi.org/10.1371/journal.pone.0062817.
19. Buric I, Farias M, Jong J, Mee C, Brazil IA. What is the molecular signature of mind-body interventions? A systematic review of gene expression changes induced by meditation and related practices. Front Immunol. 2017;8:670. https://doi.org/10.3389/fimmu.2017.00670.
20. Fjorback LO. Mindfulness and bodily distress. Dan Med J. 2012;59(11):B4547.
21. Guddeti RR, Dang G, Williams MA, Alla VM. Role of yoga in cardiac disease and rehabilitation. J Cardiopulm Rehabil Prev. 2018; https://doi.org/10.1097/hcr.0000000000000372.
22. Cooper RS, Forrester TE, Plange-Rhule J, Bovet P, Lambert EV, Dugas LR, et al. Elevated hypertension risk for African-origin populations in biracial societies: modeling the Epidemiologic Transition Study. J Hypertens. 2015;33(3):473–80.; discussion 480-471. https://doi.org/10.1097/hjh.0000000000000429.
23. Cruickshank JK, Silva MJ, Molaodi OR, Enayat ZE, Cassidy A, Karamanos A, et al. Ethnic differences in and childhood influences on early adult pulse wave velocity: the determinants of adolescent, now young adult, social wellbeing, and health longitudinal study. Hypertension. 2016;67(6):1133–41. https://doi.org/10.1161/hypertensionaha.115.07079.
24. Faerstein E, Chor D, Werneck GL, de Souza Lopes C, Kaplan G. Race and perceived racism, education, and hypertension among Brazilian civil servants: the Pro-Saude Study. Rev Bras Epidemiol. 2014;17(Suppl 2):81–7. https://doi.org/10.1590/1809-4503201400060007.
25. Michaels EK, Reeves AN, Thomas MD, Price MM, Hasson RE, Chae DH, Allen AM. Everyday racial discrimination and hypertension among midlife African American women: disentangling the role of active coping dispositions versus active coping behaviors. Int J Environ Res Public Health. 2019;16(23) https://doi.org/10.3390/ijerph16234759.
26. Orom H, Sharma C, Homish GG, Underwood W 3rd, Homish DL. Racial discrimination and stigma consciousness are associated with higher blood pressure and hypertension in minority men. J Racial Ethn Health Disparities. 2016; https://doi.org/10.1007/s40615-016-0284-2.
27. Taylor JY, Sun YV, Barcelona de Mendoza V, Ifatunji M, Rafferty J, Fox ER, et al. The combined effects of genetic risk and perceived discrimination on blood pressure among African Americans in the Jackson Heart Study. Medicine (Baltimore). 2017;96(43):e8369. https://doi.org/10.1097/md.0000000000008369.
28. Beatty Moody DL, Waldstein SR, Tobin JN, Cassells A, Schwartz JC, Brondolo E. Lifetime racial/ethnic discrimination and ambulatory blood pressure: the moderating effect of age. Health Psychol. 2016;35(4):333–42. https://doi.org/10.1037/hea0000270.
29. Brown C, Matthews KA, Bromberger JT, Chang Y. The relation between perceived unfair treatment and blood pressure in a racially/ethnically diverse sample of women. Am J Epidemiol. 2006;164(3):257–62. https://doi.org/10.1093/aje/kwj196.
30. Gabriel AC, Bell CN, Bowie JV, Hines AL, LaVeist TA, Thorpe RJ Jr. The association between perceived racial discrimination and hypertension in a low-income, racially integrated urban community. Fam Community Health. 2020;43(2):93–9. https://doi.org/10.1097/fch.0000000000000254.
31. Maraboto C, Ferdinand KC. Update on hypertension in African-Americans. Prog Cardiovasc Dis. 2020;63(1):33–9. https://doi.org/10.1016/j.pcad.2019.12.002.
32. Taylor HA Jr. Establishing a foundation for cardiovascular disease research in an African-American community—the Jackson Heart Study. Ethn Dis. 2003;13(4):411–3.
33. Okhomina VI, Seals SR, Anugu P, Adu-Boateng G, Sims M, Marshall GD Jr. Adherence and retention of African Americans in a randomized controlled trial with a yoga-based intervention: the effects of health promoting programs on cardiovascular disease risk study. Ethn Health. 2018;25:1–13. https://doi.org/10.1080/13557858.2018.1458073.
34. Johnson CC, Taylor AG, Anderson JG, Jones RA, Whaley DE. Feasibility and acceptability of an

internet-based, African dance-modified yoga program for African-American women with or at risk for metabolic syndrome. J Yoga Phys Ther. 2014;4:174. https://doi.org/10.4172/2157-7595.1000174.

35. Palta P, Page G, Piferi RL, Gill JM, Hayat MJ, Connolly AB, Szanton SL. Evaluation of a mindfulness-based intervention program to decrease blood pressure in low-income African-American older adults. J Urban Health. 2012;89(2):308–16. https://doi.org/10.1007/s11524-011-9654-6.
36. Moreno-Castro C, Lopera-Pareja EH. Comparative study of the frequency of use of natural therapies among the Spanish population and their public image on digital media. In: Paper presented at the 14th international conference on public communication of science and technology (PCST). Estambul; 2016. Retrieved from https://pcst.co/archive/paper/2623
37. Flores A, Lopez M, Krogstad J. US Hispanic population reached new high in 2018, but growth has slowed. Pew Research Center; 2019. Retrieved 22 July 2019.
38. Friedman JD. The future of yoga is in Spanish. Yoga J. 2017. Updated: Apr 5, 2017. https://www.yogajournal.com/lifestyle/future-yoga-spanish. Accessed 5-1-20.
39. Park J, Newman D, McCaffrey R, Garrido JJ, Riccio ML, Liehr P. The effect of chair yoga on biopsychosocial changes in English- and Spanish-speaking community-dwelling older adults with lower-extremity osteoarthritis. J Gerontol Soc Work. 2016;59(7–8):604–26. https://doi.org/10.1080/01634372.2016.1239234.
40. Shah AJ, Ostfeld RJ. Attitudes of inner city patients with cardiovascular disease towards meditation. J Integr Cardiol. 2016;2(2) https://doi.org/10.15761/jic.1000152.
41. Parker EA, McArdle PF, Gioia D, Trilling A, Bahr-Robertson M, Costa N, et al. An onsite fitness facility and integrative wellness program positively impacted health-related outcomes among teachers and staff at an urban elementary/middle school. Glob Adv Health Med. 2019;8:2164956119873276. https://doi.org/10.1177/2164956119873276.
42. Sarkissian M, Trent NL, Huchting K, Singh Khalsa SB. Effects of a kundalini yoga program on elementary and middle school students' stress, affect, and resilience. J Dev Behav Pediatr. 2018;39(3):210–6. https://doi.org/10.1097/dbp.0000000000000538.
43. Hernandez R, Daviglus ML, Martinez L, Durazo-Arvizu RA, Huffman JC, Ramirez F, et al. "iAlegrate!"—a culturally adapted positive psychological intervention for Hispanics/Latinos with hypertension: rationale, design, and methods. Contemp Clin Trials Commun. 2019;14:100348. https://doi.org/10.1016/j.conctc.2019.100348.
44. Clark LT, Watkins L, Pina IL, Elmer M, Akinboboye O, Gorham M, et al. Increasing diversity in clinical trials: overcoming critical barriers. Curr Probl Cardiol. 2019;44(5):148–72. https://doi.org/10.1016/j.cpcardiol.2018.11.002.
45. Spadola CE, Rottapel R, Khandpur N, Kontos E, Bertisch SM, Johnson DA, et al. Enhancing yoga participation: a qualitative investigation of barriers and facilitators to yoga among predominantly racial/ethnic minority, low-income adults. Complement Ther Clin Pract. 2017;29:97–104. https://doi.org/10.1016/j.ctcp.2017.09.001.
46. Chen KW, Berger CC, Manheimer E, Forde D, Magidson J, Dachman L, Lejuez CW. Meditative therapies for reducing anxiety: a systematic review and meta-analysis of randomized controlled trials. Depress Anxiety. 2012;29(7):545–62. https://doi.org/10.1002/da.21964.
47. Cramer H, Lauche R, Langhorst J, Dobos G. Yoga for depression: a systematic review and meta-analysis. Depress Anxiety. 2013;30(11):1068–83. https://doi.org/10.1002/da.22166.
48. da Silva TL, Ravindran LN, Ravindran AV. Yoga in the treatment of mood and anxiety disorders: a review. Asian J Psychiatr. 2009;2(1):6–16. https://doi.org/10.1016/j.ajp.2008.12.002.
49. Chu P, Gotink RA, Yeh GY, Goldie SJ, Hunink MG. The effectiveness of yoga in modifying risk factors for cardiovascular disease and metabolic syndrome: a systematic review and meta-analysis of randomized controlled trials. Eur J Prev Cardiol. 2016;23(3):291–307. https://doi.org/10.1177/2047487314562741.
50. Ziv A, Vogel O, Keret D, Pintov S, Bodenstein E, Wolkomir K, et al. Comprehensive Approach to Lower Blood Pressure (CALM-BP): a randomized controlled trial of a multifactorial lifestyle intervention. J Hum Hypertens. 2013;27(10):594–600. https://doi.org/10.1038/jhh.2013.29.
51. Brown RP, Gerbarg PL. Sudarshan Kriya yogic breathing in the treatment of stress, anxiety, and depression: part I-neurophysiologic model. J Altern Complement Med. 2005;11(1):189–201. https://doi.org/10.1089/acm.2005.11.189.
52. Kjellgren A, Bood SA, Axelsson K, Norlander T, Saatcioglu F. Wellness through a comprehensive yogic breathing program—a controlled pilot trial. BMC Complement Altern Med. 2007;7:43. https://doi.org/10.1186/1472-6882-7-43.
53. Qu S, Olafsrud SM, Meza-Zepeda LA, Saatcioglu F. Rapid gene expression changes in peripheral blood lymphocytes upon practice of a comprehensive yoga program. PLoS One. 2013;8(4):e61910. https://doi.org/10.1371/journal.pone.0061910.
54. Diamantidis CJ, Davenport CA, Lunyera J, Bhavsar N, Scialla J, Hall R, et al. Low use of routine medical care among African Americans with high CKD risk: the Jackson Heart Study. BMC Nephrol. 2019;20(1):11. https://doi.org/10.1186/s12882-018-1190-0.
55. Lor M, Koleck TA, Bakken S, Yoon S, Dunn Navarra AM. Association between health literacy and medication adherence among Hispanics with hypertension. J Racial Ethn Health Disparities. 2019;6(3):517–24. https://doi.org/10.1007/s40615-018-00550-z.
56. Nahin RL, Barnes PM, Stussman BJ, Bloom B. Costs of complementary and alternative medi-

cine (CAM) and frequency of visits to CAM practitioners: United States, 2007. Natl Health Stat Rep. 2009;30(18):1–14.
57. Snyderman R, Weil AT. Integrative medicine: bringing medicine back to its roots. Arch Intern Med. 2002;162(4):395–97. Retrieved from http://archinte.jamanetwork.com/article.aspx?articleid=211225; http://archinte.jamanetwork.com/data/Journals/InteMed/5313/isa10029.pdf
58. Jackson JE. The cross-cultural evidence on "extreme behaviors": what can it tell us? Ann N Y Acad Sci. 2009;1172:270–7. https://doi.org/10.1111/j.1749-6632.2009.04536.x.
59. Loizzo J, Charlson M, Peterson J. A program in contemplative self-healing: stress, allostasis, and learning in the Indo-Tibetan tradition. Ann N Y Acad Sci. 2009;1172:123–47. https://doi.org/10.1111/j.1749-6632.2009.04398.x.

Yoga in the Management of Arterial Hypertension

23

Laura Tolbaños-Roche, Praseeda Menon, and Subodh Tiwari

23.1 Epidemiology of Hypertension

Hypertension occurs when blood pressure (BP) is high as measured on two different days. Blood pressure or BP, the force exerted by circulating blood against the walls of the body's arteries, is reflected in two parameters: systolic, the pressure in the arteries when the heart contracts or beats, and diastolic, the pressure in the arteries when the heart rests between beats. Hypertension is diagnosed when systolic blood pressure (SBP) $\geq$ 140 mmHg and/or diastolic blood pressure (DBP) $\geq$ 90 mmHg.

According to the World Health Organization [1], arterial hypertension affects 40% of adults aged 25 and above, worldwide. A pooled analysis of 1479 population-based measurement studies from 200 countries revealed that the number of people with hypertension doubled from 594 million in 1975 to 1.13 billion in 2015 worldwide with the increase largely in low- and middle-income countries [2]. A recent review by Mills et al. [3] confirmed that the prevalence of hypertension among adults was higher in low- and middle-income countries (31.5%, 1.04 billion people) than in high-income countries (28.5%, 349 million people). However, fewer than 1 in 5 people with hypertension have the problem under control [4]. Complications of hypertension accounted for 9.4 million global deaths every year [1]. In fact, hypertension is behind 45% of deaths due to heart disease and 51% of deaths due to stroke [1]. However, its prevalence is difficult to estimate since most hypertensive people don't perceive any symptoms at all, which is why it is called a "silent killer." Hypertension is a serious public health problem not only due to its high prevalence, but also because it is the most important risk factor for cardiovascular diseases (CVDs; [1]), which is the number one cause of death globally [5].

When arterial hypertension is not well controlled, it can cause very serious pathologies such as myocardial infarction, ventricular hypertrophy, and heart failure. High BP can also cause aneurysms, increasing the possibility of blockage and rupture of the blood vessels and the risk of suffering a stroke. Arterial hypertension can also lead to renal failure, blindness, and cognitive impair-

L. Tolbaños-Roche (✉)
Faculty of Health Sciences, Section of Psychology, Department of Clinical Psychology, Psychobiology and Methodology, Universidad de La Laguna, San Cristóbal de La Laguna, Santa Cruz de Tenerife, Spain

P. Menon
Scientific Research Department, Kaivalyadhama Yoga Institute, Swami Kuvalayananda Marg, Lonavala, Maharashtra, India

S. Tiwari
S. A. D. T. Gupta Yogic Hospital and Health Care Centre, Kaivalyadhama Yoga Institute, Swami Kuvalayananda Marg, Lonavala, Maharashtra, India
e-mail: subodh@kdham.com

I. Basu-Ray, D. Mehta (eds.), *The Principles and Practice of Yoga in Cardiovascular Medicine*,
https://doi.org/10.1007/978-981-16-6913-2_23

ment. In many cases, arterial hypertension converges with other risk factors such as smoking, obesity, hypercholesterolemia, or diabetes mellitus, complicating health consequences, and augmenting the likelihood of suffering from all the mentioned pathologies. Since arterial hypertension is an asymptomatic disorder, early detection, treatment, and self-care are essential to reduce the risk of suffering from all these disorders.

The WHO [1] classified the risk factors of suffering arterial hypertension into behavioral, metabolic, socioeconomic, and other factors. Behavioral factors comprise consumption of food containing too much salt and fat, lack of enough fruits and vegetables in the diet, alcohol consumption, smoking, sedentary lifestyle, and poor stress management. Metabolic factors are obesity, cholesterol, and diabetes mellitus. Regarding socioeconomic factors, arterial hypertension is related to income, education, and housing; these factors have an impact on behavioral risk factors and can also delay early detection and treatment. Genetic factors and age can also play a role in the development of hypertension. Finally, other risk factors of hypertension are preeclampsia (hypertension during pregnancy) and "white coat syndrome" (anxiety experienced during visit to a clinic). The growth in the world's population, aging, and risk factors related to lifestyle, such as unhealthy diet, harmful and abusive use of alcohol, sedentary lifestyle, overweight, and stress are the main causes of the significant increase of hypertensive cases in recent years [1].

Complications of hypertension, including heart attack, stroke, and kidney failure lead to high spending for households on hospitalization and healthcare, driving millions into poverty [6]. According to the report on Global Economic Burden of Non-communicable Diseases [7], prepared by the World Economic Forum and the Harvard School of Public Health, over the period 2011–2025, the annual loss due to major noncommunicable diseases for low- and middle-income countries is projected to be approximately US$500 billion and amounts to approximately 4% of their gross domestic product. CVDs including hypertension account for 51% of this annual loss [1].

23.2 Pathophysiology of Hypertension

Arterial hypertension is classified as essential (primary) or secondary. Between 90 and 95% of cases are essential hypertension in which there is no identifiable cause [8], while secondary hypertension represents only 5–10% of cases and it is due to known organic factors such as chronic kidney disease, renal artery stenosis, excessive aldosterone secretion, pheochromocytoma, and sleep apnea [9].

In the pathophysiological mechanism of hypertension, kidney, sodium-water balance, and the state of vasoconstriction of the arteries play an important role. The pathogenesis is multifactorial and not yet sufficiently clear. However, the influence of genetics and the over-activation of the sympathetic nervous and renin-angiotensin-aldosterone systems are generally accepted.

Mental and psychosocial stress is one of the major risk factors of hypertension. The reactivity of the cardiovascular system to psychological stress has been extensively associated with the development of arterial hypertension. Carroll et al. [10], in a 5-year longitudinal study with a sample of 453 Dutch participants, found a significant relationship between systolic reactivity to stressful tasks and the establishment of arterial hypertension disorder. The study of Phillips [11] also confirms the relationship between high cardiovascular stress reactivity and the development of arterial hypertension, systemic atherosclerosis, and cardiovascular disease markers, together with contribution from the interaction of genetic and environmental factors.

Gawlik et al. [12] carried out an online cross-sectional survey on 59,798 adult participants, who completed a Million Hearts community cardiovascular screening between 2013 and 2018, in order to estimate the effects of stress on hypertension and high cholesterol (parameters of cardiovascular health). The authors reported that higher stress was associated with higher prevalence of pre-hypertension/hypertension and elevated total cholesterol among all race/ethnic groups as well as all age groups. The estimation of the effect of stress on cardiovascular health, adjusting for other relevant confounders (age, sex, race/ethnicity, smoking status, BMI, total cholesterol—for the model on pre-hypertension/hypertension, and blood pressure—for the model on elevated cholesterol), showed that compared to those with low stress, high stress was associated with significant higher odds of having pre-hypertension/hypertension and elevated cholesterol.

The stress response implies an activation of the Sympathetic Nervous System (SNS) with the corresponding secretion of adrenaline and norepinephrine. This neuroendocrine response accelerates the heart rate (HR) in order to supply more blood to the muscles. When the cardiovascular stress response is maintained over time, the cardiovascular system deteriorates substantially. The maintenance of high BP leads to the development of arterial hypertension, and subsequently, this deterioration may result in different cardiovascular pathologies such as atherosclerosis, ischemic heart disease, heart attack, and cerebrovascular accidents. Another hypothesis in the pathology of essential hypertension is rooted in the concept of allostasis, referring to the ability of our body in maintaining stability when facing stressful challenges through bodily change, adapting, and achieving a dynamic balance [13]. The persistence of high BP causes gradual adaptation in terms of arterial smooth muscle cells, thereby hypertrophy, thickening of the carotid sinus wall, and increase in the production rate of hormones related to BP, viz., renin, norepinephrine, cortisol, etc. [14].

The Polyvagal Theory [15] represents an interesting explanation about the role of the physiological activation process in the development of cardiovascular diseases. This theory exposed a complex and integrative vision of the Autonomic Nervous System (ANS) beyond the intervention of only the SNS in physiological activation. This theory proposes the Parasympathetic Nervous System (PNS) as a modulator of stress vulnerability and reactivity. According to this theory, the ANS consists of three hierarchically organized subsystems that support three different behavioral and emotional adaptation strategies as given below.

1. The dorsal branch of the vagus nerve (myelinated), called the "social engagement system" [16], regulates areas of the body related to social communication (facial expression, vocalization, listening, etc.). This system is the most recent and sophisticated, in evolutionary terms.
2. The sympathetic-adrenal system is related to mobilization behaviors and physiological activation (fight and flight behavior). This system is more primitive and less flexible than the dorsal branch of the vagus nerve.
3. The ventral branch of the vagus nerve is the most primitive neuronal circuit. This branch is activated because of hypoxia and enables immobilization related to survival (feigning death, vaso-vagal syncope, and behavioral shutdown).

First, the newest circuits come into play, and when these are insufficient, the older ones intervene. The myelinated vagus acts as a heart level inhibitor of the SNS, functioning as an active vagal brake and contributing to the modulation of cardiac output. This vagal brake provides a neural mechanism to rapidly change the visceral state, increasing or decreasing the HR, and thereby supporting either the metabolic needs of mobilization, communication behaviors or behaviors leading to the development of a calm state. Under stress conditions the SNS is activated and the social engagement system is inhibited. Therefore, the myelinated vagus becomes less active, and vagal tone decreases. In a situation of chronic stress, when the vagal brake does not work properly, the sympathetic-adrenal system, phylogenetically older than the myelinated vagus, would regulate the metabolic response facing the environmental challenges. Therefore, the cardiovascular system would be more exposed to the SNS activation with corresponding elevation of BP [15, 17].

23.3 Mechanisms of Yoga in Hypertension Management

23.3.1 Psycho-physiological Mechanisms

Yoga focuses on the attainment and maintenance of psycho-physiological balance, making available to the practitioner a set of techniques for coping with stress, reducing psycho-physiological activation, and facilitating mental calmness as a naturally positive state of mind. Besides that, yoga offers a holistic approach, which takes into consideration all the constitutive aspects of an integral health regimen, including aspects of healthy lifestyle, viz., a healthy diet, physical activity, invigorating breathing, a healthy thought process, the practice of conscious awareness in every daily activity, being surrounded by a healthy and natural environment, etc. In addition, yoga promotes a general attitude of respect, commitment, and personal responsibility in the care and maintenance of one's health.

The beneficial action of yoga practice in the prevention and management of arterial hypertension could be based on two main pathways: (1) Health behaviors: yoga practice is itself a physical activity and is based on maintaining healthy habits and lifestyle; and (2) Stress management: yoga involves a set of techniques to prevent and cope with stress.

Firstly, the practice of regular physical activity is generally associated with the reduction of BP. The protective effect of physical activity on the risk of developing hypertension was demonstrated in a prospectively-conducted study in Finland with a very large sample (8302 men and 9139 women) aged 25 to 64, during a mean follow-up of 11 years [18]. The practice of yoga too can be considered a healthy form of physical activity; however, the scope of yoga goes beyond the health benefits of a physical or sports training program. The practice of aerobic exercise has been compared with conscious activities, such as yoga and Feldenkrais Method, where the latter were more effective in reducing anxiety and increasing positive mood [19]. Besides that, the practice of yoga supports a holistic approach toward life and is associated with adopting and maintaining a healthy lifestyle. This was demonstrated in a study by Satish and Kumar [20] on the relationship between lifestyle and yoga practice with a sample of 870 young Indian people from Chennai (India), of which 368 were yoga practitioners for at least 6 months and 502 were non-practitioners. The researchers found that yoga practitioners scored higher on protective health factors and showed more control over risk behaviors than non-practitioners. Yoga practitioners also reported greater physical and psychological well-being. Likewise, the findings of the study by Butzer et al. [21], wherein the effect of yoga on prevention of adolescent substance use risk factors in a middle school setting was evaluated, suggested that school-based yoga can prevent willingness to smoke cigarettes in both males and females as well as improve emotional self-control in females.

There is further evidence about yoga leading to healthy behavior. Speroni et al. [22] carried out an intervention program based on yoga practice, healthy habits, and nutrition education to reduce extra weight and promote a healthier lifestyle with a total of 217 nurses, self-selected to the intervention ($n = 108$) or control (no intervention; $n = 109$) groups. The intervention group experienced significant decreases in Body Mass Index and waist circumference measurement and also stated an increase in their level of physical activity as well as an improvement in eating habits after the program. Watts et al. [23] used data collected as part of wave 4 of Project EAT (Eating and Activity in Teens and Young Adults), a population-based cohort study in Minnesota (USA). A sample of 1820 young adults completed the Project EAT survey and a food frequency questionnaire, and a subset, who reported practicing yoga additionally, participated in semi-structured interviews ($n = 46$). Young adult yoga practitioners reported healthier eating behaviors and higher levels of physical activity than non-practitioners. Yoga also supported healthy eating through motivation to eat in a healthier manner, greater mindfulness, management of emotional eating, more healthy food cravings, and the influence of the yoga community, as assessed by the interviews. Additionally, yoga supported physical activity through activity as part of yoga practice, motivation to do other forms of activity, increased capacity to be active, and by complementing an active lifestyle.

Secondly, stress leads to alterations in the regulation of the hypothalamic-pituitary-adrenal (HPA) system, which gets reflected in various psycho-neuro-endocrinological processes, such as an increase in cortisol levels and decrease in serotonergic activity [24, 25]. In addition, stress also reduces the Gamma Aminobutyric Acid (GABA) and Parasympathetic Nervous System (PNS) activity. A reduction in brain GABA levels and an increase in cortisol levels are biologic markers of stress [26]. Impairments in serotonin neurotransmission have been strongly linked to stress and depression [27, 28] and a meta-analysis revealed that serotonergic activity moderates the relationship between stress and depression [29]. There is also evidence of the relation between low levels of GABA and depression and anxiety [30]. The reduction in the PNS activity leads to decreased heart rate variability (HRV) and reduced cardiac control by the vagal brake. Reduced PNS activity also creates a higher dependence on the Sympathetic Nervous System (SNS) led excitation of the cardiovascular system among other systems, and thereby negative cardiovascular health consequences such as arterial hypertension [31]. Yoga practices serve to reduce the effects of stress through increasing the PNS and GABA activity, reducing the reactivity of the HPA system and the allostatic load, in turn, balancing the Autonomic Nervous System (ANS) [31, 32]. Streeter et al. [33] additionally demonstrated that yoga practices decreased depressive symptoms in participants with major depressive disorder.

The positive effect of yoga practice on stress management has been demonstrated in healthy population as well as in chronic disease patients. A systematic review of 1469 studies, published between 2104 and 2018, selected from the databases of PubMed and Scopus, investigated the effect of different types of yoga (e.g., Hatha Yoga, Bikram Yoga, Kundalini Yoga, Sudarshan Kriya Yoga, Kripalu Yoga, Yin Yoga) on stress in healthy population. After a step-by-step thorough filtration process, only 12 studies were finally included in the review, which, in turn, revealed that most types of yoga reduced stress in healthy population [34]. Likewise, a rigorous systematic review and meta-analysis examined the benefits of yoga interventions on psychological distress among people living with HIV/AIDS (PLWHA). Seven studies sampling 396 PLWHA met inclusion criteria. The review showed that PLWHA who followed yoga interventions reported significant improvements in perceived stress, positive affect, and anxiety compared to controls [35].

Innes et al. [36] hypothesized primarily two mechanistic pathways underlying the beneficial effects of yoga interventions on cardiovascular risk profiles after conducting a systematic review of yoga therapy publications on CVD risk indices including hypertension. According to the authors, in the action of the first pathway, yoga may alleviate the effects of stress and foster multiple positive downstream effects on neuroendocrine status, metabolic function, and related inflammatory responses by reducing the activation and reactivity of the sympatho-adrenal system and the HPA axis, and promoting feelings of well-being. In the action of the second pathway, yoga may enhance parasympathetic output by directly stimulating the vagus nerve, and thereby shift the autonomic nervous system balance from primarily sympathetic to parasympathetic, leading to positive changes in cardiac-vagal function, in mood and energy state, and in related neuroendocrine, metabolic, and inflammatory responses.

23.3.2 Psychological and Neurocognitive Mechanisms

Perception is personal and subjective. During perception, reality is filtered and determined by "top-down" processing [37], or what Siegel [38] calls the "construction" function, as opposed to a "bottom-up" or "conduction" function of the mind. According to Siegel [38], "top-down" processing refers to how we have experienced things in the past and created mental models and schemas of those experiences. Therefore, our perceptions are shaped by top-down learning from prior experience. However, in the "bottom-up" processing, the sensory experience is conducted as an energy flow. The senses capture the energy of the body and the outside world and send the information to the brain. Although the senses have limitations, the conduction process provides information closest to the objective and actual reality. In this way, we can experience the subjective sense of energy flow before it is transformed into structured information, living in the "here and now," seeing and perceiving with beginner's eyes and mind.

Once the sensation reaches the brain, the "construction" or "top-down" processing comes into play, resulting in perception, awareness of what is being perceived and, subsequently, construction and narration of the experience. This process connects the perceived information with some previous experiences, "labeling" them and creating models that fit those past experiences and transforms the energy of the primary and original perception (the more objective one) to a secondary one, one that is more subjective and processed. The reinterpretations of experiences shape the "own stories" of living reality, which are stored in memory and, in turn, determine new experiences and provide new sources of distortion of perceived reality, which in a kind of vicious circle, reinforces and perpetuates internal dissonance and imbalance. According to the yogic and meditative philosophies this state of dissonance is called *dvandva* (in Sanskrit) or *klesa* (in Pali) and in modern science is understood as stress [39].

In general, the "construction" or "top-down" processing predominates in the human being. In fact, the brain circuit associated with this process has been called the "default mode network" because of activation without performing any specific task [40]. Therefore, promoting the development of the "conduction" function and achieving a balance between both functions could be fundamental in personal integration and that with the outside world, as well as in establishing and maintaining well-being [38].

Yoga and meditative practices propose coming fully into contact with the sensation, the experience derived from the pure experience of what is actually being felt and perceived, and feeling and perceiving without interpretations or explanations, without categorizations or evaluations, or in other words, without any conceptualization. In neurofunctional terms, this means to reinforce the "conduction" manner of processing of the mind. This process of awareness of actual experience would facilitate a more objective knowledge of the reality and a harmonious and balanced integration of the internal experience, in all corporeal, cognitive, and relational (with others and the environment) aspects.

Through observation and development of awareness, yoga practices, including meditation, provide a greater understanding of the nature of internal thoughts and representations, and enable one to detect physical, mental, and emotional habits. Continued yoga practice and the development of awareness of the present moment help to avoid or minimize judgments and assessments, thereby approaching the true nature of experience. When the experience is observed in an objective way, one realizes that everything is in a continuous process of change, and sensations, emotions, and thoughts are continuously transforming. The understanding of this impermanent nature of everything (within and outside oneself) allows oneself to overcome identification with what is happening, reduces reactivity, and improves acceptance. As a consequence, a state of internal equilibrium can be achieved, feeling more independent of changing external circumstances and potential internal fluctuations, and when these happen, being more able to understand and accept them.

Specifically, yoga practices involve a process of integration of perceptions, feelings and thoughts, leading to restoration of the psychophysiological balance. The capacity for integration has been proposed as the central mechanism that underlies adaptive regulation and health [41, 42]. Starting from a visceral, sensorial, and motor awareness, through an embodiment process, yoga practices act on emotional and cognitive levels in a "bottom-up" process. Likewise, awareness of the body and its related processes would act from the cognitive to the emotional and physiological levels in a "top-down" awareness pathway, facilitating not only the control of certain autonomic processes, but also the integration of physiological, emotional, and cognitive levels of experience and its interaction with the environment.

Furthermore, neuroplasticity is the inherent ability of the central nervous system (CNS) to adapt and reorganize its structure and function in response to internal and/or external stimuli. The high-level of plasticity of the CNS suggests that it is modifiable by any sort of training or intervention, and this neuroplastic ability can be leveraged in a clinical sample as well [43]. In this regard, yoga interventions have shown a positive impact, improving systemic biomarkers of neuroplasticity in healthy [44] and stressed individuals [45], as well as in major depressive disorder [43]. Although no study has as yet been undertaken on the role of yoga and neuroplasticity in essential arterial hypertension, taking a cue from the Tolahunase et al. [43] study on a clinical sample, it may be possible to hypothesize that yoga interventions carry the potential to capitalize on brain plasticity in hypertension as well.

23.4 Types of Yoga Studied

The modality, dosage, and duration of the yoga interventions in the study of the effect of yoga on management of arterial hypertension vary widely. The variety of the types of yoga used in the interventions has been a difficulty to compare the studies in most of the rigorous reviews. Although interventions based on different types of yoga have demonstrated their effectiveness, a combination of methods such as *asana, pranayama*, and relaxation practices (mainly *Shavasana*) has been proven to be more efficacious [46].

Despite the diversity in the type of yoga used in the interventions, in a systematic review conducted subsequently, the same authors reported that, among all the reviewed studies mentioning different types of yoga (*Hatha Yoga*, yoga with supervised exercise, unspecified yoga, yoga consisting of *asana* and *pranayama*), the emphasis on mind-body therapies reinforcing meditative states and breathing-focused techniques (in addition to other mind-body practices) was similar throughout [47].

In a comprehensive bibliometric analysis of publications about yoga therapy research inclinical populations, Jeter, Slutsky, Singh, and Khalsa [48] pointed out the need for standardized yoga protocols in randomized controlled trials to determine efficacy/effectiveness. This expressed need may conflict with the clinical practice of yoga, wherein yoga as a form of therapy needs to be tailored to individual needs, specific symptoms and severity of disease.

There exist limited studies comparing the effectiveness of different types of yoga on management of hypertension. In a three-armed randomized controlled trial (RCT) comparing the BP-lowering effect of yoga interventions with and without yoga postures in patients with arterial hypertension, Cramer et al. [49] found that a yoga intervention even without postures (comprising breathing, meditation, relaxation techniques, and some educational-interactive activities) was successful in lowering the ambulatory systolic blood pressure (short-term) significantly better than the controlled condition as well as the condition of yoga intervention with postures. The authors concluded that their obtained results were in accordance with the findings of earlier studies, that yoga is safe and effective in patients taking medications for arterial hypertension, and therefore, can be recommended as an additional treatment in this condition.

Tolbaños-Roche et al. [50] analyzed the differential effectiveness of three yoga interventions, specifically designed for essential arterial hypertension treatment: (1) "Yoga Practice" which included *asana*, *pranayama,* and relaxation, (2) only "*Pranayama*" and, (3) only "Meditation." Although a clinically significant decrease in BP was found in all the yoga interventions, the results showed a differential effect of improvement in self-regulation and emotional symptomatology, as well as a decrease in physiological parameters related to essential hypertension, specifically in the "Meditation" intervention.

Pranayama practices used in the management of hypertension have also demonstrated a significant decrease of SBP and DBP parameters, as well as an enhancement of HRV [51–55]. Meditation interventions (transcendental meditation and mindfulness techniques) have shown more effectiveness in decreasing BP in patients above 60 years, whereas yoga (mainly focused on postural and breathing practices but also including meditative physical relaxation) contributed to the decrease in BP of patients aged less than 60 years [56].

23.5 Evidence About the Efficacy of Yoga in Hypertension Management

23.5.1 Efficacy of Yoga and Allied Interventions

The practice of yoga induces a coordinated psycho-physiological response that can be considered the antithesis of the stress response. This relaxation response consists of a reduction in cognitive and somatic excitation that involves a modification in the activity of the HPA axis and of the ANS [57], with reduction in SNS activity and a corresponding improvement in PNS activity, resulting in decreased systolic blood pressure (SBP), diastolic blood pressure (DBP), heart rate (HR), and increased heart rate variability (HRV) [58, 59]. Furthermore, a reduction in cardiovascular reactivity to stress induced by physical activity, with better recovery in the cardiovascular parameters of SBP, DBP, and HR was found after a 2-month yoga training program [60].

The effect of yoga interventions in reduction of BP in hypertension patients has also been widely confirmed [60–64]. Patel [65] also demonstrated the efficacy of yoga practice in hypertensive patients, with significant decreases in BP, and reduced intake of antihypertensive medication. Compared to treatment with antihypertensive drugs, the greater efficacy of yoga therapy in the reduction of SBP and HR opens the doors for considering yoga therapy as a substitute for pharmacological therapy (see [66]). Likewise, a 21-day naturopathy and yoga intervention program in hypertensive patients taking antihypertensive medication significantly lowered SBP and DBP, improved blood lipid profile, and reduced body weight. After withdrawing medication in the most favorable cases, who reached normal BP values, approximately 26% of them maintained BP within these normal limits even after 1 year without medication [67]. In a review of studies conducted (1972–2012) on the efficacy of yoga in arterial hypertension, with a total of 19 studies analyzed, 12 of them reported significant decreases in the BP of the participants [46]. Another study by Metri et al. [68] carried out a 1-week residential yoga-based lifestyle program (Integrated Approach of Yoga Therapy, IAYT), with 20 hypertensive patients in India, which consisted of sessions of *asana*, breathing practices, meditation and relaxation techniques, low salt, low-calorie diet, devotional session, and counselling. A significant improvement in SBP, baroreflex sensitivity and total peripheral vascular resistance was found in the study group after the intervention compared to the control group. This study revealed the relevance of the holistic approach of yoga in the management of hypertension.

A recent systematic review and meta-analysis of RCTs assessed the efficacy and safety of yoga by comparing it with usual care or nonpharmacological interventions in secondary prevention of CVD. Results from 7 finally shortlisted RCTs comprising 4671 participants revealed that although no mortality benefits of yoga in CVD patients were observed, it could be a promising alternative for CVD patients as it significantly improved health-related quality of life, BP, BMI, triglycerides, and high-density lipoprotein cholesterol (HDL) without causing severe adverse events, and was associated with a lesser number of composite cardiovascular events [69].

In the Park and Han [56] systematic review (mentioned earlier), which included 510 indexed publications (1946–2014) on the effect of mindfulness meditation and yoga on hypertensive patients, only 13 studies qualified the rigorous selection criteria when the Cochrane risk-of-bias tool was applied to assess the validity of the studies. The meta-analysis indicated that the practice of meditation and yoga significantly decreased SBP and DBP in patients with similar baseline BP ranges. However, they found different results depending on the baseline range of BP and age of participants; the practice of meditation was more effective in decreasing BP in patients above 60 years, while the practice of yoga was more effective in patients below 60 years. Despite these differences, the authors concluded that both practices proved to be effective alternatives to pharmacotherapy. Further, the practice of yoga can also reduce the impact of age on cardiovascular function. Significantly lower BP and HR were found in yoga practitioners over 40 years with 5 years of experience in yoga, compared to a control group [70].

In yet another systematic review (mentioned earlier) by Innes et al. [36], 70 eligible original studies (1970–2004; including 22 RCTs, 21 non-randomized controlled clinical trials, 26 uncontrolled clinical trials, and 1 observational study) evaluating the effects of yoga on CVD or CVD risk indices associated with insulin resistance syndrome (IRS) were identified. Despite methodological and other limitations, these authors reported that the results of these reviewed studies indicated beneficial changes overall in several IRS-related indices of CVD risk, including glucose tolerance and insulin sensitivity, lipid profiles, anthropometric characteristics, BP, oxidative stress, coagulation profiles, sympathetic activation, and cardiovagal function, as well as improvement in several clinical endpoints.

23.5.2 Efficacy of Pranayama-Specific Interventions

Pranayama practices, which involve voluntary slow and deep yogic breathing, can significantly contribute to the management of hypertension. This was confirmed by a systematic review and meta-analysis, which investigated the efficacy of yoga as an antihypertensive lifestyle therapy and included 49 qualifying controlled trials. In this study, Wu et al. [71] compared interventions which included yogic breathing techniques and meditation/mental relaxation with those that did not, and demonstrated that yoga is a viable antihypertensive lifestyle therapy that produces the greatest BP benefits when yogic breathing techniques are included together with meditation/mental relaxation.

Pranayama practices have also shown a balancing effect on the ANS activity. The practice of various *pranayama* practices increases HRV [72] and decreases BP [73]. Some research has focused on analyzing the effects of yogic breathing techniques based on the use of a single nostril (*surya pranayama*—breathing through the right nostril; *chandra pranayama*—breathing through the left nostril), as well as both nostrils alternatively (*anuloma-viloma pranayama*). The function of naturally occurring nasal respiratory cycles had been analyzed in *Shivasvarodaya*, the ancient Indian text which deals with the relation between a person's mental state and the accompanying breath [74]. The left *swara* (the flow of air as well as *prana*, the subtle aspect of breath) through the left nostril presides over mental actions (*soumya karya*—quieter activities; [51]), the right *swara* through the right nostril presides over physical actions (*roudra karya*—exertional activities; [52]), and both *swara* through both nostrils together preside over spiritual actions (meditative activities) [75]. *Shivasvarodaya* states that the *swara* changes at regular intervals in a person, and advises correct action for the appropriate *swara* [75].

In healthy subjects, right nostril breathing increases SBP and DBP, while left and alternate nostril breathing decreases BP. There is also a greater increase in HR when breathing through the right nostril than with the other two practices. The effects of right nostril breathing may be due to sympathetic activity increasing, while the BP and HR decreasing in left and alternate nostril breathing may be due to a combination of effects, such as changes in cardiac output and peripheral vascular resistance [54]. In essential arterial hypertension patients, a statistically significant decrease of SBP and HR and a slight decrease of DBP (statistically non-significant) with left nostril breathing were found [51]. The authors attribute the statistically significant results to the normalization of autonomic cardiovascular rhythms, with an increase of vagal modulation and/or a decrease of sympathetic activity. The authors reasoned that the non-significant change in the DBP may have been because the DBP was maintained within normal values by the medication, rendering little possibility for a significant change after performing these *Pranayama* practices. In another study with essential arterial hypertension patients, Bhavanani et al. [52] found a non-significant decrease in SBP and HR after right nostril breathing, attributing this small improvement to the role of yogic practices in restoration of homeostasis. In healthy subjects, right nostril breathing increases BP and HR; however, as sympathetic reactivity is already higher than normal in hypertensive patients, right nostril breathing would contribute to bringing the cardiovascular parameters to normal, in a kind of homeostatic or balancing effect.

Recent studies have demonstrated the effect of specific *Pranayama* practices such as *Shitali Pranayama* (yogic breathing with the tongue curled up like a bird's beak) as a solitary intervention on cardiovascular and autonomic changes in hypertension with a significant reduction in blood pressure as well as an improvement in HRV [55]. Similarly, a single short session of *Bhramari Pranayama* (yogic breathing with the sound of a bumble-bee) significantly augmented the parasympathetic tone as indicated by a significant improvement in HRV parameters, with a significant increase in the HF (high frequency) power and decrease in the LF (low frequency) power values immediately after the practice [53]. This practice, however, did not demonstrate a significant reduction in BP.

23.5.3 Efficacy of Yoga in Other Psycho-physiological Parameters Associated with Hypertension

Some studies have focused on the effect of yoga on the psychological parameters associated with hypertension along with the BP parameters [50, 76]. These authors found an increase in interoceptive awareness and improvements in emotional symptomatology related to hypertension, such as anxiety and depression symptoms, distress, and perceived stress, as well as perception of happiness and satisfaction with life along with statistical or clinical improvements in SBP, DBP, and HR in a group of Spanish hypertensive patients, who followed a yoga intervention, compared with a control group.

Carlson et al. [77] demonstrated that mindfulness-based interventions have other positive physiological effects, viz., improvements in immune function and cortisol levels, along with a reduction in BP. Positive emotional changes such as reduction in the degree of stress [78] and improvement in anxiety and depression symptoms [79] have also been found. A brief mindfulness training session was also shown to be effective, with reductions in BP, fatigue and anxiety symptoms, and improvement in visuospatial processing and memory in the participants compared to a control group, who listened to a book recording [80].

23.5.4 Feasibility of Yoga as an Adjuvant Therapy in Hypertension Management

It is important to note that, although BP is usually well controlled by antihypertensive drugs, some studies have questioned the risks and damages that pharmacotherapy can cause in patients with mild hypertension. A Cochrane systematic review [81] based on four randomized controlled trials revealed that the total mortality of 8912 hypertensive patients, who were treated with antihypertensive drugs for 4–5 years, was not lowered when compared to a control group. Also, drug treatment did not reduce the incidence of coronary heart disease, stroke, and general cardiovascular problems in 7080 participants compared to the control group. Moreover, the study reported that the withdrawal rate of patients from medication substantially increased as a consequence of adverse effects of drug therapy.

The growing interest in nonpharmacological interventions to treat blood pressure in hypertensive and pre-hypertensive patients at low cardiac risk led Chaddha et al. [82] to carry out the recent meta-analysis of RCTs which assessed the impact of device-guided and non-device-guided slow breathing on blood pressure reduction in hypertensive and pre-hypertensive patient populations. The review included 17 studies from 103 citations eligible for full-text review searching PubMed, EMBASE, CINAHL, Cochrane CENTRAL, Cochrane Database of Systematic Reviews, Web of Science, BIOSIS (Biological Abstracts) Citation Index and Alt HealthWatch. Although the included studies showed high heterogeneity, slow breathing showed reductions in SBP and DBP in this patient population. The authors concluded that it may be a reasonable first treatment for low-risk hypertensive and pre-hypertensive patients, who are reluctant to start medication.

A recent RCT by Sharma et al. [83] analyzed the feasibility of introducing the integrated approach of yoga therapy (IAYT) in a cardiac rehabilitation center in Bengaluru in southern India. This study was conducted to determine the efficacy of yoga in improving cardiac conditions and managing the cardiac risk factors in patients aged 30–65 years having acute myocardial infarction with left ventricular dysfunction. The results revealed that, compared to the standard cardiac care treatment, although the 12-week yoga intervention provided no added benefit in improving the primary outcome measure of left ventricular ejection fraction (LVEF; a powerful predictor of cardiac mortality), the yoga group was not significantly different on the LVEF parameter from the control group. The authors reasoned that significant improvement in the LVEF parameter is more likely when yoga therapy is coupled with standard medical therapy in patients with cardiac failure. Further, the cardiac patients practicing yoga demonstrated a favorable profile compared to controls in terms of reduced cardiac depression, anxiety, and improved quality of life and metabolic equivalents. Additionally, the authors reported the integration of yoga practice in a cardiac rehabilitation (CR) program to be feasible, thereby offering support to the feasibility of yoga as an adjuvant therapy in cardiovascular conditions.

Exercise is routinely prescribed to cardiac patients for its multiple benefits. Cardiac patients may typically have co-morbidities that prevent them from participating in traditional exercise. The lower metabolic demand of yoga is flexible, ranging from chair based to continuous flow, presenting an option for cardiac patients to participate in an exercise intervention with a sense of mastery, rather than difficulty [84]. The implementation of yoga practices in the management of arterial hypertension may also have cost savings, both for patients and health systems. On the one hand, direct cost savings due to reduction in the need for medication and in hospitalizations arising out of complications, and on the other hand, savings on indirect cost due to loss of productivity, can both be achieved by implementing evidence-based yoga practice modules along with adopting yoga's holistic approach to an individual and the environment [85].

23.6 Clinical Practice of Yoga in Hypertension Management

As was explained earlier, evidence about the efficacy and beneficial effects of lifestyle changes (yoga and allied practices) in the treatment of chronic diseases like hypertension either in combination with drugs and surgery or as an alternative therapy has been accumulating over the past years. This led Dr. Dean Ornish, founder and president of the Preventive Medicine Research Institute and a Clinical Professor of Medicine at the University of California (San Francisco, USA), to study the clinical application of lifestyle interventions in coronary heart disease and related conditions along with risk factors such as high levels of cholesterol, BP, and blood sugar. For the last four decades, Dr. Ornish and colleagues have been developing a lifestyle program based on wholefoods and plant-based diet, stress-management techniques including yoga and meditation, moderate exercise, and social support

[86]. The Ornish Lifestyle Medicine program [87] offers intensive cardiac rehabilitation (CR) based on the model of a structured class at different centers across the USA. The program is conducted by a multidisciplinary team which includes a nurse, exercise physiologist, stress management specialist (such as a certified meditation/yoga teacher, psychologist or clinical social worker), and a dietitian. All therapeutic decisions (e.g., medications, revascularization) are under the clinical supervision of a referring physician [88].

A systematic review from the American Heart Association (AHA) on the potential benefits of meditation on cardiovascular risk concluded that, given the low costs and low risks of this intervention, meditation may be considered as an adjunct to guideline-directed cardiovascular risk reduction [89]. However, the AHA stated that the benefits of such interventions will have to be better established as the reviewed studies on the effect of meditation on BP in the clinical context were inconclusive. The HARMONY (Hypertension Analysis of Stress Reduction Using Mindfulness Meditation and Yoga) trial also could not find benefit to patients in the initial stage of hypertension, who had followed an 8-week mindfulness-based stress reduction program, compared to wait-list controls [90]. In contrast, in the pilot study of Palta et al. [91], wherein an 8-week RCT on BP-control was conducted on female hypertensives with mindfulness-based versus social support interventions, a 11/4 mmHg decrease in SBP/DBP was observed in the mindfulness intervention group. These interventions were provided in residence for lowincome, urban, African-American predominantly hypertensive females aged 62 years or older. Multivariate regression analysis revealed significantly lower SBP (21.92 mmHg) and DBP (16.70 mmHg) in the mindfulness group compared to the social support control group.

Raghuram et al. [92] investigated the long-term effects of a yoga-based CR intervention versus a physiotherapy-based active control condition, in addition to conventional CR provided to both groups after coronary artery bypass grafting (CABG). Results demonstrated improvements in LVEF (cardiac mortality predictor), BMI, serum glucose, and lipid profile, and a decrease in perceived stress, anxiety, and depression. This RCT done with a total of 250 males, aged 35–65 years, over a period of 1 year at a CR center in Bengaluru, South India, demonstrated the importance of a long-term yoga intervention to produce a significant effect in LVEF (cf. [83]) and other hypertension-associated risk factors. The authors also concluded that the addition of yoga-based relaxation to conventional post-CABG CR can help in better management of risk factors in those with abnormal baseline values and may help in preventing recurrence.

The Advanced Centre for Yoga Therapy Education and Research (ACYTER), a collaborative venture between Jawaharlal Institute of Postgraduate Medical Education and Research (JIPMER; Puducherry, India) and Morarji Desai National Institute of Yoga (MDNIY; New Delhi, India) has been focusing primarily on the role of yoga in the prevention and management of cardiovascular disorders and diabetes mellitus since 2008. Between 2008 and 2012, more than 36,000 patients attended individual and group therapy sessions for these two conditions [93]. A study with 130 heart-failure patients recruited from the cardiology outpatient department of JIPMER, examined the effects of a 12-week yoga therapy program on BP, HR, HRV, and rate pressure product (RPP). After a total of 36 supervised yoga sessions over 12 weeks, the yoga intervention group showed a significant decrease in HR, BP, and RPP compared to a control group of heart-failure patients, who were only on the standard-of-care treatment. Also, normalized Low Frequency power (LFnu) and LF:HF ratio decreased significantly and normalized High Frequency power (HFnu) increased significantly in the yoga group compared to the control group, showing a significant improvement in the parasympathetic activity and reduction in the sympathetic activity in heart-failure patients [94].

From 2010 onwards, the Center for Yoga Therapy, Education and Research (CYTER) of Sri Balaji Vidyapeeth (SBV), a reputed private university in southern India, has been training and helping medical educators and administrators for setting up integrative health centers in their respective institutions. CYTER has also been conducting a scientifically established Yoga Therapy program offered by Dr. Ananda Balayogi Bhavanani (a certified medical doctor as well as a yoga therapist) and team. This team has been developing individualized therapeutic yoga protocols for patients with various medical conditions such as diabetes, hypertension, musculoskeletal and psychiatric disorders, and also receiving excellent feedback from the program's participants [95, 96].

Other Indian medical institutions offer integrative yoga programs for the management of chronic diseases including arterial hypertension. An observational cohort study involving pre–post-comparative analysis of patients, enrolled between April and July 2015, was carried out in a hospital in South India, which has been offering an "Integrated Naturopathy and Yoga" (INY) program. The INY program includes a highly structured 15-day routine of natural-food diet, daily yogic exercises, meditation, relaxation, and patient counselling and health education. Among the 80 patients, who underwent a 3-month follow-up, 79 (99%) achieved the recommended clinical BP target (<140/90 mmHg), 45 (56%) achieved normal BP (<120/80 mmHg), 66 (83%) achieved more than 50% reduction in the dosage of antihypertensive medication, and 8 patients (10%) showed remarkable recovery with all medications withdrawn while maintaining normal BP. In addition, the patients achieved significant reductions in body weight, BMI, percentage of body fat, blood triglycerides, and mild increase in HDL cholesterol. Additionally, in patients with diabetes as a co-morbidity, there was a significant reduction in glycosylated hemoglobin levels [85].

Recently, the International Society of Hypertension (ISH) developed worldwide practice guidelines for the management of hypertension in a practical format that is easy-to-use particularly in low, but also in high resource settings—by clinicians, but also nurses and community health workers, as appropriate. These guidelines have included yoga (under regular physical activity) and meditation/mindfulness practices (for stress reduction) as a part of lifestyle modifications in the management of hypertension [97]. This inclusion in the ISH guidelines may provide added impetus for yoga and meditation practices to be adopted in mainstream healthcare. Safety and benefits considered, yoga is a promising alternative and complementary choice for conventional CR programs in patients with CVD, especially for patients in low- and middle-income countries where such programs may be unavailable or too expensive [69].

23.7 Conclusion

Yoga and meditative practice have proved effective not only in regulation of high BP but also in the improvement of related emotional symptomatology. As has been argued, yoga practice is a process of integration and attunement of the systemic unity of the organism: body, mind, and environment. This integrative capacity has been proposed as the central mechanism underlying adaptive regulation and health. In addition, yoga leads to changes in lifestyle, promoting healthy behaviors and habits that include a healthy diet, avoiding consuming toxic substances, and a general attitude of care for one's health, and respect, commitment, and personal responsibility in health maintenance, as well. Consequently, it provides a framework within which patients can learn new ways to take care of themselves and their health, complementing medication intake, or at times, having the opportunity to avoid dependence on medication.

The attitude of self-awareness offers patients the possibility of a new way of being with themselves. By learning to be aware, they come into contact with the experience arising from physical and mental stillness, being able to generate a non-judgmental and non-reactive space, that is, a space of acceptance. Beyond the physical practice, yoga is a practice of awareness in every daily activity, self-observation, and recognition of own feelings, thoughts and emotions, and the links between them. Through specific yoga practices, patients learn to reduce their psychophysiological activation, promote a state of mental calmness, as well as that of positive and healthy changes in their body postures, emotions, attitudes, and relationship with the environment. In this way, the awareness process itself could act as a process of transformation for the patients.

The result of a systematized and continual yoga intervention could lead to the regulation and, even to the normalization of BP in these patients, with corresponding health benefits and decrease in demand for medical treatments, as well as a probable reduction or cessation of medication intake. More broadly, these positive effects of yoga could be extended to the prevention and treatment of many other pathologies related to stress and psycho-physiological imbalances. Therefore, the time is ripe to implement evidence-based yoga practices accompanied with yoga's holistic approach in mainstream healthcare.

References

1. World Health Organization. A global brief on hypertension: silent killer, global public health crisis; 2013. Retrieved from https://www.who.int/cardiovascular_diseases/publications/global_brief_hypertension/en/
2. Zhou B, Bentham J, Di Cesare M, Bixby H, Danaei G, Cowan MJ, Paciorek CJ, Singh G, Hajifathalian K, Bennett JE, Taddei C, Bilano V, Carrillo-Larco RM, Djalalinia S, Khatibzadeh S, Lugero C, Peykari N, Zhang WZ, Lu Y, et al. Worldwide trends in blood pressure from 1975 to 2015: a pooled analysis of 1479 population-based measurement studies with 19· 1 million participants. Lancet. 2017;389(10064):37–55.
3. Mills KT, Stefanescu A, He J. The global epidemiology of hypertension. Nat Rev Nephrol. 2020;16(4):223–37.
4. World Health Organization. Hypertension; 2019. Retrieved from https://www.who.int/news-room/fact-sheets/detail/hypertension
5. World Health Organization. Cardiovascular diseases (CVDs); 2017. Retrieved from https://www.who.int/news-room/fact-sheets/detail/cardiovascular-diseases-(cvds)
6. World Health Organization. Impact of out-of-pocket payments for treatment of non-communicable diseases in developing countries: a review of literature; 2011. Retrieved from https://www.who.int/health_financing/documents/cov-dp_e_11_02-ncd_finburden/en/
7. Bloom DE, Cafiero ET, Jané-Llopis E, Abrahams-Gessel S, Bloom LR, Fathima S, Feigl AB, Gaziano T, Hamandi A, Mowafi M, O'Farrell D, Ozaltin E, Pandya A, Prettner K, Rosenberg L, Seligman B, Stein A, Weinstein C, Weiss J. The global economic burden of noncommunicable diseases; 2012. Retrieved from http://www3.weforum.org/docs/WEF_Harvard_HE_GlobalEconomicBurdenNonCommunicableDiseases_2011.pdf
8. Yaxley JP, Thambar SV. Resistant hypertension: an approach to management in primary care. J Family Med Prim Care. 2015;4(2):193.
9. Weber MA, Schiffrin EL, White WB, Mann S, Lindholm LH, Kenerson JG, Flack JM, Carter BL, Materson BJ, Ram CVS, Cohen DL, Cadet J-C, Jean-Charles RR, Taler S, Kountz D, Townsend RR, Chalmers J, Ramirez AJ, Bakris GL, Wang J. Clinical practice guidelines for the management of hypertension in the community: a statement by the American Society of Hypertension and the International Society of Hypertension. J Clin Hypertens. 2014;16(1):14–26.
10. Carroll D, Ginty AT, Painter RC, Roseboom TJ, Phillips AC, de Rooij SR. Systolic blood pressure reactions to acute stress are associated with future hypertension status in the Dutch Famine Birth Cohort Study. Int J Psychophysiol. 2012;85(2):270–3.
11. Phillips AC. Stress and cardiovascular reactivity. In: Alvarenga M, Byrne D, editors. Handbook of psychocardiology. Singapore: Springer; 2016. p. 163–77.
12. Gawlik KS, Melnyk BM, Tan A. Associations between stress and cardiovascular disease risk factors among million hearts priority populations. Am J Health Promot. 2019;33(7):1063–6.
13. Sapolsky RM. Why zebras don't get ulcers: a guide to stress, stress related diseases, and coping. New York, NY: W.H. Freeman; 1994.
14. Wang Y, Winters JM. Modeling the adaptive pathophysiology of essential hypertension. In: Proceedings of the engineering in medicine and biology society 2011 annual international conference of the IEEE; 2011. p. 1029–32. https://doi.org/10.1109/IEMBS.2011.6090239
15. Porges SW. The polyvagal theory: phylogenetic substrates of a social nervous system. Int J Psychophysiol. 2001;42(2):123–46.
16. Porges SW. Social engagement and attachment. Ann N Y Acad Sci. 2003;1008(1):31–47.
17. Porges SW. The polyvagal perspective. Biol Psychol. 2006;74(2):116–43.
18. Hu G, Barengo NC, Tuomilehto J, Lakka TA, Nissinen A, Jousilahti P. Relationship of physical activity and body mass index to the risk of hypertension: a prospective study in Finland. Hypertension. 2004;43(1):25–30.
19. Netz Y, Lidor R. Mood alterations in mindful versus aerobic exercise modes. J Psychol Interdiscip Appl. 2003;137(5):405–19.
20. Satish L, Kumar BS. Lifestyle survey of urban youth: an analysis of healthy behaviour in relation to yoga practice. Indian J Commun Psychol. 2013;9(2):230–44.

21. Butzer B, LoRusso A, Shin SH, Khalsa SBS. Evaluation of yoga for preventing adolescent substance use risk factors in a middle school setting: a preliminary group-randomized controlled trial. J Youth Adolesc. 2017;46(3):603–32.
22. Speroni KG, Williams DA, Seibert DJ, Gibbons MG, Earley C. Helping nurses care for self, family, and patients through the nurses living fit intervention. Nurs Adm Q. 2012;37(4):286–94.
23. Watts AW, Rydell SA, Eisenberg ME, Laska MN, Neumark-Sztainer D. Yoga's potential for promoting healthy eating and physical activity behaviors among young adults: a mixed-methods study. Int J Behav Nutr Phys Act. 2018;15(1):42.
24. Douglass L. Yoga as an intervention in the treatment of eating disorders: does it help? Eat Disord. 2009;17:126–39.
25. Tafet GE, Bernardini R. Psychoneuroendocrinological links between chronic stress and depression. Prog Neuro-Psychopharmacol Biol Psychiatry. 2003;27(6):893–903.
26. Streeter CC, Whitfield TH, Owen L, Rein T, Karri SK, Yakhkind A, Perlmutter R, Prescot A, Renshaw PF, Ciraulo DA, Jensen JE. Effects of yoga versus walking on mood, anxiety, and brain GABA levels: a randomized controlled MRS study. J Altern Complement Med. 2010;16(11):1145–52.
27. Firk C, Markus CR. Serotonin by stress interaction: a susceptibility factor for the development of depression? J Psychopharmacol. 2007;21(5):538–44.
28. Mahar I, Bambico FR, Mechawar N, Nobrega JN. Stress, serotonin, and hippocampal neurogenesis in relation to depression and antidepressant effects. Neurosci Biobehav Rev. 2014;38:173–92.
29. Karg K, Burmeister M, Shedden K, Sen S. The serotonin transporter promoter variant (5-HTTLPR), stress, and depression meta-analysis revisited: evidence of genetic moderation. Arch Gen Psychiatry. 2011;68(5):444–54.
30. Brambilla P, Pérez J, Barale F, Schettini G, Soares JC. GABAergic dysfunction in mood disorders. Mol Psychiatry. 2003;8:721–37.
31. Streeter CC, Gerbarg PL, Saper RB, Ciraulo DA, Brown RP. Effects of yoga on the autonomic nervous system, gamma-aminobutyric-acid, and allostasis in epilepsy, depression, and post-traumatic stress disorder. Med Hypotheses. 2012;78(5):571–9.
32. Streeter CC, Jensen JE, Perlmutter RM, Cabral HJ, Tian H, Terhune DB, Renshaw PF. Yoga asana sessions increase brain GABA levels: a pilot study. J Altern Complement Med. 2007;13(4):419–26.
33. Streeter CC, Gerbarg PL, Brown RP, Scott TM, Nielsen GH, Owen L, Sakai O, Sneider JT, Nyer MB, Silveri MM. Thalamic gamma aminobutyric acid level changes in major depressive disorder after a 12-week iyengar yoga and coherent breathing intervention. J Altern Complement Med. 2020;26(3):190–7.
34. Wang F, Szabo A. Effects of yoga on stress among healthy adults: a systematic review. Altern Ther Health Med. 2020;26(4):AT6214.
35. Dunne EM, Balletto BL, Donahue ML, Feulner MM, DeCosta J, Cruess DG, Salmoirago-Blotcher E, Wing RR, Carey MP, Scott-Sheldon LAJ. The benefits of yoga for people living with HIV/AIDS: a systematic review and meta-analysis. Complement Ther Clin Pract. 2019;34:157–64.
36. Innes KE, Bourguignon C, Taylor AG. Risk indices associated with the insulin resistance syndrome, cardiovascular disease, and possible protection with yoga: a systematic review. J Am Board Fam Pract. 2005;18(6):491–519.
37. Engel AK, Fries P, Singer W. Dynamic predictions: oscillations and synchrony in top-down processing. Nat Rev Neurosci. 2001;2:704–16.
38. Siegel DJ. Mind: a journey to the heart of being human. New York, NY: WW Norton & Company; 2016.
39. Pradhan B. Yoga and mindfulness based cognitive therapy: a clinical guide. Berlin: Springer; 2014.
40. Fair DA, Cohen AL, Dosenbach NU, Church JA, Miezin FM, Barch DM, Raichle ME, Petersen SE, Schlaggar BL. The maturing architecture of the brain's default network. Proc Natl Acad Sci. 2008;105(10):4028–32.
41. Siegel DJ. The developing mind: how relationships and the brain interact to shape who we are. New York, NY: Guilford Press; 1999.
42. Siegel DJ. The mind in psychotherapy: an interpersonal neurobiology framework for understanding and cultivating mental health. Psychol Psychother Theory Res Pract. 2019;92(2):224–37.
43. Tolahunase MR, Sagar R, Faiq M, Dada R. Yoga-and meditation-based lifestyle intervention increases neuroplasticity and reduces severity of major depressive disorder: a randomized controlled trial. Restor Neurol Neurosci. 2018;36(3):423–42.
44. Tolahunase M, Sagar R, Dada R. Impact of yoga and meditation on cellular aging in apparently healthy individuals: a prospective, open-label single-arm exploratory study. Oxidative Med Cell Longev. 2017;2017:7928981. https://doi.org/10.1155/2017/7928981.
45. Harkess KN, Ryan J, Delfabbro PH, Cohen-Woods S. Preliminary indications of the effect of a brief yoga intervention on markers of inflammation and DNA methylation in chronically stressed women. Transl Psychiatry. 2016;6:e965. https://doi.org/10.1038/tp.2016.234.
46. Sharma M, Haider T. Yoga as an alternative and complementary treatment for hypertensive patients: a systematic review. J Evid Based Complement Altern Med. 2012;17(3):199–205.
47. Haider T, Sharma M, Branscum P. Yoga as an alternative and complimentary therapy for cardiovascular disease: a systematic review. J Evid Based Complementary Altern Med. 2017;22(2):310–16.
48. Jeter PE, Slutsky J, Singh N, Khalsa SBS. Yoga as a therapeutic intervention: a bibliometric analysis of published research studies from 1967 to 2013. J Altern Complement Med. 2015;21(10):586–92.

49. Cramer H, Sellin C, Schumann D, Dobos G. Yoga in arterial hypertension: a three-armed, randomized controlled trial. Dtsch Arztebl Int. 2018;115(50):833.
50. Tolbaños-Roche L, Miró-Barrachina MT, Ibáñez-Fernández I, Betancort M. YOGA and self-regulation in management of essential arterial hypertension and associated emotional symptomatology: a randomized controlled trial. Complement Ther Clin Pract. 2017;29:153–61.
51. Bhavanani AB, Madanmohan, Sanjay Z. Immediate effect of chandra nadi pranayama (left unilateral forced nostril breathing) on cardiovascular parameters in hypertensive patients. Int J Yoga. 2012;5(2):108–111. https://doi.org/10.4103/0973-6131.98221
52. Bhavanani AB, Madanmohan, Sanjay Z. Suryanadi pranayama (right unilateral nostril breathing) may be safe for hypertensives. J Yoga Phys Ther. 2012;2:118. https://doi.org/10.4172/2157-7595.1000118.
53. Ghati N, Killa A, Sharma G, Karunakaran B, Agarwal A, Mohanty S, Nivethitha L, Siddharthan D, Pandeyet RM. A randomized trial of the immediate effect of bee-humming breathing exercise on blood pressure and heart rate variability in patients with essential hypertension. Explore (New York, N.Y.). 2020;17(4):312–9.
54. Raghuraj P, Telles S. Immediate effect of specific nostril manipulating yoga breathing practices on autonomic and respiratory variables. Appl Psychophysiol Biofeedback. 2008;33:65–75.
55. Thanalakshmi J, Maheshkumar K, Kannan R, Sundareswaran L, Venugopal V, Poonguzhali S. Effect of Sheetali pranayama on cardiac autonomic function among patients with primary hypertension—a randomized controlled trial. Complement Ther Clin Pract. 2020;39:101138.
56. Park SH, Han KS. Blood pressure response to meditation and yoga: a systematic review and meta-analysis. J Altern Complement Med. 2017;23(9):685–95.
57. Benson H. The relaxation response. New York: Morrow; 1975.
58. Patki RA, Makwana JJ, Karmarkar G, Wadikar SS. Effect of regular yogic practice on autonomic functions. Indian Practitioner. 2003;56:9–11.
59. Udupa K, Bhavanani AB, Vijayalakshmi P, Krishnamurthy N. Effect of pranayam training on cardiac function in normal young volunteers. Indian J Physiol Pharmacol. 2003;47(1):27–33.
60. Madanmohan, Udupa K, Bhavanani AB, Shatapathy CC, Sahai A. Modulation of cardiovascular response to exercise by yoga training. Indian J Physiol Pharmacol. 2004;48(4):461–5.
61. Aivazyan TA. Psychological relaxation therapy in essential hypertension: efficacy and its predictors. Yoga Mimamsa. 1990;29:27–39.
62. Broota A, Varma R, Singh A. Role of relaxation in hypertension. J Indian Acad Appl Psychol. 1995;21:29–36.
63. Cohen DL, Bloedon LT, Rothman RL, Farrar JT, Galantino ML, Volger S, Mayor C, Szapary PO, Townsend RR. Iyengar yoga versus enhanced usual care on blood pressure in patients with prehypertension to stage I hypertension: a randomized controlled trial. Evid Based Complement Altern Med. 2011;2011:546428. https://doi.org/10.1093/ecam/nep130.
64. Latha AU, Kaliappan KV. Yoga, pranayama, thermal biofeedback techniques in the management of stress and high blood pressure. J Indian Psychol. 1991;9:36–46.
65. Patel C. Stress management and hypertension. Acta Physiol Scand. 1997;161:155–7.
66. Murugesan R, Govindarajulu N, Bera TK. Effect of selected yogic practices on the management of hypertension. Indian J Physiol Pharmacol. 2000;44(2):207–10.
67. Murthy SN, Rao NSN, Nandkumar B, Kadam A. Role of naturopathy and yoga treatment in the management of hypertension. Complement Ther Clin Pract. 2011;17(1):9–12.
68. Metri KG, Pradhan B, Singh A, Nagendra HR. Effect of 1-week yoga-based residential program on cardiovascular variables of hypertensive patients: a Comparative Study. Int J Yoga. 2018;11(2):170.
69. Li J, Gao X, Hao X, Kantas D, Mohamed EA, Zheng X, Xu H, Zhang L. Yoga for secondary prevention of coronary heart disease: a systematic review and meta-analysis. Complement Ther Med. 2020;57:102643. https://doi.org/10.1016/j.ctim.2020.102643.
70. Bharshankar JR, Bharshankar RN, Deshpande VN, Kaore SB, Gosavi GB. Effect of yoga on cardiovascular system in subjects above 40 years. Indian J Physiol Pharmacol. 2003;47(2):202–6.
71. Wu Y, Johnson BT, Acabchuk RL, Chen S, Lewis HK, Livingston J, Park CL, Pescatello LS. Yoga as antihypertensive lifestyle therapy: a systematic review and meta-analysis. Mayo Clin Proc. 2019;94(3):432–46.
72. Khattab K, Khattab AA, Ortak J, Richardt G, Bonnemeier H. Iyengar yoga increases cardiac parasympathetic nervous modulation among healthy yoga practitioners. Evid Based Complement Alternat Med. 2007;4(4):511–7.
73. Harinath K, Malhotra AS, Pal K, Prasad R, Kumar R, Kain TC, Sawhney RC. Effects of Hatha yoga and Omkar meditation on cardiorespiratory performance, psychologic profile, and melatonin secretion. J Altern Complement Med. 2004;10(2):261–8.
74. Maheshananda S, Sharma BR, Bodhe R, Bhat R, Satapathy B, Mukherjee R. Sivasvarodayah. Pune: Kaivalayadhma Publications; 2015.
75. Muktibodhananda S. Swara yoga: the tantric science of brain breathing. Munger: Bihar School of Yoga; 1984.
76. Tolbaños-Roche L, Mas-Hesse B. Application of an integrative yoga therapy programme in cases of essential arterial hypertension in public healthcare. Complement Ther Clin Pract. 2014;20(4):285–90.
77. Carlson LE, Speca M, Faris P, Patel KD. One year pre–post intervention follow-up of psychological, immune, endocrine and blood pressure outcomes of mindfulness-based stress reduction (MBSR) in breast

and prostate cancer outpatients. Brain Behav Immun. 2007;21(8):1038–49.
78. Garland EL, Gaylord SA, Fredrickson BL. Positive reappraisal mediates the stress-reductive effects of mindfulness: an upward spiral process. Mindfulness. 2011;2(1):59–67.
79. Hofmann SG, Sawyer AT, Witt AA, Oh D. The effect of mindfulness-based therapy on anxiety and depression: a meta-analytic review. J Consult Clin Psychol. 2010;78(2):169.
80. Zeidan F. The effects of brief mindfulness meditation training on mood, cognitive, and cardiovascular variables. Doctoral dissertation, The University of North Carolina at Charlotte, North Carolina; 2009. Retrieved from https://libres.uncg.edu/ir/uncc/f/Zeidan_uncc_0694D_10079.pdf
81. Diao D, Wright JM, Cundiff DK, Gueyffier F. Pharmacotherapy for mild hypertension. Sao Paulo Med J. 2012;130(6):417–8.
82. Chaddha A, Modaff D, Hooper-Lane C, Feldstein DA. Device and non-device-guided slow breathing to reduce blood pressure: a systematic review and meta-analysis. Complement Ther Med. 2019;45:179–84.
83. Sharma KS, Pailoor S, Choudhary NR, Bhat P, Shrestha S. Integrated yoga practice in cardiac rehabilitation program: a randomized control trial. J Altern Complement Med. 2020;26(10):918–27.
84. Pullen PR. The benefits of yoga therapy for heart failure patients (doctoral dissertation). Atlanta, GA: Georgia State University; 2009.
85. Edla SR, Kumar AM, Srinivas B, Raju MS, Gupta V. 'Integrated Naturopathy and Yoga' reduces blood pressure and the need for medications among a cohort of hypertensive patients in South India: 3-months follow-up study. Adv Integr Med. 2016;3(3):90–7.
86. Ornish D. It's time to embrace lifestyle medicine. Time. 2015;185(6–7):97.
87. Ornish D, Scherwitz LW, Billings JH, Gould KL, Merritt TA, Sparler S, Armstrong WT, Ports TA, Kirkeeide RL, Hogeboom C, Brand RJ. Intensive lifestyle changes for reversal of coronary heart disease. JAMA. 1998;280(23):2001–7.
88. Freeman AM, Taub PR, Lo HC, Ornish D. Intensive cardiac rehabilitation: an underutilized resource. Curr Cardiol Rep. 2019;21(4):1–11.
89. Levine GN, Lange RA, Bairey-Merz CN, Davidson RJ, Jamerson K, Mehta PK, Michos ED, Norris K, Ray IB, Saban KL, Shah T, Stein R, Smith SC. Meditation and cardiovascular risk reduction. J Am Heart Assoc. 2017;6(10):e002218.
90. Bloom K, Baker B, How M, Dai M, Abbey S, Myers M, Abramson BL, Irvine J, Perkins N, Tobe SW. Hypertension analysis of stress reduction using mindfulness meditation and yoga: results from the harmony randomized controlled trial. Am J Hypertens. 2014;27(1):122–9.
91. Palta P, Page G, Piferi RL, Gill JM, Hayat MJ, Connolly AB, Szanton SL. Evaluation of a mindfulness-based intervention program to decrease blood pressure in low-income African-American older adults. J Urban Health. 2012;89(2):308–16.
92. Raghuram N, Parachuri VR, Swarnagowri MV, Babu S, Chaku R, Kulkarni R, Bhuyan B, Bhargav H, Nagendra HR. Yoga based cardiac rehabilitation after coronary artery bypass surgery: one-year results on LVEF, lipid profile and psychological states—a randomized controlled study. Indian Heart J. 2014;66(5):490–502.
93. Bhavanani AB, Zeena S, Jayasettiaseelon E, Dayanidy G, Vithiyalakshmi L. A review of selected yoga research findings from ACYTER, JIPMER in 2008–12. Int Yoga J Sense. 2012;2(2):203–13.
94. Krishna BH, Pal P, Pal GK, Balachander J, Jayasettiaseelon E, Sreekanth Y, Sridhar MG, Gaur GS. Effect of yoga therapy on heart rate, blood pressure and cardiac autonomic function in heart failure. J Clin Diagn Res. 2014;8(1):14–6.
95. Bhavanani AB. Role of yoga in prevention and management of lifestyle disorders. Yoga Mimamsa. 2017;49(2):42.
96. Bhavanani AB, Ramanathan M, Balaji R, Pushpa D. Differential effects of uninostril and alternate nostril pranayamas on cardiovascular parameters and reaction time. Int J Yoga. 2014;7(1):60–5.
97. Unger T, Borghi C, Charchar F, Khan NA, Poulter NR, Prabhakaran D, Ramirez A, Schlaich M, Stergiou GS, Tomaszewski M, Wainford RD, Williams B, Schutte AE. 2020 International Society of Hypertension global hypertension practice guidelines. Hypertension. 2020;75(6):1334–57.

24 Meditation in Prevention and Treatment of Cardiovascular Disease: An Evidence-Based Review

Robert H. Schneider, Komal Marwaha, and John Salerno

24.1 Introduction

Cardiovascular disease (CVD) remains the number one cause of death, accounting for over 30% of all deaths worldwide [1, 2]. Despite recent health care advances, over 17 million people die annually due to CVD and this worldwide death rate is predicted to rise to 23 million by 2023 [1]. Poorer countries are most adversely affected, accounting for 80% of CVD mortality [1]. The estimated annual economic burden in the US for CVD is $555 billion and this exorbitant cost is expected to increase to $1.1 trillion by 2035 [3]. By 2030 it is estimated that the total worldwide cost of CVD will rise from approximately US$863 billion to over US$1 trillion US [4]. To reverse CVD trends, there is a need to consider novel interventions for the prevention and management of CVD that may be less expensive and have fewer side effects than conventional pharmacologic and surgical interventions.

Since psychosocial stress has been identified as an important risk factor for cardiovascular morbidity and mortality [5] in patients with established cardiovascular disease [6, 7] and non-diseased individuals [8, 9], stress reduction could potentially be an important behavioral intervention in the management of CVD.

Numerous studies have reported the use of stress reduction techniques such as meditation, progressive muscle relaxation, and yoga in the prevention and management of CVD [10–12]. The American Heart Association (AHA) in its 2017 scientific statement on Cardiovascular Risk Reduction proposed the practice of meditation as a potential cost-effective supplement to more conventional medical therapies for CVD risk reduction [13].

Growing evidence from the scientific literature indicates a positive impact of meditation practice on CVD but different meditation practices vary widely in technique and so are their physiological and clinical effects as described below. As elaborated in this review, findings shown for one type of meditation may not be extrapolated to all types of meditation. This review will focus on, meta-analyses, systematic reviews and randomized trials for cardiovascular effects of each type of meditation technique separately.

R. H. Schneider (✉)
Department of Physiology and Health, College of Integrative Medicine, Maharishi International University, Fairfield, IA, USA

Institute for Prevention Research, Maharishi Vedic City, IA, USA
e-mail: RSchneider@miu.edu

K. Marwaha
Department of Physiology and Health, College of Integrative Medicine, Maharishi International University, Fairfield, IA, USA

J. Salerno
Institute for Prevention Research, Maharishi Vedic City, IA, USA

I. Basu-Ray, D. Mehta (eds.), *The Principles and Practice of Yoga in Cardiovascular Medicine*,
https://doi.org/10.1007/978-981-16-6913-2_24

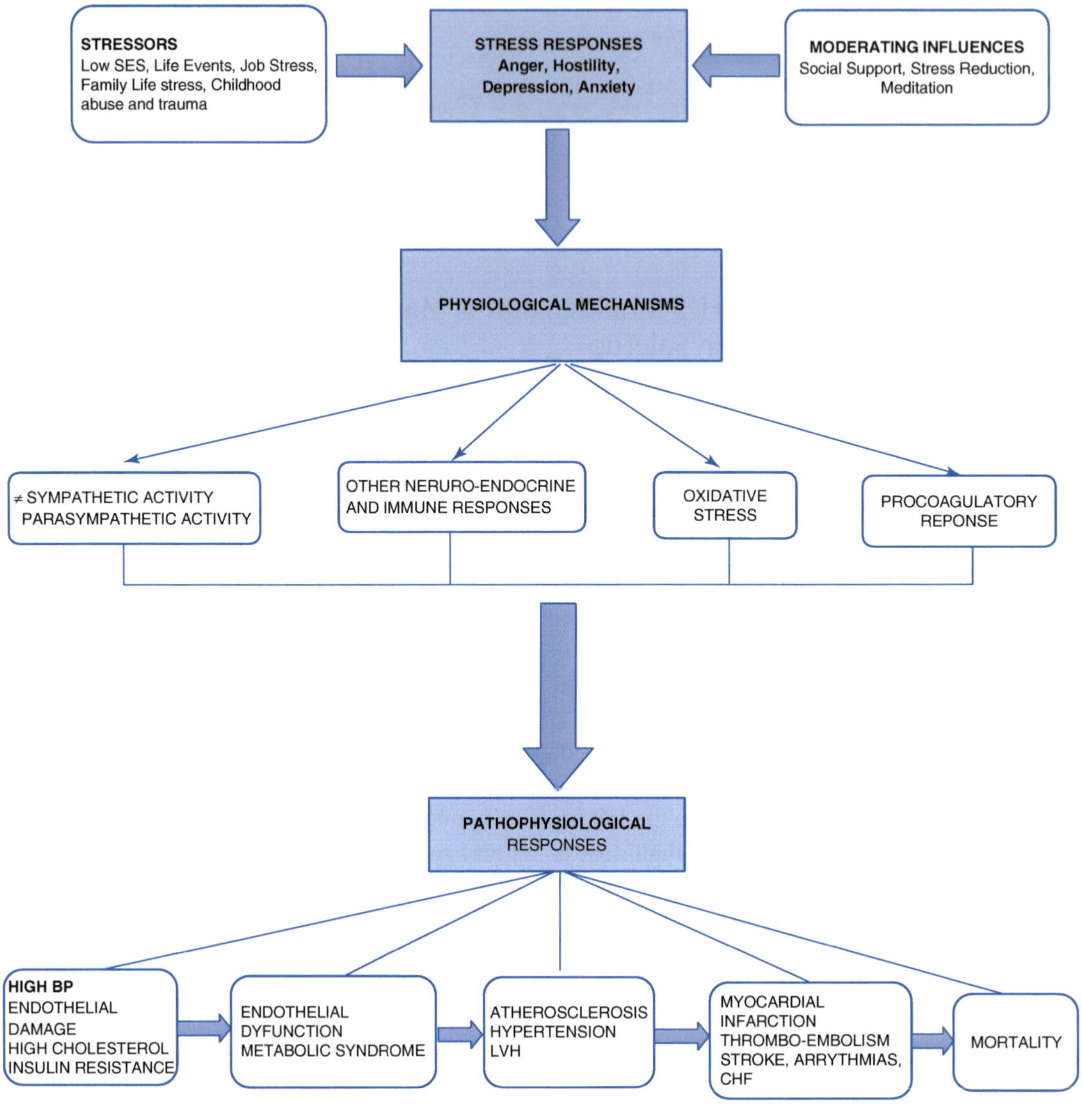

Fig. 24.1 Stress and stress response mechanisms leading to cardiovascular diseases

This narrative review updates previous reviews of the evidence for widely practiced and extensively researched meditation techniques on clinical CVD and its risk factors (e.g., hypertension, left ventricular hypertrophy, smoking, hypercholesterolemia, diabetes, metabolic syndrome, depression, anxiety, anger, and social distress); CVD surrogate markers (e.g., carotid intima-media thickness, exercise tolerance); cardiovascular clinical events (e.g., all-cause mortality, CVD mortality, myocardial infarction, stroke, acute coronary syndrome, revascularization). Since psychological stress appears to contribute to all recognized mechanisms underlying cardiac events [14] (see Fig. 24.1), we will also briefly review the available evidence of pathophysiological mechanisms affected by different meditation techniques.

24.2 The Transcendental Meditation (TM) Technique

The TM technique is a meditation modality restored from the ancient Vedic tradition of Yoga by Maharishi Mahesh Yogi and taught worldwide since 1957. TM practice is described as a simple and easy technique for reducing psychophysiological stress and gaining deep relaxation and rest [15, 16]. It is practiced twice daily for 20 min while sitting in a comfortable position with closed eyes and allowing the mind to effortlessly experience quieter levels of the thinking process until it transcends or goes beyond the state of ordinary thinking. This has been described as the least excited state of awareness or pure consciousness or in the traditional language of Yoga, *Samadhi* [15–17]. In this settled mind-body state, mental activity is quiet but the mind is fully awake and simultaneously, the body is deeply rested. Neuroscientists describe this psychophysiological state as a wakeful hypometabolic state of physiology [18].

Effect of TM Practice on the Pathophysiological Pathways of CVD A meta-analysis of 31 studies on TM demonstrated that during TM practice significant reductions in several indicators of autonomic activity including reduced respiratory rate, reduced plasma lactate, and increased galvanic skin response (a measure of sympathetic tone) compared to quietly resting with closed eyes [19]. Other studies have reported decreased sympathetic activity [20, 21], decreased plasma catecholamine levels [22], decreased adrenergic receptor sensitivity [23], and reduced plasma cortisol [24] with TM practice.

In a study conducted with at-risk adolescents for hypertension, TM practice was found both to reduce cardiovascular reactivity and to enhance autonomic recovery from laboratory stressors [25]. Cardiovascular reactivity to stress has been thought to contribute to hypertension long-term, as well as vascular damage and accelerated atherosclerosis [26]. Reduced cardiovascular reactivity with TM practice may explain reduced blood pressure (BP) and the reduction of clinical events discovered in long-term meditators.

Long-term TM practitioners are also found to have reduced total peripheral resistance—indicating decreased vasoconstriction which is a function of sympathetic tone. These findings suggest that declines in sympathetic nervous system activity during TM practice may be the responsible mechanism underlying the beneficial influence on high BP and cardiovascular health [27].

Another important risk factor for coronary heart disease (CHD) is elevated levels of plasma cortisol. In the Edinburgh study which included 919 patients with type 2 diabetes, elevated levels of plasma cortisol were associated with increased fasting glucose and total cholesterol levels along with prevalent ischemic heart disease, independent of conventional risk factors [28]. TM practice has been found to decrease cortisol response to a metabolic stressor [29]. In a study of postmenopausal women who were long-term practitioners of TM, Walton et al. compared their cortisol levels in participants with participants who were not TM practitioners. The 16 women who practiced TM for an average of 23 years were matched to 14 control women. The cortisol response to a metabolic stressor (75 g of glucose, orally) was tested in both saliva and urine. Findings showed that post glucose cortisol rose significantly faster in the control group than in the TM group. In addition, urinary excretion of cortisol was 3 times higher in the control group than the TM group [29].

In another study that examined cortisol levels in 16 patients randomized to either TM or control groups, TM did not demonstrate acute inhibitory effects on renin, aldosterone, or cortisol levels in the unstressed state [30]. However, in the stressed state following venipuncture, a consistently significant rise in cortisol was observed in the controls, while TM patients did not show such an effect. The investigators concluded that longer-term practice of TM may not directly influence cortisol in the unstressed state but suggested that TM practice could blunt the response to stress [30].

24.2.1 Effect of TM on CVD Risk Factors

Hypertension TM practice has demonstrated blood pressure lowering effects similar to some primary antihypertensive medications [31]. There have been 12 randomized controlled trials (RCTs) of TM on BP—totaling more than 1000 subjects that demonstrated the efficacy of TM in lowering BP [25, 32–39].

In a study on the longer-term effects of TM on hypertension, 102 participants were randomized to either one of three groups: TM, progressive muscular relaxation (PMR), or a health education program. All groups were followed over a 12-month period. TM was found to be twice as effective as PMR in reducing BP with no significant change observed in the health education group [40].

In April 2013, the American Heart Association (AHA) Scientific Statement on Alternative Treatments to Lower Blood Pressure recommended TM for consideration in clinical practice for the treatment of hypertension [12]. It also concluded that TM was the only meditation with sufficient evidence for consideration in clinical practice for lowering BP [12].

A series of systematic reviews, meta-analyses, and RCTs have verified TM efficacy in reducing BP and other CVD risk factors. A meta-analysis of nine RCTs totaling 711 subjects reported a significant reduction in systolic blood pressure (SBP) (−4.7 mm Hg) and diastolic blood pressure (DBP) (−3.2 mm Hg) with TM compared to control arms [41]. The BP reduction in the hypertensive subgroup was −5.1/−2.1 mm Hg and in high-quality studies was −6.4/−3.4 mm Hg [41].

Another systematic review and meta-analysis that included only high-quality RCTs on stress reduction for BP reported an average change of −5.0/−2.8 mm Hg with TM [42].

Recent meta-analyses that were published after the 2013 AHA scientific statement also found TM effective for clinical use in reducing BP [43, 44]. In 2015, Bai et al. conducted a systematic review and meta-analysis of 12 studies that included 996 participants. They found a −4.26 mm Hg reduction in SBP and −2.33 mm Hg reduction in DBP with TM practice compared with control groups [43].

More recently Ooi et al. conducted an overview of eight systematic reviews and meta-analyses that comprised a report by the Agency for Healthcare Research and Quality, a Cochrane systematic review, four independent reviews, and two additional reviews [44]. The authors found a clear trend of increasing evidence over the years supporting the effectiveness of TM in lowering BP [44].

Left Ventricular Mass Higher left ventricular mass is an indicator of hypertensive heart disease and a major risk factor for cardiovascular mortality [45]. In an RCT on 86 adult hypertensive subjects, after a 7-month intervention, the left ventricular mass index was 7.55 gm/m^2 lower in the TM group compared to the health education participants ($P = 0.040$) [46].

In another RCT conducted in African American adolescents with high normal blood pressure, Barnes et al. reported significantly reduced LVM in patients randomized to TM compared to HE group, after 4 months of intervention [47]. In a pilot study conducted in 34 mildly hypertensive adults, investigators found a 1-year intervention of TM led to significant LVMI reduction from the baseline in both the health education and TM groups [48].

Psychosocial Stress Factors There is an extensive body of research connecting psychosocial stress factors [49–52] such as depression and anxiety through disturbance of physiological mechanisms to CVD [53–56] (see Fig. 24.1).

Meta-analyses have suggested a strong association between myocardial infarction incidence and acute experiences of anger, anxiety, sadness, grief, and distress [57, 58]. Related research on the TM technique has shown significant reductions in psychological distress [38] including anxiety [59], posttraumatic stress [60, 61], and depression [62, 63].

In a recent RCT at the Department of Veterans Affairs San Diego Healthcare System, 203 veterans with a current diagnosis of PTSD resulting from active military service were randomly assigned to a TM group or prolonged exposure therapy (PE) group, or an active control group of health education (HE) [60]. Each treatment provided 12 sessions over 12 weeks, with daily home practice. TM and HE were mainly given in a group setting and PE was given individually. The primary outcome was change in PTSD symptom severity over 3 months, assessed by the Clinician-Administered PTSD Scale (CAPS). TM was found significantly non-inferior to PE on change in CAPS score from baseline to 3-month post-test (the difference between groups in mean change −5.9, 95% CI −14.3 to

2.4, $P = 0.0002$). In standard superiority comparisons, significant reductions in CAPS scores for PTSD were found for TM versus HE ($P = 0.0009$), and PE versus HE ($P = 0.041$). Clinically significant improvements on the CAPS score were shown in 61% of those receiving TM, 42% of those receiving PE, and 32% of those receiving HE [60].

In a randomized controlled study, 300 university students assigned to either TM or wait-list control, over a 3-month treatment period, demonstrated significant improvements in anxiety, depression, anger, hostility, and coping in those practicing TM compared to the waitlist control [38].

A meta-analysis of 143 studies found TM twice as effective as placebo in reducing trait anxiety while most meditation and relaxation techniques were no better than placebo [64]. This report was updated in 2013 by a meta-analysis of 16 randomized controlled trials on TM totaling 1295 subjects [59] that assessed the effects of initial anxiety level, age, duration of practice, the regularity of practice, research quality, author affiliation, and type of control group on effect sizes. TM practice was found to be more effective than treatment as usual as well as most alternative treatments [59]. The strongest TM effects were observed in individuals under high stress, such as veterans suffering from a posttraumatic stress disorder and prison inmates. Studies using repeated measures analyses showed substantial reductions during the first 2 weeks and sustained effects at 3 years [59].

Another meta-analysis compared the effect of TM, mindfulness, and other meditation on a composite index of trait anxiety, negative emotion, neuroticism, perception, self-concept, and self-realization. It found an effect size of 0.24 for mindfulness and for other meditation techniques compared to 0.37 for TM [65].

Insulin Resistance and Metabolic Syndrome Psychological stress is linked with impaired glycemic control in diabetics and increased risk of diabetes mellitus and CVD [66]. An RCT involving 103 subjects with chronic heart disease exhibited a reduction in insulin resistance (-0.75 ± 2.04 vs. 0.52 ± 2.84; $P = 0.01$) and HR variability (0.10 ± 0.17 vs. -0.50 ± 0.17 high-frequency power; $P = 0.07$) after 16 weeks' practice of TM compared with the control group [31]. This study indicated that stress reduction using TM may help in the management of metabolic syndrome and may prevent the development of diabetes which are both important risk factors for coronary heart disease (CHD). This effect on insulin resistance may also be the biochemical mechanism for the regression of carotid atherosclerosis found with TM and its clinical cardiovascular effects.

Smoking Cigarette smoking is another key risk factor of CVD. A meta-analysis of 131 studies [67] found TM was more effective than standard rehabilitation programs and other self-development techniques, in reducing tobacco usage [67]. As there was no attempt to change health habits during the course of TM instruction, this spontaneous and positive lifestyle modification could possibly be related to brain integration [68] and normalization of the neurochemistry upon regular TM practice [69–71].

However, another study of TM in 295 college students found no significant reduction in cigarette smoking at a 3-month follow-up between those randomized to TM and those in a waitlist control group but TM instruction significantly lowered drinking rates among males but not female students [72].

24.2.2 Effect of TM on Surrogate Markers of CVD

Carotid Atherosclerosis Carotid intima-media thickness is one of the stronger non-invasive measures of atherosclerosis, a precursor to heart attacks and stroke. An RCT studied the effect of TM practice on the carotid artery intima-media thickness measured by B mode ultrasound on 138 hypertensive subjects randomized to either the TM group or a health education group. After 7 months intervention period, carotid intima-media thickness in the TM group was significantly lower than the control group [34].

Exercise Tolerance in Coronary Heart Disease Patients A controlled trial of 16 subjects with chronic stable angina awaiting revascularization surgery showed significant improvement on exercise stress testing after 7.6 months of TM practice. This effect was found with all functional measures including significant increases in exercise duration, improved maximal exercise workload compared with waitlisted controls, as well as lower rate-pressure products at given workloads and significantly delayed onset of ST depression [73].

In an RCT that analyzed 23 Black patients hospitalized for heart failure who were randomly assigned to either TM or routine health education [74] after 6 months, the TM group had a significant increase in their 6-min walk distance as well as improvement in depression scores and quality of life measures compared to the health education group [74].

24.2.3 Effect of TM on CV Clinical Events and Mortality

Hospitalization for CVD A cohort study of 2000 TM practitioners compared to 600,000 matched controls found an 87% reduction in hospitalization for heart disease and a 56% reduction in hospitalization for all major categories of disease [75]. There was no difference in the hospitalization for childbirth—indicating that the TM practitioners attended hospitals when needed [75].

CVD and All Cause Mortality In a study of 201 patients with coronary heart disease, after an average follow-up of 5.4 years, there was a 48% reduction (hazard ratio 0.52; 95% CI, 0.29–0.92) in the composite of all-cause mortality, myocardial infarction, or stroke in the TM practitioners compared to health education controls [76]. There was also a dose-response relationship. This indicates—the more regular the subjects were in their meditation practice, the greater was their disease-free survival. For those that practiced with high regularity, i.e., towards 20 mins twice daily, the risk reduction was 66%. The majority of people in this study were regular in their practice (i.e., at least once a day) [76].

In another study that included 202 older hypertensive patients randomly assigned to TM or controls, a 23% reduction in all-cause mortality and a 30% decrease in cardiovascular mortality were found in TM participants compared to combined controls [77]. TM practice effect on mortality reduction is on par with, or greater than, those observed in long-term intervention, large-scale, primary prevention studies of cholesterol therapy [78] and of blood pressure reduction [79, 80].

In another study, mortality and cause of death were assessed over 8 years of follow-up in 109 older African American participants who had participated in a hypertension study. Participants were randomly assigned to either TM or progressive muscle relaxation or to a health education group for 3 months. The adjusted relative risk for CVD mortality was significantly reduced by 81% in the TM group when compared with the control group [81].

Summary Several independently conducted systematic reviews, meta-analyses, and scientific statements indicate the effectiveness of the TM technique in BP reduction prevention, comparable to lifestyle modification therapies recommended by AHA and European Society of Hypertension guidelines (e.g., sodium restriction, weight loss, aerobic exercise) [82]. TM practice has been shown to beneficially effect other cardiovascular risk factors including psychological stress, anxiety, depression, posttraumatic stress, anger, hostility, insulin resistance, left ventricular mass, surrogate markers; carotid intima-media thickness and exercise tolerance. In long-term RCTs, TM practice was found to decrease mortality rates, myocardial infarction and stroke, and CVD hospitalization.

24.3 Mindfulness-Based Stress Reduction (MBSR)

MBSR is a multicomponent intervention providing systematic training of informal mindfulness meditation practices and the informal application of mindfulness in daily life. It also includes gentle stretching and mindful yoga, as well as psychoeducation about the applications of mindfulness to support improved health, health-enhancing behaviors, and stress reduction [83].

MBSR is another widely practiced stress reduction program that employs an 8-week structured mindfulness meditation program to ease mental and physical suffering associated with physical, psychosomatic, and psychiatric disorders [84]. The individual learns the capacity to live with an open and non-judgmental awareness of all experiences within the present moment [84]. The technique assumes that greater awareness of the here-and-now will provide a clearer and more accurate perception, reduce negative affect, and improve energy and coping [85, 86].

Pathophysiological Mechanisms of CVD The mechanisms of possible BP-lowering or cardiovascular effects by MBSR have not been fully elucidated, but it is proposed that MBSR reduces psychological stress and its psychological correlates. One study of 15 participants with hypertension and chronic kidney disease reported a decrease in muscle sympathetic nerve activity and BP during mindfulness meditation [87]. There are few studies that have assessed changes in catecholamines and cortisol, though results are heterogeneous.

One study found a decrease in catecholamine levels with MBSR compared to the control group [88]. A few other studies reported a significant decrease in stress biomarkers [89] including cortisol levels [90–93] while several did not find any change in catecholamine or cortisol levels with MBSR compared to the control group [94–100]. Studies also suggest that MBSR reduces pro-inflammatory markers [101] and gene expression in older adults [102].

24.3.1 Effect of MBSR on CVD Risk Factors Hypertension

There was no meta-analysis available before 2013 and the available randomized and nonrandomized studies reported varied results of BP-lowering efficacy of MBSR, ranging from decrease in SBP only [90] or DBP only [103], or both [104, 105] or no significant reduction in either SBP or DBP with MBSR compared to the control group [106, 107]. Because of the negative or mixed results of studies, AHA did not recommend the use of MBSR in clinical practice to reduce BP and ascribed Class III, no benefit, Level of Evidence C to MBSR [12].

Since the AHA 2013 scientific statement, more RCTs have been published that assessed BP-lowering efficacy of MBSR. Some found MBSR effective in reducing BP [104, 108] while others did not [95, 109]. In 2014, Abbott et al. conducted a systematic review and meta-analysis to determine the effectiveness of MBSR in patients with vascular disease [110]. For assessing the efficacy of MBSR on BP reduction, they pooled the results of 4 RCTs and found moderate effect sizes of MBSR for SBP, SMD −0.78 (95% CI −1.46 to −0.09, P = 0.03), and DBP, SMD −0.67 (95% CI −1.26 to −0.08, P = 0.03) compared to control group [110].

However, the authors did not report the change of BP in standard clinical units, i.e., mmHg. In order to determine BP reduction in mmHg with MBSR, we calculated the weighted mean difference in BP by including all the RCTs published in the English language including those in the Abbott et al. review plus RCTs published subsequently that had assessed the effects of MBSR on BP. There were seven RCTs published through 2017 [95, 103–105, 107–109]. The calculated weighted means of these trials showed −2.99 mm Hg in SBP and −1.03 mm Hg in DBP with MBSR (Table 24.1) compared to the control group [111].

Of the seven RCTs, the small study by Palta et al. [105] reported markedly different effects from the other six studies and had the smallest sample size (N = 20). Therefore, in a sensitivity analysis, the weighted mean difference was recalculated without this study. The results showed a weighted mean difference of −2.36 mm Hg in SBP and −0.52 mm Hg in DBP with MBSR (Table 24.2) compared to the control groups [111].

Left Ventricular Function A non-randomized study investigated the impact of 8 weeks MBSR on left ventricular (LV) function in 34 female patients with microvascular angina on anti-anginal medication. The authors reported signifi-

Table 24.1 Weighted mean of BP reduction with MBSR

	RCT	ΔSBP (mm Hg)	ΔDBP (mm Hg)	Sample size	Weight
1.	Hughes, 2013	−4.1	−3.1	56	0.089
2.	Hartman, 2012	−6.4	−3.5	110	0.175
3.	Blom, 2014	0	0.4	101	0.161
4.	Palta, 2012	−21.92	−16.7	20	0.031
5.	Momeni, 2016	−13	−2.1	60	0.095
6.	Daubenmier, 2017	1	1.5	194	0.309
7.	RajaKhan, 2017	0.9	0.4	86	0.137
	Mean change in BP (mm Hg)	−6.217	−3.3		
	Weighted mean	−2.99	−1.03	627	

RCT randomized controlled trial, Δ*SBP* change in systolic blood pressure, Δ*DBP* change in diastolic blood pressure

Table 24.2 Weighted mean of BP reduction with MBSR excluding study by Palta et al.

	RCT	ΔSBP (mm Hg)	ΔDBP (mm Hg)	Sample size	Weight
1.	Hughes, 2013	−4.1	−3.1	56	0.092
2.	Hartman, 2012	−6.4	−3.5	110	0.181
3.	Blom, 2014	0	0.4	101	0.166
4.	Momeni, 2016	−13	−2.1	60	0.098
5.	Daubenmier, 2017	1	1.5	194	0.319
6.	RajaKhan, 2017	0.9	0.4	86	0.141
	Mean change in BP (mm Hg)	−3.6	−1.06		
	Weighted mean	−2.364	−0.522	607	

RCT randomized controlled trial, Δ*SBP* change in systolic blood pressure, Δ*DBP* change in diastolic blood pressure

cantly reduced global longitudinal strain (GLS) of the left ventricle after 8 weeks of MBSR practice [112].

24.3.2 Psychosocial Stress and Negative Emotional States

Studies suggest positive effects of mindfulness-based practices (meditation or therapy) on depression and anxiety symptoms [113–115] and perceived stress [116].

In 2010, Hofmann et al. conducted a meta-analysis of 39 randomized controlled studies totaling 1140 participants receiving mindfulness-based therapy for a range of conditions, including cancer, generalized anxiety disorder, depression, and other psychiatric or medical conditions. They reported moderate effect size estimates for reducing anxiety symptoms (Hedges' $g = 0.63$) and depressive symptoms (Hedges' $g = 0.59$) [113].

Similarly, in 2012 a meta-analysis of 22 (13 non-randomized and 9 RCTs) studies found MBSR associated with significantly reduced symptoms of anxiety (Hedges' 0.60) and depression (Hedges' g 0.42) in pre- to post-analysis. For controlled analysis, the pooled effect sizes (Hedges' g 0.37) for anxiety symptoms ($P < 0.001$) and 0.44 for symptoms of depression ($P < 0.001$) [114].

The similar effect size of MBSR was found on stress and anxiety in pre-post analyses (Hedge's $g = 0.55$) and between-group analyses (Hedge's $g = 0.53$). The obtained results were maintained at an average of 19 weeks of follow-up [115].

For depression also, a recent meta-analysis of 18 RCTs reported the moderate effect of MBSR in reducing depression in young people at post-test (Hedges' $g = -0.45$) but effects were not found statistically significant in follow-up

(Hedges' $g = -0.24$) due to a lack of statistical power [117].

Insulin Resistance A small prospective observational study that estimated the changes in glycemic control in 14 type-2 diabetic patients found a reduction in glycated hemoglobin - HbA1c after I month MBSR practice in 11 patients completing the program [118].

An RCT that evaluated the cardiometabolic effects of MBSR in 86 obese women randomized to 8 weeks of MBSR or health education and followed them for 16 weeks did not find change in insulin resistance, BP or weight in the MBSR group but fasting glucose at 8 weeks and at 16 weeks significantly decreased in MBSR group compared to baseline [95].

A recent RCT of 60 patients randomized to MBSR and control group investigated the effect of MBSR intervention on emotion regulation and glycemic control of patients with type 2 diabetes. After 3 months as a follow-up, the MBSR intervention group showed a significant reduction in all outcome measures including FBS, HbA1C, anxiety, and depression scores in comparison with the control group [119].

Smoking A meta-analysis of four randomized, controlled trials of mindfulness training involving a total of 474 patients found MBSR more effective than group counseling, with 25% of mindfulness training participants remaining abstinent from smoking for >4 months, compared with 14% of those receiving more-traditional cessation instruction [120].

In another study of volunteers wishing to reduce stress, half of whom were smokers, who were randomized to either a 2-week program of mindfulness meditation or relaxation training, a 60% reduction in smoking was observed among those instructed in mindfulness, with no reduction in those instructed in relaxation training. In this study, the meditation group brain scan in resting-state showed increased activity in the anterior cingulate and prefrontal cortex areas that are related to self-control but not the relaxation training group [121].

There are other small studies that have also shown the efficacy of mindfulness training in increasing abstinence rates when compared with more-traditional intervention programs [122–125].

24.3.3 Effects of MBSR on Surrogate Markers of CVD

Effect of MBSR on Exercise Capacity in Cardiac Patients An RCT examined the physiological and psychological outcomes of 12 weeks online mindfulness training program ($N = 215$) compared to usual care ($N = 109$) in patients with existing diagnosed heart disease (ischemic, valvular, congenital heart disease, or cardiomyopathy). The primary outcome was exercise capacity as measured by a 6 min-walk test. On a 12-month follow-up, compared to the control group, participants in the online MBSR program demonstrated significantly improved exercise capacity (effect size; 13.2, 95% CI: −0.02–26.4, $P = 0.050$) [126].

Effect of MBSR on Endothelial Function A non-randomized study investigated the impact of 8 weeks MBSR on endothelial function in 34 female patients with microvascular angina on anti-anginal medication. The study reported significantly improved reactive brachial flow-mediated dilatation from baseline after 8 weeks of programmed MBSR treatment [112].

24.3.4 Effect of MBSR on CVD Clinical Events

CVD Morbidity and Mortality An RCT of online mindfulness training program ($n = 215$) and usual care ($n = 109$) in cardiac disease patients for 12 weeks did not find any difference in the composite end-point (all-cause mortality, heart failure, symptomatic arrhythmia, cardiac surgery, and percutaneous cardiac intervention) in MBSR group compared to usual care [127].

To the best of our knowledge, no other RCTs have reported significant effects of MBSR meditation on major adverse cardiovascular clinical events.

Summary Systemic reviews and meta-analyses have suggested the efficacy of MBSR in reducing smoking, insulin resistance, depression, anxiety, psychological stress, but the effect on physiological correlates of stress has been heterogeneous. The weighted mean BP change derived from all the randomized controlled trials published in the English language through 2017 on MBSR found a modest decrease in SBP ~2 mm Hg and DBP ~1 mm Hg. No long-term effects on CVD clinical events have been documented.

24.4 Yoga

The practice of yoga is historically intertwined with meditative and contemplative aspects [128]. However, the forms of Yoga most commonly practiced in the West are largely physical postures or exercises, called asanas and to a lesser extent, breathing exercises (pranayama) or meditation alone [128]. Most of the available studies on yoga have physical components included as intervention and results cannot be completely attributed to the meditation component of yoga only. Since this chapter focuses on the effects of meditation on CVD and CVD risk factors, we would mention if studies included postures/exercises or if they employed meditation as a primary intervention.

Pathophysiological Mechanisms of CVD Results of randomized control trial on Rajyoga [129] and systemic review of studies suggest that yoga (asana and breathing or meditation) possibly balance the autonomic activity to parasympathetic side [129] and thus reduces BP [130]. Investigators have reported significant improvement of all inflammatory biomarkers (interleukin-6, C-reactive protein, and extracellular superoxide dismutase) after 8-week of yoga training as compared to the control group [131]. Whether additional pathways are involved requires future investigation.

24.4.1 Effects of Yoga on CVD Risk Factors

Hypertension In 2013, the AHA review committee [12] assigned a Class III, no benefit, Level of Evidence C to yoga for BP-lowering effectiveness due to the lack of available meta-analysis, methodically weak qualitative reviews [132, 133], and the mixed findings of RCTs [12, 134, 135]. But since then several meta-analyses and systemic reviews have demonstrated significant BP reduction with yoga [136, 137].

A recent meta-analysis by Chu et al. (22 RCTs and 768 participants) found a −5.21 mmHg decrease in SBP and −4.98 mmHg decrease in DBP in the yoga group compared to the control group [138]. Similar results are reported by Park and Hans in 2017 in the meta-analysis of 6 RCTs (394 participants) and found a −4.59 mm Hg decrease in SBP and −3.65 mm Hg reduction in DBP with yoga [139]. All these meta-analysis and reviews have included studies with both postures and meditation included in yoga practice.

24.4.2 Effect of Yoga on Left Ventricle Function

An RCT evaluated the effect of yoga training in addition to standard medical therapy on cardiac function and N terminal pro B-type natriuretic peptide (NT -pro-BNP) in 130 heart failure patients randomized to control Group or Yoga Group. After 12 weeks, improvement in left ventricular ejection fraction, myocardial performance index, and reduction in NT pro-BNP were statistically significant in both the groups. The between-group comparisons from pre to post 12 weeks were significant for Yoga group improvements (LVEF, $P < 0.01$, Tei index, $P < 0.01$, NT pro-BNP, $P < 0.01$) [140].

Another RCT compared the long-term effects of a yoga-based cardiac rehabilitation program with only a physiotherapy-based program as an add-on to conventional rehabilitation after coronary artery bypass grafting (CABG) on risk factors in 250 male participants (35–65 years). The study reported significant improvement in LVEF in the Yoga group ($P = 0.001$) than the control group in those with abnormal baseline EF (<53%) after 1 year [141].

24.4.3 Psychological Stress and Negative Affective States

A prospective randomized control study measured the short-term effect of Raj yoga on 150 patients undergoing elective coronary artery bypass surgery randomized to either Raja yoga group or Control Group. Anxiety and serum cortisol levels were measured before the start of Raja yoga training or patient counseling on the morning of the day of surgery, on the second postoperative day, and on the fifth postoperative day. The results showed that on the second and on the fifth postoperative days, the patients who underwent Raja yoga training had significantly lower anxiety levels in comparison with the control group. The serum cortisol level was also favorably modulated by the practice of Raja yoga meditation [142].

A systemic review on the effect of yoga on stress was conducted by including 17 studies published from 2011 to May 2013. Of the 17 studies, 12 demonstrated positive changes in psychological or physiological outcomes related to stress but many studies showed decreased perceived stress, the intervention was clubbed with mindfulness [143].

Insulin Resistance Clinical trials have demonstrated the benefits of yoga in diabetes; improving blood glucose [144, 145], insulin-glucose ratios, glycosylated hemoglobin [145], and requirement for oral hypoglycemics and insulin [144].

A systematic review of published literature (22 RCTs, 21 nonrandomized controlled trials, 26 uncontrolled (pre and post) clinical trials, and 1 cross-sectional study) from 1970 to 2004, studied the effects of yoga on anthropometric and physiologic indices of CVD risk and on related clinical endpoints. The review reported beneficial changes overall in insulin resistance syndrome (IRS)-related indices of CVD risk, including glucose tolerance and insulin sensitivity, lipid profiles, anthropometric characteristics, BP, oxidative stress, coagulation profiles, sympathetic activation, and cardiovagal function, as well as improvement in several clinical endpoints. The results of this review indicate that yoga may reduce many IRS-related risk factors for CVD, improve clinical outcomes, and may aid in the management of CVD and other IRS-related conditions [130].

In a randomized control trial 101 subjects diagnosed with metabolic syndrome were randomly assigned to usual care versus usual care plus yoga group for 12 weeks. After 12 weeks significant improvement in waist circumference, BP, blood glucose, HbA1c, triglycerides, and HDL-C in Yoga group was observed [146].

Cramer et al. in a meta-analysis reported that yoga improved HbA1c (MD = −0.45%; 95% CI = −0.87, −0.02) and insulin resistance (MD = −0.19; 95% CI = −0.30, −0.08) relative to usual care or no intervention [147].

But a more recently (2017) published systematic review and random-effects meta-analysis of 32 RCTs did not find fasting blood glucose or glycosylated hemoglobin difference between yoga and non-exercise or exercise controls [138]. More systemic reviews and meta-analyses are needed to substantiate the beneficial effects of yoga on insulin resistance and diabetes. Most of the studies included in reviews and meta-analyses had yogic exercises in their interventions [138, 144–146]. Hence, the results cannot be attributed to meditation only.

Smoking A review of the impact of evidence-based yoga intervention on smoking cessation that included studies (2 pre-post tests and 8 RCTs) in the English language published between 2004 and 2013 reported that most studies indicated that yoga-based interventions were effective in reducing craving and number of cigarettes smoked during smoking cessation. Most of the interventions included rhythmic breathing besides physically gentle movement and had shown improvement in quitting smoking [148].

24.4.4 Effect of Yoga on Surrogate Markers of CVD

Carotid Atherosclerosis In a pre-post study that included 123 individuals with angiographically documented moderate to severe CAD, the effect of Raja yoga meditation for stress management, healthy diet (low fat, high fiber vegetarian diet) and moderate aerobic exercise were assessed by angiography for change in severity. After 2 years follow-up, it was found that the decline in absolute % diameter of coronary stenosis and cardiac events were correlated with percent adherence to the intervention. In patients with the highest adherence, percent diameter stenosis regressed by 18.2 ± 12.0 absolute percentage points (29% relative improvement, $P < 0.0001$). Least adherence had a progression of 10.6 ± 13.2 absolute percentage points (23% relative worsening, $P < 0.0001$) Cardiac events were also significantly less in most adherence compared to least adherence participants [149]. The results of this study cannot be attributed to the meditation component of yoga only as intervention also involved diet and moderate aerobic exercise [149].

Cramer et al. in a meta-analysis reported that yoga improved total cholesterol (MD = −13.09 mg/dl; 95% CI = −19.60, −6.59), HDL (MD = 2.94 mg/dl; 95% CI = 0.57, 5.31), VLDL (MD = −5.70 mg/dl; 95% CI = −7.36, −4.03), triglycerides (MD = −20.97 mg/dl; 95% CI = −28.61, −13.32) relative to usual care or no intervention [147].

A systematic review and random-effects meta-analysis of 32 RCTs compared the effect of yoga to non-exercise controls and exercise controls. The results found significant improvement in total cholesterol, low-density lipoprotein cholesterol, and high-density lipoprotein cholesterol with yoga compared with non-exercise control, but results were not different between yoga and exercise controls [138].

Exercise Capacity To the best of our knowledge, no RCTs have reported the effect of yoga on exercise tolerance in CVD patients, as of this writing.

An RCT investigated the effect of an 8-week regimen of yoga ($n = 9$) compared to standard medical therapy ($n = 10$) on exercise capacity (graded exercise test (GXT) to VO_2max), inflammatory markers; interleukin-6, high-sensitivity C-reactive protein, extracellular superoxide dismutase, and quality of life in patients with New York Heart Association Class I-III heart failure. Investigators reported significant improvement of all biomarkers and functional capacity in the yoga group after 8-week of yoga training as compared to the control group [131]. Meta-analysis of two trials also suggested that yoga compared with control had a positive impact on peak VO_2 in patients with congestive heart failure [150].

24.4.5 Effect of Yoga on Cardiovascular Clinical Events

Little published literature is available on the effect of the meditation component of yoga on left ventricular mass or cardiovascular clinical events [151].

Summary Clinical trials have suggested the benefits of yoga in hypertension, coronary artery disease, dyslipidemia, diabetes, and improving the insulin-glucose ratio. However, these studies on yoga mostly have a physical component of yoga included in the intervention and results cannot be completely attributed to meditation component of yoga. There is no current evidence for efficacy in reducing cardiovascular mortality [152].

24.5 Other Meditation Techniques

Other meditation techniques such as Samantha meditation, Zen meditation, Qigong, etc. have not been extensively researched as compared to meditation techniques mentioned in the chapter. Limited studies that are available demonstrate some efficacy in effecting CVD risk factors.

24.6 Qigong

Qigong is a mind-body integrative intervention (consisting of both inner focus and a concentration on breathing and physicial practices) from traditional Chinese medicine used to prevent and cure ailments, to improve health and energy levels through regular practice [153].

Findings from limited studies available suggest the use of qigong programs for reducing stress, anxiety, and depression and improving associated health outcomes, including the promotion of adequate sleep [153]. A meta-analysis of two trials suggested benefits of qigong in reducing blood pressure [weighted mean difference, SBP −12.1 mmHg, 95% confidence interval (CI) −17.1 to −7.0; DBP −8.5 mmHg, 95% CI −12.6 to −4.4] compared to waitlist controls [153]. More trials are needed to substantiate these findings.

A systematic literature review of qigong intervention studies published in English or Chinese since 1980 found statistically significant positive associations between participation in qigong and fasting and 2-h oral glucose tolerance test results [154].

An RCT of 29 participants did not find a significant difference in cholesterol, HDL, LDL, or triglycerides between the experimental and control groups after 1 month of daily qigong training [155] but a systemic review of studies published the same year found statistically significant positive associations between participation in qigong and triglycerides and total cholesterol [154]. Results of studies on qigong results cannot be attributed to meditation only because it also involves concentration on breathing, and physical practices also.

24.7 Zen Meditation

In Zen meditation, one focuses one's awareness on one's breath and observes thoughts and experiences as they pass through the mind and environment but with an emphasis on a focus of the breath at the level of the belly and on posture while sitting [13]. Data from a small observational study suggest that there is a change in autonomic activity with Zen meditation [156]. A study of 59 elderly participants with stage I hypertension randomized to Zen meditation (20 min twice daily for 3 months) or a waitlist found significant improvement in psychological facets and overall quality of life [157]. A meta-analysis of 65 intervention studies that examined the therapeutic effect of five different meditation practices found Zen Buddhist meditation significantly reduced blood pressure [158].

For other types of meditation techniques, there isn't sufficient literature available to substantiate efficacy in CVD and CVD risk factors.

Conclusion A review of systematic reviews, meta-analyses, scientific statements, and recent randomized controlled clinical trials demonstrates the efficacy of meditation in the prevention and treatment of CVD but with distinct heterogeneity; that is, clinical effects vary with the type of meditation practiced. The Transcendental Meditation technique has substantial published evidence for efficacy in reducing stress, BP, LVM, insulin resistance, carotid intima-media thickness, CVD hospitalization, and clinical events and mortality. There are signs that this form of meditation is moving from alternative status to a mainstream healthcare approach.

MBSR has been found effective in reducing stress and smoking in many studies. MBSR has some positive effects on reducing BP, but TM and Yoga have more substantial evidence for efficacy in high blood pressure.

Studies on Yoga have shown promising results on insulin resistance and carotid atherosclerotic disease as well, but these effects are due to yoga as an intervention as a whole including postures (asanas) and breathing techniques (pranayama). These results cannot be attributed to meditation component of yoga alone, which itself is heterogenous. There is no current evidence for efficacy in reducing cardiovascular morbidity and mortality [151].

There is insufficient evidence to comment on the effectiveness of other meditation techniques, e.g., Zen and Qigong in cardiovascular disease.

CVD risk factors					
	TM	MBSR	Yoga	Zen	Qigong
Blood pressure	4 meta-analysis, 12 RCTs reported a decrease in SBP and DBP (−5/−3 mm Hg) [41–43]	From 7 RCTs, the reported decrease in SBP and DBP (WMD −2.5/−0.5 mmHg) [111]	A meta-analysis reported a decrease in SBP and DBP (−5/−4 mm Hg) [136, 137]	A meta-analysis reported a decrease in SBP and DBP (WMD = −3.67/−6.08 mm Hg) [158]	A meta-analysis of two RCTs reported a decrease in SBP and DBP (WMD −12.1/−8.5 mmHg)
Left ventricular mass or function	A decrease in left ventricular mass [46–48]	Reduced global longitudinal strain (GLS) of the left ventricle after 8 weeks of MBSR practice [112]	Improved left ventricular ejection fraction (LVEF) [140, 141], myocardial performance index [140]		
Psychosocial stress and negative affective states	Significant reductions in psychological distress [38, 65]. Anxiety [59], posttraumatic stress [60, 61] depression, [62, 63] anger, and hostility [38]	A decrease in depression anxiety [113–115], distress, perceived stress [116]	Decreased anxiety [142], perceived stress [143]	Improvement in psychological facets of and overall quality of life [157]	Reduces stress, anxiety, and depression
Insulin resistance and metabolic syndrome	Significant reduction in insulin resistance [31]	Two RCTs reported a significant reduction in insulin resistance [118, 119], while others did not [95]	Improved blood glucose [144, 145], insulin-glucose ratio [144], glycosylated hemoglobin [145, 147], and requirement for oral hypoglycemics and insulin [144] But a more recently (2017) published systematic review and random-effects meta-analysis of 32 RCTs did not find fasting blood glucose or glycosylated hemoglobin difference between yoga and non-exercise or exercise controls [138]		Significant positive associations between participation in qigong and fasting and 2-h oral glucose tolerance test results [154]
Smoking	Meta-analysis of 131 studies reported TM more effective than standard rehabilitation programs and other self-development techniques, in reducing smoking [67]	A meta-analysis of 4 randomized, controlled trials of mindfulness training demonstrated 25% of participants remaining abstinent from smoking for >4 months [120]	Most studies indicate that yoga-based interventions were effective in reducing craving and the number of cigarettes smoked during smoking cessation [148]		

Surrogate markers of CVD					
Carotid atherosclerosis or endothelial functions	Reduced carotid intima-media compared to controls [34]	Improved reactive brachial flow-mediated dilatation from baseline after 8 weeks of programmed MBSR treatment [112]	Reduction in serum cholesterol, LDL, and triglycerides [147] A systematic review and random-effects meta-analysis of 32 RCTs compared the effect of yoga to non-exercise controls and exercise controls found significant improvement in total cholesterol, low-density lipoprotein cholesterol, and high-density lipoprotein cholesterol with yoga compared with non-exercise control but results were not different between yoga and exercise controls [138]		A systemic review of studies published the same year found statistically significant positive associations between participation in qigong and triglycerides and total cholesterol [154]
Exercise tolerance in coronary heart disease patients	Significantly improved exercise stress testing; increases in exercise duration, improved maximal exercise workload, lower rate-pressure products at given workloads and significantly delayed onset of ST depression compared with waitlisted controls [73]				
Exercise capacity in cardiac patients	Significant increase in 6-min walk distance in CHF patients [74]	Significantly improved exercise capacity as measured by a 6 min-walk test. After 12-month mindfulness training compared to the control group [126]	An 8-week regimen of yoga compared to standard medical therapy on exercise capacity, in patients with New York Heart Association Class I-III heart failure. Investigators reported significant improvement in functional capacity in the yoga group after 8-week of yoga training as compared to the control group [131]		

CVD risk factors					
	TM	MBSR	Yoga	Zen	Qigong
Clinical events					
Hospitalization for CVD	87% reduction in hospitalization for heart disease and a 56% reduction in hospitalization for all major categories of disease [75]				
CVD mortality	48% reduction in the composite of all-cause mortality, myocardial infarction, or stroke compared to health education controls in coronary heart disease patients [76] Risk reduction was 66% for those that practiced with high regularity, i.e., towards 20 mins twice daily [76] In older hypertensive patients 23% reduction in all-cause mortality, a 30% decrease in cardiovascular mortality in TM participants compared to combined control [77] In older patients who participated in hypertensive studies, the adjusted relative risk for CVD mortality significantly reduced by 81% in the TM group when compared with the control group over 8 years of follow-up [81]	No difference in the composite end-point (all-cause mortality, heart failure, symptomatic arrhythmia, cardiac surgery, and percutaneous cardiac intervention) in the MBSR group compared to usual care [127]	No effect on all-cause mortality found in meta-analysis on yoga (7 RCTs, 4871 participants) 153		

Pathophysiological mechanisms of CVD					
Autonomic activity	Decreases autonomic activity [19] decreases sympathetic activity [20, 21]	Decrease in muscle sympathetic nerve activity during mindfulness meditation [87]	Balance the autonomic activity to parasympathetic side [129]	Peripheral sympathetic-nervous-system activity	
Catecholamines	Decreased plasma catecholamine levels [22], decreased adrenergic receptor sensitivity [23]	Some studies reported a significant decrease in stress biomarkers [89] including catecholamine levels [88], cortisol levels [90–93] while several did not find any change in catecholamine or cortisol levels with MBSR compared to the control group [94–100]			
Cortisol	Reduced plasma cortisol [24] Decreased cortisol response to a metabolic stressor [29, 30]	Some studies reported a significant decrease in stress biomarkers [89] including catecholamine levels [88], cortisol levels [90–93] while several did not find any change in catecholamine or cortisol levels with MBSR compared to the control group [94–100]			
Inflammatory markers		Results of some studies suggest a reduction in pro-inflammatory markers [101] and gene expression in older adults [102] while others found no significant change between groups in regard to cortisol, IL-5 [98]	Investigators reported significant improvement of all biomarkers (interleukin-6, C-reactive protein, and extracellular superoxide dismutase) and functional capacity in the yoga group after 8-week of yoga training as compared to the control group [131]		

References

1. WHF. Cardiovascular diseases (CVDs)—Global facts and figures. 2017. https://www.world-heart-federation.org/resources/cardiovascular-diseases-cvds-global-facts-figures/. Accessed 17 Nov 2017.
2. WHO. Cardiovascular Diseases Global Facts and Figures. 2017. https://www.who.int/en/news-room/fact-sheets/detail/cardiovascular-diseases-(cvds). Accessed 17 Nov 2018.
3. AHA. Cardiovascular disease: a costly burden for America projections through 20352017.
4. AHA. Heart disease and stroke statistics 2017. At-a-Glance. 2017.
5. Öhlin B, Nilsson PM, Nilsson JÅ, Berglund G. Chronic psychosocial stress predicts long-term cardiovascular morbidity and mortality in middle-aged men. Eur Heart J. 2004;25(10):867–73.
6. Frasure-Smith N. In-hospital symptoms of psychological stress as predictors of long-term outcome after acute myocardial infarction in men. Am J Cardiol. 1991;67(2):121–7.
7. Ruberman W, Weinblatt E, Goldberg JD, Chaudhary BS. Psychosocial influences on mortality after myocardial infarction. N Eng J Med. 1984;311(9):552–9.
8. Rosengren A, Tibblin G, Wilhelmsen L. Self-perceived psychological stress and incidence of coronary artery disease in middle-aged men. Am J Cardiol. 1991;68(11):1171–5.
9. Cohen BE, Edmondson D, Kronish IM. State of the art review: depression, stress, anxiety, and cardiovascular disease. Am J Hypertens. 2015;28(11):1295–302.
10. Bennett P, Carroll D. Stress management approaches to the prevention of coronary heart disease. Br J Clin Psychol. Feb 1990;29(Pt 1):1–12.
11. Ray IB, Menezes AR, Malur P, Hiltbold AE, Reilly JP, Lavie CJ. Meditation and coronary heart disease: a review of the current clinical evidence. Ochsner J. Winter 2014;14(4):696–703.
12. Brook RD, Appel LJ, Rubenfire M, et al. Beyond medications and diet: alternative approaches to lowering blood pressure: a scientific statement from the American Heart Association. Hypertension (Dallas, TX: 1979). 2013;61(6):1360–83.
13. Levine GN, Lange RA, Bairey-Merz CN, et al. Meditation and cardiovascular risk reduction: a scientific statement from the American Heart Association. J Am Heart Assoc. 2017;6(10):e002218.
14. Bairey Merz CN, Dwyer J, Nordstrom CK, Walton KG, Salerno JW, Schneider RH. Psychosocial stress and cardiovascular disease: pathophysiological links. Behav Med (Washington, D.C.). 2002;27(4):141–7. Winter
15. Rosenthal NE. Transcendence: healing and transformation through transcendental meditation. New York: TarcherPerigee; 2012.
16. Roth B. Strength in stillness: the power of transcendental meditation. New York: Simon & Schuster; 2018.
17. Nader T, editor. One unbounded ocean of consciousness. Barcelona: Aguilar Publishing; 2021.
18. Jevning R, Wallace RK, Beidebach M. The physiology of meditation: a review. A wakeful hypometabolic integrated response. Neurosci Biobehav Rev. 1992;16(3):415–24. Fall
19. Dillbeck M, Orme-Johnson D. Physiological differences between transcendental meditation and rest. Am Psychol. 1987;42:879–81.
20. Alexander CN, Swanson GC, Rainforth MV, Carlisle TW, Todd CC, Oates RM Jr. Effects of the transcendental meditation program on stress reduction, health, and employee development: a prospective study in two occupational settings. Anxiety Stress Coping. 1993;6(3):245–62.
21. Gaylord C, Orme-Johnson D, Travis F. The effects of the transcendental meditation technique and progressive muscle relaxation on EEG coherence, stress reactivity, and mental health in black adults. Int J Neurosci. 1989;46(1–2):77–86.
22. Infante JR, Torres-Avisbal M, Pinel P, et al. Catecholamine levels in practitioners of the transcendental meditation technique. Physiol Behav. 2001;72(1):141–6.
23. Mills PJ, Schneider RH, Hill D, Walton KG, Wallace RK. Beta-adrenergic receptor sensitivity in subjects practicing transcendental meditation. J Psychosom Res. 1990;34(1):29–33.
24. Jevning R, Wilson AF, Davidson JM. Adrenocortical activity during meditation. Horm Behav. Feb 1978;10(1):54–60.
25. Barnes VA, Treiber FA, Davis H. Impact of transcendental meditation on cardiovascular function at rest and during acute stress in adolescents with high normal blood pressure. J Psychosom Res. 2001;51(4):597–605.
26. Lovallo WR. Cardiovascular reactivity: mechanisms and pathways to cardiovascular disease. Int J Psychophysiol. 2005;58(2–3):119–32.
27. Barnes VA, Treiber FA, Turner JR, Davis H, Strong WB. Acute effects of transcendental meditation on hemodynamic functioning in middle-aged adults. Psychosom Med. 1999;61(4):525.
28. Reynolds RM, Labad J, Strachan MW, et al. Elevated fasting plasma cortisol is associated with ischemic heart disease and its risk factors in people with type 2 diabetes: the Edinburgh type 2 diabetes study. J Clin Endocrinol Metab. Apr 2010;95(4):1602–8.
29. Walton KG, Fields JZ, Levitsky DK, Harris DA, Pugh ND, Schneider RH. Lowering cortisol and CVD risk in postmenopausal women: a pilot study using the transcendental meditation program. Ann N Y Acad Sci. 2004;1032:211–5.
30. Michaels RR, Parra J, McCann DS, Vander AJ. Renin, cortisol, and aldosterone during transcendental meditation. Psychosom Med. 1979;41(1):50–4.
31. Paul-Labrador M, Polk D, Dwyer J, et al. Effects of a randomized controlled trial of transcendental meditation on components of the metabolic syndrome in subjects with coronary heart disease. Arch Intern Med. 2006;166(11):1218–24.
32. Bagga OP, Gandhi A. A comparative study of the effect of transcendental meditation (T.M.) and

Shavasana practice on cardiovascular system. Indian Heart J. 1983;35(1):39–45.
33. Alexander CN, Langer EJ, Newman RI, Chandler HM, Davies JL. Transcendental meditation, mindfulness, and longevity: an experimental study with the elderly. J Pers Soc Psychol. 1989;57(6):950–64.
34. Castillo-Richmond A, Schneider RH, Alexander CN, et al. Effects of stress reduction on carotid atherosclerosis in hypertensive African Americans. Stroke. 2000;31(3):568–73.
35. Barnes VT, Johnson FA, MH. Impact of transcendental meditation on ambulatory blood pressure in African-American adolescents. Am J Hypertens. 2004;17(4):366–9.
36. Barnes VA, Davis HC, Murzynowski JB, Treiber FA. Impact of meditation on resting and ambulatory blood pressure and heart rate in youth. Psychosom Med. 2004;66(6):909–14.
37. Schneider RH, Alexander CN, Staggers F, et al. A randomized controlled trial of stress reduction in African Americans treated for hypertension for over one year*. Am J Hypertens. 2005;18(1):88–98.
38. Nidich SI, Rainforth MV, Haaga DAF, et al. A randomized controlled trial on effects of the transcendental meditation program on blood pressure, psychological distress, and coping in young adults. Am J Hypertens. 2009;22(12):1326–31.
39. Wenneberg SR, Schneider RH, Walton KG, et al. A controlled study of the effects of the transcendental meditation program on cardiovascular reactivity and ambulatory blood pressure. Int J Neurosci. 1997;89(1–2):15–28.
40. Schneider RH, Staggers F, Alexander CN, et al. A randomized controlled trial of stress reduction for hypertension in older African Americans. Hypertension. 1995;26(5):820–7.
41. Anderson JW, Liu C, Kryscio RJ. Blood pressure response to transcendental meditation: a meta-analysis. Am J Hypertens. 2008;21(3):310–6.
42. Rainforth MV, Schneider RH, Nidich SI, Gaylord-King C, Salerno JW, Anderson JW. Stress reduction programs in patients with elevated blood pressure: a systematic review and meta-analysis. Curr Hypertens Rep. 2007;9(6):520–8.
43. Bai Z, Chang J, Chen C, Li P, Yang K, Chi I. Investigating the effect of transcendental meditation on blood pressure: a systematic review and meta-analysis. J Hum Hypertens. 2015;29(11):653–62.
44. Ooi SL, Giovino M, Pak SC. Transcendental meditation for lowering blood pressure: an overview of systematic reviews and meta-analyses. Complement Ther Med. 2017;34:26–34.
45. Levy D, Garrison RJ, Savage DD, Kannel WB, Castelli WP. Prognostic implications of echocardiographically determined left ventricular mass in the Framingham Heart Study. N Engl J Med. 1990;322(22):1561–6.
46. Schneider RH, Myers HF, Marwaha K, et al. Stress reduction in the prevention of left ventricular hypertrophy: a randomized controlled trial of transcendental meditation and health education in hypertensive African Americans. Ethn Dis. 2019;29(4):577–86.
47. Barnes VA, Kapuku GK, Treiber FA. Impact of Transcendental Meditation on left ventricular mass in African American adolescents. Evid Based Complement Altern Med. 2012;2012:923153.
48. Kondwani K, Schneider R, Alexander CN, et al. Left ventricular mass regression with the Transcendental Meditation technique and a health education program in hypertensive African Americans. J Soc Behav Pers. 2005;17(1):181.
49. Rozanski A. Psychosocial risk factors and cardiovascular disease: epidemiology, screening, and treatment considerations. Cardiov Innov Appl. 2016;1:417–31.
50. Compare A, Zarbo C, Manzoni GM, et al. Social support, depression, and heart disease: a ten year literature review. Front Psychol. 2013;4:384.
51. Hamer M. Psychosocial stress and cardiovascular disease risk: the role of physical activity. Psychosom Med. 2012;74(9):896–903.
52. Albus C. Psychological and social factors in coronary heart disease. Ann Med. 2010;42(7):487–94.
53. Nemeroff CB, Vale WW. The neurobiology of depression: inroads to treatment and new drug discovery. J Clin Psychiatry. 2005;66:5–13.
54. Nicholson A, Kuper H, Hemingway H. Depression as an aetiologic and prognostic factor in coronary heart disease: a meta-analysis of 6362 events among 146 538 participants in 54 observational studies. Eur Heart J. 2006;27(23):2763–74.
55. Ford CD, Sims M, Higginbotham JC, et al. Psychosocial factors are associated with blood pressure progression among African Americans in the Jackson Heart Study. Am J Hypertens. 2016;29(8):913–24.
56. Glozier N. Screening, referral and treatment for depression in patients with coronary heart disease. Med J Aust. 2013;198(9):1–7.
57. Nawrot TS, Perez L, Kunzli N, Munters E, Nemery B. Public health importance of triggers of myocardial infarction: a comparative risk assessment. Lancet. 2011;377(9767):732–40.
58. Culic V, Eterovic D, Miric D. Meta-analysis of possible external triggers of acute myocardial infarction. Int J Cardiol. 2005;99(1):1–8.
59. Orme-Johnson DW, Barnes VA. Effects of the transcendental meditation technique on trait anxiety: a meta-analysis of randomized controlled trials. J Altern Complement Med. 2014;20(5):330–41.
60. Nidich S, Mills PJ, Rainforth M, et al. Non-trauma-focused meditation versus exposure therapy in veterans with post-traumatic stress disorder: a randomised controlled trial. Lancet Psychiatry. 2018;5(12):975–86.
61. Herron RE, Rees B. The transcendental meditation program's impact on the symptoms of post-traumatic stress disorder of veterans: an uncontrolled pilot study. Mil Med. 2018;183(1–2):e144–50.

62. Elder C, Nidich S, Moriarty F, Nidich R. Effect of transcendental meditation on employee stress, depression, and burnout: a randomized controlled study. Perm J. 2014;18(1):19–23. Winter
63. Nidich S, O'Connor T, Rutledge T, et al. Reduced trauma symptoms and perceived stress in male prison inmates through the transcendental meditation program: a randomized controlled trial. Perm J. 2016;20(4):43–7. Fall
64. Eppley KR, Abrams AI, Shear J. Differential effects of relaxation techniques on trait anxiety: a meta-analysis. J Clin Psychol. 1989;45(6):957–74.
65. Orme-Johnson DW, Dillbeck MC. Methodological concerns for meta-analyses of meditation: comment on Sedlmeier et al. (2012). Psychol Bull. 2014;140(2):610–6.
66. Isomaa B, Almgren P, Tuomi T, et al. Cardiovascular morbidity and mortality associated with the metabolic syndrome. Diabetes Care. 2001;24(4):683–9.
67. Alexander CN, Robinson P, Rainforth M. Treating and preventing alcohol, nicotine, and drug abuse through transcendental meditation: a review and statistical meta-analysis. Alcohol Treat Q. 1994;11(1–2):13–87.
68. Travis F, Arenander A. Cross-sectional and longitudinal study of effects of transcendental meditation practice on interhemispheric frontal asymmetry and frontal coherence. Int J Neurosci. 2006;116(12):1519–38.
69. Bujatti M, Riederer P. Serotonin, noradrenaline, dopamine metabolites in transcendental meditation-technique. J Neural Transm. 1976;39(3):257–67.
70. Elias AN, Wilson AF. Serum hormonal concentrations following transcendental meditation—potential role of gamma aminobutyric acid. Med Hypotheses. 1995;44(4):287–91.
71. MacLean CR, Walton KG, Wenneberg SR, et al. Effects of the transcendental meditation program on adaptive mechanisms: changes in hormone levels and responses to stress after 4 months of practice. Psychoneuroendocrinology. 1997;22(4):277–95.
72. Haaga DA, Grosswald S, Gaylord-King C, et al. Effects of the transcendental meditation program on substance use among university students. Cardiol Res Pract. 2011;2011:537101.
73. Zamarra JW, Schneider RH, Besseghini I, Robinson DK, Salerno JW. Usefulness of the transcendental meditation program in the treatment of patients with coronary artery disease. Am J Cardiol. 1996;77(10):867–70.
74. Jayadevappa R, Johnson JC, Bloom BS, et al. Effectiveness of transcendental meditation on functional capacity and quality of life of African Americans with congestive heart failure: a randomized control study. Ethn Dis. 2007;17(1):72–7. Winter
75. Orme-Johnson D. Medical care utilization and the transcendental meditation program. Psychosom Med. 1987;49(5):493–507.
76. Schneider RH, Grim CE, Rainforth MV, et al. Stress reduction in the secondary prevention of cardiovascular disease: randomized, controlled trial of transcendental meditation and health education in blacks. Circ Cardiovasc Qual Outcomes. 2012;5(6):750–8.
77. Schneider RH, Alexander CN, Staggers F, et al. Long-term effects of stress reduction on mortality in persons > or = 55 years of age with systemic hypertension. Am J Cardiol. 2005;95(9):1060–4.
78. Shepherd J, Cobbe SM, Ford I, et al. Prevention of coronary heart disease with pravastatin in men with hypercholesterolemia. West of Scotland Coronary Prevention Study Group. N Engl J Med. 1995;333(20):1301–7.
79. Wright JT Jr, Williamson JD, Whelton PK, et al. A randomized trial of intensive versus standard blood-pressure control. N Engl J Med. 2015;373(22):2103–16.
80. ALLHAT Officers and Coordinators for the ALLHAT Collaborative Research Group. The Antihypertensive and Lipid-Lowering Treatment to Prevent Heart Attack Trial. Major outcomes in high-risk hypertensive patients randomized to angiotensin-converting enzyme inhibitor or calcium channel blocker vs diuretic: the Antihypertensive and Lipid-Lowering Treatment to Prevent Heart Attack Trial (ALLHAT). JAMA. 2002;288(23):2981–97.
81. Barnes VA, Schneider RH, Alexander CN, Rainforth M. Impact of the transcendental meditation program on mortality in older African Americans with hypertension-eight-year follow-up. J Soc Behav Pers. 2005;17(1):201.
82. Williams B, Mancia G, Spiering W, et al. 2018 ESC/ESH guidelines for the management of arterial hypertension: the task force for the management of arterial hypertension of the European Society of Cardiology and the European Society of Hypertension: the task force for the management of arterial hypertension of the European Society of Cardiology and the European Society of Hypertension. J Hypertens. 2018;36(10):1953–2041.
83. Segal ZV, Williams J, Teasdale JD. Mindfulness-based cognitive therapy for depression: a new approach to preventing relapse. New York: The Guilford Press; 2002.
84. Kabat-Zinn J. An outpatient program in behavioral medicine for chronic pain patients based on the practice of mindfulness meditation: theoretical considerations and preliminary results. Gen Hosp Psychiatry. 1982;4(1):33–47.
85. Grossman P, Niemann L, Schmidt S, Walach H. Mindfulness-based stress reduction and health benefits: a meta-analysis. J Psychosom Res. 2004;57(1):35–43.
86. Kerr CE, Jones SR, Wan Q, et al. Effects of mindfulness meditation training on anticipatory alpha modulation in primary somatosensory cortex. Brain Res Bull. 2011;85(3–4):96–103.
87. Park J, Lyles RH, Bauer-Wu S. Mindfulness meditation lowers muscle sympathetic nerve activ-

ity and blood pressure in African-American males with chronic kidney disease. Am J Physiol. 2014;307(1):R93–R101.
88. Kopf S, Oikonomou D, Hartmann M, et al. Effects of stress reduction on cardiovascular risk factors in type 2 diabetes patients with early kidney disease—results of a randomized controlled trial (HEIDIS). Exp Clin Endocrinol Diabetes. 2014;122(6):341–9.
89. Dada T, Mittal D, Mohanty K, et al. Mindfulness meditation reduces intraocular pressure, lowers stress biomarkers and modulates gene expression in glaucoma: a randomized controlled trial. J Glaucoma. 2018;27(12):1061–7.
90. Carlson LE, Speca M, Faris P, Patel KD. One year pre-post intervention follow-up of psychological, immune, endocrine and blood pressure outcomes of mindfulness-based stress reduction (MBSR) in breast and prostate cancer outpatients. Brain Behav Immun. 2007;21(8):1038–49.
91. Lengacher CA, Kip KE, Barta M, et al. A pilot study evaluating the effect of mindfulness-based stress reduction on psychological status, physical status, salivary cortisol, and interleukin-6 among advanced-stage cancer patients and their caregivers. J Holist Nurs. 2012;30(3):170–85.
92. Jensen CG, Vangkilde S, Frokjaer V, Hasselbalch SG. Mindfulness training affects attention—or is it attentional effort? J Exp Psychol Gen. 2012;141(1):106–23.
93. Witek-Janusek L, Albuquerque K, Chroniak KR, Chroniak C, Durazo-Arvizu R, Mathews HL. Effect of mindfulness based stress reduction on immune function, quality of life and coping in women newly diagnosed with early stage breast cancer. Brain Behav Immun. 2008;22(6):969–81.
94. Robert McComb JJ, Tacon A, Randolph P, Caldera Y. A pilot study to examine the effects of a mindfulness-based stress-reduction and relaxation program on levels of stress hormones, physical functioning, and submaximal exercise responses. J Altern Complement Med. 2004;10(5):819–27.
95. Raja-Khan N, Agito K, Shah J, et al. Mindfulness-based stress reduction in women with overweight or obesity: a randomized clinical trial. Obesity. 2017;25(8):1349–59.
96. Klatt MD, Buckworth J, Malarkey WB. Effects of low-dose mindfulness-based stress reduction (MBSR-ld) on working adults. Health Educ Behav. 2009;36(3):601–14.
97. Cash E, Salmon P, Weissbecker I, et al. Mindfulness meditation alleviates fibromyalgia symptoms in women: results of a randomized clinical trial. Ann Behav Med. 2015;49(3):319–30.
98. Malarkey WB, Jarjoura D, Klatt M. Workplace based mindfulness practice and inflammation: a randomized trial. Brain Behav Immun. 2013;27(1):145–54.
99. Rosenkranz MA, Davidson RJ, Maccoon DG, Sheridan JF, Kalin NH, Lutz A. A comparison of mindfulness-based stress reduction and an active control in modulation of neurogenic inflammation. Brain Behav Immun. 2013;27(1):174–84.
100. Nyklicek I, Mommersteeg PM, Van Beugen S, Ramakers C, Van Boxtel GJ. Mindfulness-based stress reduction and physiological activity during acute stress: a randomized controlled trial. Health Psychol. 2013;32(10):1110–3.
101. Bower JE, Crosswell AD, Stanton AL, et al. Mindfulness meditation for younger breast cancer survivors: a randomized controlled trial. Cancer. 2015;121(8):1231–40.
102. Creswell JD, Irwin MR, Burklund LJ, et al. Mindfulness-based stress reduction training reduces loneliness and pro-inflammatory gene expression in older adults: a small randomized controlled trial. Brain Behav Immun. 2012;26(7):1095–101.
103. Hartmann M, Kopf S, Kircher C, et al. Sustained effects of a mindfulness-based stress-reduction intervention in type 2 diabetic patients: design and first results of a randomized controlled trial (the Heidelberger diabetes and stress-study). Diabetes Care. 2012;35(5):945–7.
104. Hughes JW, Fresco DM, Myerscough R, van Dulmen MH, Carlson LE, Josephson R. Randomized controlled trial of mindfulness-based stress reduction for prehypertension. Psychosom Med. 2013;75(8):721–8.
105. Palta P, Page G, Piferi RL, et al. Evaluation of a mindfulness-based intervention program to decrease blood pressure in low-income African-American older adults. J Urban Health. 2012;89(2):308–16.
106. Campbell TS, Labelle LE, Bacon SL, Faris P, Carlson LE. Impact of mindfulness-based stress reduction (MBSR) on attention, rumination and resting blood pressure in women with cancer: a waitlist-controlled study. J Behav Med. 2012;35(3):262–71.
107. Blom K, Baker B, How M, et al. Hypertension analysis of stress reduction using mindfulness meditation and yoga: results from the HARMONY randomized controlled trial. Am J Hypertens. 2014;27(1):122–9.
108. Momeni J, Omidi A, Raygan F, Akbari H. The effects of mindfulness-based stress reduction on cardiac patients' blood pressure, perceived stress, and anger: a single-blind randomized controlled trial. J Am Soc Hypertens. 2016;10(10):763–71.
109. Daubenmier J, Moran PJ, Kristeller J, et al. Effects of a mindfulness-based weight loss intervention in adults with obesity: a randomized clinical trial. Obesity. 2016;24(4):794–804.
110. Abbott RA, Whear R, Rodgers LR, et al. Effectiveness of mindfulness-based stress reduction and mindfulness based cognitive therapy in vascular disease: a systematic review and meta-analysis of randomised controlled trials. J Psychosom Res. 2014;76(5):341–51.
111. Marwaha K, Schneider RH. Stress, stress reduction and hypertension: an updated review. In: Giuseppe M, Guido G, Konstantinos T, Anna D, Enrico A-R, editors. Manual of hypertension of the european

society of hypertension. 3rd ed. Boca Raton, FL: CRC Press; 2019. p. 109–17.
112. Kim BJ, Cho IS, Cho KI. Impact of mindfulness based stress reduction therapy on myocardial function and endothelial dysfunction in female patients with microvascular angina. J Cardiovasc Ultrasound. 2017;25(4):118–23.
113. Hofmann SG, Sawyer AT, Witt AA, Oh D. The effect of mindfulness-based therapy on anxiety and depression: a meta-analytic review. J Consult Clin Psychol. 2010;78(2):169–83.
114. Piet J, Wurtzen H, Zachariae R. The effect of mindfulness-based therapy on symptoms of anxiety and depression in adult cancer patients and survivors: a systematic review and meta-analysis. J Consult Clin Psychol. 2012;80(6):1007–20.
115. Khoury B, Sharma M, Rush SE, Fournier C. Mindfulness-based stress reduction for healthy individuals: a meta-analysis. J Psychosom Res. Jun 2015;78(6):519–28.
116. Omidi A, Zargar F. Effects of mindfulness-based stress reduction on perceived stress and psychological health in patients with tension headache. J Res Med Sci. 2015;20(11):1058–63.
117. Chi X, Bo A, Liu T, Zhang P, Chi I. Effects of mindfulness-based stress reduction on depression in adolescents and young adults: a systematic review and meta-analysis. Front Psychol. 2018;9:1034.
118. Rosenzweig S, Reibel DK, Greeson JM, et al. Mindfulness-based stress reduction is associated with improved glycemic control in type 2 diabetes mellitus: a pilot study. Altern Ther Health Med. 2007;13(5):36–9.
119. Armani KA, Vahdani B, Noorbala AA, et al. The impact of mindfulness-based stress reduction on emotional wellbeing and glycemic control of patients with type 2 diabetes mellitus. J Diabetes Res. 2018;2018:1986820.
120. Oikonomou MT, Arvanitis M, Sokolove RL. Mindfulness training for smoking cessation: a meta-analysis of randomized-controlled trials. J Health Psychol. 2017;22(14):1841–50.
121. Tang YY, Tang R, Posner MI. Brief meditation training induces smoking reduction. Proc Natl Acad Sci USA. 2013;110(34):13971–5.
122. Davis JM, Mills DM, Stankevitz KA, Manley AR, Majeskie MR, Smith SS. Pilot randomized trial on mindfulness training for smokers in young adult binge drinkers. BMC Complement Altern Med. 2013;13:215.
123. Davis JM, Goldberg SB, Anderson MC, Manley AR, Smith SS, Baker TB. Randomized trial on mindfulness training for smokers targeted to a disadvantaged population. Subst Use Misuse. 2014;49(5):571–85.
124. Brewer JA, Mallik S, Babuscio TA, et al. Mindfulness training for smoking cessation: results from a randomized controlled trial. Drug Alcohol Depend. 2011;119(1–2):72–80.
125. Davis JM, Manley AR, Goldberg SB, Smith SS, Jorenby DE. Randomized trial comparing mindfulness training for smokers to a matched control. J Subst Abus Treat. 2014;47(3):213–21.
126. Gotink RA, Younge JO, Wery MF, et al. Online mindfulness as a promising method to improve exercise capacity in heart disease: 12-month follow-up of a randomized controlled trial. PLoS One. 2017;12(5):e0175923.
127. Younge JO, Wery MF, Gotink RA, et al. Web-based mindfulness intervention in heart disease: a randomized controlled trial. PLoS One. 2015;10(12):–e0143843.
128. De Michelis E. A history of modern yoga: Patanjali and western esotericism. London: Continuum International; 2005.
129. Bharshankar JR, Mandape AD, Phatak MS, Bharshankar RN. Autonomic functions in Raja-yoga meditators. Indian J Physiol Pharmacol. 2015;59(4):396–401.
130. Innes KE, Bourguignon C, Taylor AG. Risk indices associated with the insulin resistance syndrome, cardiovascular disease, and possible protection with yoga: a systematic review. J Am Board Fam Pract. 2005;18(6):491–519.
131. Pullen PR, Nagamia SH, Mehta PK, et al. Effects of yoga on inflammation and exercise capacity in patients with chronic heart failure. J Card Fail. 2008;14(5):407–13.
132. Yang K. A review of yoga programs for four leading risk factors of chronic diseases. Evid Based Complement Altern Med. 2007;4(4):487–91.
133. Okonta NR. Does yoga therapy reduce blood pressure in patients with hypertension? An integrative review. Holist Nurs Pract. 2012;26(3):137–41.
134. Cohen DL, Bloedon LT, Rothman RL, et al. Iyengar yoga versus enhanced usual care on blood pressure in patients with prehypertension to stage I hypertension: a randomized controlled trial. Evid Based Complement Altern Med. 2011;2011:546428.
135. Cade WT, Reeds DN, Mondy KE, et al. Yoga lifestyle intervention reduces blood pressure in HIV-infected adults with cardiovascular disease risk factors. HIV Med. 2010;11(6):379–88.
136. Hagins M, Selfe T, Innes K. Effectiveness of yoga for hypertension: systematic review and meta-analysis. Evid Based Complement Alternat Med. 2013;2013:649836.
137. Cramer H, Lauche R, Haller H, Steckhan N, Michalsen A, Dobos G. Effects of yoga on cardiovascular disease risk factors: a systematic review and meta-analysis. Int J Cardiol. 2014;173(2):170–83.
138. Chu P, Gotink RA, Yeh GY, Goldie SJ, Hunink MG. The effectiveness of yoga in modifying risk factors for cardiovascular disease and metabolic syndrome: a systematic review and meta-analysis of randomized controlled trials. Eur J Prev Cardiol. 2016;23(3):291–307.
139. Park S-H, Han KS. Blood pressure response to meditation and yoga: a systematic review and meta-analysis. J Altern Complement Med. 2017;23(9):685–95.

140. Krishna BH, Pal P, Pal G, et al. A randomized controlled trial to study the effect of yoga therapy on cardiac function and N terminal pro BNP in heart failure. Integr Med Insights. 2014;9:1–6.
141. Raghuram N, Parachuri VR, Swarnagowri MV, et al. Yoga based cardiac rehabilitation after coronary artery bypass surgery: one-year results on LVEF, lipid profile and psychological states--a randomized controlled study. Indian Heart J. 2014;66(5):490–502.
142. Kiran U, Ladha S, Makhija N, et al. The role of Rajyoga meditation for modulation of anxiety and serum cortisol in patients undergoing coronary artery bypass surgery: a prospective randomized control study. Ann Card Anaesth. 2017;20(2):158–62.
143. Sharma M. Yoga as an alternative and complementary approach for stress management: a systematic review. J Evid Based Complement Altern Med. 2014;19(1):59–67.
144. Sahay BK. Yoga and diabetes. J Assoc Physicians India. 1986;34(9):645–8.
145. Singh S, Malhotra V, Singh KP, Madhu SV, Tandon OP. Role of yoga in modifying certain cardiovascular functions in type 2 diabetic patients. J Assoc Physicians India. 2004;52:203–6.
146. Khatri D, Mathur KC, Gahlot S, Jain S, Agrawal RP. Effects of yoga and meditation on clinical and biochemical parameters of metabolic syndrome. Diabetes Res Clin Pract. 2007;78(3):e9–10.
147. Cramer H, Lauche R, Haller H, Steckhan N, Michalsen A, Dobos G. Effects of yoga on cardiovascular disease risk factors: a systematic review and meta-analysis. International J Cardiol. 2014;173(2):170–83.
148. Dai CL, Sharma M. Between inhale and exhale: yoga as an intervention in smoking cessation. J Evid-Based Complement Altern Med. 2014;19(2):144–9.
149. Gupta SK, Sawhney RC, Rai L, et al. Regression of coronary atherosclerosis through healthy lifestyle in coronary artery disease patients—Mount Abu Open Heart Trial. Indian Heart J. 2011;63(5):461–9.
150. Gomes-Neto M, Rodrigues ES Jr, Silva WM Jr, Carvalho VO. Effects of yoga in patients with chronic heart failure: a meta-analysis. Arq Bras Cardiol. 2014;103(5):433–9.
151. Prabhakaran D, Chandrasekaran AM, Singh K, et al. Yoga-Based cardiac rehabilitation after acute myocardial infarction: a randomized trial. J Am College Cardiol. 2020;75(13):1551–61.
152. Li J, Gao X, Hao X, et al. Yoga for secondary prevention of coronary heart disease: a systematic review and meta-analysis. Complement Ther Med. 2021;57:102643.
153. Lee MS, Chen KW, Sancier KM, Ernst E. Qigong for cancer treatment: a systematic review of controlled clinical trials. Acta Oncol. 2007;46(6):717–22.
154. Xin L, Miller YD, Brown WJ. A qualitative review of the role of qigong in the management of diabetes. J Altern Complement Med. 2007;13(4):427–33.
155. Vera FM, Manzaneque JM, Maldonado EF, et al. Biochemical changes after a qigong program: lipids, serum enzymes, urea, and creatinine in healthy subjects. Med Sci Monit. 2007;13(12):Cr560–6.
156. Fiorentini A, Ora J, Tubani L. Autonomic system modification in Zen practitioners. Indian J Med Sci. 2013;67(7–8):161–7.
157. de Fatima Rosas Marchiori M, Kozasa EH, Miranda RD, Monezi Andrade AL, Perrotti TC, Leite JR. Decrease in blood pressure and improved psychological aspects through meditation training in hypertensive older adults: a randomized control study. Geriatr Gerontol Int. 2015;15(10):1158–64.
158. Ospina M. Meditation practices for health state of the research. Darby, PA: DIANE Publishing; 2007.

25 Yoga for Heart Failure

Paula R. Seffens (aka Pullen), Aneesha Thobani, William S. Seffens, Senait Asier, and Puja K. Mehta

25.1 Introduction

A 62-year-old African American male with chronic congestive heart failure with reduced ejection fraction (HFrEF) of 20% who had maintained an active lifestyle prior to the diagnosis of his hypertensive cardiomyopathy presented with complaints of exercise intolerance. Despite being optimized on all goal-directed medical therapies and in euvolemic state, he complained of feeling weak and having the inability to tolerate moderate-level aerobic exercise. The dyspnea and fatigue from exercise experienced by patients with heart failure (HF) is a common clinical problem. The patient was experiencing intolerance to aerobic exercise even though he did not have evidence of volume overload and his blood pressure was well controlled. Exercise intolerance remains a major complaint among patients with HF in those with HFrEF as well as those with heart failure with preserved EF (HFpEF). Yoga therapy (YT) may be a helpful modality for these patients. Yoga may improve cardiovascular risk by positively influencing sympathetic/parasympathetic balance, the hypothalamic–pituitary–adrenal (HPA) axis, and vascular reactivity. Yoga may be particularly helpful for those who cannot undergo traditional cardiac rehabilitation exercises due to limitations.

25.2 Exercise Intolerance in Heart Failure

Exercise intolerance in HF stems from several factors: a decreased cardiac output, low muscle blood flow during exercise, skeletal muscle dysfunction, and physical deconditioning (Fig. 25.1). Peak oxygen uptake (VO2) is often used to assess exercise capacity and is directly related to peak exercise cardiac output and muscle blood flow. When comparing patients with HF and normal subjects, the peak VO2 achieved during exercise is much lower in HF than in normal patients [1]. Patients with HF also have impaired leg blood flow and lower levels of oxygen consumption [2, 3]. Several studies have looked at using inotropic and vasodilator therapies such as dobutamine, hydralazine, angiotensin converting enzyme

P. R. Seffens (aka Pullen) (✉)
Department of Kinesiology, University of North Georgia, Dahlonega, GA, USA
e-mail: Paula.seffens@ung.edu

A. Thobani
J. Willis Hurst Internal Medicine Residency Program, Emory University School of Medicine, Atlanta, GA, USA

W. S. Seffens
Department of Biology, University of North Georgia, Dahlonega, GA, USA

S. Asier · P. K. Mehta
Emory Women's Heart Center and Emory Clinical Cardiovascular Research Institute, Emory University School of Medicine, Atlanta, GA, USA

I. Basu-Ray, D. Mehta (eds.), *The Principles and Practice of Yoga in Cardiovascular Medicine*,
https://doi.org/10.1007/978-981-16-6913-2_25

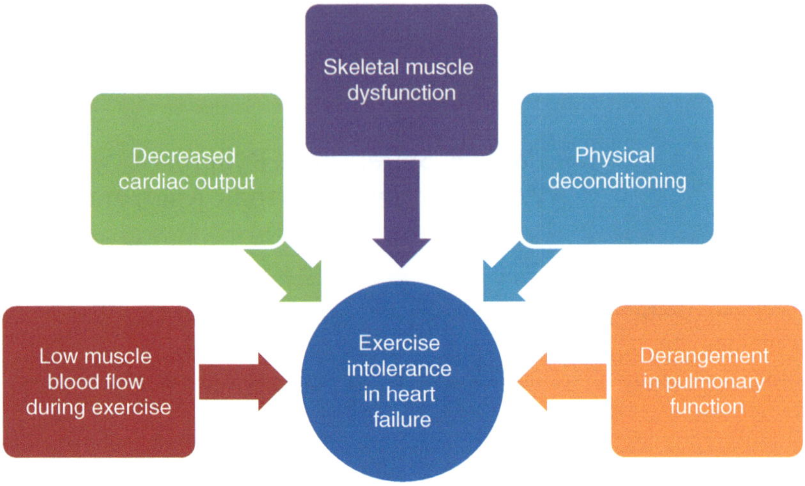

Fig. 25.1 Exercise intolerance in heart failure. There are many factors that contribute to exercise intolerance in heart failure that encompass multiple organ systems

inhibitors, nitrates, and prazosin, and have revealed no significant improvement in exercise tolerance in the acute setting despite stabilization of hemodynamics [4–6]. Since acute therapies that increase cardiac output transiently do not have an improvement in patients with HF, it is important to consider deconditioning and skeletal muscle dysfunction as contributors of exercise intolerance. HF results in a chronic hypoperfusion state which in turn leads to further skeletal muscle dysfunction resulting in poor oxygen utilization, delayed recovery of muscles after exercise, and even muscle wasting; all of which contribute to further fatigue for the patient [3, 7, 8]. Furthermore, derangements in pulmonary function and respiratory muscles also are contributors to exercise intolerance in patients with HF [1, 9].

25.3 Benefits of Exercise and Cardiac Rehabilitation in Heart Failure

Exercise training and physical activity in compensated HF patients help improve functional status, clinical outcomes, and quality of life [10]. Multiple clinical trials have shown that exercise training in patients with compensated HFrEF decreases cardiovascular mortality and HF-related hospitalizations [11, 12]. Exercise training has also been shown to reduce symptoms of depression in HF patients [13]. For patients with stable New York Heart Association (NYHA) functional class II to III for both HFrEF and HFpEF patients, current guidelines recommend an exercise-training program such as cardiac rehabilitation [14, 15]. A cardiac rehabilitation (CR) program for patients with HF should consist of a combination of aerobic training, resistance training, and inspiratory muscle training. However, patients with HF face several barriers to attending CR including decreased referrals from physicians, only being referred when HF is secondary to myocardial infarction, or lack of resources at the rehabilitation center [16]. Many rehabilitation programs do not have a tailored program specifically for patients with HF. Other challenges to attending CR include lack of awareness of the benefits of a CR program, cost and insurance issues, lack of time, limited locations and access, transportation issues, or even embarrassment of exercising in front of others. Traditionally, women are less likely to be referred to CR, and less likely to participate in CR program even if referred [17–19].

25.4 Complementary and Integrative Strategies

For many patients with HF, standard CR programs are not suitable. Eastern medicine's integrative methods such as Tai Chi, Yoga, meditation, biofeedback, and acupuncture have been investigated to varying degrees in HF population to assess the impact on physiological parameters, biomarkers, psychological symptoms of anxiety and depression, and QoL [20]. A systemic review of randomized controlled trials on these mind-body therapies in HF concluded small-to-moderate benefits of these methods [20].

Yoga is an ancient practice based on Ayurvedic medicine from the Indian subcontinent. Yoga combines various body movements and postures known as *asanas* with breathing techniques known as *pranayama* along with meditation to improve physical functioning and well-being. The *asanas* are ancient postures, often modified to fit individual levels of ability ranging from simple to moderate to more complex postures [21]. Due to the varying exertional abilities of HF patients, they may choose to practice an individualized form of Yoga. Many medical centers in the United States offer Yoga classes to cardiac patients [11]. Typically, a Yoga session will include a balanced combination of breathing techniques, relaxing postures, and a meditation component. The recently published American Heart Association's scientific statement on the benefits of meditation on cardiovascular disease states: "Overall, studies of meditation suggest a possible benefit on cardiovascular risk, although the overall quality and, in some cases, quantity of study data are modest" [22]. Complementary and integrative strategies may be beneficial in cardiovascular disease treatment and thus more rigorous, randomized, and adequately powered clinical trials are needed to further validate these benefits.

25.5 Benefits of Yoga in Heart Failure

Recent research has shown objective improvements in patients with HF who practice Yoga. N terminal pro B-type natriuretic peptide (NT-pro BNP) is a marker used in the clinic and hospital settings to risk stratify, detect, and assess the severity of HF. The NT-pro BNP is a cardiac neurohormone that is secreted from the myocardium in response to increased cardiac stress and stretch, from increased pressure or volume. A study by Krishna et al. [23] revealed that Yoga therapy (YT) in addition to standard medical therapy actually improved cardiac function and decreased NT-pro BNP levels. The study consisted of 130 patients randomized into two groups: a control group and a group that received yoga therapy for 12 weeks. At the end of the 12 weeks, left ventricular ejection fraction (LVEF) increased 36.88% in the YT group and 16.9% in the control group ($p < 0.01$), and NT-pro BNP was reduced 63.75% in the Yoga group and 10.77% in the control group ($p < 0.01$) [23]. The authors further studied the effect of YT on heart rate, blood pressure, and cardiac autonomic function. In the HF group with NYHA I and II symptoms who were treated with 12 weeks of YT in addition to medical therapy there was a significant 15.53 ± 3.34% decrease in heart rate ($p < 0.001$), 6.12 ± 3.70% decrease in systolic blood pressure ($p < 0.001$), 13.25 ± 5.22% decrease in diastolic blood pressure ($p < 0.001$), and 20.73 ± 3.80% decrease in myocardial oxygen consumption ($p < 0.001$) as measured by the rate pressure product (HR*SBP) when compared to the control group only [24].

HF is a condition of neurohormonal and sympathetic activation [25, 26].

In another study, Yoga increased parasympathetic activity and decreased sympathetic activity in patients with HF [24]. There is a clinical trial ongoing to test the effects of yoga and breathing techniques on cardiorespiratory function in patients with HF with preserved ejection fraction [27]. Furthermore, the Yoga-CaRe trial by Prabhakaran et al. [28] demonstrated that in 4014 post-myocardial infarction patients, Yoga-based cardiac rehabilitation improved self-reported quality of life (QoL) and was safe, although there were no major differences in major adverse cardiac events (MACE) in those who were in the Yoga group compared to usual cardiac rehabilitation [28]. There remains a need for large cardiovascular disease trials to demonstrate the impact on cardiopulmonary reserve and physical functioning. Whether or not Yoga should be a "prescribed" exercise form in all patients with HF who undergo CR remains a question.

Currently, Yoga as a primary or therapeutic alternative to traditional CR programs is not part of any published management guidelines for HF therapy. As recent as 2014 [29], CR became an option for all stable patients with HF to improve exercise tolerance and QoL in the United States. This development was primarily due to the positive results of the HF-ACTION study which reported that exercise training was associated with reductions in all-cause mortality or hospitalization and cardiovascular mortality or HF hospitalization [11]. Pullen et al. [30] examined the effects of Yoga on stable patients with HF in an outpatient setting where patients were randomized to either Yoga treatment or to standard medical care. The treatment group received 60-min, biweekly yoga classes led by a qualified Yoga instructor at a hospital-based vascular research laboratory for an 8-week period [30]. The measurements included exercise capacity, QoL, flexibility, and inflammatory biomarkers. At the end of the 8-week period, in the Yoga group there was a significant improvement in all biomarkers (interleukin-6, C-reactive protein, and extracellular superoxide dismutase). Furthermore, the Yoga group had a higher functional capacity as compared to the standard medical care control group [30]. In another study, the patients that attended supervised Yoga sessions reported significant body weight loss and reduced severity of depression [31].

25.6 Implicated Mechanisms in Yoga

The benefits of Yoga stem from three main mechanisms: vagal nerve stimulation, reduction in perceived stress, and musculoskeletal stimulation. By massaging the vagal nerve directly, Yoga promotes parasympathetic activation thus leading to decreased heart rate (HR), blood pressure, improved HR variability (HRV), and metabolic and psychological benefits resulting in improved outcomes [30, 32, 33]. Scientific analysis of the mechanisms of Yoga and its effects on physiological systems are beginning to emerge rapidly in medical literature. Innes et al. [34] conducted an in-depth systematic review to demonstrate the benefits of Yoga, the authors pooled 70 studies that met specific inclusion criteria between 1970 and 2004 [34]. All the studies looked at the role of Yoga in the reduction of insulin resistance, metabolic syndrome, and cardiovascular diseases. The authors found that Yoga improved cardiovascular risk profile by exerting a mechanical massaging effect to stimulate the vagal nerve [34]. Furthermore, the underlying physiology by which the practice of Yoga can improve cardiovascular disease-related outcomes may involve direct parasympathetic activation and/or release of extracellular factors such as extracellular vesicles (EVs) (Figs. 25.2 and 25.3). Several studies have examined the effects of various exercise protocols on circulating EVs, some focusing on larger particles reflecting apoptotic bodies and microvesicles (MVs). These studies revealed that platelet and monocyte-derived particles transiently increased in response to strenuous exercise [35, 36]. The impact of physical activity on the level of small EVs with characteristic features of exosomes in the circulation has been analyzed and found that the levels of small EVs increased in response to cycling exercise and dropped during the early recovery phase [37]. Intriguingly, the dynamics of small EVs in peripheral blood differed between cycling and running exercise protocols, suggesting that small EVs may be implicated in long-distance signaling during exercise-mediated adaptation processes that could include yoga. Typically these MVs contain proteins, enzymes, RNAs, and microRNAs that have significant effects on target cells that uptake these packages [38]. However, it remains unclear if newly synthesized factors or existing factors that are released from mechanical stretch are causing the observed outcomes. The third mechanism involves musculoskeletal massage from the direct mechanical effects of stretching on affected connective tissue [39]. Studies have shown that low amplitude static stretching may have beneficial antifibrotic and anti-inflammatory effects [40].

Endothelial dysfunction is associated with adverse cardiovascular outcomes [41]. One study showed that brachial artery reactivity improved

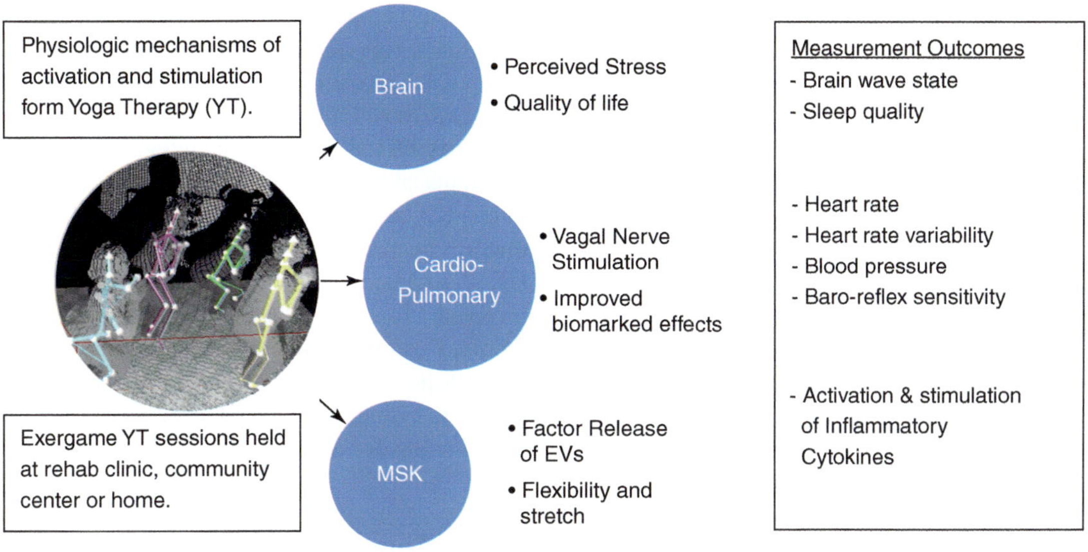

Fig. 25.2 Multisystem effects of Yoga. The point skeleton indicates the effects of Yoga on the brain, cardiopulmonary, and musculoskeletal systems. *EV* Extracellular Vesicles, *MSK* Musculoskeletal

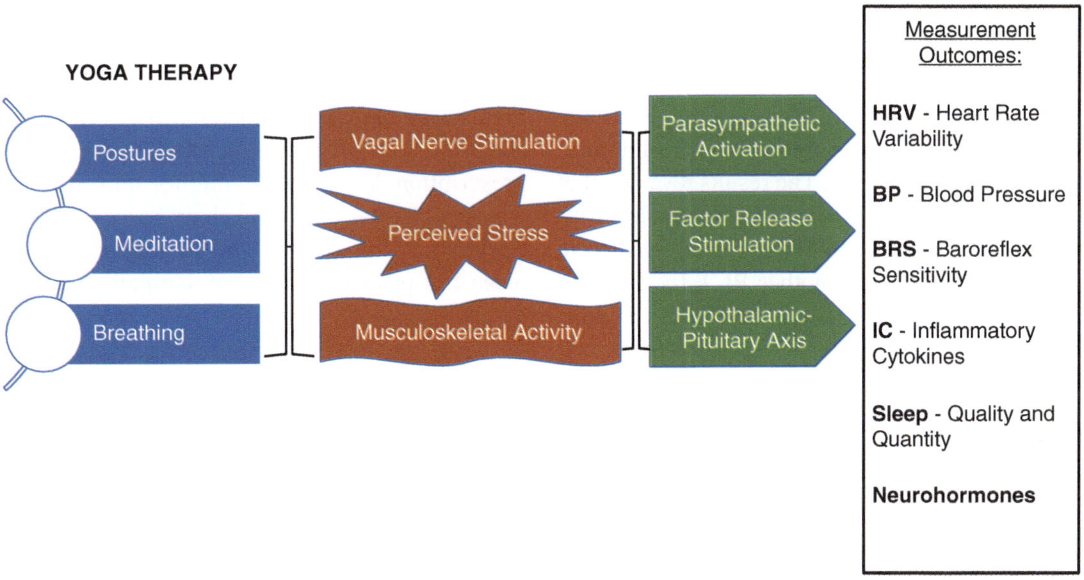

Fig. 25.3 Mechanisms implicated in Yoga. Yoga therapy leads to parasympathetic activation, factor release stimulation, and impacts the hypothalamic–pituitary axis with measurable outcomes

after a 6-week yoga treatment intervention for patients with coronary artery disease (CAD) [42]. Another group studied the underlying mechanisms of blunted vasodilatation in HF patients and concluded that sympathetic activation modulated the blunted muscle endothelium-mediated vasodilatation during mental stress [43]. These studies elucidate the role of Yoga on various sympathetic downregulation mechanisms. Additional physiological mechanisms of Yoga that have been the subject of scientific inquiry are improvement in baroreflex sensitivity, increased heart rate variability (HRV), and decreased catecholamine response to hypoxia and hypercapnia [44–46].

These studies concluded that parasympathetic activity improved, sympathetic stimulation decreased, and NT-pro BNP production was decreased in patients with HF that participated in a 12-week yoga intervention, as opposed to standard medical therapy alone [46]. Collectively, these anthropometric, psychological, and metabolic changes may lead to improved coagulation and inflammatory profiles. Yoga, therefore, may promote increased fibrinolysis, decreased free-radical production, decreased oxidative stress, and improved endothelial function [47]. The literature suggests that Yoga may be a helpful addition in management of patients with cardiac risk factors. Whether Yoga improves outcomes beyond traditional exercise and optimal current medical therapy remains unknown.

Patients with HF can incorporate Yoga into their lives to improve disease management and symptoms. Additional randomized controlled trials (RCT) have been published that examined cardiac function, pulmonary function, and QoL in cardiac patients who received Yoga interventions. Yadav et al. [48] conducted a 3-month RCT of various Yoga postures, breathing techniques, and relaxation exercises. The results revealed that forced vital capacity (FVC) increased by 24% and systolic blood pressure decreased by 11% in the Yoga group [48]. Another RCT focusing on traditional exercise methods revealed a significant improvement in left ventricular diameter and ejection fraction in HF patients that received 24 weeks of aerobic exercise training [49]. There is limited research for the benefits of Yoga therapy directly on left ventricular function.

In order to make Yoga widely available, Exergame-style technologies based on personal computers or smartphones to augment could be utilized. Efforts using 3-Dimensional room sensors like Microsoft Kinect for qualitative analysis of Yoga postures could lead to wide-scale adoption through inexpensive channels. These low-cost hardware and software platforms are programed to collect patient performance measures to assess therapeutic outcomes such as stretch, compliance to ideal postures, respiration, or energy expenditure. These applications can engage multiple participants for motivation and adherence, and provide healthcare providers with assessment reports. The data and outcomes studied thus far reveal that Yoga and breathing practices can have multiple beneficial effects for patients with HF, and could be integrated into CR programs and/or performed as a home therapy. A pilot study tested the use of Tele-Yoga and found that it is an acceptable modality for patients with HF. Participants in the intervention group that received bi-weekly 1-h Tele-Yoga classes reported enjoying Yoga and enjoyed the home-based aspect. However, further research is warranted to refine this type of technology and its effectiveness for delivery [50].

25.7 Conclusion

Cardiac patients are encouraged to exercise and stay active for a beneficial impact on morbidity and mortality, as well as positive impact on psychological factors and quality of life. Patients with HF typically have limitations that prevent them from participating in traditional exercise programs and require a personalized exercise prescription. Yoga is a flexible form of exercise therapy that ranges from chair based to more rigorous postures that can be individualized. Yoga has positive effects on sympathetic/parasympathetic balance and the HPA axis, as well as beneficial effects on reducing risk factors. Options for delivery of Yoga to patients with HF may range from participation in a CR facility or a supervised home-based program using smart and connected technology [33]. Published research to date supports that Yoga is a safe and effective addition to the management of patients with HF and results in an improved QoL. The benefits of Yoga, either in conjunction with or as an alternative to traditional exercise requires further investigation for efficacy. Multicenter randomized trials and long-term studies designed to specify the type, amount, and delivery of Yoga and to inform guidelines recommendations are needed.

Conflicts Pullen: none; Thobani: none; Seffens: none; Mehta: none.

References

1. Sullivan MJ, Higginbotham MB, Cobb FR. Increased exercise ventilation in patients with chronic heart failure: intact ventilatory control despite hemodynamic and pulmonary abnormalities. Circulation. 1988;77(3):552–9.
2. Reddy HK, et al. Hemodynamic, ventilatory and metabolic effects of light isometric exercise in patients with chronic heart failure. J Am Coll Cardiol. 1988;12(2):353–8.
3. Harrington D, et al. Skeletal muscle function and its relation to exercise tolerance in chronic heart failure. J Am Coll Cardiol. 1997;30(7):1758–64.
4. Franciosa JA, Goldsmith SR, Cohn JN. Contrasting immediate and long-term effects of isosorbide dinitrate on exercise capacity in congestive heart failure. Am J Med. 1980;69(4):559–66.
5. Wilson JR, Ferraro N. Effect of the renin-angiotensin system on limb circulation and metabolism during exercise in patients with heart failure. J Am Coll Cardiol. 1985;6(3):556–63.
6. Wilson JR, Martin JL, Ferraro N. Impaired skeletal muscle nutritive flow during exercise in patients with congestive heart failure: role of cardiac pump dysfunction as determined by the effect of dobutamine. Am J Cardiol. 1984;53(9):1308–15.
7. Belardinelli R, et al. Skeletal muscle oxygenation and oxygen uptake kinetics following constant work rate exercise in chronic congestive heart failure. Am J Cardiol. 1997;80(10):1319–24.
8. Clark AL, Poole-Wilson PA, Coats AJ. Exercise limitation in chronic heart failure: central role of the periphery. J Am Coll Cardiol. 1996;28(5):1092–102.
9. Walsh JT, et al. Inspiratory muscle endurance in patients with chronic heart failure. Heart. 1996;76(4):332–6.
10. Ades PA, et al. Cardiac rehabilitation exercise and self-care for chronic heart failure. JACC Heart Fail. 2013;1(6):540–7.
11. O'Connor CM, et al. Efficacy and safety of exercise training in patients with chronic heart failure: HF-ACTION randomized controlled trial. JAMA. 2009;301(14):1439–50.
12. Taylor RS, et al. Exercise-based rehabilitation for heart failure. Cochrane Database Syst Rev. 2014;4:CD003331.
13. Tu RH, et al. Effects of exercise training on depression in patients with heart failure: a systematic review and meta-analysis of randomized controlled trials. Eur J Heart Fail. 2014;16(7):749–57.
14. Pina IL, et al. Exercise and heart failure: a statement from the American Heart Association Committee on exercise, rehabilitation, and prevention. Circulation. 2003;107(8):1210–25.
15. Yancy CW, et al. 2013 ACCF/AHA guideline for the management of heart failure: a report of the American College of Cardiology Foundation/American Heart Association task force on practice guidelines. J Am Coll Cardiol. 2013;62(16):e147–239.
16. Dalal HM, et al. Why do so few patients with heart failure participate in cardiac rehabilitation? A cross-sectional survey from England, Wales and Northern Ireland. BMJ Open. 2012;2(2):e000787.
17. Wenger NK. Current status of cardiac rehabilitation. J Am Coll Cardiol. 2008;51(17):1619–31.
18. Sandesara PB, et al. Cardiac rehabilitation and risk reduction: time to "rebrand and reinvigorate". J Am Coll Cardiol. 2015;65(4):389–95.
19. Boden WE, et al. Exercise as a therapeutic intervention in patients with stable ischemic heart disease: an underfilled prescription. Am J Med. 2014;127(10):905–11.
20. Gok Metin Z, et al. Mind-body interventions for individuals with heart failure: a systematic review of randomized trials. J Card Fail. 2018;24(3):186–201.
21. Carroll J, Blansit A, Otto RM, Wygand JW. The metabolic requirements of vinyasa yoga. Med Sci Sports Exerc. 2003; https://doi.org/10.1097/00005768-200305001-00856.
22. Levine GN, et al. Meditation and cardiovascular risk reduction: a scientific statement from the American Heart Association. J Am Heart Assoc. 2017;6(10):e002218.
23. Krishna BH, et al. A randomized controlled trial to study the effect of yoga therapy on cardiac function and N terminal pro BNP in heart failure. Integr Med Insights. 2014;9:1–6.
24. Krishna BH, et al. Effect of yoga therapy on heart rate, blood pressure and cardiac autonomic function in heart failure. J Clin Diagn Res. 2014;8(1):14–6.
25. Floras JS. Sympathetic nervous system activation in human heart failure: clinical implications of an updated model. J Am Coll Cardiol. 2009;54(5):375–85.
26. Hartupee J, Mann DL. Neurohormonal activation in heart failure with reduced ejection fraction. Nat Rev Cardiol. 2017;14(1):30–8.
27. Lopes CP, et al. Yoga and breathing technique training in patients with heart failure and preserved ejection fraction: study protocol for a randomized clinical trial. Trials. 2018;19(1):405.
28. Dorairaj Prabhakaran MD, D.E.D., CCDC & Vice-President, PHFI. Effectiveness of a yoga-based cardiac rehabilitation (Yoga-CaRe) program: a multi-centre randomised controlled trial of patients with acute myocardial infarction from India. 2018.
29. (CMS), C.f.M.M.S. Decision memo for cardiac rehabilitation (cr) programs - chronic heart failure (CAG-00437N).
30. Pullen PR, et al. Benefits of yoga for African American heart failure patients. Med Sci Sports Exerc. 2010;42(4):651–7.
31. Kubo A, Hung YY, Ritterman J. Yoga for heart failure patients: a feasibility pilot study with a multiethnic population. Int J Yoga Therap. 2011;21:77–83.
32. Pullen PR, et al. Effects of yoga on inflammation and exercise capacity in patients with chronic heart failure. J Card Fail. 2008;14(5):407–13.

33. Pullen PR, Seffens WS, Thompson WR. Yoga for heart failure: a review and future research. Int J Yoga. 2018;11(2):91–8.
34. Innes KE, Bourguignon C, Taylor AG. Risk indices associated with the insulin resistance syndrome, cardiovascular disease, and possible protection with yoga: a systematic review. J Am Board Fam Pract. 2005;18(6):491–519.
35. Wahl P, et al. Effects of high intensity training and high volume training on endothelial microparticles and angiogenic growth factors. PLoS One. 2014;9(4):e96024.
36. Lovett JAC, Durcan PJ, Myburgh KH. Investigation of circulating extracellular vesicle MicroRNA following two consecutive bouts of muscle-damaging exercise. Front Physiol. 2018;9:1149.
37. Fruhbeis C, et al. Physical exercise induces rapid release of small extracellular vesicles into the circulation. J Extracell Vesicles. 2015;4:28239.
38. Hartjes TA, et al. Extracellular vesicle quantification and characterization: common methods and emerging approaches. Bioengineering (Basel). 2019;6(1):7.
39. Berrueta L, et al. Stretching impacts inflammation resolution in connective tissue. J Cell Physiol. 2016;231(7):1621–7.
40. Corey SM, et al. Stretching of the back improves gait, mechanical sensitivity and connective tissue inflammation in a rodent model. PLoS One. 2012;7(1):e29831.
41. Siasos G, et al. Role of local coronary blood flow patterns and shear stress on the development of microvascular and epicardial endothelial dysfunction and coronary plaque. Curr Opin Cardiol. 2018;33(6):638–44.
42. Sivasankaran S, et al. The effect of a six-week program of yoga and meditation on brachial artery reactivity: do psychosocial interventions affect vascular tone? Clin Cardiol. 2006;29(9):393–8.
43. Santos AC, et al. Sympathetic activation restrains endothelium-mediated muscle vasodilatation in heart failure patients. Am J Physiol Heart Circ Physiol. 2005;289(2):H593–9.
44. Bernardi L, et al. Slow breathing increases arterial baroreflex sensitivity in patients with chronic heart failure. Circulation. 2002;105(2):143–5.
45. Madanmohan, et al. Effect of six weeks of shavasan training on spectral measures of short-term heart rate variability in young healthy volunteers. Indian J Physiol Pharmacol. 2004;48(3):370–3.
46. Spicuzza L, et al. Yoga and chemoreflex response to hypoxia and hypercapnia. Lancet. 2000;356(9240):1495–6.
47. Sinha S, et al. Improvement of glutathione and total antioxidant status with yoga. J Altern Complement Med. 2007;13(10):1085–90.
48. Yadav A, et al. Effect of yoga regimen on lung functions including diffusion capacity in coronary artery disease patients: a randomized controlled study. Int J Yoga. 2015;8(1):62–7.
49. Hassanpour Dehkordi A, Khaledi Far A. Effect of exercise training on the quality of life and echocardiography parameter of systolic function in patients with chronic heart failure: a randomized trial. Asian J Sports Med. 2015;6(1):e22643.
50. Selman L, et al. Appropriateness and acceptability of a Tele-Yoga intervention for people with heart failure and chronic obstructive pulmonary disease: qualitative findings from a controlled pilot study. BMC Complement Altern Med. 2015;15:21.

Yoga for Mental Health and Comorbidities

26

Praerna Hemant Bhargav, Hemant Bhargav, Rashmi Arsappa, and Shivarama Varambally

26.1 Introduction

Cardiovascular diseases (CVDs) comprise a group of disorders affecting the heart or blood vessels. These include diseased vessels, structural problems and blood clots. CVDs rank first amongst various causes of death globally, causing approximately 17.9 million premature deaths each year, contributing to 31% of global mortality [1].

It has been a long-standing notion that mental health status affects physical health state, and this mind-body connection plays an important role in multiple aspects to the pathogenesis of CVDs. Currently, there is sufficient research evidence conferring that mental health comorbidities such as depression, anxiety disorders (generalized anxiety disorder and panic anxiety disorder) and post-traumatic stress disorder are important risk factors for development, progression, and poor prognosis of CVDs [2, 3]. In addition, they affect the quality of life adversely, and impact the success of effective prevention, detection, evaluation, and treatment of cardiovascular events [3]. The American Heart Association identified depression as a risk factor contributing to poor prognosis among patients suffering from acute coronary syndromes [4]. Also, as per European guidelines, depression, anxiety, and psycho-social stressors such as work-related stress or poor social support are potential risk factors for increasing the incidence of CVD and adverse outcomes in patients with existing CVD [5]. Thus, failure in the detection of underlying mental disorders may lead to an underestimation of overall CVD risk and, importantly, may lead to suboptimal quality health care. In order to recognize and address the damaging impact of psychological stress and mental disorders on physical health in CVD, adoption of appropriate screening methods is essential, following which implementation of mind-body strategies such as Yoga programs may be beneficial [6].

P. H. Bhargav · H. Bhargav (✉)
Department of Integrative Medicine, National Institute of Mental Health and Neurosciences (NIMHANS), Bengaluru, India

R. Arsappa
Department of Psychiatry, National Institute of Mental Health and Neurosciences (NIMHANS), Bengaluru, India

S. Varambally
Department of Integrative Medicine, National Institute of Mental Health and Neurosciences (NIMHANS), Bengaluru, India

Department of Psychiatry, National Institute of Mental Health and Neurosciences (NIMHANS), Bengaluru, India

I. Basu-Ray, D. Mehta (eds.), *The Principles and Practice of Yoga in Cardiovascular Medicine*,
https://doi.org/10.1007/978-981-16-6913-2_26

26.2 Common Mental Health Co-Morbidities in CVDs: Epidemiology Burden and Clinical Symptoms

26.2.1 Depression and CVD

Depression is a common mental health co-morbidity in cardiovascular disease patients with a prevalence ranging from 15% to 30% [7]. In patients with coronary heart disease (CHD), one in five suffers from depression which is three times more often than in the general population [8]. Although the prevalence of depression in established CHD is higher in women than men, depression is more strongly related to a worse cardiac prognosis in men than in women [9]. Patients of CHD with depressive symptoms are at a significantly higher risk for recurrent cardiovascular events and mortality as both the disorders share a syndemic relationship, each worsening the prognosis of the other [10, 11]. A meta-analysis of over 25 years of research to investigate the relationship between post-MI depression and cardiac prognosis showed that post-MI depression was associated with a 1.6–2.7-fold increased risk of impaired outcomes within 24 months [12]. Also, it has been a consistent observation that co-morbid depressive symptoms are an important hindrance in effective cardiac care, preventing improvement despite continued cardiac interventions, medications, and supportive care [11, 12].

26.2.2 Anxiety and CVD

Anxiety is another common co-morbid negative psychological state with CVDs [13]. Generalized anxiety disorder and panic disorder are the commonest type of anxiety disorders in CVDs. Anxiety leads to the development and progression of CHD and heart failure, thereby substantially increasing cardiovascular morbidity and mortality [14, 15]. According to a recent meta-analysis, anxiety is associated with a 41% higher risk of developing CHD [16]. Kubzansky et al. assessed independent contributions of non-overlapping symptoms of anxiety, depression, and general distress on the incidence of CHD in a prospective study of 11 years of follow-up in 1300 men (161 events). They found that anxiety was independently associated with the incidence of CHDs [17].

26.2.3 Post-Traumatic Stress Disorder and CVD

Post-Traumatic Stress Disorder (PTSD) can develop as a result of potential trauma caused by sudden cardiac events or may develop following an intrusive experience of treatments such as coronary surgery [18]. PTSD has been found to be associated with decreased myocardial blood flow, and it can increase the risk of developing CHD or cardiac-specific mortality by 27% in individuals initially free of CHD [19]. PTSD symptoms are found to be present in 10–25% of patients with ACS [20, 21], these symptoms double the risk of recurrent ACS or mortality due to ACS (highest within 1–3 years) as compared to those patients who do not have PTSD [22].

26.3 Syndemic Relation Between CVDs and Mental Disorders

There is a bi-directional association between CVDs and mental health disorders: people with CVD are at greater risk of developing depression and anxiety, and people with mental disorders like anxiety and depression are at greater risk of developing cardiovascular diseases, and both the disorders worsen the prognosis of the other. Co-occurring non-communicable diseases (NCDs) such as CVDs (associated with mental health diseases as well as due to side effects of psychiatric medications) in fact are one of the prominent causes of death for people with mental disorders [23, 24]. The end result is that people with mental disorders live 8–20 years lesser on an average than the general population, and co-occurring CVDs are often the cause of death [25, 26].

26.3.1 Cardiac Disorders and Stress

Stress is defined as the disruption of an individual's biological, psychological, and social domains as a result of environmental challenges or perceived threats [27]. Psychological stress adversely affects both physical and mental health. Accumulating evidence shows that chronic exposure to daily stressors and/or severe psychological trauma increases the risk of morbidity and mortality in patients with existing CVDs. Stress also reduces compliance with conventional care and lifestyle modification programs. Various behavioral factors such as poor diet and sedentary lifestyles are associated with chronic stress and are important risk factors for CVD [28, 29]. Stressors such as loneliness and work-related stress are found to be associated with increased risk of CVD events by 50% and 40%, respectively [30]. A study demonstrated that 30–70% of patients with existing coronary artery disease develop acute myocardial ischemia in response to psychological stressors as measured by perfusion imaging or echocardiography [31]. Such stress-induced ischemia are often un-associated with chest pain or other typical ischemic symptoms, but they have been shown to increase the risk of recurrent CVD events and mortality [32, 33].

26.3.2 The Heart-Brain Connection

The interaction of the heart and psyche is bi-directional. Stressful life experiences and exaggerated emotions affect the heart directly through the autonomic nervous system and indirectly through neuroendocrine pathways. On the other hand, change in cardiac activity and function affects conscious awareness and may get experienced as symptoms. Most of the time, psychological aspects of organic illnesses get usually ignored, or underdiagnosed and such somatic complaints of fatigue, lethargy, insomnia, and loss of appetite are generally attributed to underlying physical conditions or medications. Also, concern regarding the use of psychotropic drugs in cardiovascular conditions among cardiac care providers leads to negligence in dealing with mental health.

In such a scenario, mind-body interventions like yoga therapy can play a significant role in the effective management of symptoms without significant adverse events. Figure 26.1 provides a schematic diagram on the relationship between CVDs and mental health disorders.

26.4 Introduction to Yoga

Yoga which literally means "union" advocates controlling of the mental state through techniques that utilize behavioral modifications (*yamas and niyamas*), bodily postures (*asanas*), breath regulation (*pranayama*), sense organ control (*prathyahara*), mental imageries and relaxations (*yoga nidra*) and meditation (*dharana, dhyana* and *samadhi*) (Patanjali Yoga Sutra 2:29). Though traditionally, yoga was developed as a tool for self-improvement to achieve the ultimate union of individual consciousness with the universal consciousness (*moksha*), research in the last two decades has demonstrated its usefulness in improving psychological health, well-being, and quality of life in both health and disease [34].

26.5 Yoga for Mental Disorders: Current Evidence

In recent years, yoga is increasingly being recognized as an effective therapy for various lifestyle disorders throughout the world. Cramer et al. in their recent systematic review and meta-analysis of 12 RCTs (randomized controlled trials) on yoga for depression, concluded that yoga leads to better improvement in short term depression than relaxation and aerobic exercise and can be considered as an ancillary treatment option for patients with depressive disorders or symptoms [35]. Another previous systematic review by the same author reported positive effects of yoga on depressive symptoms which were comparable to other evidence-based interventions [36]. A couple of controlled studies have explored the use of Yoga intervention as monotherapy in mild to moderate depression as compared to the attentional control group and anti-depressant medications, respectively, and found the effect of yoga

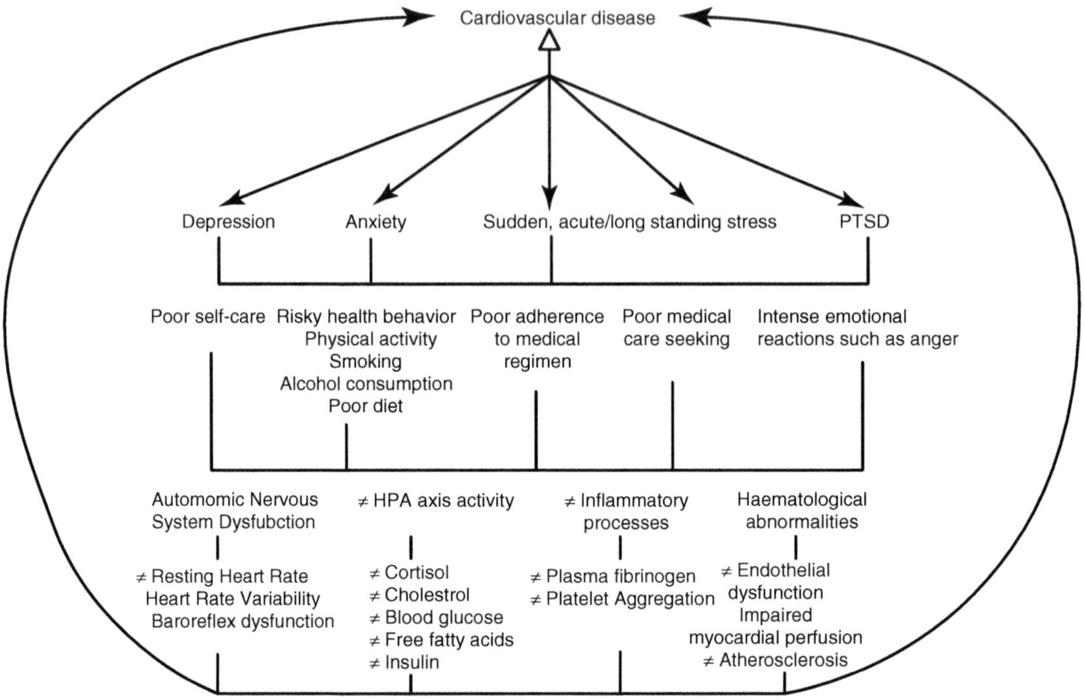

Fig. 26.1 Flow diagram depicting the relationship between mental health disorders and heart diseases

to be comparable to anti-depressant medications [37, 38]. Though there is a need for more studies in anxiety disorders, a recent meta-analysis concluded that yoga might be effective and safe for individuals with high levels of anxiety [39]. Similarly, a number of studies have reported positive effects with yoga in PTSD as well. A recent meta-analysis on seven studies found statistically significant and potentially relevant clinical effects of yoga on symptoms of PTSD though authors stressed upon the need for more robust studies in this area [40].

26.6 Yoga for Mental Health Co-Morbidities in CVDs: Current Evidence

As discussed before, it is important to enhance well-being, reduce stress and promote psychological health in patients with CVD for better disease-related outcomes. Yoga has been reported to improve mental disorders independently and in association with CVDs, and has a potential role to play in improving long-term cardiovascular health and well-being.

Yoga has shown promising outcomes for the treatment of a myriad number of psycho-somatic diseases and NCDs, including depression, anxiety, post-traumatic stress disorder, heart diseases and hypertension [41]. A recent meta-analysis of 49 trials concluded that yoga (includes breathing techniques and meditation/mental relaxation) is a viable standalone anti-hypertensive lifestyle therapy when it is practiced for at least three sessions per week [42]. Thus, an array of scientific evidence supports the benefits of yoga in both physical health and mental health co-morbidity in CVDs. Some of the individual studies showing the usefulness of yoga in improving cardiac health as well as mental health conditions in CVD patients are described in Table 26.1.

Table 26.1 Overview of Yoga Researches on Mental Health Conditions and Cardiac Health in Patients with CVDs

S. no.	Title, journal name	Author, year of publication	Sample	Intervention groups	Duration of intervention	Results/conclusion
1.	Yoga-based cardiac rehabilitation after coronary artery bypass surgery: One-year results on LVEF, lipid profile and psychological states—A randomized controlled study [43]	Raghuram N, Venkateshwara Rao Parachuri, M V Swarnagowri, Suresh Babu 2014	250 male participants, to undergo CABG	Yoga Group (YG)—Yoga-based lifestyle modification program Control Group (CG)—Physiotherapy based lifestyle modification program	Pre-op day to 6 weeks 6 weeks–6 months 6 months–12 months	Significantly better improvement in LVEF in YG than CG in those with abnormal baseline EF (<53%) after 1 year. Also, perceived stress, anxiety, depression, and negative affect reduced significantly in YG while only anxiety scores reduced in CG
2.	Effect of yoga on arrhythmia burden, anxiety, depression, and quality of life in paroxysmal atrial fibrillation [44]	Dhanunjaya Lakkireddy, Donita Atkins, Jayasree Pillarisetti, Kay Ryschon, et al. 2013	49 patients with paroxysmal atrial fibrillation	Self as control First 3 months—no intervention Next 3 months—Yoga	Yoga—60 min session twice/week for 3 months	In patients with paroxysmal AF, yoga improved symptoms, arrhythmia burden, heart rate, blood pressure, anxiety and depression scores, and several domains of QoL on SF-36
3.	Effects of yoga in patients with paroxysmal atrial fibrillation—a randomized controlled study [45]	Maria Wahlstrom, Monica Rydell Karlsson, Jörgen Medin, Viveka Frykman. 2016	80 patients with paroxysmal atrial fibrillation	Control Group—Standard treatment Yoga Group—Standard treatment + Yoga	12 weeks	Yoga with light movements and deep breathing led to improved QoL, lower blood pressure and lower heart rate in patients with PAF compared to a control group
4.	Five-week yin yoga-based interventions decreased plasma adrenomedullin and increased psychological health in stressed adults: A randomized controlled trial [46]	Daiva Daukantait, Una Tellhed, Rachel E. Maddux1, Thomas Svensson, Olle Melander. 2018	105 adults	Control Group Yin Yoga group YOMI group—Yin yoga with psychoeducation and mindfulness	5 weeks	The five-week Yin yoga-based interventions appeared to reduce both the physiological and psychological risk factors known to be associated with NCDs. The study suggests that incorporating Yin yoga could be an easy and low-cost method of limiting the negative health effects associated with high stress

(continued)

Table 26.1 (continued)

S. no.	Title, journal name	Author, year of publication	Sample	Intervention groups	Duration of intervention	Results/conclusion
5.	"More than I expected:" Perceived benefits of yoga practice among older adults at risk for cardiovascular disease [47]	Gina K Alexander, Kim E Innes, Terry K Selfe, Cynthia J Brown 2013	42 old adults on CVD risk	Yoga Group—Iyengar Yoga	8 weeks–90 min sessions for 2 days with 30 min daily home practice for 5 days	Practicing yoga (a) Improved overall physical function and capacity; (b) Reduced stress/anxiety and enhanced calmness (83% of participants); (c) Enriched the quality of sleep (d) Supported efforts toward dietary improvements
6.	Randomized controlled trial of yoga for chronic poststroke hemiparesis: motor function, mental health, and quality of life outcomes [48]	Maarten AI, Susan H, John P 2014	22 persons with chronic poststroke hemiparesis	Yoga Group—Yoga Control Group—No treatment	10 weeks	Promising results in addressing mental health and quality of life in persons with stroke-related activity limitations

26.7 Probable Mechanisms

Various studies have reported yoga to have immunomodulatory effect, and it predominantly works through down-regulation of hypo–thalamo–pituitary (HPA) axis, modulation of expression of several inflammatory mediators, thereby restoring homeostasis and physiological functions of systems related to immune responses [49]. Yoga seems to work on the autonomic nervous system and the endocrine system through correction and improved balance. Thirdly, yoga may enhance psychological health, which would indirectly improve outcomes by reducing risk factors such as poor diet, bad habits, sedentary lifestyle through better compliance with lifestyle regulation.

26.8 Role of Lifestyle in Mental Health Co-Morbidities in CVDs

Psychosocial factors such as smoking, alcohol consumption, diet, or physical activity can affect behavior which in turn can influence the risk of CVDs. There is evidence to show that patients with co-morbid depression with CHD have lower adherence to treatments [50] and recommended lifestyle changes such as smoking cessation, exercise, or practicing self-management (e.g., weight monitoring in heart failure) [51]. Improvement in mental health conditions such as depression, anxiety is associated with better self-reported adherence to medications and secondary prevention lifestyle measures [52].

26.9 Clinical Yoga Practices for Mental Health Disorders in CVDs

NIMHANS has developed scientifically validated yoga therapy modules for anxiety and depression, which include specific practices that address the clinical symptoms of anxiety and depression. As per the module, practices which open up the chest and increase energy such as *Ardhachakrasana, Ustrasana, Bhujangasana, anuloma-viloma, Ujjayi, Bhastrika, Kapalbhati, Suryaanuloma-viloma (Right nostril breathing), Pranvajapa* (Om chanting) and Yogic counseling are useful in depression [53]; cooling and calming practices such as hands in and out breathing, hands stretch breathing, *Shashankasana breathing, Pavanmuktasana breathing, Bharamari* (Humming breath) *and* Chandra anuloma-viloma (left nostril breathing) are helpful in ameliorating anxiety symptoms. *Om* chanting may also help in improving concentration. *Savasana* at the end helps in regaining energy and removing fatigue. Yogic counseling, on the other hand, helps alleviate intellectual conflicts and develops better understanding of one's own thoughts and emotions.

26.9.1 Tentative Yoga Module for Management of Mental Health Co-Morbidities in CVDs

When a patient has CVD, it is very important to avoid contra-indicated yogic practices. Thus, practices that improve mental health but are not contra-indicated for the heart should be prescribed.

Following is the list of yoga practices that should not be taught to patients having CVDs, as they may increase the venous return/workload on the heart and raise blood pressure:

1. Dynamic practices involve raising the hands above head levels such as *Suryanamakara* (Sun Salutations) and *Padahastasana (Hand to feet pose).*
2. Fast breathing practices such as dynamic *Kapalabhati* (Skull shining breath) and *Bhastrika* (Bellows breathing).
3. Inverted poses such *Sarvangasana* (Shoulder stand), *viparitkarini* (Half-shoulder stand), *ardha-sirsasana* (Half head stand) and *purna sirsasana* (full head stand).

Following is the list of practices that should be emphasized more in patients with CVD and co-morbid depression:

1. Loosening practices (total 10 min)
   (a) Slow jogging
   (b) Spine twisting
   (c) Tiger breathing
   (d) Toe bending: 1 min
   (e) Ankle movements (flexion, extension & rotation)
   (f) Knee bending (flexion & extension)
   (g) Loosening of finger and wrist joint
   (h) Loosening of elbow
   (i) Shoulder rotation
   (j) Neck movements (up and down, sideways)
2. Asanas (total 5 min)
   (a) *Ardhachakrasana*
   (b) *Ardha-ustrasana*
   (c) *Bhujangasana*
   (d) *Makarasana*
   (e) *Setubandhasana*
3. Pranayama (total 5 min)
   (a) *Vibhagiya* pranayama
   (b) *Anuloma-viloma* (Alternate nostril breathing)
   (c) Very slow gentle *Kapalabhati* (20 strokes per minute)
   (d) *Ujjayi* breathing
4. Meditation (total 10 min)
   (a) Om Chanting
   (b) Shavasana

Following is the list of practices which should be emphasized more in patients with CVD and co-morbid anxiety:

1. Loosening practices (total 10 min)
   (a) Hands in and out breathing
   (b) Hand stretch breathing
   (c) Shashankasana breathing
   (d) Spine twisting
   (e) Shoulder rotation
   (f) Neck movements (up and down, sideways)
2. Asanas (total 5 min)
   (a) *Janu-sirshasana*
   (b) *Shashankasana*
   (c) *Vakrasana*
   (d) *Makarasana*
   (e) *Pavanmuktasana*
3. Pranayama (total 5 min)
   (a) *Vibhagiya pranayama*
   (b) *Chandra Anuloma-viloma* (Left nostril breathing)
   (c) *Bhramari* (Humming breath)
   (d) Cooling pranayama: *Sitali* and *Sadanta*
4. Meditation (total 10 min)
   (a) Yoga nidra
   (b) Shavasana with deep abdominal breathing

26.10 Future Directions

Researchers have reported wide variations in the yoga methods adopted in different cardiac conditions with varying frequency of sessions. Some studies used physical postures along with breathing practices [44, 47], while some used breathing practices with meditation [46], and others imparted a holistic package comprising of all the three (physical postures, breathing practices, and meditation) together [43, 45, 48]. This heterogeneity in yoga interventions is a major hindrance to generalization of yoga practices in clinical settings. Thus, future studies should focus on the standardization of yoga programs and try to understand the underlying mechanisms of the practices. The modules should also incorporate systematic lifestyle suggestions as per yogic literature. Evidence suggests that yoga is a safe and useful tool to manage mental health co-morbidities in CVDs. More rigorous studies with objective variables, robust design and long-term follow-up are recommended in future to further establish the clinical utility of yoga.

References

1. World Health Organization. Cardiovascular diseases (CVDs) fact sheet. World Health Organization; 2017.
2. Cohen BE, Edmondson D, Kronish IM. State of the art review: depression, stress, anxiety, and cardiovascular disease. Am J Hypertens. 2015;28(11):1295–302.

3. Mensah GA, Collins PY. Understanding mental health for the prevention and control of cardiovascular diseases. Glob Heart. 2015;10(3):221–4. https://doi.org/10.1016/j.gheart.2015.08.003.
4. Lichtman JH, Froelicher ES, Blumenthal JA, Carney RM, Doering LV, Frasure-Smith N, Freedland KE, Jaffe AS, Leifheit-Limson EC, Sheps DS, Vaccarino V, Wulsin L, American Heart Association Statistics, Committee of the Council on Epidemiology and Prevention and the Council on Cardiovascular and Stroke Nursing. Depression as a risk factor for poor prognosis among patients with acute coronary syndrome: systematic review and recommendations: a scientific statement from the American Heart Association. Circulation. 2014;129:1350–69.
5. Perk J, De Backer G, Gohlke H, Graham I, Reiner Z, Verschuren M, Albus C, Benlian P, Boysen G, Cifkova R, Deaton C, Ebrahim S, Fisher M, Germano G, Hobbs R, Hoes A, Karadeniz S, Mezzani A, Prescott E, Ryden L, Scherer M, Syvänne M, Scholte op Reimer WJ, Vrints C, Wood D, Zamorano JL, Zannad F, European Association for Cardiovascular Prevention & Rehabilitation (EACPR), ESC Committee for Practice Guidelines (CPG). European guidelines on cardiovascular disease prevention in clinical practice (version 2012). The fifth joint task force of the European Society of Cardiology and other societies on cardiovascular disease prevention in clinical practice (constituted by representatives of nine societies and by invited experts). Eur Heart J. 2012;33:1635–701.
6. Duan-Porter W, Coeytaux RR, McDuffie JR, et al. Evidence map of yoga for depression, anxiety, and posttraumatic stress disorder. J Phys Act Health. 2016;13(3):281–8. https://doi.org/10.1123/jpah.2015-0027.
7. Lane D, Carroll D, Ring C, Beevers DG, Lip GY. The prevalence and persistence of depression and anxiety following myocardial infarction. Br J Health Psychol. 2002;7:11–21.
8. Rutledge T, Reis VA, Linke SE, Greenberg BH, Mills PJ. Depression in heart failure a meta-analytic review of prevalence, intervention effects, and associations with clinical outcomes. J Am Coll Cardiol. 2006;48:1527–37.
9. Doyle F, McGee H, Conroy R, et al. Systematic review and individual patient data meta-analysis of sex differences in depression and prognosis in persons with myocardial infarction: a MINDMAPS study. Psychosom Med. 2015;77(4):419–28.
10. Fiedorowicz JG. Depression and cardiovascular disease: an update on how course of illness may influence risk. Curr Psychiatry Rep. 2014;16(10):492.
11. Frasure-Smith N, Lespérance F. Reflections on depression as a cardiac risk factor. Psychosom Med. 2005;67:S19–25.
12. Meijer A, Conradi HJ, Bos EH, Thombs BD, van Melle JP, de Jonge P. Prognostic association of depression following myocardial infarction with mortality and cardiovascular events: a meta-analysis of 25 years of research. Gen Hosp Psychiatry. 2011;33(3):203–16.
13. Martens EJ, de Jonge P, Na B, Cohen BE, Lett H, Whooley MA. Scared to death? Generalized anxiety disorder and cardiovascular events in patients with stable coronary heart disease: the heart and soul study. Arch Gen Psychiatry. 2010;67:750–8.
14. Roest AM, Martens EJ, de Jonge P, Denollet J. Anxiety and risk of incident coronary heart disease: a meta-analysis. J Am Coll Cardiol. 2010;56(1):38–46.
15. Celano CM, Millstein RA, Bedoya CA, Healy BC, Roest AM, Huffman JC. Association between anxiety and mortality in patients with coronary artery disease: a meta-analysis. Am Heart J. 2015;170(6):1105–15.
16. Emdin CA, Odutayo A, Wong CX, Tran J, Hsiao AJ, Hunn BH. Meta-analysis of anxiety as a risk factor for cardiovascular disease. Am J Cardiol. 2016;118(4):511–9.
17. Kubzansky L, Cole S, Kawachi I, Vokonas P, Sparrow D. Shared and unique contributions of anger, anxiety, and depression to coronary heart disease: a prospective study in the normative aging study. Ann Behav Med. 2006;31:21–9.
18. Vilchinsky N, Ginzburg K, Fait K, Foa EB. Cardiac-disease-induced PTSD (CDI-PTSD): a systematic review. Clin Psychol Rev. 2017;55:92–106.
19. Edmondson D, Kronish IM, Shaffer JA, Falzon L, Burg MM. Posttraumatic stress disorder and risk for coronary heart disease: a meta-analytic review. Am Heart J. 2013;166(5):806–14.
20. Edmondson D, Rieckmann N, Shaffer JA, et al. Posttraumatic stress due to an acute coronary syndrome increases risk of 42-month major adverse cardiac events and all-cause mortality. J Psychiatr Res. 2011;45(12):1621–6.
21. Levine AB, Levine LM, Levine TB. Posttraumatic stress disorder and cardiometabolic disease. Cardiology. 2014;127(1):1–19.
22. Edmondson D, Richardson S, Falzon L, Davidson KW, Mills MA, Neria Y. Posttraumatic stress disorder prevalence and risk of recurrence in acute coronary syndrome patients: a meta-analytic review. PLoS One. 2012;7(6):e38915.
23. Walker ER, McGee RE, Druss BG. Mortality in mental disorders and global disease burden implications: a systematic review and meta-analysis. JAMA Psychiatry. 2015;72(4):334–41.
24. Riba M, Wulsin L, Rubenfire M. Psychiatry and heart disease: the mind, brain and heart. Wiley-Blackwell; 2011. p. 272.
25. Wahlbeck K, Westman J, Nordentoft M, Gissler M, Laursen TM. Outcomes of Nordic mental health systems: life expectancy of patients with mental disorders. Br J Psychiatry. 2011;199(6):453–8.
26. Druss BG, Zhao L, Von ES, Morrato EH, Marcus SC. Understanding excess mortality in persons with mental illness: 17-year follow up of a nationally representative US survey. Med Care. 2011;49(6):599–604.

27. Lewith GT, Jonas WB, Walach H, editors. Clinical research in complementary therapies: principles, problems and solutions. London: Churchill Livingston; 2012.
28. Sabzmakan L, Morowatisharifabad MA, Mohammadi E, Mazloomy-Mahmoodabad SS, Rabiei K, Naseri MH, Shakibazadeh E, Mirzaei M. Behavioral determinants of cardiovascular diseases risk factors: a qualitative directed content analysis. ARYA Atheroscler. 2014;10:71–81.
29. Carroll C, Naylor E, Marsden P, Dornan T. How do people with type 2 diabetes perceive and respond to cardiovascular risk? Diabet Med. 2003;20: 355–60.
30. Steptoe A, Kivimäki M. Stress and cardiovascular disease: an update on current knowledge. Annu Rev Public Health. 2013;34:337–54.
31. Krantz DS, Burg MM. Current perspective on mental stress-induced myocardial ischemia. Psychosom Med. 2014;76:168–70.
32. Jiang W, Samad Z, Boyle S, Becker RC, Williams R, Kuhn C, Ortel TL, Rogers J, Kuchibhatla M, O'Connor C, Velazquez EJ. Prevalence and clinical characteristics of mental stress-induced myocardial ischemia in patients with coronary heart disease. J Am Coll Cardiol. 2013;61:714–22.
33. Strike PC, Steptoe A. Systematic review of mental stress-induced myocardial ischaemia. Eur Heart J. 2003;24:690–703.
34. Rao NP, Varambally S, Gangadhar BN. Yoga school of thought and psychiatry: therapeutic potential. Indian J Psychiatry. 2013;55(Suppl 2):S145–9.
35. Cramer H, Lauche R, Langhorst J, Dobos G. Yoga for depression: a systematic review and meta-analysis. Depress Anxiety. 2013;30(11):1068–83.
36. Cramer H, Anheyer D, Lauche R. A systematic review of yoga for major depressive disorder. J Affect Disord. 2017;213:70–7.
37. Prathikanti S, Rivera R, Cochran A. Treating major depression with yoga: a prospective, randomized controlled trial. PLoS One. 2017;12:1–36.
38. Janakiramaiah N, Gangadhar BN, Naga VenkateshaMurthy PJ, Harish MG, Subbakrishna DK, Vedamurthachara A. Antidepressant efficacy of Sudarshan Kriya Yoga (SKY) in melancholia: a randomized comparison with electroconvulsive therapy (ECT) and imipramine. J Affect Disord. 2000;57:255–9.
39. Cramer H, Lauche R, Anheyer D, Pilkington K, de Manincor M, Dobos G, Ward L. Yoga for anxiety: a systematic review and meta-analysis of randomized controlled trials. Depress Anxiety. 2018;35(9):830–43.
40. Cramer H, Anheyer D, Saha FJ, Dobos G. Yoga for posttraumatic stress disorder - a systematic review and meta-analysis. BMC Psychiatry. 2018;18(1):72. https://doi.org/10.1186/s12888-018-1650-x.
41. Mishra SK, Singh P, Bunch SJ, Zhang R. The therapeutic value of yoga in neurological disorders. Ann Indian Acad Neurol. 2012;15:247–54.
42. Wu Y, Johnson BT, Acabchuk RL, et al. Yoga as antihypertensive lifestyle therapy: a systematic review and meta-analysis. Mayo Clin Proc. 2019;94(3):432–46. https://doi.org/10.1016/j.mayocp.2018.09.023.
43. Raghuram N, Parachuri VR, Swarnagowri MV, Babu S, Chaku R, Kulkarni R, Bhuyan B, Bhargav H, Nagendra HR. Yoga based cardiac rehabilitation after coronary artery bypass surgery: one-year results on LVEF, lipid profile and psychological states--a randomized controlled study. Indian Heart J. 2014;66(5):490–502. https://doi.org/10.1016/j.ihj.2014.08.007.
44. Lakkireddy D, Atkins D, Pillarisetti J, et al. Effect of yoga on arrhythmia burden, anxiety, depression, and quality of life in paroxysmal atrial fibrillation: the YOGA my heart study. J Am Coll Cardiol. 2013;61(11):1177–82. https://doi.org/10.1016/j.jacc.2012.11.060.
45. Wahlstrom M, Rydell Karlsson M, Medin J, Frykman V. Effects of yoga in patients with paroxysmal atrial fibrillation - a randomized controlled study. Eur J Cardiovasc Nurs. 2017;16(1):57–63. https://doi.org/10.1177/1474515116637734.
46. Daukantaitė D, Tellhed U, Maddux RE, Svensson T, Melander O. Five-week yin yoga-based interventions decreased plasma adrenomedullin and increased psychological health in stressed adults: a randomized controlled trial. PLoS One. 2018;13(7):e0200518. https://doi.org/10.1371/journal.pone.0200518.
47. Alexander GK, Innes KE, Selfe TK, Brown CJ. "More than I expected": perceived benefits of yoga practice among older adults at risk for cardiovascular disease. Complement Ther Med. 2013;21(1):14–28. https://doi.org/10.1016/j.ctim.2012.11.001.
48. Immink MA, Hillier S, Petkov J. Randomized controlled trial of yoga for chronic poststroke hemiparesis: motor function, mental health, and quality of life outcomes. Top Stroke Rehabil. 2014;21(3):256–71. https://doi.org/10.1310/tsr2103-256.
49. Venkatesh HN, Ravish H, Delphine Silvia CRW, Srinivas H. Molecular signature of the immune response to yoga therapy in stress-related chronic disease conditions: an insight. Int J Yoga. 2020;13(1):9–17.
50. Gehi A, Haas D, Pipkin S, Whooley MA. Depression and medication adherence in outpatients with coronary heart disease: findings from the heart and soul study. Arch Intern Med. 2005;165:2508–13.
51. Rumsfeld JS, Ho PM. Depression and cardiovascular disease: a call for recognition. Circulation. 2005;111:250–3.
52. Bauer LK, Caro MA, Beach SR, Mastromauro CA, Lenihan E, Januzzi JL, Huffman JC. Effects of depression and anxiety improvement on adherence to medication and health behaviors in recently hospitalized cardiac patients. Am J Cardiol. 2012;109: 1266–71.
53. Naveen GH, Thirthahalli J, Rao MG, Varambally S, Christopher R, Gangadhar BN. Positive therapeutic and neurotropic effects of yoga in depression: a comparative study. Indian J Psychiatry. 2013;55(3):S400–4.

Role of Yoga and Meditation in Palliative Care

27

Dibbendhu Khanra, Anindya Mukherjee, Shishir Soni, and Indranill Basu-Ray

27.1 Core Concept

Palliative care focuses on improving quality of life for persons of any age who are living with any serious illness and for their families [1]. Patients and their relatives usually seek for new approaches to mental well-being that can help in dealing with psychological and emotional aspects of adapting to the life-changing illness.

Various arguments in the past had tried to put role of meditation as a means of purifying the mind by allowing state of wholeness, integrity, and perfection while few considered it as a means of moving someone either emotionally or intellectually [2]. However, in terms of health benefits it is a means of producing a state of physical and mental relaxation which produces a sense of wellbeing that reduces anxiety and stress as well as allows people to look beyond life's difficulties. Life situations or health problems where the magnitude of anxiety and stress is greater, meditation is thought to provide more relief beyond the usual therapy and has been the subject of debate for researchers around the world especially for patients with terminal illness receiving palliative care. Other theories supporting the role of meditation include "crisis of faith in terminally ill" and "weak belief associated with depression" where role of meditation was thought to build up faith by self-realization and curb depression [2]. It has also been connected with spirituality that is being reflected in different forms of meditation including transcendental (associated with Hinduism) and mindfulness (Buddhism), this has an additional advantage of implementing this practice of relaxation exercise in those who believe in spirituality, moreover spiritual aspects of care is an important domain of palliative care [1, 2].

27.2 Magnitude of the Problem

Conventionally palliation has been linked with cancer, but with betterment and progression of cardiovascular disease (CVD) management, people with cardiovascular diseases are living

D. Khanra
Heart and Lung Centre, New Cross Hospital, Royal Wolverhampton NHS Trust, Wolverhampton, UK

A. Mukherjee
Department of Cardiology, Nilratan Sircar Medical College, Kolkata, India

S. Soni
Department of Cardiology, All India Institute of Medical Sciences, Rishikesh, India

I. Basu-Ray (✉)
Department of Cardiology, All India Institute of Medical Sciences, Rishikesh, India

Department of Cardiology, Memphis Veteran Administration Hospital, Memphis, TN, USA

School of Public Health, The University of Memphis, Memphis, TN, USA
e-mail: ibr@ibasuray.com

I. Basu-Ray, D. Mehta (eds.), *The Principles and Practice of Yoga in Cardiovascular Medicine*, https://doi.org/10.1007/978-981-16-6913-2_27

longer and hence the need for palliation is growing in later parts of their life. Age-adjusted CVD mortality is 170/100,00 among males and 108/100,000 among females in the United States of America (USA) [3]. The rates are 2–3 times higher in India with 349/100,000 among males and 265/100,000 among women [3]. Psychological stress has got an immense effect on heart health [4]. After an acute myocardial infarction (AMI) the uncertainty, helplessness, and unable to control the flow of events leads to immense psychological stress and impairs the patients' mental health as well as cardiovascular health [5]. Similarly, in patients with heart failure (HF), complexities of self-management, progressive functional limitations, and exacerbations leading to hospitalizations lead to high levels of stress resulting in increased risk of adverse situations, diminished quality of life, and more burdensome disease course [6]. Thus, maintaining mental and emotional wellbeing poses additional challenges to all the CVD patients that may be in different stages of the disease progression.

Palliative care is challenging for physicians to offer as well as for patients to receive. The experience of accepting this challenge at the end of the life for a patient may raise various questions such as why did it happen? Why me? Why now? Why continue if it is going to end someday? In this situation, answers to these questions may not help and the only solution seems to adapt to the situation and to maintain mental and emotional wellbeing to continue to receive palliative care [7].

27.3 Physiological Rationale for the Use of Yoga and Meditation

Perceived stress can affect intrinsic and extrinsic cardiovascular disease process like plaque formation, progression, and platelet reactivity. It also delays care seeking. It also induces negative responses like anger and hostility which increases the risk and adversities of CVD [5]. Increased sympathetic drive and withdrawal of parasympathetic tone leads to mechanical and electrical adversities which can amount to sudden cardiac death or fatal arrhythmias [8]. Thus, physiological rationale behind behavioral interventions such as yoga and meditation is improving CVD outcomes by decreasing stress and disrupting its detrimental effects on CVD pathophysiology [9].

In CVD, including coronary artery disease (CAD), heart failure, and arrhythmias, various studies have shown beneficial effects in prevention and cardiac rehabilitation [10–15]. The possible physiological bases have been proposed to be stress reduction, decreased sympathetic activity, neurohormonal, neuroendocrine, and metabolic alterations as discussed above [10, 13, 15] (see Fig. 27.1).

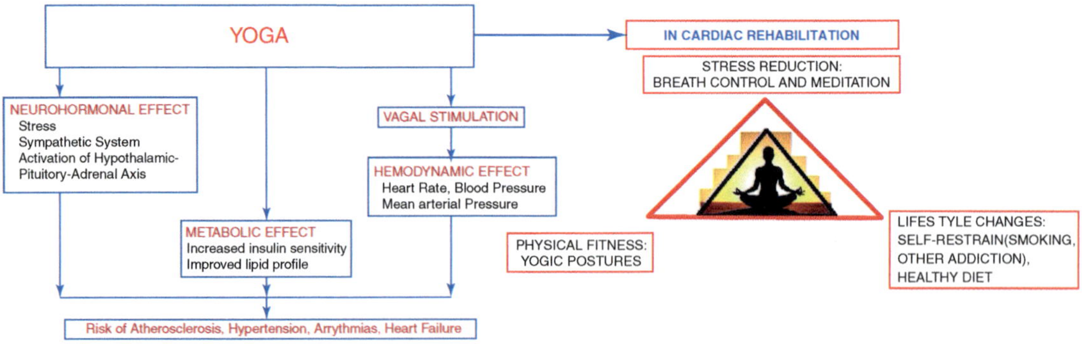

Fig. 27.1 Illustrating pathophysiologic rationale for usefulness of Yoga in palliative care by reducing stress, positive cardiovascular effects, and its role in cardiac rehabilitation

27.4 Yoga and Meditation for Palliative Care Need of Transition from "Cafeteria Approach" to "Tailor Made Approach"

Palliative care physicians along with yoga-meditation trainers can provide "tailor made" therapy for an individual patient with special emphasis on involving those yoga exercises, which are easy to perform and are not likely discomfort or harmful in anyways [16]. The past decades have seen individual patients seeking alternative therapy with a basket of choices that include Yoga, meditation, aromatherapy, massage, acupuncture, and various other therapies but with recent emerging evidences and trials' results, tailor-made yoga, and meditation may be a useful alternative, as some difficult yoga exercises may not be feasible for a particular patient and treating physician can guide in advising them which is feasible and useful thus conceptualizing "tailor made yoga" [16–18]. Some of the Yoga practices are compiled in Table 27.1 and Fig. 27.2.

Table 27.1 Description of various yoga and meditation practices that can be adapted in palliative care

Serial no.	Yoga and meditation practice	Description	Caution
1	Yogic small movements (Sukshma Vyayamas) [18]	Small movements involving neck, shoulder, trunk, and knee	Should be avoided if painful on initiation
2	Yoga body postures (Asanas) [19, 20]	Stretching exercises involving different muscles in different postures	Avoid if arthritis or neurogenic pain/ sciatica
3.	Regulated breathing practices (PRANAYAMA) [16, 18]	Different forms of breathing exercises with varying timing and duration of inhalation and exhalation	Physician consultation is required in particular lung diseases and should be avoided in acute lung diseases with breathlessness and those at risk of pneumothorax
4.	Meditation (Dhyan) [16]	An act of continuous contemplation "Internalized awareness"	Prolonged act of just relaxation may not be useful

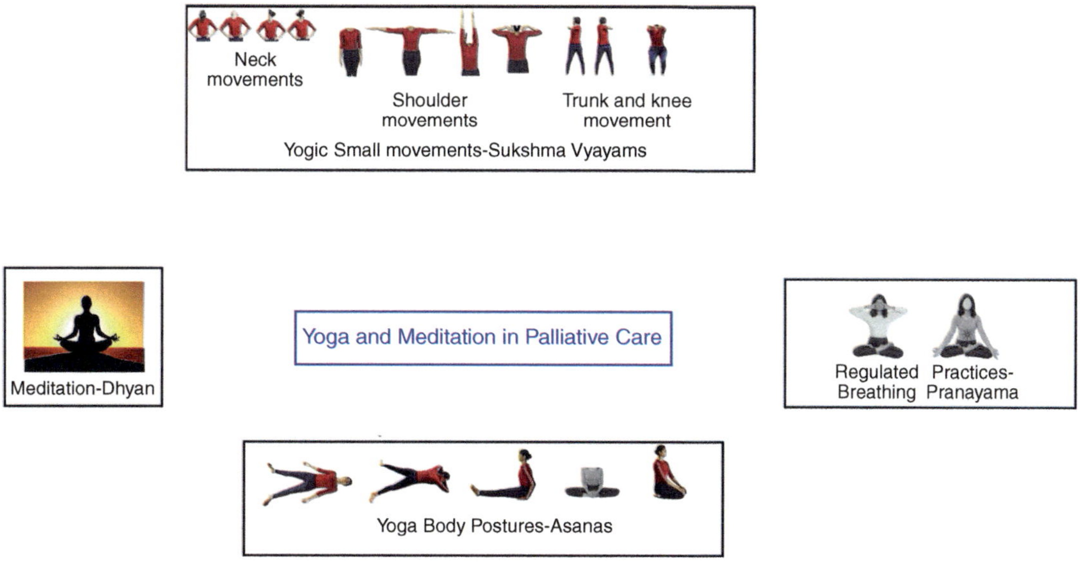

Fig. 27.2 Illustrating different simplest forms of Yoga that can be selectively practiced by a patient taking palliative care under physician guidance

27.5 Evidence Supporting Yoga and Meditation in Palliative Care

Various studies have been published in past to find conclusive evidence of the usefulness of yoga and meditation in palliative care [19]. Prabhakaran et al. reported that in patients of AMI randomized to yoga in cardiac rehabilitation and enhanced standard care, self-rated health was better in the yoga group (baseline-adjusted mean difference in favor of yoga 1.5; 95% CI: 0.5 to 2.5). Major adverse cardiac events (MACE) were lesser in the yoga group (hazard ratio: 0.90; 95% confidence interval [CI]: 0.71 to 1.15). More patients in yoga group returned to pre-infarct activities [9]. Tobacco cessation or treatment adherence did not differ among the groups [9]. Better quality of life, lesser cardiac events, and functional improvement have been reported much earlier by Ornish et al. and Manchanda et al. in patients of CAD practicing yoga and lifestyle modifications [20, 21]. Christa et al. reported improved parasympathetic activity and heart rate variability in optimally medicated post-infarct patients [8]. The YOGA My Heart Study pointed out the role of yoga in paroxysmal atrial fibrillation (AF) reducing both symptomatic ($p < 0.001$) and asymptomatic AF ($p < 0.001$) and improving anxiety, depression ($p < 0.001$), and several domains of quality of life [22]. A meta-analysis of two studies found yoga to enhance exercise capacity (peak VO2 weighted mean difference 3.87 95% CI: 1.95 to 5.80) and health-related quality of life (standardized mean difference −12.46 95% CI: −22.49 to −2.43) in patients of congestive HF [23].

27.6 Evidence Gaps and Future Directions

Key research needs to be performed if Yoga and meditation in palliative care are going to achieve their potential to enhance value throughout the health care system. Moreover, important gaps in clinical evidence need to be addressed so that persons with serious illnesses can be offered care that is more useful rather than just focusing on improving psychosocial aspects. Thus optimal, and randomized, controlled trials of interventions are needed to identify benefits of yoga and meditation in palliative care.

Conflicts of Interest None.

References

1. Kelley AS, Morrison RS. Palliative care for the seriously ill. N Engl J Med. 2015;373:747–55.
2. Ball MS, Vernon B. A review on how meditation could be used to comfort the terminally ill. Palliat Support Care. 2015;13:1469–72.
3. World health organization. Global status report on non-communicable diseases 2014. Geneva: World Health Organization; 2014.
4. Dimsdale JE. Psychological stress and cardiovascular disease. J Am Coll Cardiol. 2008;51(13):1237–46. https://doi.org/10.1016/j.jacc.2007.12.024.
5. Xu X, Bao H, Strait KM, Edmondson DE, Davidson KW, Beltrame JF, Bueno H, Lin H, Dreyer RP, Brush JE, Spertus JA, Lichtman JH, D'Onofrio G, Krumholz HM. Perceived stress after acute myocardial infarction: a comparison between young and middle-aged women versus men. Psychosom Med. 2017;79(1):50–8. https://doi.org/10.1097/PSY.0000000000000429.
6. Harris KM, Jacoby DL, Lampert R, Soucier RJ, Burg MM. Psychological stress in heart failure: a potentially actionable disease modifier. Heart Fail Rev. 2020; https://doi.org/10.1007/s10741-020-10056-8.
7. Candy B, Jones L, Varagunam M, Speck P, Tookman A, King M. Spiritual and religious interventions for well-being of adults in the terminal phase of disease. Cochrane Database Syst Rev. 2012;16:CD007544.
8. Christa E, Srivastava P, Chandran DS, Jaryal AK, Yadav RK, Roy A, Deepak KK. Effect of yoga-based cardiac rehabilitation on heart rate variability: randomized controlled trial in patients post-MI. Int J Yoga Ther. 2019;29(1):43–50. https://doi.org/10.17761/2019-00019.
9. Prabhakaran D, Chandrasekaran AM, Singh K, Mohan B, Chattopadhyay K, Chadha DS, Yoga-CaRe Trial Investigators, et al. Yoga-based cardiac rehabilitation after acute myocardial infarction: a randomized trial. J Am Coll Cardiol. 2020;75(13):1551–61. https://doi.org/10.1016/j.jacc.2020.01.050.
10. Yeung A, Kiat H, Denniss AR, Cheema BS, Bensoussan A, Machliss B, et al. Randomised controlled trial of a 12 week yoga intervention on negative affective states, cardiovascular and cognitive function in post-cardiac rehabilitation patients. BMC Complement Altern Med. 2014;14:411.

11. Pullen PR, Seffens WS, Thompson WR. Yoga for heart failure: a review and future research. Int J Yoga. 2018;11:91–8.
12. Deutsch SB, Krivitsky EL. The impact of yoga on atrial fibrillation: a review of the yoga my heart study. J Arrhythm. 2015;31:337–8.
13. Chandrasekaran AM, Kinra S, Ajay VS, Chattopadhyay K, Singh K, Singh K, et al. Effectiveness and cost-effectiveness of a yoga-based cardiac rehabilitation (Yoga-CaRe) program following acute myocardial infarction: study rationale and design of a multi-center randomized controlled trial. Int J Cardiol. 2019;280:14–8.
14. Manchanda SC. Yoga – a promising technique to control cardiovascular disease. Indian Heart J. 2014;66:487–9.
15. Chattopadhyay K, Chandrasekaran AM, Praveen PA, Manchanda SC, Madan K, Ajay VS, et al. Development of a yoga-based cardiac rehabilitation (Yoga-CaRe) programme for secondary prevention of myocardial infarction. Evid Based Complement Alternat Med. 2019;2019:7470184.
16. Deshpande A. Yoga for palliative care. Integr Med Res. 2018;7:211–3.
17. Shafto K, Gouda S, Catrine K, Brown ML. Integrative approaches in pediatric palliative care. Children (Basel). 2018;5:75.
18. Ministry of AYUSH. Common yoga protocol 2019. http://ayush.gov.in/booklets-common-yoga-protocol-0.
19. Rathore S, Kumar B, Tehrani S, Khanra D, Duggal B, Chandra PD. Cardiac rehabilitation: appraisal of current evidence and utility of technology aided home-based cardiac rehabilitation. Indian Heart J. 2020;72(6):491–9. https://doi.org/10.1016/j.ihj.2020.08.013.
20. Manchanda SC, Narang R, Reddy KS, et al. Retardation of coronary atherosclerosis with yoga lifestyle intervention. J Assoc Phys India. 2000;48:687–94.
21. Ornish D, Scherwitz LW, Billings JH, et al. Intensive lifestyle changes for reversal of coronary heart disease. J Am Med Assoc. 1998;280:2001–7.
22. Lakkireddy D, Atkins D, Pillarisetti J, Ryschon K, Bommana S, Drisko J, et al. Effect of yoga on arrhythmia burden, anxiety, depression, and quality of life in paroxysmal atrial fibrillation: the YOGA my heart study. J Am Coll Cardiol. 2013;61(11):1177–82. https://doi.org/10.1016/j.jacc.2012.11.060.
23. Gomes-Neto M, Rodrigues ES Jr, Silva WM Jr, Carvalho VO. Effects of yoga in patients with chronic heart failure: a meta-analysis. Arq Bras Cardiol. 2014;103(5):433–9. https://doi.org/10.5935/abc.20140149.

Yoga-Based Cardiac Rehabilitation Program for Cardiovascular Health

28

Ambalam M. Chandrasekaran,
Dorairaj Prabhakaran, and Sanjay Kinra

28.1 Introduction

Cardiovascular diseases (CVDs) are a leading cause of death and disability worldwide and are increasing rapidly in much of the developing world. It accounted for 17 million deaths in 2016 with atherosclerotic diseases accounting for about 15 million deaths. Also, CVDs were responsible for 320 million years of life lost in 2016 most of which were premature [1, 2].

One of the greatest successes in reducing CVD mortality in high-income countries is secondary prevention [3]. Secondary prevention has the potential to reduce by almost 75% adverse CV outcomes in patients who suffer an acute coronary syndrome (ACS) or develop coronary artery disease (CAD). Thus, there is a vital need for effective secondary prevention interventions, aimed at improving both the duration and the quality of life of those affected. The psychosocial and economic aspects of CVD management are particularly important, not only in the high- and middle-income countries with its ageing population, but also in low and low-middle income countries, where acute myocardial infarction (AMI) increasingly occurs in the 30s and 40s, in previously healthy adults who experience considerable difficulty in accepting their new health status, with implications for enthusiasm and readiness to re-engage with the family and return to economically productive activity [4]. Cardiac rehabilitation has been demonstrated to achieve secondary prevention goals as well as improve the psychosocial status of individuals who have suffered ACS or have undergone coronary artery bypass surgery. However, it is not available in most LMICs because it is expensive and alternate ways of CR need to be explored [5].

Yoga is an ancient Indian system of philosophy; a mind–body discipline encompassing an array of philosophical precepts, mental attitudes and physical practices. Hatha yoga, the most commonly recognised form of yoga incorporates elements of physical poses, breath control and meditation, and self-restraint. As such, it covers most of the elements of a comprehensive CR programme: improved physical fitness, stress reduction and lifestyle. The structure of a yoga training programme is also similar to CR and

A. M. Chandrasekaran
Centre for Chronic Disease Control,
New Delhi, Delhi, India
e-mail: chandrasekaran@ccdcindia.org

D. Prabhakaran (✉)
Research and Policy, Public Health Foundation of India, Gurgaon, National Capital Region, Haryana, India
e-mail: dprabhakaran@phfi.org; dprabhakaran@ccdcindia.org

S. Kinra
Non-Communicable Disease Epidemiology, London School of Hygiene and Tropical Medicine, London, UK
e-mail: sanjay.kinra@lshtm.ac.uk

I. Basu-Ray, D. Mehta (eds.), *The Principles and Practice of Yoga in Cardiovascular Medicine*,
https://doi.org/10.1007/978-981-16-6913-2_28

offers cardiovascular benefits. Yoga, therefore, simulates the cardiac rehabilitation programme and encompasses core components of CR [6].

In this chapter, we will discuss the benefits and limitations of cardiac rehabilitation; the current state of evidence of cardiovascular benefits of yoga and relevance of Yoga-based cardiac rehabilitation programme in cardiovascular conditions.

28.2 Cardiac Rehabilitation

The World Health Organization defines cardiac rehabilitation as "*the sum of activities required to influence favorably the underlying cause of the disease, as well as to ensure the patient the best possible physical, mental and social conditions, so that they may, by their own efforts, preserve or resume when lost, as normal a place as possible in the life of the community*" [7]. It is also defined as a coordinated and structured programme designed to remove or reduce the underlying causes of cardiovascular disease, as well as to provide the best possible physical, mental and social conditions, so that people can, by their own efforts, continue to play a full part in their community [8]. Several professional organisations provided several definitions of CR. All these definitions always stressed CR as various activities aimed at improving the health outcomes following a cardiac illness.

1. *History of Cardiac Rehabilitation programme*
   The benefits of exercise in angina pectoris were documented in the 1700s. However, it was largely ignored for more than two centuries. In the 1930s, bed rest for 6 weeks was the norm after acute myocardial infarction. Later in the 1940s, sitting in chair was introduced and in the 1950s, a short walking of 3–5 min was introduced after acute myocardial infarction [9]. Soon, the benefits of early mobilisation were observed with benefits in reduction of hospital stay, reduction in mortality and morbidity. Further, several studies on exercise training added evidence base for the beneficial effects of early mobilisation and introduction of physical activity after a cardiac event.
   Later, as the research evolves over the importance of dietary approaches, behavioural modifications to manage stress and re-orient to normal and healthy life, these components were included in the recovery after cardiac event. In the post PCI era, the comprehensive rehabilitation programme evolved further to include various components including tailored behavioural modification and lifestyle risk factor management, psychosocial health, medical risk factor management, cardioprotective therapies in a long-term perspective with regular clinical audits and evaluation.
2. *Benefits of Cardiac rehabilitation programmes*
   Cardiac rehabilitation is associated with numerous benefits. Recent Cochrane review reported that, in patients with coronary artery disease, exercise-based cardiac rehabilitation reduced cardiovascular mortality and hospital admissions [10]. In addition, exercise-based cardiac rehabilitation programme is found to be cost-effective and improve quality of life [11]. Another Cochrane review found that cardiac rehabilitation may reduce all-cause mortality in the long term and reduce hospital admissions, heart failure specific admissions and improved quality of life in patients with heart failure [12].
   Physiologically, exercise training may improve myocardial oxygen demand, endothelial function, autonomic tone, coagulation and clotting factors, inflammatory markers, and the development of coronary collateral vessels [13–15]. In addition, exercise training may improve risk factors of atherosclerotic cardiovascular diseases such as reduction in lipids, blood pressure, heart rate, tobacco cessation, etc. [16]. Dietary approaches may also aid in risk factor control. Psychological interventions may reduce depression and anxiety.
3. *Essential components of CR programmes*
   Recent comprehensive cardiac rehabilitation programme includes various components such as health behaviour change and educa-

tion, lifestyle risk factor management including physical activity and exercise, healthy eating and body composition, tobacco cessation, psychosocial health, medical risk management, long term strategies and audit and evaluation [17, 18].

However, the quintessential components of cardiac rehabilitation programme are improving physical fitness, reducing stress and improving lifestyle including dietary changes in addition to pharmacological management.

4. *Current models of CR*

   Hospital-based cardiac rehabilitation may involve four phases. The first phase is delivered during hospital stay which may comprise of early mobilisation and health education. The second phase of CR is the post-discharge pre-exercise period where the support and education will be provided through telephonic calls and or home visits. The third phase of cardiac rehabilitation is the crucial part of cardiac rehabilitation. It includes regular outpatient based care involving supervised exercise training, behavioural change programmes and nutritional counselling. These may be spread over 13 sessions to 36 sessions. The fourth phase is the long-term self-care at home which involves inculcating healthy habits such as prescribed dietary changes and regular physical activity over the long term [17, 19].

   Increasingly, home-based cardiac rehabilitation programmes are becoming popular. It may have all the components of the hospital-based CR programme without any hospital visits by the patients. Hybrid CR programmes involving both home and hospital based are also increasingly becoming popular [20].

5. *Indications and contra-indications of CR*

   CR is indicated in recent myocardial infarction, acute coronary artery syndrome, chronic stable angina, congestive heart failure, after coronary artery bypass surgery, after a percutaneous coronary intervention, valvular surgery and cardiac transplantation [9].

   It is contraindicated in unstable angina, acute decompensated congestive heart failure, complex ventricular arrhythmias, severe pulmonary hypertension (right ventricular systolic pressure > 60 mm Hg), intracavitary thrombus, recent thrombophlebitis with or without pulmonary embolism, severe obstructive cardiomyopathies, severe or symptomatic aortic stenosis, uncontrolled inflammatory or infectious pathology and any musculoskeletal condition that prevents adequate participation in exercise.

6. *Limitations of CR*

   Although CR programme has numerous benefits, there are several limitations.

   (a) *Validity of scientific evidence:* Most of the evidence supporting the use of cardiac rehabilitation stemmed from the pre-PCI era where mortality and morbidity were higher following a cardiac event. With the advancement in pharmacological management and interventional strategies, need for exercise-based CR has been often questioned [21]. While, there is a consensus to involve various approaches in comprehensive cardiac rehabilitation programmes, efficacy and effectiveness of various approaches are not often backed by sufficient evidence from randomised controlled trials [22–24]. This limits the prescription of CR or referral by cardiologists and further limits uptake of CR among patients.

   (b) *Need for multidisciplinary team:* Cardiac rehabilitation programme as recommended by western professional societies demands a multidisciplinary team which are often resource intensive. This jeopardises the availability and access of CR to the needy population and hence, availability of CR programmes is virtually non-existent in resource constraint settings [5, 25–27].

   (c) Low participation rate: Participation in CR programme is very low even in the high-income countries due to various reasons such as problems with commuting and lack of social and family support etc. [28] Difficulties in commuting to the centre offering CR programme was very often quoted as a barrier to participation.

This could be because of the aggregation of CR centres in cities and inadequate essential CR services at the primary care level. Another major barrier in the uptake of CR is the lack of social and family support especially in women and the elderly population who often require additional support in availing the CR services [29–31].

28.3 Yoga-Based Cardiac Rehabilitation Programme

Yoga is an ancient Indian system of philosophy; a mind–body discipline encompassing an array of philosophical precepts, mental attitudes and physical practices. Of the seven major branches of yoga, Hatha yoga, which itself includes many different styles (e.g. Iyengar, Ashtanga, etc.), is probably the most commonly recognised and incorporates elements of physical poses, breath control and meditation, and self-restraint (including that of diet, smoking, alcohol intake and sleep patterns) [6]. As such, it covers most of the elements of a comprehensive CR programme: improved physical fitness, stress reduction and lifestyle (Fig. 28.1). The philosophical aspects of yoga may be particularly beneficial in engendering healthy mental attitudes for engagement with society, potentially of great benefit following a life-threatening event that results in considerable introspection. The structure of a yoga training programme is also similar to CR (a series of exercise-cum-education sessions) but requires considerably fewer resources (a yoga teacher). Yoga, therefore, simulates cardiac rehabilitation programme and encompasses core components of CR.

While yoga may not be as physically intensive as a physical activity or exercise programme, it has its own merits [32]. Near dozen of randomised controlled trials evaluating the effects of Yoga versus on exercise on various outcomes related to cardiovascular health, general health and other biomarkers. Most of these studies have reported that, except for outcomes related to energy expenditure and metabolic equivalents, yoga programme is not different from exercise programme in improving these outcomes and in most cases, yoga outperformed exercise programmes [32].

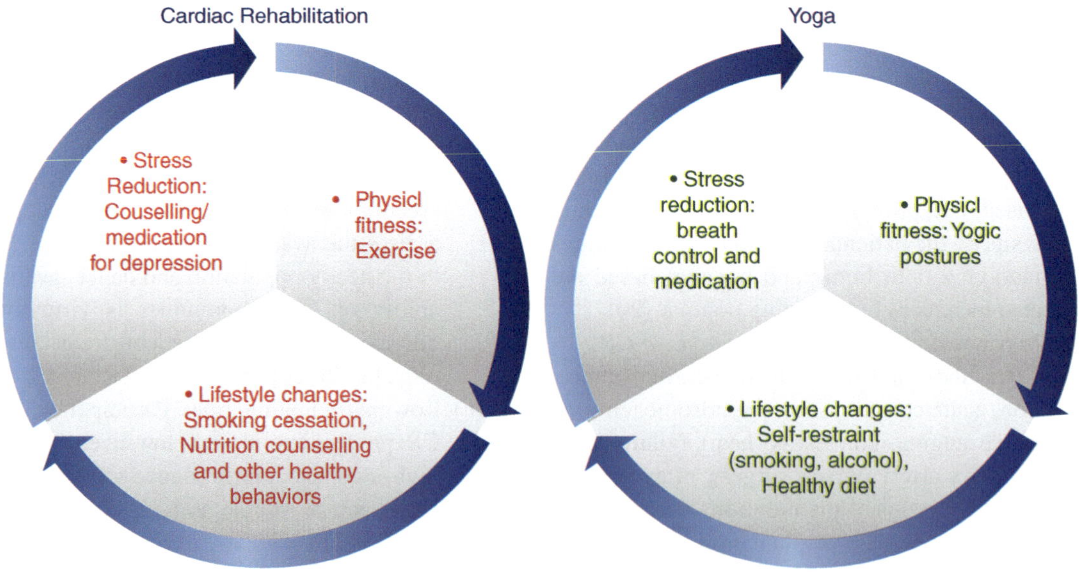

Fig. 28.1 Similarities between Cardiac Rehabilitation and Yoga programme

28.4 Yoga in Cardiac Health

Cardiovascular benefits of yoga have been explored extensively in the last five decades. It has been demonstrated that yoga could act at multiple levels including changes at subtler levels, i.e., genetic and molecular mechanisms, risk factor management and at psychological level. Evidence from these studies strongly suggest the evaluation of yoga programmes in patients with established cardiovascular diseases.

28.4.1 Underlying Mechanisms

1. *Yoga in cardiovascular biology*
   Cardiovascular benefits of Yoga are primarily mediated through the autonomic nervous system and hypothalamic-pituitary-adrenal (HPA) axis [33–36]. Yoga has been shown to induce parasympathetic predominance which in turn may increase heart rate variability and improve vascular tone reducing blood pressure. On the other hand, through HPA axis, yoga acts on endocrine pathway reducing cortisol and renin activity and also acts on neurotransmitters reducing dopamine and increasing serotonin.
2. *Yoga in cardiovascular risk factor control*
   Recent meta-analysis of 44 RCTs (n = 3168) has demonstrated that yoga improved most of the modifiable cardiovascular risk factors such as systolic blood pressure, diastolic blood pressure, heart rate, respiratory rate, waist circumference, waist/hip ratio, total cholesterol, HDL, VLDL, triglycerides, HbA1c and insulin resistance. However, the studies included in the meta-analysis have mostly unclear or high risk of bias [37, 38].
3. *Yoga in improving quality of life and mental health outcomes*
   Yoga has been shown to improve quality of life and several mental health outcomes across patients with different age group, different morbidities, etc. Meta-analysis of RCTs evaluating yoga on cancer patients, elderly population, chronic pelvic pain, rheumatic diseases reported yoga improve quality of life (Lin K, Tulloch A, Sivaramakrishnan D) and several mental health outcomes such as depression, anxiety, etc. [39–42]. However, most of the results of these meta-analyses are limited by an unclear or high risk of bias in included studies. Despite the limitations, Yoga has been often recommended to improve the quality of life in various pathologies.

28.5 Yoga-Based Cardiac Rehabilitation Programme in Patients with Established Cardiovascular Diseases

The first-ever study of effects of yoga in patients with ischemic heart disease patients was reported from India in 1971 by Tulpule et al. The authors reported that patients doing yoga postures and pranayama have 8% cumulative mortality in comparison with 21% cumulative mortality over a 5-year follow-up. Since then, numerous studies have reported the effects of yoga-based programmes in atherosclerotic cardiovascular diseases and also in heart failure.

28.5.1 Effects of Yoga in Cardiovascular Events

Ornish et al. reported that the control group had a higher risk of any cardiovascular event (composite of death, recurrent myocardial infarction, cardiac hospitalisations and revascularisation procedures) than the lifestyle intervention (45/78.81 person-years of follow-up vs. 25/108.04 person-years of follow-up, risk ratio—2.47, $p < 0.001$) at 5 years of follow-up [43].

Stress reduction based on transcendental meditation was reported to reduce cardiovascular events (composite of all-cause mortality, non-fatal myocardial infarction and non-fatal stroke) in those who were randomised to stress reduction than the control who received health education (20 vs. 32, Hazards Ratio—0.52 [0.29–0.92], p = 0.025) at a median follow-up of 5.4 years after adjusting for age, gender and lipid-lowering medications [44].

Recent Yoga-CaRe trial by Prabhakaran et al. reported a non-significant reduction of cardiovascular events (composite of death, recurrent myocardial infarction, non-fatal stroke and emergency cardiac hospital admissions) in patients who underwent Yoga-based cardiac rehabilitation programme (Yoga-CaRe) than enhanced standard care (131/1970 vs. 146/1989, Hazard Ratio—0.90 [0.71–1.15], $p = 0.41$) at a median follow-up of 22 months (Fig. 28.2). However, those who attended more than ten direct number contact sessions of intervention had a lower incidence of major adverse cardiovascular events (Hazards ratio—0.57 [0.39–0.82]) as compared to the enhanced standard care group. The incidence of major adverse cardiovascular events was also lower among those who self-practiced for more than the median duration (30 min a day) than those at or below the median, when compared to standard care [45].

The earlier trials by Ornish et al. and Schneider et al. had more frequent training sessions and follow-up sessions than the Yoga-CaRe trial which had only 13 training sessions after which the participant has to continue home practice as the latter has been planned as an effectiveness trial to mimic real-life settings.

28.5.2 Effects of Yoga on Revascularisation

Studies by Ornish et al., Manchanda et al. reported a reduction in the need for revascularisation in patients randomised to yoga lifestyle intervention than the control group whereas Schneider et al. and Prabhakaran et al. found no difference in need revascularisation between the stress reduction group and the control group [43, 44, 46].

28.5.3 Effects of Yoga in Coronary Atherosclerosis

Two studies have reported the effects of yoga in coronary atherosclerosis and both studies demonstrated that yoga-based programme could reverse coronary atherosclerosis. The study by Ornish and colleagues reported that at 1 year, comprehensive lifestyle changes including stress management (yoga-based stretching and relaxation practices), dietary changes, tobacco cessation and exercise training reduced diameter stenosis from 40.0 (16.9)% to 37.8(16.5)% whereas it progressed in the control group from

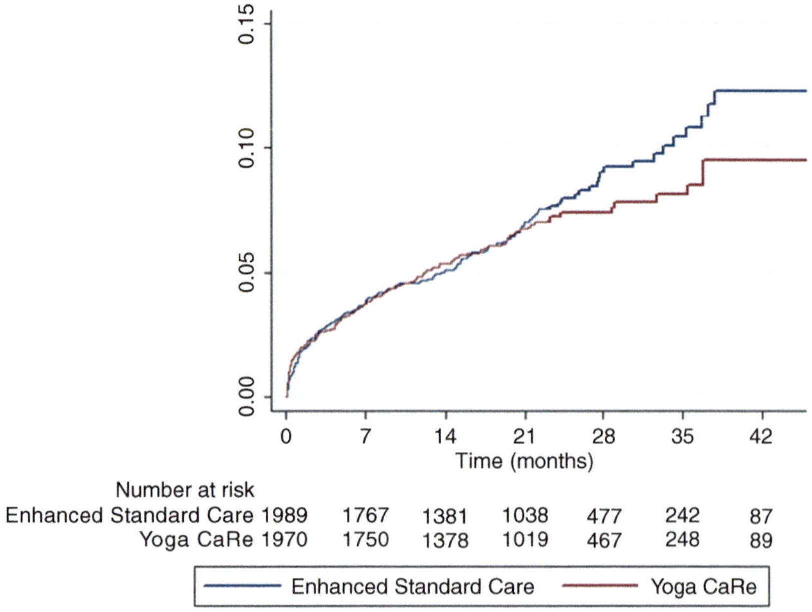

Fig. 28.2 Kaplan–Meier plot of cardiovascular events in Yoga-CaRe trial Source Prabhakaran et al., AHA 2018

42.7 (15.5)% to 46.1 (18.5)%. Overall, 82% of participants in lifestyle management group showed regression without the use of lipid-lowering drugs. In addition, the 5-year follow-up of participants reported further reductions in stenosis [43].

Similarly, the second study by Manchanda and colleagues demonstrated that at 1 year, more lesions regressed in Yoga lifestyle intervention (20 vs. 2%) and less lesions progressed (5 vs. 37%) than the control group. The yoga lifestyle intervention received a similar intervention as the earlier study and the control group received the American Heart Association step I diet [46].

28.5.4 Effects of Yoga on Angina

Angina frequency was reported to reduce in patient who underwent Yoga-based cardiac rehabilitation in RCTs by Manchanda et al. and Ornish et al. (1983) whereas no difference was reported in Ornish et al. (1998) and Toobert DJ (2000). The effect on angina could have been masked by higher rates of revascularisation in the later trials [43, 46–48].

28.5.5 Effects of Yoga on Cardiovascular Risk Factors

Several studies reported the beneficial effects of Yoga in cardiovascular risk factors in patients with cardiovascular diseases. In a nutshell, Yoga increased left ventricular ejection fraction and high-density lipoproteins and reduced systolic and diastolic blood pressure, heart rate, total cholesterol, low-density lipoproteins, triglycerides, body weight and body mass index (Table 28.1) [44, 46–65].

28.5.6 Effects of Yoga on Patient-Reported Outcomes

Few studies on patients with heart failure and coronary artery disease reported that yoga improves the quality of life. Recent Yoga-CaRe trial found Yoga-CaRe programme reduced the odds of having poor quality of life by 27%. Also, it has been shown to reduce the odds of poor re-integration to normal activities at 12 weeks (unpublished).

28.6 Landmark Trials Evaluating Yoga-Based Comprehensive Programmes in Coronary Atherosclerosis

Few landmark trials evaluating yoga-based comprehensive programmes in patients with coronary artery disease reported its potential in this patient group. These trials are discussed in the following section.

28.6.1 Lifestyle Heart Trial

Ornish et al. investigated the effects of residential rehabilitation involving stress management training (yogic poses), meditation, applied meditation and vegan diet (1400 Kcal, 5.2 mg cholesterol devoid of sugar, salt, alcohol and caffeine) in a rural environment for 24 days. The control group continued usual care (n = 24 in each arm). The immediate benefits noted include an increase in the mean duration of exercise, improved left ventricular regional wall motion, left ventricular ejection fraction and a decrease in cholesterol and angina episodes. In continuation, the Lifestyle Heart trial evaluated the same intervention components in a different model in 48 patients and moderate aerobic exercise and tobacco cessation were additionally included in the intervention. Patients in the intervention group underwent training in a week-long residential patient retreat followed by twice-weekly 4 h sessions. At 1 year, the intervention group showed regression of atherosclerosis, reduction in angina frequency, duration and severity, reduction in total and LDL cholesterol. At 5 years, changes in regression continued in the intervention group and control group had a higher risk of any cardiovascular events (odds ratio—2.47 [1.48–4.20]). The trial also reported that comprehensive inten-

Table 28.1 Summary of cardiovascular outcomes in meta-analysis

Outcome or subgroup	Studies	Participants	Statistical method	Effect estimate
Any cardiovascular events				
Revascularisation	3	291	Risk ratio (M-H, random, 95% CI)	0.49 [0.17, 1.39]
Anginal episodes/week	4	145	Mean difference (IV, random, 95% CI)	−5.42 [−7.01, −3.82]
Left ventricular ejection fraction (LVEF) [%]	5	445	Mean difference (IV, random, 95% CI [%])	2.48 [−2.33, 7.29]
Systolic blood pressure [mm of Hg]	12	1189	Mean difference (IV, random, 95% CI [mm of hg])	−4.63 [−6.27, −2.99]
Diastolic blood pressure [mm of Hg]	7	599	Mean difference (IV, random, 95% CI)	−4.76 [−8.03, −1.49]
Heart rate [beats/minute]	5	539	Mean difference (IV, random, 95% CI)	−7.01 [−10.73, −3.30]
Total cholesterol [mg/dl]	8	636	Mean difference (IV, random, 95% CI)	−16.08 [−35.65, 3.50]
LDL cholesterol [mg/dl]	7	590	Mean difference (IV, random, 95% CI)	−6.38 [−23.87, 11.11]
HDL cholesterol [mg/dl]	8	636	Mean difference (IV, random, 95% CI)	2.38 [0.35, 4.42]
Triglycerides [mg/dl]	8	636	Mean difference (IV, random, 95% CI)	−28.31 [−37.98, −18.63]
Weight [kg]	6	436	Mean difference (IV, random, 95% CI [kg])	−2.73 [−5.40, −0.05]
Body mass index [kg/m^2]	3	691	Mean difference (IV, random, 95% CI)	−0.85 [−1.85, 0.15]
Depression	3	330	Std. mean difference (IV, random, 95% CI)	−0.44 [−0.91, 0.03]
Anxiety	3	310	Std. mean difference (IV, random, 95% CI)	−0.05 [−0.28, 0.17]

sive lifestyle modification involving yogic poses, meditation and other lifestyle changes improved myocardial perfusion and stenosis flow reserve, etc. Also, stress management through yoga poses, meditation and applied meditation was associated with a reduction in body weight, total and LDL cholesterol at 1 year and regression. Its association with regression of atherosclerosis strengthened at 5 years [43, 48, 53, 66].

28.6.2 Indian Lifestyle Heart Trial

Manchanda et al., randomised 42 patients with stable coronary artery disease patients into a yoga group or a control group. The yoga intervention includes yogic practices, dietary approach and moderate aerobic exercises. The intervention was delivered in a residential centre for 4 days and further followed every fortnight for monitoring and evaluation. The control group received AHA step-I diet. At 1 year, the Yoga group showed regression in atherosclerosis. In addition, improvements were noted in NYHA functional class, angina episodes, weight, total and LDL cholesterol, triglycerides, exercise duration and ST segment depression [46].

28.6.3 Trial of Stress Reduction by Transcendental Meditation

Schneider et al. reported the beneficial effects of transcendental meditation in coronary heart disease patients. In this trial, 201 patients were randomised to receive either transcendental meditation or health education. The intervention involves six 1.5–2 h individual and group sessions. Thereafter, follow-up and maintenance meetings were scheduled every week for the first month, twice monthly in the next month and once a month till the end of the study. The control group intervention was matched for time spent by intervention group participants in all aspects.

The trial demonstrated that transcendental meditation reduces the risk of cardiovascular events by 48% at the end of 5.4 years of follow-up. Also, improvements were noted in systolic blood pressure [44].

28.6.4 Yoga-CaRe Trial

Yoga-CaRe trial is one of the largest trials of cardiac rehabilitation and also of yoga in cardiac patients. In this trial, Prabhakaran et al. randomised near 4000 patients (recruited through 24 hospitals in India) into a yoga-based cardiac rehabilitation programme or to enhanced standard care [67]. Firstly, the team developed a Yoga-based cardiac rehabilitation programme through a structured rehabilitation programme involving a review of yogic texts, systematic review and an expert consensus to identify heart-friendly and healthy yoga practices. The practices were fitted into the four-phase model of cardiac rehabilitation programme comprising of 13 sessions spread over 12 weeks. See Tables 28.2 and 28.3 for details of Yoga-CaRe programme. The enhanced standard care received lifestyle advice over three sessions [68].

The primary outcomes of the study are major cardiovascular events (composite of all-cause mortality, non-fatal myocardial infarction, non-fatal stroke and emergency cardiac admissions) and self-rated health as measured by Visual analogue scale of the European Quality of Life questionnaire (EQ-5DD-5L). At a median follow-up of 22 months, Yoga-CaRe programme showed a non-significant reduction in cardiovascular events. However, adherence-based analysis showed Yoga-CaRe reduced the incidence of MACE among those with high adherence to either direct contact sessions or home practice. The self-rated health at 12 weeks improved in Yoga-CaRe group than the enhanced standard care. Also, the odds of poor quality of life reduced in Yoga-CaRe group.

Table 28.2 Four phases of the Yoga-CaRe programme

Phase		During week (post-myocardial infarction)	Type of care
I	Inpatient care	1 (Session 1)	Face-to-face individual session—education
II	Formal outpatient session-I	3 (Session 2)	Face-to-face individual session—yoga (supervised)
III	Formal outpatient session-II	5–7 (Sessions 3–8; twice/ week) 8–12 (Sessions 9–13; once/ week)	Face-to-face group sessions—yoga (supervised) and education; during the rest of the week, self-practice of yoga at home using the booklet and DVD provided
IV	Long-term maintenance of lifestyle changes and self-practice of yoga at home	13+	Maintenance of lifestyle changes and self-practice of yoga at home on most days using the booklet and DVD provided

Among the secondary outcomes, the Yoga-CaRe improved return to pre-infarct activities whereas other outcomes such as tobacco cessation, adherence to drugs did not differ at 12 weeks [45] and unpublished data.

28.7 Demonstration Projects of Comprehensive Rehabilitation Programmes Involving Yoga

Ornish et al. demonstrated that the results he found in the Lifestyle Heart Trial can be implemented successfully in multi-centre approaches in two consecutive studies. The Multisite Lifestyle Demonstration Study (MLDS), the first demon-

Table 28.3 Components of the formal outpatient session-I

	Items	Time
Breathing exercises	1. Anulom vilom/ nadishodhana pranayam (without kumbhak) (alternate nostril breathing) 2. Bhramari pranayama (bee breathing) 3. Ujjayi pranayam (loud breathing)	Around 15 min for 3—each one for about 5 min
Meditation and relaxation practices	1. Chanting 2. Mindfulness meditation 3. Shavasana (relaxation training)	Around 15 min for 3—each one for about 5 min in a darkened room

stration study reported that comprehensive rehabilitation involving yoga can improve significantly improve medical and psychosocial outcomes. In the same study, the intervention group could avoid revascularisation for 3 years and demonstrated improvements in angina. These changes were observed regardless of the LVEF [69].

The second demonstration study in 24 sites reported similar improvements in cardiovascular outcomes at 3 months and 12 months. Similarly, the intervention is also reported to be cost-effective [70].

In the Mount Abu Open Heart trial, 123 patients with coronary artery disease underwent a lifestyle modification programme including rajyoga meditation, low-fat high-fibre vegetarian diet and moderate aerobic exercise. The intervention was delivered in a 7-day in-house programme followed by home practice and 6 monthly refresher programmes. 91% of patients showed a trend towards regression, 51% reported a reduction by 10 absolute points. The risk ratio of cardiac events between most and least adherence was 4.32 (1.69–11.70) [71].

28.8 Components and Structure of Yoga-Based Cardiac Rehabilitation Programme

Due to the wide heterogeneity in the branches of yoga and various practices prescribed under each of these practices, it is essential to use only those which has been tested to be safe or agreed to be safe for use by patients with cardiovascular diseases. Several yogic postures, breathing practices, meditative and relaxation practices have been tested in cardiovascular practices. Based on these components and an expert consensus, Yoga-CaRe programme was developed. These practices were fitted in a four-phase model of cardiac rehabilitation (Table 28.2). The various components prescribed in these phases and duration of their practices are tabulated (Tables 28.3 and 28.4). In addition, as like in the various landmark trials (except Yoga-CaRe trial), wherever feasible 1 week of residential/in-patient Yoga-based cardiac rehabilitation may also be offered in addition to the formal outpatient session-II. Also, transcendental meditation and rajyoga meditation are specialised meditative techniques may not be known to all yoga professionals. Hence, we have included simple meditative practices and wherever feasible these specialised meditative techniques may be provided.

Table 28.4 Components of the formal outpatient session-II

	Core items (select 2 out of 3)[a]	Elective items (select 1 out of 2)	Time
Health rejuvenating exercises	1. Shoulder exercises 2. Chest exercises 3. Abdomen exercises		Around 9 min for 3—each one for about 3 min
Yoga poses-standing	1. Katichakrasana (waist wheel pose) 2. Tadasana (palm tree pose) 3. Urdhvahastottanasana (up stretched arms pose)	1. Ardha-katichakrasana (lateral arc pose) 2. Trikonasana (triangle pose)	Around 25 min for 9 (3 standing, 3 sitting and 3 lying)—2-sided poses for about 3 min (1.5 min on each side—right and left), and central-positioned poses for about 1.5 min
Yoga poses—sitting	4. Gomukhasana (cow face pose) 5. Janushirsasana (head on the knee pose) 6. Vakrasana (twisted pose)	1. Ardha-padmasana (half lotus pose) 2. Vajrasana (adamant pose)	
Yoga poses—lying	1. Ekpadottanasana (half-leg raise pose) 2. Naukasana (boat pose) 3. Ardha-pavanamuktasana (wind releasing pose)	1. Markatasana (monkey pose) 2. Merudandasana (spinal cord pose)	
Breathing exercises	1. Anulom vilom/nadishodhana pranayam (without kumbhak) (alternate nostril breathing) 2. Bhramari pranayama (bee breathing) 3. Ujjayi pranayam (loud breathing)	1. Sitali pranayam (tongue hissing) 2. Sitkari pranayam (teeth hissing)	Around 15 min for 3—each one for about 5 min
Meditation and relaxation practices	1. Chanting 2. Mindfulness meditation 3. Shavasana (relaxation training)	1. Dirghasvasa preksha (perception of deep breathing) 2. Antaranga trataka (internal concentrated gazing)	Around 15 min for 3—each one for about 5 min in a darkened room
Moderated discussion	1. Lifestyle changes 2. Self-practice of yoga at home 3. Any life issues (common problems, issues or crises)		Around 10 min

[a]Health rejuvenating exercises and discussion—all the three core items are to be selected

28.9 Conclusion

Yoga-based cardiac rehabilitation programme may act through its effect on cardiovascular biology, i.e., hypothalamic–pituitary–adrenal axis and autonomic nervous system; cardiovascular risk factor control and behavioural and psyschosocial changes including an improvement in quality of life. Structured, comprehensive yoga-based cardiac rehabilitation programme has demonstrated similar improvements in several intermediary outcomes, quality of life and in some trials even on cardiovascular events. It may be a potential low-cost cardiac rehabilitation tool in places where conventional exercise-based comprehensive cardiac rehabilitation is not feasible and may reduce unmet needs of cardiac rehabilitation in resource constraint settings.

References

1. GBD 2016 DALYs and HALE Collaborators. Global, regional, and national disability-adjusted life-years (DALYs) for 333 diseases and injuries and healthy life expectancy (HALE) for 195 countries and territories, 1990–2016: a systematic analysis for the Global Burden of Disease Study 2016. Lancet (London, England). 2017;390(10100):1260–344. Available from http://www.ncbi.nlm.nih.gov/pubmed/28919118
2. Naghavi M, Abajobir AA, Abbafati C, Abbas KM, Abd-Allah F, Abera SF, et al. Global, regional, and national age-sex specific mortality for 264 causes of death, 1980–2016: a systematic analysis for the Global Burden of Disease Study 2016. Lancet. 2017;390(10100):1151–210.
3. Piepoli MF, Corrà U, Adamopoulos S, Benzer W, Bjarnason-Wehrens B, Cupples M, et al. Secondary prevention in the clinical management of patients with cardiovascular diseases. Core components, standards and outcome measures for referral and delivery: a policy statement from the cardiac rehabilitation section of the European Association for Cardiovascular Prevention & Rehabilitation. Endorsed by the Committee for Practice Guidelines of the European Society of Cardiology. Eur J Prev Cardiol. 2014 [cited 2019 Apr 18];21(6):664–81. Available from http://journals.sagepub.com/doi/10.1177/2047487312449597
4. Ajay VS, Prabhakaran D. Coronary heart disease in Indians: implications of the INTERHEART study. Indian J Med Res. 2010;132:561–6.
5. Shanmugasegaram S, Perez-Terzic C, Jiang X, Grace SL. Cardiac rehabilitation services in low- and middle-income countries: a scoping review. J Cardiovasc Nurs. 2014 [cited 2019 Apr 18];29(5):454–63. Available from http://content.wkhealth.com/linkback/openurl?sid=WKPTLP:landingpage&an=00005082-201409000-00011
6. Feuerstein G, editor. The deeper dimensions of yoga: theory and practice. Boston: Shambhala Publications; 2003.
7. World Health Organisation. Needs and action priorities in cardiac rehabilitation and secondary prevention in patients with coronary heart disease. Geneva; 1993.
8. NICE. MI—secondary prevention. Secondary prevention in primary and secondary care for patients following a myocardial infarction. NICE Guidel. 2013;(November). Available from https://www.nice.org.uk/guidance/cg172/evidence/myocardial-infarction-secondary-prevention-full-guideline-pdf-248682925%0Ahttps://guideline.gov/summaries/summary/47700%0Ahttp://www.nice.org.uk/nicemedia/live/14302/65691/65691.pdf
9. Mampuya WM. Cardiac rehabilitation past, present and future: an overview. Cardiovasc Diagn Ther. 2012;2(1):38–49.
10. Anderson L, Thompson DR, Oldridge N, Zwisler A-D, Rees K, Martin N, et al. Exercise-based cardiac rehabilitation for coronary heart disease. Cochrane Database Syst Rev. 2016;1:CD001800.
11. Shepherd CW, While AE. Cardiac rehabilitation and quality of life: a systematic review. Int J Nurs Stud. 2012;49(6):755–71.
12. Long L, Mordi IR, Bridges C, Sagar VA, Davies EJ, Coats AJ, et al. Exercise-based cardiac rehabilitation for adults with heart failure. Cochrane Database Syst Rev. 2019 [cited 2019 Jul 31];1:CD003331. Available from http://www.ncbi.nlm.nih.gov/pubmed/30695817
13. Vogiatzis I, Zakynthinos S. The physiological basis of rehabilitation in chronic heart and lung disease. J Appl Physiol. 2013 [cited 2019 Dec 30];115(1):16–21. Available from https://www.physiology.org/doi/10.1152/japplphysiol.00195.2013
14. Sadeghi M, Khosravi-Broujeni H, Salehi-Abarghouei A, Heidari R, Roohafza H. Effect of cardiac rehabilitation on inflammation: a systematic review and meta-analysis of controlled clinical trials. ARYA Atheroscler. 2018;14(2):85–94.
15. Bruning RS, Sturek M. Benefits of exercise training on coronary blood flow in coronary artery disease patients. Prog Cardiovasc Dis. 2015;57(5):443–53.
16. Gielen S, Laughlin MH, O'Conner C, Duncker DJ. Exercise training in patients with heart disease: review of beneficial effects and clinical recommendations. Prog Cardiovasc Dis. 2015;57(4):347–55.
17. BACPR. The BACPR standards and core components for cardiovascular disease prevention and rehabilitation 2012. London: BACPR; 2012.
18. Aacvpr. Cardiac rehabilitation: an underutilized class I treatment for cardiovascular disease. Available from https://www.aacvpr.org/Portals/0/resources/professionals/CRupdate2.06.12.pdf
19. Buckingham SA, Taylor RS, Jolly K, Zawada A, Dean SG, Cowie A, et al. Home-based versus centre-based cardiac rehabilitation: abridged Cochrane systematic review and meta-analysis. Open Hear. 2016;3(2):e000463.
20. Clark RA, Conway A, Poulsen V, Keech W, Tirimacco R, Tideman P. Alternative models of cardiac rehabilitation: A systematic review. Eur J Prev Cardiol. 2015 [cited 2019 Apr 18];22(1):35–74. Available from http://www.ncbi.nlm.nih.gov/pubmed/23943649
21. Sandesara PB, Lambert CT, Gordon NF, Fletcher GF, Franklin BA, Wenger NK, et al. Cardiac rehabilitation and risk reduction: time to "rebrand and reinvigorate.". J Am Coll Cardiol. 2015;65(4):389–95.
22. Price KJ, Gordon BA, Bird SR, Benson AC. A review of guidelines for cardiac rehabilitation exercise programmes: is there an international consensus? Eur J Prev Cardiol. 2016;23:1715–33.
23. Thomas RJ, Balady G, Banka G, Beckie TM, Chiu J, Gokak S, et al. 2018 ACC/AHA clinical performance and quality measures for cardiac rehabilitation: a report of the American College of Cardiology/American Heart Association Task Force on Performance Measures. J Am Coll Cardiol. 2018;71(16):1814–37.

24. Ibanez B, James S, Agewall S, Antunes MJ, Bucciarelli-Ducci C, Bueno H, et al. 2017 ESC guidelines for the management of acute myocardial infarction in patients presenting with ST-segment elevation. Eur Heart J. 2018;39(2):119–77.
25. Turk-Adawi K, Sarrafzadegan N, Grace SL. Global availability of cardiac rehabilitation. Nat Rev Cardiol. 2014 [cited 2018 Dec 12];11(10):586–96. Available from http://www.ncbi.nlm.nih.gov/pubmed/25027487
26. Ragupathi L, Stribling J, Yakunina Y, Fuster V, McLaughlin MA, Vedanthan R. Availability, use, and barriers to cardiac rehabilitation in LMIC. Glob Heart. 2017;12(4):323–334.e10.
27. Madan K, Babu AS, Contractor A, Sawhney JPS, Prabhakaran D, Gupta R. Cardiac rehabilitation in India. Prog Cardiovasc Dis. 2014;56(5):543–50.
28. Dalal HM, Wingham J, Palmer J, Taylor R, Petre C, Lewin R. Why do so few patients with heart failure participate in cardiac rehabilitation? A cross-sectional survey from England, Wales and Northern Ireland. BMJ Open. 2012;2(2):1–8.
29. Ruano-Ravina A, Pena-Gil C, Abu-Assi E, Raposeiras S, van't Hof A, Meindersma E, et al. Participation and adherence to cardiac rehabilitation programs. A systematic review. Int J Cardiol. 2016;223:436–43.
30. Pack QR, Squires RW, Lopez-Jimenez F, Lichtman SW, Rodriguez-Escudero JP, Lindenauer PK, et al. Participation rates, process monitoring, and quality improvement among cardiac rehabilitation programs in the United States. J Cardiopulm Rehabil Prev. 2015 [cited 2018 Dec 12];35(3):173–80. Available from http://www.ncbi.nlm.nih.gov/pubmed/25763922
31. Ades PA, Keteyian SJ, Wright JS, Hamm LF, Lui K, Newlin K, et al. Increasing cardiac rehabilitation participation From 20% to 70%: a road map from the million hearts cardiac rehabilitation collaborative. Mayo Clin Proc. 2017 [cited 2018 Dec 12];92(2):234–42. Available from https://linkinghub.elsevier.com/retrieve/pii/S0025619616306486
32. Ross A, Thomas S. The health benefits of yoga and exercise: a review of comparison studies. J Altern Complement Med. 2010 [cited 2014 Nov 30];16(1):3–12. Available from http://www.ncbi.nlm.nih.gov/pubmed/20105062.
33. Riley KE, Park CL. How does yoga reduce stress? A systematic review of mechanisms of change and guide to future inquiry. Health Psychol Rev. 2015 [cited 2019 Jul 31];9(3):379–96. Available from http://www.ncbi.nlm.nih.gov/pubmed/25559560
34. Pascoe MC, Bauer IE. A systematic review of randomised control trials on the effects of yoga on stress measures and mood. J Psychiatr Res. 2015 [cited 2018 Jan 4];68:270–82. Available from http://www.ncbi.nlm.nih.gov/pubmed/26228429
35. Ross A, Thomas S. The health benefits of yoga and exercise: a review of comparison studies. J Altern Complement Med. 2010;16(1):3–12.
36. Harte JL, Eifert GH, Smith R. The effects of running and meditation on beta-endorphin, corticotropin-releasing hormone and cortisol in plasma, and on mood. Biol Psychol. 1995;40(3):251–65. Available from http://www.ncbi.nlm.nih.gov/pubmed/7669835
37. Cramer H, Lauche R, Haller H, Steckhan N, Michalsen A, Dobos G. Effects of yoga on cardiovascular disease risk factors: a systematic review and meta-analysis. Int J Cardiol. 2014 [cited 2014 Nov 28];173(2):170–83. Available from http://www.ncbi.nlm.nih.gov/pubmed/24636547
38. Chu P, Gotink RA, Yeh GY, Goldie SJ, Hunink MGM. The effectiveness of yoga in modifying risk factors for cardiovascular disease and metabolic syndrome: a systematic review and meta-analysis of randomized controlled trials. Eur J Prev Cardiol. 2016;23(3):291–307. Available from http://www.embase.com/search/results?subaction=viewrecord&from=export&id=L607786965
39. Patel NK, Newstead AH, Ferrer RL. The effects of yoga on physical functioning and health related quality of life in older adults: a systematic review and meta-analysis. J Altern Complement Med. 2012;18(10):902–17. Available from https://login.proxy.library.emory.edu/login?url=http://search.ebscohost.com/login.aspx?direct=true&db=cin20&AN=104426406&site=ehost-live&scope=site
40. Cramer H, Lauche R, Langhorst J, Dobos G. Yoga for depression: a systematic review and meta-analysis. Depress Anxiety. 2013 [cited 2015 Jan 23];30(11):1068–83. Available from http://www.ncbi.nlm.nih.gov/pubmed/23922209
41. Wu Y, Johnson BT, Acabchuk RL, Chen S, Lewis HK, Livingston J, et al. Yoga as Antihypertensive Lifestyle Therapy: A Systematic Review and Meta-analysis. Mayo Clin Proc. 2019 [cited 2019 Apr 22];94(3):432–46. Available from: http://www.ncbi.nlm.nih.gov/pubmed/30792067
42. Cramer H, Lauche R, Klose P, Lange S, Langhorst J, Dobos GJ. Yoga for improving health-related quality of life, mental health and cancer-related symptoms in women diagnosed with breast cancer. Cochrane database Syst Rev. 2017 [cited 2018 Mar 28];1(1):CD010802. Available from: http://www.ncbi.nlm.nih.gov/pubmed/28045199
43. Ornish D, Scherwitz LW, Billings JH, Brown SE, Gould KL, Merritt TA, et al. Intensive lifestyle changes for reversal of coronary heart disease. JAMA. 1998;280(23):2001–7.
44. Schneider RH, Grim CE, Rainforth MV, Kotchen T, Nidich SI, Gaylord-King C, et al. Stress reduction in the secondary prevention of cardiovascular disease: randomized, controlled trial of transcendental meditation and health education in blacks. Circ Cardiovasc Qual Outcomes. 2012;5(6):750–8. Available from http://www.embase.com/search/results?subaction=viewrecord&from=export&id=L368317765
45. Prabhakaran D, Chandrasekaran A, Singh K, et al. Effectiveness of a yoga-based cardiac rehabilitation (yoga-care) program: a multi-centre randomised controlled trial of 4,014 patients with acute myocardial infarction from india. In: Circulation. New Delhi: Lippincott Williams & Wilkins Hagerstown,

MD; 2018 [cited 2019 Mar 14]. p. e756. Available from: https://www.ahajournals.org/doi/10.1161/CIR.0000000000000636
46. Manchanda SC, Narang R, Reddy KS, Sachdeva U, Prabhakaran D, Dharmanand S, et al. Retardation of coronary atherosclerosis with yoga lifestyle intervention. J Assoc Physicians India. 2000;48(7):687–94.
47. Toobert DJ, Glasgow RE, Radcliffe JL. Physiologic and related behavioral outcomes from the Women's Lifestyle Heart Trial. Ann Behav Med. 2000;22(1):1–9.
48. Ornish D, Scherwitz LW, Doody RS, Kesten D, McLanahan SM, Brown SE, et al. Effects of stress management training and dietary changes in treating ischemic heart disease. JAMA. 1983;249(1):54–9. Available from: http://www.ncbi.nlm.nih.gov/pubmed/6336794
49. Ades PA, Savage PD, Cress ME, Brochu M, Lee NM, Poehlman ET. Resistance training on physical performance in disabled older female cardiac patients. Med Sci Sport Exerc. 2003;35(8):1265–70. Available from https://login.proxy.library.emory.edu/login?url=http://search.ebscohost.com/login.aspx?direct=true&db=cin20&AN=106720372&site=ehost-live&scope=site
50. Curiati JA, Bocchi E, Freire JO, Arantes AC, Braga M, Garcia Y, et al. Meditation reduces sympathetic activation and improves the quality of life in elderly patients with optimally treated heart failure: a prospective randomized study. J Altern Complement Med. 2005;11(3):465–72. Available from https://login.proxy.library.emory.edu/login?url=http://search.ebscohost.com/login.aspx?direct=true&db=cin20&AN=106513804&site=ehost-live&scope=site
51. Hari Krishna B, Pal P, Pal GK, Balachander J, Jayasettiaseelon E, Sreekanth Y, et al. Yoga improves quality of life and functional capacity in heart failure patients. Biomed Res Int. 2014;25(2):178–82. Available from http://biomedres.info/yahoo_site_admin/assets/docs/178-182-Bandi_Hari_Krishna.70223308.pdf
52. Raghuram N, Parachuri VR, Swarnagowri MV, Babu S, Chaku R, Kulkarni R, et al. Yoga based cardiac rehabilitation after coronary artery bypass surgery: one-year results on LVEF, lipid profile and psychological states—a randomized controlled study. Indian Heart J. 2014;66(5):490–502. Available from http://www.ncbi.nlm.nih.gov/pubmed/25443601
53. Gould KL, Ornish D, Scherwitz L, Brown S, Edens RP, Hess MJ, et al. Changes in myocardial perfusion abnormalities by positron emission tomography after long-term, intense risk factor modification. Jama. 1995;274(11):894–901. Available from http://jama.jamanetwork.com/article.aspx?articleid=389631
54. Hägglund E, Hagerman I, Dencker K, Strömberg A. Effects of yoga versus hydrotherapy training on health-related quality of life and exercise capacity in patients with heart failure: a randomized controlled study. Eur J Cardiovasc Nurs. 2017 [cited 2018 Jan 16];16(5):381–9. Available from http://journals.sagepub.com/doi/10.1177/1474515117690297
55. Pal A, Srivastava N, Narain VS, Agrawal GG, Rani M. Effect of yogic intervention on the autonomic nervous system in the patients with coronary artery disease: a randomized controlled trial. East Mediterr Heal J. 2013;19(5):452–8. Available from: http://www.embase.com/search/results?subaction=viewrecord&from=export&id=L373932475
56. Parswani MJ, Sharma MP, Iyengar S. Mindfulness-based stress reduction program in coronary heart disease: a randomized control trial. Int J Yoga. 2013;6(2):111–7. Available from https://www.ncbi.nlm.nih.gov/pmc/articles/PMC3734636/
57. Paul-Labrador M, Polk D, Dwyer JH, Velasquez I, Nidich S, Rainforth M, et al. Effects of a randomized controlled trial of transcendental meditation on components of the metabolic syndrome in subjects with coronary heart disease. Arch Intern Med. 2006;166(11):1218–24. Available from: http://www.embase.com/search/results?subaction=viewrecord&from=export&id=L43877632
58. Wahlstrom M, Rydell Karlsson M, Medin J, Frykman V. Effects of yoga in patients with paroxysmal atrial fibrillation—a randomized controlled study. Eur J Cardiovasc Nurs. 2017;16(1):57–63. Available from http://journals.sagepub.com/doi/abs/10.1177/1474515116637734
59. Yadav A, Singh S, Singh KP, Pai P. Effect of yoga regimen on lung functions including diffusion capacity in coronary artery disease patients: a randomized controlled study. Int J Yoga. 2015;8(1):62–7. Available from http://www.ncbi.nlm.nih.gov/pmc/articles/PMC4278137/
60. Younge JO, Wery MF, Gotink RA, Utens EMWJ, Michels M, Rizopoulos D, et al. Web-Based Mindfulness Intervention in Heart Disease: A Randomized Controlled Trial. Quinn TJ, editor. PLoS One. 2015;10(12):e0143843. Available from http://dx.plos.org/10.1371/journal.pone.0143843
61. Jatuporn S, Sangwatanaroj S, Saengsiri A-O, Rattanapruks S, Srimahachota S, Uthayachalerm W, et al. Short-term effects of an intensive lifestyle modification program on lipid peroxidation and antioxidant systems in patients with coronary artery disease. Clin Hemorheol Microcirc. 2003;29(3–4):429–36. Available from http://www.ncbi.nlm.nih.gov/pubmed/14724371
62. Mahajan AS, Reddy KS, Sachdeva U. Lipid profile of coronary risk subjects following yogic lifestyle intervention. Indian Heart J. 1999;51(1):37–40. Available from http://www.ncbi.nlm.nih.gov/pubmed/10327777
63. Pullen PR, Thompson WR, Benardot D, Brandon LJ, Mehta PK, Rifai L, et al. Benefits of yoga for African American heart failure patients. Med Sci Sports Exerc. 2010;42(4):651–7. Available from http://www.ncbi.nlm.nih.gov/pubmed/19952833
64. Jayadevappa R, Johnson JC, Bloom BS, Nidich S, Desai S, Chhatre S, et al. Effectiveness of transcen-

dental meditation on functional capacity and quality of life of African Americans with congestive heart failure: a randomized control study. Ethn Dis. 2007;17(1):72–7. Available from http://www.embase.com/search/results?subaction=viewrecord&from=export&id=L46231367
65. Toise SCF, Sears SF, Schoenfeld MH, Blitzer ML, Marieb MA, Drury JH, et al. Psychosocial and cardiac outcomes of yoga for ICD patients: a randomized clinical control trial: yoga trial for ICD patients. Pacing Clin Electrophysiol. 2014;37(1):48–62. https://doi.org/10.1111/pace.12252.
66. Ornish D, Brown SE, Billings JH, Scherwitz LW, Armstrong WT, Ports TA, et al. Can lifestyle changes reverse coronary heart disease? The Lifestyle Heart Trial. Lancet. 1990;336(8708):129–33. Available from http://www.sciencedirect.com/science/article/pii/014067369091656U
67. Chandrasekaran AM, Kinra S, Ajay VS, Chattopadhyay K, Singh K, Singh K, et al. Effectiveness and cost-effectiveness of a yoga-based cardiac rehabilitation (Yoga-CaRe) program following acute myocardial infarction: study rationale and design of a multi-center randomized controlled trial. Int J Cardiol. 2019;280:14–8.
68. Chattopadhyay K, Chandrasekaran AM, Praveen PA, Manchanda SC, Madan K, Ajay VS, et al. Development of a yoga-based cardiac rehabilitation (Yoga-CaRe) programme for secondary prevention of myocardial infarction. Evid Based Complement Alternat Med. 2019;2019:7470184.
69. Ornish D. Avoiding revascularization with lifestyle changes: the multicenter lifestyle demonstration project. Am J Cardiol. 1998 [cited 2019 Mar 12];82(10):72–6. Available from https://www--sciencedirect-com.proxy.library.emory.edu/science/article/pii/S0002914998007449
70. Silberman A, Banthia R, Estay IS, Kemp C, Studley J, Hareras D, et al. The effectiveness and efficacy of an intensive cardiac rehabilitation program in 24 sites. Am J Health Promot. 2010;24(4):260–6.
71. Gupta SK, Sawhney RC, Rai L, Chavan VD, Dani S, Arora RC, et al. Regression of coronary atherosclerosis through healthy lifestyle in coronary artery disease patients—Mount Abu Open Heart Trial. Indian Heart J. 2011;63(5):461–9.

29 Yoga as a Potential Intervention for Preventing Cardiac Complications in COVID-19: Augmenting Immuno-Modulation and Bolstering Mental Health

Indranill Basu-Ray and Kashinath Metri

Abbreviations

ACE	Angiotensin-converting enzyme
BDNF	Brain-derived neurotrophic factor
COVID-19	Coronavirus disease
HIV	Human immunodeficiency virus
HPA	Hypothalamic-pituitary-adrenal
IFN	Interferon
IgA	Immunoglobulin A
IL	Interleukin
TNF	Tumor necrosis factor

29.1 Introduction

Coronavirus disease (COVID-19) is a highly contagious viral disease caused by the severe acute respiratory syndrome coronavirus (SARS-CoV-2). Initially reported in Wuhan, Hubei Province, China in 2019 [1, 2], COVID-19 quickly attained pandemic status, having affected more than 30 million people and caused more than 950,000 deaths worldwide as of late September 2020 [3]. Given the novelty of the disease and the lack of immediate treatments or vaccines, early protective measures to prevent extensive spread of infection have been limited to quickly accessible ploys, such as social distancing, hand washing, wearing of facial coverings, and the "lockdown" of businesses considered to be nonessential to ongoing daily living. Months into the pandemic, these lockdowns have been relaxed in varying degrees across the globe because of their deleterious economic effects, but many experts argue that easing social restrictions has contributed to spikes in the number of cases.

Despite the fact that different vaccines and drugs are available for treating infected persons but prevention remains the corner stone for management of this epidemic. While vaccination is a powerful preventive mechanism. It is important to understand the importance of integrative approaches to prevention of this disease that has either killed or maimed millions and continue to do so. Drug treatment for the disease remains a poor alternative only for the very sick to prevent them from dying as reckless use of medication will create more resistant strain with acclerated devastation compared to what has been seen in recent years. In the context of integrative medicine, yoga is a mind–body discipline that promotes healthy living through the practice of

I. Basu-Ray (✉)
Memphis VA Medical Center, Memphis, TN, USA

The University of Memphis, Memphis, TN, USA

All India Institute of Medical Sciences, Rishikesh, Uttarakhand, India
e-mail: ibr@ibasuray.com

K. Metri
Department of Yoga, Central University of Rajasthan, Bandar Seendri, Rajasthan, India

I. Basu-Ray, D. Mehta (eds.), *The Principles and Practice of Yoga in Cardiovascular Medicine*,
https://doi.org/10.1007/978-981-16-6913-2_29

postures (asana), breathing techniques (pranayama), meditation (dhyana), and concentration (dharana) [4]. Its numerous benefits for physical health include its proven ability to help prevent chronic conditions such as hypertension, diabetes, and heart failure by lowering associated risk factors [5]; yoga can attenuate cardiac arrhythmia, congestive cardiac failure, and ischemic heart disease [6–10]. Numerous randomized clinical trials have demonstrated the role of yoga in preventing and managing various chronic communicable and noncommunicable disorders [11]. Consistent practice of yoga strengthens innate and adaptive immunity [12, 13] and helps to enhance physiological functions, such as respiration, digestion, circulation, and hormone production [14–16]. Within the realm of mental health, yoga plays a significant role in reducing depression [17, 18], stress, and anxiety [19, 20] and promotes feelings of wellbeing, calm, and self-control [20–23].

In this chapter, we discuss various inflammatory, infectious, and psychosocial aspects of COVID-19 and explore yoga's anti-inflammatory and immune-modulating capabilities, along with its role in reducing risk for immune dysfunction and impaired mental health.

29.2 SARS-COV-2 Infection

SARS-CoV-2 enters the body through the respiratory system. Given that droplet (and possibly aerosolized) transmission is thought to be the primary mode of viral spread, a person can become infected when his or her mucus membrane (within the nose, eyes, or mouth) comes into contact with the respiratory secretions of an actively infected person. Having entered the body, the SARS-CoV-2 virus uses its S-spike to bind to the angiotensin-converting enzyme (ACE)2 receptors as an entry point into the cell. The ACE2 receptor is expressed primarily in both type I and type II pneumocytes but also in other types of cells, including endothelial cells. Thus, it plays a vital role in vascular integrity and hemodynamic regulation [24–26].

29.2.1 The Role of Immunity

The human immune system comprises vast, effective network of multiple organs, including the spleen, thymus, lymph nodes, tonsils, and bones. Immune cells and their products destroy intruding infective organisms and neutralize them. The immune system can mount two different lines of defense: innate immunity and adaptive immunity.

Innate immunity is the rapid-acting first line of defense that effectively inhibits infective agents and novel pathogens, such as SARS-CoV-2, from entering the body. This elaborate immunological cascade appropriately arrests the disease and helps to initiate the repair mechanism, thus ensuring satisfactory resolution of the infection and generating targeted resistance to defend the body against reinfection by the same organism [27]. A response of this nature is thought to occur in approximately 80% of individuals who become infected but who either are asymptomatic or develop mild symptoms that abate and culminate in an uneventful recovery. Thus, an optimal innate immune response may play a vital role in the prevention and early disposal of most COVID-19 infections.

Should this first line of defense fail, the immune system activates adaptive immunity, which, along with fighting the infection, "remembers" it, so as to prevent reentry of such invaders [28]. The adaptive immune system involves T lymphocytes, B lymphocytes, and pathogen-specific antibodies in addition to the proinflammatory cytokines and chemokines that help to eliminate the pathogen [29]. Although these processes are highly effective, they are also very potent and can render bystander damage to the body's own cells and organs.

COVID-19 manifests in three different ways: (1) some patients are asymptomatic, suggesting that their innate immunity is functioning adequately; (2) some patients are only mildly symptomatic and achieve spontaneous recovery, suggesting that their innate immunity detected and restricted the infection and that their adap-

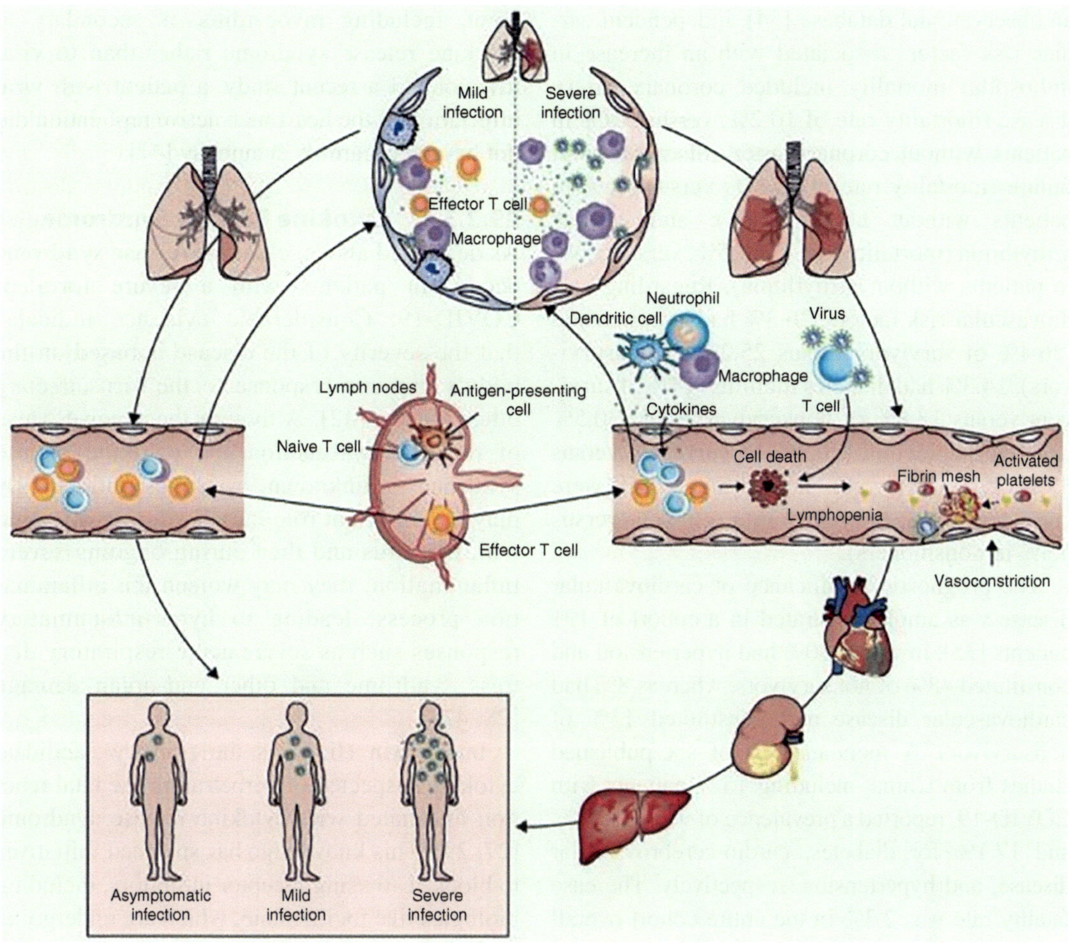

Fig. 29.1 Pathological changes in lungs in early and severe stages of COVID-19 [31] COVID-19, coronavirus disease 2019

tive immunity got rid of the virus; and (3) other patients develop moderate-to-severe illness and either recover or die from the infection [30]. For those who die, the immune system becomes overwhelmed and produces a massive, cascading release of cytokines. This so-called "cytokine release syndrome" initiates widespread tissue destruction and multiorgan failure, leading to death [28]. In this scenario, the resources harnessed by the body to kill the virus largely outweigh the appropriate levels needed; in other words, the body's immunological reaction is ultimately what kills, rather than the virus (Fig. 29.1).

29.2.2 Cardiovascular Effects

Cardiac involvement appears to be pervasive in patients with COVID-19, particularly in those ill enough to be hospitalized [26]. Patients with established cardiovascular disease or cardiac risk factors are more vulnerable, have worse morbidity profiles, and are at higher risk for mortality if they contract COVID-19. In various studies, nearly 30% of afflicted patients had hypertension, and 15% had preexisting cardiovascular disease [32, 33].

In an analysis of the in-hospital deaths of 8910 COVID-19 patients from 169 hospitals tracked in an observational database [34], independent cardiac risk factors associated with an increase in in-hospital mortality included coronary artery disease (mortality rate of 10.2%, versus 5.2% in patients without coronary artery disease), heart failure (mortality rate of 15.3%, versus 5.6% in patients without heart failure), and cardiac arrhythmia (mortality rate of 11.5%, versus 5.6% in patients without arrhythmia). Regarding cardiovascular risk factors, 26.3% had hypertension (26.4% of survivors versus 25.2% of nonsurvivors), 14.3% had diabetes mellitus (14% of survivors versus 18.8% of nonsurvivors), and 30.5% had hyperlipidemia (30.2% of survivors versus 35% of nonsurvivors). In addition, 5.5% were current smokers (mortality rate of 9.4%, versus 5.3% in nonsmokers).

The prognostic significance of cardiovascular disease was amply illustrated in a cohort of 191 patients [35], in which 30% had hypertension and constituted 48% of nonsurvivors, whereas 8% had cardiovascular disease and constituted 13% of nonsurvivors. A meta-analysis of six published studies from China, including 1527 patients with COVID-19, reported a prevalence of 9.7%, 16.4%, and 17.1% for diabetes, cardio-cerebrovascular disease, and hypertension, respectively. The case fatality rate was 2.3% in the entire cohort overall but was significantly higher in patients with hypertension, diabetes, or cardiovascular disease (6%, 7.3%, and 10.5%, respectively) [36, 37].

29.2.3 Mechanisms of Cardiac Damage

Accumulating evidence indicates that COVID-19 is frequently associated with cardiac involvement and, often, cardiac inflammation [38]. What is more sobering is the finding that this ubiquitous cardiac involvement is rampant even in healthy young patients who have minimal symptoms not requiring hospitalization [38]. Multiple mechanisms for cardiac damage have been proposed, on the basis of studies conducted during the previous SARS and Middle East respiratory syndrome epidemics and the currently ongoing COVID-19 epidemic [25, 26, 39, 40]. Some evidence from autopsy studies suggests that cardiac involvement, including myocarditis, is secondary to cytokine release syndrome rather than to viral invasion: In a recent study, a patient with viral infiltration of the heart with active replication did not have myocarditis at autopsy [41].

29.2.3.1 Cytokine Release Syndrome

As described above, cytokine release syndrome occurs in patients with a severe form of COVID-19. Considerable evidence indicates that the severity of the disease is based on the body's immune response to the virus, among other factors [42]. Although the precise cause of immune dysfunction and cytokine release syndrome is unknown, cytokines undoubtedly play an important role initially during infection with the virus and then during ongoing severe inflammation; they may worsen the inflammation process, leading to hyper-inflammatory responses such as severe acute respiratory distress syndrome and other end-organ damage [28, 43].

Interleukin (IL)-6 is the primary candidate cytokine suspected of perpetrating the fatal reaction associated with cytokine release syndrome [27, 29]. This knowledge has spawned initiatives to block IL-6 using receptor inhibitors, including biologics like tocilizumab, which are undergoing trials in moderately to severely ill patients with COVID-19 [29]. Other proinflammatory cytokines are significantly elevated in severe cases, including IL-2 receptor, IL-10, IL-8, and tumor necrosis factor (TNF)-α [28, 39].

29.2.3.2 Direct Myocardial Cell Injury

The interaction of SARS-CoV-2 with ACE2 can result in changes to the ACE2 pathways, leading to acute injury of the lung, heart, and endothelial cells [39]. In a cardiac biopsy performed on a 50-year-old COVID-19 patient, infiltration of cardiac myocytes by interstitial mononuclear inflammatory cells was noticed [25, 39]. Also noted is a mismatch between myocardial oxygen supply and demand: Increased cardiometabolic demand associated with the systemic infection and ongoing hypoxia caused by severe pneumonia or acute respiratory distress syndrome can lead to increased demand in the face of inadequate supply, producing myocardial damage [39].

29.2.3.3 Acute Coronary Syndrome

Acute plaque rupture leading to acute coronary syndrome is part of the systemic inflammation and catecholamine surge inherent in this disease; increased plaque vulnerability could be associated [39, 44]. Coronary thrombosis was also identified as a possible cause of acute coronary syndrome in COVID-19 patients [45].

29.3 Pandemics, Immunity, and Mental Health

As of September 2020, no effective vaccines were yet available, and remdesivir, the sole antiviral agent effective against COVID-19 thus far, shortens the illness timetable by only 33% [46]. Although many vaccines are in development, none has cleared Phase III clinical trials; many potential candidates have been found to be ineffective or have significant side effects leading to their demise. This lack of a highly effective treatment or vaccine means that preventive measures—including hygiene, social distancing, and personal protective equipment—are the few available means of attempting to manage the spread of COVID-19. However, the partial or complete lockdowns needed for social distancing have produced job losses and financial hardships that have led to myriad psychological issues, including stress, anxiety, depression, and panic attacks—all of which downregulate the immune system and, consequently, worsen disease manifestations [47, 48]; suicides, opioid overdoses, and domestic violence also have increased during this time of isolation and economic downturn. Further, stress and anxiety levels appear to worsen in households with vulnerable persons, such as children, pregnant women, or elderly relatives, given the higher disease severity and mortality rates in these groups.

29.3.1 Stress

Chronic and subacute stress negatively affect the immune system [49]. Whereas the ability to cope with stress helps preserve immune function, persons with higher stress levels and poor coping mechanisms have subpar immunity. Elevated stress levels associated with extended lockdowns, accompanied by fear, anxiety, and depression, lead to weakened immunity that opens the floodgates of infection [50]. Moreover, people who have stressful life events appear to have a greater risk for respiratory infections [51].

Stress affects immune function by increasing the secretion of glucocorticoids and catecholamines. Stress also attenuates the parasympathetic system [52], inducing chronic sympathetic overdrive with its attendant hormonal milieu (including cortisol excess and a robust catecholaminergic drive) that attenuate the immune system's effectiveness [53]. The pathophysiology at play under such conditions is increased inflammation and decreased protection against invading microorganisms [53]. Elevated glucocorticoid levels dysregulate cytokine production, thereby affecting natural-killer cell activity and reducing immunoglobulin A (IgA) production [53]. Poor antibody response and decreased natural-killer cell activity are associated with less resilience during stressful situations [54, 55]. Elevated cortisol potentiates glucose intolerance and diabetes and thus further increases the risk for infection [56].

The paradox of amplified inflammation during stress despite higher serum corticosteroid levels is not well described. Although chronic stressors should ameliorate the symptoms of inflammation-related diseases, this is at odds with the excess morbidity and mortality documented in chronically stressed individuals. Miller and colleagues [57] have hypothesized that macrophage resistance to cortisol negative feedback develops under conditions of chronic stress, due to compensatory downregulation at the immune cell (glucocorticoid) receptor. Early life stress can give rise to blunted cortisol negative feedback of the innate inflammatory response [58]. This may set the stage for the stress-related chronic inflammation thought to lower the threshold for stress-related noncommunicable disease [59]. Further research is needed to discern the probable mechanism for this phenomenon.

29.3.2 Anxiety

Pandemics are associated with heightened anxiety, both individually and collectively. The highly contagious nature of COVID-19 and the lack of treatment options are a threat to survival and may trigger or aggravate existing anxiety and panic disorders.

Anxiety dysregulates the hypothalamic–pituitary–adrenal (HPA) axis, which in turn contributes to significant immune dysfunction [60, 61]. In a study of 42 patients with panic disorder and 42 healthy individuals, Koh and Lee observed significantly lower IL-2 production and lymphocyte proliferation levels in patients with anxiety disorder than in those without [62]. Complex changes in the inflammation milieu related to aberrant cytokines, particularly IL-1β, IL-6, TNF-α, and interferon (IFN)-γ, have been documented in anxiety-based disorders [63]. Further, persons with anxiety disorder exhibit lower CD4+ cell counts, compared with healthy controls. Studies have also documented the elevation of suppressor CD8+ cells in these conditions, along with a potentiated cytokine response [64].

29.3.3 Depression

During lockdowns, social isolation and lack of physical activity are two prominent risk factors for depression. Depression is known to downregulate immunity, thereby increasing susceptibility to COVID-19-related morbidity and mortality [65]. As with anxiety, depression can induce the body's immunological system to respond abnormally, contributing to heightened infection and mishandling of severe infection and leading to a magnified, self-damaging cytokine response [66].

Individuals with depression were found to have a 60% higher risk for infection, in comparison with nondepressed cohorts [67]. Depression is correlated with disrupted T-cell function and elevated levels of cytokines, such as TNF-α, IL-1, and IL-6 [68], along with alteration in immune markers, including decreases in mitogen proliferation, natural-killer cell activity, and the types and respective quantities of antibodies produced [69]. Depression also dysregulates the neuroendocrine system [70] and consequently increases inflammation, altering the immune system's effectiveness while simultaneously increasing bystander damage [68].

29.4 Yoga and Immunity

Yoga has been found to have a positive impact on the immune system [71–73] and inflammation pathways (Table 29.1 [13]). Multiple studies have substantiated yoga's beneficial effect on

Table 29.1 Studies on yoga and immunity

Author/year	Intervention	Results	Conclusion
Agnihotri et al., 2014 [61]	6-week yoga intervention (30 min/day, 5 days/week of asana and pranayama)	Decreased eosinophil and neutrophil counts among patients with asthma in yoga group	Asana and pranayama help to improve hemoglobin counts and to decrease bronchial inflammation
Chen et al., 2017 [74]	20-week yoga intervention (60 min/day, twice a week of asana and pranayama)	Significantly lower cortisol levels; high IgA; improvement in CD3+ and CD4+ cell counts in yoga group	Asana and pranayama bolster immune response by reducing cortisol levels and increasing IgA and CD3/4+ counts
Naoroibam et al., 2016 [71]	1-month yoga intervention (60 min/day, 6 days/week of asana and pranayama)	Significantly higher CD4+ cell counts in yoga group	Asana and pranayama improve immunity in HIV-1–infected adults
Kiloor et al., 2019 [75]	8-week yoga intervention (60 min/day, 5 days/week of asana and pranayama)	Significantly lower rates of anxiety, stress, and depression in yoga group	Asana and pranayama help lower stress, anxiety, and depression levels of HIV-positive patients
Yadav et al., 2012 [76]	10-day yoga intervention (asana and pranayama)	Decreased levels of cortisol, IL-6, and TNF-α; increased β-endorphin levels	Asana and pranayama reduce inflammation and stress levels over a short span of intervention
Rao et al., 2008 [60]	1-month yoga intervention (pranayama)	Increased CD56+ cell counts in yoga group	Pranayama bolsters innate immunity after surgery

IgA denotes immunoglobulin A, *IL* interleukin, *TNF* tumor necrosis factor

Table 29.2 Studies on yoga and inflammation

Author/year	Intervention	Results	Conclusion
Kiecolt-Glaser et al., 2014 [77]	12-week yoga intervention (twice weekly) among breast cancer survivors	Significant decrease in IL-6, TNF-α, and IL-1β	Yoga practice helps reduce inflammation
Chen et al., 2016 [78]	8-week Hatha yoga intervention (twice weekly) among healthy females	Significant decrease in IL-6, IL-8, IL-1β, and TNF-α	Yoga intervention improves risk for metabolic disorder and inflammatory cytokine dysregulation
Rajbhoj et al., 2016 [79]	12-week yoga intervention among healthy male participants	Significant decrease in IL-10 and IL-1β	Yoga practices could reduce pro- and anti-inflammatory cytokines

IL denotes interleukin, *TNF* tumor necrosis factor

inflammation and have shown that it reduces, and may even inhibit, cytokine release syndrome (Table 29.2 [13]).

The unregulated cytokine storm unleashed by the body in response to SARS-CoV-2 damages multiple organs, resulting in high morbidity and mortality. Cytokine profiles in patients diagnosed with COVID-19 showed marked elevation of T-helper lymphocyte type 1, IFN-γ, and inflammatory cytokines IL-1β, IL-6, and IL-12 for at least 2 weeks after disease onset [80]. Evidence indicates that yoga practice helps to reduce inflammation by downregulating a vast array of initiators and modulators that perpetuate chronic inflammation, including IL-6, TNF-α, and IL-1β [12, 13, 76, 77, 81].

Among these, IL-6 is a mortality predictor in COVID-19 patients, which may explain why primary evidence suggests that IL-6 inhibitors have shown promise as treatments [82]. Randomized controlled trials have documented a significant reduction in IL-6 levels in yoga groups versus controls [83]. In one study of breast cancer patients, researchers observed a significant reduction in IL-6 at the 3-month follow-up for patients who practiced yoga, compared with a non-yoga control group [84]. Moreover, increasing the amount of yoga practice led to a more pronounced decrease in IL-6, suggesting a dose-response effect. Another randomized trial showed significantly lower IL-6 secretion after yoga practice in healthy individuals and significantly lower secretion of IL-6 when cultured blood was challenged with a toll-like receptor agonist [78].

Besides attenuating inflammation, yoga increases the number and activity of natural-killer cells [21, 60, 85], thus enhancing cell-mediated cytotoxicity of invading infective agents. Evidence shows that yoga practice is associated with improvement in CD3+ and CD4+ cell counts, salivary cortisol levels, and IgA [74], a dominant player in innate immunity that is present on body linings, such as those of the lungs and the gastrointestinal tract [86]. Yoga increases IgA levels at the exposed lung border, where type II pneumocytes are prevalent. Additionally, cortisol, which dampens the body's ability to fight infection, is decreased by practicing yoga.

Yoga was shown to be effective in immunocompromised conditions such as HIV, contributing to improvements in CD4+ counts and anxiety, depression, and stress [71, 75]. It has been found to be equally effective in improving CD56+ cell count, anxiety, and depression in chronic disorders such as cancer [60].

29.5 Yoga and Psychosocial Health

Clinical trials have revealed a significant role for yoga practice in reducing depression and its associated variables (Table 29.3 [13]), promoting a positive attitude during stress, and enhancing self-awareness and coping ability (Fig. 29.2 [12, 13]). Yoga (asana, pranayama, and meditation) improves calmness and mindfulness and increases an individual's awareness and self-control [21].

Multiple studies have confirmed that yoga practice reduces depression and improves mood

Table 29.3 Studies on yoga and stress, anxiety, and depression

Author/year	Intervention	Results	Conclusion
West et al., 2004 [87]	90-min Hatha yoga session	Significant reduction in titers, negative affect, and cortisol	Hatha yoga reduces both cortisol and perceived stress level
Michalsen et al., 2005 [17]	3-month Iyengar yoga intervention among mentally distressed women	Compared to the control groups significant reduction in perceived stress was observed	Yoga helps to improve perceived stress among distressed women
Janakiramaiah et al., 2000 [88]	Sudarshan Kriya for 4 weeks among patients with melancholic depression	Significant reduction in depression score	Sudarshan Kriya demonstrated its antidepressant effects in depression
Smith et al., 2007 [20]	10-week Hatha yoga intervention	Significant improvement in SF-36 scores was observed in yoga group	Hatha yoga intervention helps to improve stress, anxiety and health status compared to relaxation
Naveen et al., 2016 [89]	3-month yoga intervention among patients with depression	Significant improvement in depression, BDNF, and serum cortisol was observed	3 month yoga intervention helped improve BDNF, cortisol, and depression in depressive patients
Streeter et al., 2012 [90]	60-min yoga intervention	27% increase in GABA levels in yoga group	Yoga could help treat disorders with low GABA levels like depression, anxiety
Shelov et al., 2009 [23]	8-week yoga intervention	Elevated levels of mindfulness, per Freiburg mindfulness inventory	Yoga increases mindfulness and potentially prevents later development of negative emotional mood states

BDNF denotes brain-derived neurotrophic factor, *GABA* γ-aminobutyric-acid

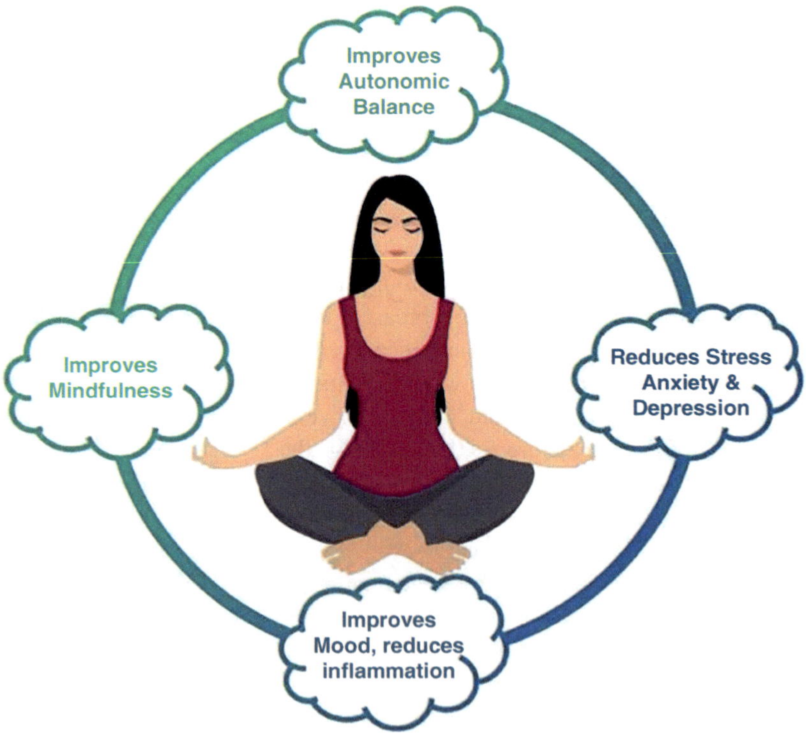
Improves Autonomic Balance
Improves Mindfulness
Reduces Stress Anxiety & Depression
Improves Mood, reduces inflammation

Fig. 29.2 Yoga helps to improve various health parameters related to immunity [Contribution by Mohammad A. Salem, MD; used with permission]

and cognitive function among patients with mild-to-moderate depression; this is achieved by enhancing the HPA axis function, increasing brain-derived neurotrophic factor and serotonin levels, and lowering cortisol and inflammatory marker levels [18, 88, 89]. Autonomic dysfunction is a hallmark of both anxiety and depression [91]; regular yoga practice of pranayama can help improve autonomic balance by decreasing sympathetic overactivity and improving parasympathetic activity [89]. Yoga also enhances the γ-aminobutyric acid system, which is implicated in anxiety and depression [89].

In particular, Hatha yoga (a variation in which only yoga postures are practiced, with little or no meditation) has been shown to improve HPA axis dysregulation, correct autonomic balance, and enhance homeostasis by hastening recovery from stress [19]. In a study among 131 participants with mild to moderate stress levels, 10 weeks of a Hatha yoga intervention significantly reduced stress and anxiety and improved relaxation [20]. In another study, 90-min Hatha yoga sessions led to a significant reduction in titers, negative affect, and cortisol levels [87].

Yoga helps to lower the allostatic load of the stress response [90]. It reduces sympathetic overactivity and improves parasympathetic tone during stressful situations, as indicated by oxygen consumption level, heart rate, and the high-frequency component of heart rate variability [92]. In one study, 16 distressed women participated in 3 months of Iyengar yoga, with another group of eight women serving as a control. After 3 months, the yoga group had significantly lower levels of perceived stress, depression, anxiety, and salivary cortisol, compared with controls; well-being also improved significantly for the women in the yoga group [17]. Outcomes from an 8-week asana, pranayama, and meditation intervention indicated that medical treatment plus yoga was more effective in reducing anxiety than was medical treatment alone [93].

Yoga improves body awareness, boosts feelings and thoughts, and allows its practitioners to experience body sensations in a nonjudgmental way [22]. Importantly, yoga promotes focusing on present experiences instead of ruminating over future or past worries [23]. Self-awareness aids the avoidance of addictive or overindulgent behaviors, including overeating and excess sleeping. Moreover, yoga improves various cognitive facets, such as attention, concentration, memory, and executive functioning [94]. During this time of pandemic-related lockdown and social isolation, yoga can help people remain active and maintain a positive attitude.

29.6 Yoga and Cardiorespiratory Protection

Patients with COVID-19 often manifest severe cardiorespiratory illness [1]. Myocarditis with severe refractory acute heart failure has been noted in patients with COVID-19 [95]. Myocarditis is possibly caused by cytokine-mediated destruction; however, the chance of direct damage from COVID-19 cannot be ignored, as both the heart and the vascular endothelium express the ACE2 receptors that are entry gates for the SARS-CoV-2 virus [25].

Yoga is known to have various positive effects on the cardiovascular and respiratory systems, such that consistent yoga practice may play a protective role. Yoga has been proven to improve various forms of cardiac arrhythmia, congestive cardiac failure, ischemic heart disease, and hypertension [6–10]. Regular yoga practice attenuates systolic and diastolic blood pressure and mean arterial pressure; it has also been credited with maintaining appropriate blood pressure with less medication [96]. Simply lying down in the Savasana yogic posture for 20 min daily was shown to lower systolic and diastolic blood pressure and to reduce the need for antihypertensive medication [97]. Yoga has also been shown to improve cardiac function in patients with congestive cardiac failure [98] and to improve baroreflex sensitivity, peripheral vascular resistance, and heart rate variability [99].

Evidence indicates that yoga offers multifaceted protection from cardiac damage mediated by aberrant cytokine release, such as that seen with COVID-19. A study in patients with heart failure found that 8 weeks of yoga intervention significantly lowered levels of IL-6, C-reactive protein, and extracellular superoxide dismutase, compared with results from non-yoga controls [100]. Yoga also helps to attenuate catecholamine secretion, which has been implicated in the development of severe cardiomyopathy and heart failure [101].

29.7 Conclusions

The present COVID-19-related lockdowns and social isolation have produced an aggregation of psychological and somatic aberrations that may well increase susceptibility to the very infection they were designed to avoid. Accumulated evidence suggests that, for many, yoga practice may attenuate these ill effects of COVID-19-induced immune dysfunction at any point along the disease trajectory [12, 13]. Long-term yoga practitioners may even be resistant to the dystrophic immune response seen in moderate-to-severe COVID-19, secondary to yoga-induced modulation of cytokine response to stress [102].

From a public health perspective, yoga represents a low-cost, noninvasive strategy for alleviating the physical and emotional toll of the COVID-19 pandemic; as an added benefit, it can be performed at home, in adherence to social distancing guidelines. We, therefore, propose that patients with COVID-19 (and even those without) should consider yoga as an intervention that may enhance innate immunity and mental health for all comers and expedite recovery for the ill. Notwithstanding, appropriate clinical trials are required to document the efficacy of this strategy.

References

1. Basu-Ray I, Almaddah N, Adeboye A, Soos MP. Cardiac manifestations of coronavirus (COVID-19). In: StatPearls. Treasure Island, FL: StatPearls Publishing LLC; 2020.
2. Weiss SR, Navas-Martin S. Coronavirus pathogenesis and the emerging pathogen severe acute respiratory syndrome coronavirus. Microbiol Mol Biol Rev. 2005;69:635–64. https://doi.org/10.1128/MMBR.69.4.635-664.2005.
3. World Health Organization. Coronavirus disease (COVID-2019) situation reports. 2020. Available online at: https://www.who.int/emergencies/diseases/novel-coronavirus-2019/situation-reports Accessed 30 June 2020.
4. Elson BD, Hauri P, Cunis D. Physiological changes in yoga meditation. Psychophysiology. 1977;14:52–7. https://doi.org/10.1111/j.1469-8986.1977.tb01155.x.
5. McCall MC, Ward A, Roberts NW, Heneghan C. Overview of systematic reviews: yoga as a therapeutic intervention for adults with acute and chronic health conditions. Evid Based Complement Alternat Med. 2013;2013:945895. https://doi.org/10.1155/2013/945895.
6. Posadzki P, Cramer H, Kuzdzal A, Lee MS, Ernst E. Yoga for hypertension: a systematic review of randomized clinical trials. Complement Ther Med. 2014;22:511–22. https://doi.org/10.1016/j.ctim.2014.03.009.
7. Bhavanani AB, Ramanathan M, Balaji R, Pushpa D. Comparative immediate effect of different yoga asanas on heart rate and blood pressure in healthy young volunteers. Int J Yoga. 2014;7:89–95. https://doi.org/10.4103/0973-6131.133870.
8. Lakkireddy D, Atkins D, Pillarisetti J, Ryschon K, Bommana S, Drisko J, et al. Effect of yoga on arrhythmia burden, anxiety, depression, and quality of life in paroxysmal atrial fibrillation: the YOGA My Heart Study. J Am Coll Cardiol. 2013;61:1177–82. https://doi.org/10.1016/j.jacc.2012.11.060.
9. Hagins M, States R, Selfe T, Innes K. Effectiveness of yoga for hypertension: systematic review and meta-analysis. Evid Based Complement Alternat Med. 2013;2013:649836. https://doi.org/10.1155/2013/649836.
10. Patel C, North WR. Randomised controlled trial of yoga and bio-feedback in management of hypertension. Lancet. 1975;2:93–5. https://doi.org/10.1016/s0140-6736(75)90002-1.
11. Desveaux L, Lee A, Goldstein R, Brooks D. Yoga in the management of chronic disease: a systematic review and meta-analysis. Med Care. 2015;53:653–61. https://doi.org/10.1097/MLR.0000000000000372.
12. Nagarathna R, Nagendra HR, Majumdar V. A perspective on yoga as a preventive strategy for coronavirus disease 2019. International Journal of Yoga. 2020;13(2):89.
13. Nadholta P, Bali P, Singh A, Anand A. Potential benefits of Yoga in pregnancy-related complications during the COVID-19 pandemic and implications for working women. Work. 2020;67(2):269–79. https://doi.org/10.3233/WOR-203277. PMID: 33044208.
14. Prinster T. Yoga for cancer: a guide to managing side effects, boosting immunity, and improving recovery for cancer survivors. Rochester, VT: Healing Arts Press; 2014. 324 p.

15. Harinath K, Malhotra AS, Pal K, Prasad R, Kumar R, Kain TC, et al. Effects of Hatha yoga and Omkar meditation on cardiorespiratory performance, psychologic profile, and melatonin secretion. J Altern Complement Med. 2004;10:261–8. https://doi.org/10.1089/107555304323062257.
16. Hagen I, Nayar US. Yoga for children and young people's mental health and well-being: research review and reflections on the mental health potentials of yoga. Front Psychiatry. 2014;5:35. https://doi.org/10.3389/fpsyt.2014.00035.
17. Michalsen A, Grossman P, Acil A, Langhorst J, Lüdtke R, Esch T, et al. Rapid stress reduction and anxiolysis among distressed women as a consequence of a three-month intensive yoga program. Med Sci Monit. 2005;11:CR555–61.
18. Cramer H, Lauche R, Langhorst J, Dobos G. Yoga for depression: a systematic review and meta-analysis. Depress Anxiety. 2013;30:1068–83. https://doi.org/10.1002/da.22166.
19. Patil SG, Aithala MR, Naregal GV, Shanmukhe AG, Chopade SS. Effect of yoga on cardiac autonomic dysfunction and insulin resistance in non-diabetic offspring of type-2-diabetes parents: a randomized controlled study. Complement Ther Clin Pract. 2019;34:288–93. https://doi.org/10.1016/j.ctcp.2019.01.003.
20. Smith C, Hancock H, Blake-Mortimer J, Eckert K. A randomised comparative trial of yoga and relaxation to reduce stress and anxiety. Complement Ther Med. 2007;15:77–83. https://doi.org/10.1016/j.ctim.2006.05.001.
21. Cook-Cottone CP. Mindfulness and yoga for self-regulation: a primer for mental health professionals. New York: Springer Publishing Company; 2015. 322 p.
22. Daubenmier JJ. The relationship of yoga, body awareness, and body responsiveness to self-objectification and disordered eating. Psychol Women Q. 2005;29:207–19. https://doi.org/10.1111/j.1471-6402.2005.00183.x.
23. Shelov DV, Suchday S, Friedberg JP. A pilot study measuring the impact of yoga on the trait of mindfulness. Behav Cogn Psychother. 2009;37:595–8. https://doi.org/10.1017/S1352465809990361.
24. Wang D, Hu B, Hu C, Zhu F, Liu X, Zhang J, et al. Clinical characteristics of 138 hospitalized patients with 2019 novel coronavirus-infected pneumonia in Wuhan, China. JAMA. 2020;323:1061–9. https://doi.org/10.1001/jama.2020.1585.
25. Xu Z, Shi L, Wang Y, Zhang J, Huang L, Zhang C, et al. Pathological findings of COVID-19 associated with acute respiratory distress syndrome. Lancet Respir Med. 2020;8:420–2. https://doi.org/10.1016/S2213-2600(20)30076-X.
26. Zheng YY, Ma YT, Zhang JY, Xie X. COVID-19 and the cardiovascular system. Nat Rev Cardiol. 2020;17:259–60. https://doi.org/10.1038/s41569-020-0360-5.
27. Cao X. COVID-19: immunopathology and its implications for therapy. Nat Rev Immunol. 2020;20:269–70. https://doi.org/10.1038/s41577-020-0308-3.
28. Shi Y, Wang Y, Shao C, Huang J, Gan J, Huang X, et al. COVID-19 infection: the perspectives on immune responses. Cell Death Differ. 2020;27:1451–4. https://doi.org/10.1038/s41418-020-0530-3.
29. Mehta P, McAuley DF, Brown M, Sanchez E, Tattersall RS, Manson JJ, et al. COVID-19: consider cytokine storm syndromes and immunosuppression. Lancet. 2020;395:1033–4. https://doi.org/10.1016/S0140-6736(20)30628-0.
30. CDC Covid-Response Team. Severe outcomes among patients with coronavirus disease 2019 (COVID-19)—United States, February 12–March 16, 2020. MMWR Morb Mortal Wkly Rep. 2020;69:343–6. https://doi.org/10.15585/mmwr.mm6912e2.
31. Li H, Liu L, Zhang D, Xu J, Dai H, Tang N, et al. SARS-CoV-2 and viral sepsis: observations and hypotheses. Lancet. 2020;395:1517–20. https://doi.org/10.1016/S0140-6736(20)30920-X.
32. Huang C, Wang Y, Li X, Ren L, Zhao J, Hu Y, et al. Clinical features of patients infected with 2019 novel coronavirus in Wuhan, China. Lancet. 2020;395:497–506. https://doi.org/10.1016/S0140-6736(20)30183-5.
33. Shi S, Qin M, Shen B, Cai Y, Liu T, Yang F, et al. Association of cardiac injury with mortality in hospitalized patients with COVID-19 in Wuhan, China. JAMA Cardiol. 2020; https://doi.org/10.1001/jamacardio.2020.0950.
34. Mehra MR, Desai SS, Kuy S, Henry TD, Patel AN. Cardiovascular disease, drug therapy, and mortality in Covid-19. N Engl J Med. 2020;382:e102. https://doi.org/10.1056/NEJMoa2007621.
35. Zhou F, Yu T, Du R, Fan G, Liu Y, Liu Z, et al. Clinical course and risk factors for mortality of adult inpatients with COVID-19 in Wuhan, China: a retrospective cohort study. Lancet. 2020;395:1054–62. https://doi.org/10.1016/S0140-6736(20)30566-3.
36. Wu Z, McGoogan JM. Characteristics of and important lessons from the coronavirus disease 2019 (COVID-19) outbreak in China: summary of a report of 72,314 cases from the Chinese Center for Disease Control and Prevention. JAMA. 2020; https://doi.org/10.1001/jama.2020.2648.
37. Li B, Yang J, Zhao F, Zhi L, Wang X, Liu L, et al. Prevalence and impact of cardiovascular metabolic diseases on COVID-19 in China. Clin Res Cardiol. 2020;109:531–8. https://doi.org/10.1007/s00392-020-01626-9.
38. Puntmann VO, Carerj ML, Wieters I, Fahim M, Arendt C, Hoffmann J, et al. Outcomes of cardiovascular magnetic resonance imaging in patients recently recovered from coronavirus disease 2019 (COVID-19). JAMA Cardiol. 2020; https://doi.org/10.1001/jamacardio.2020.3557.
39. Xiong TY, Redwood S, Prendergast B, Chen M. Coronaviruses and the cardiovascular sys-

tem: acute and long-term implications. Eur Heart J. 2020;41:1798–800. https://doi.org/10.1093/eurheartj/ehaa231.
40. Clerkin KJ, Fried JA, Raikhelkar J, Sayer G, Griffin JM, Masoumi A, et al. COVID-19 and cardiovascular disease. Circulation. 2020;141:1648–55. https://doi.org/10.1161/CIRCULATIONAHA.120.046941.
41. Lindner D, Fitzek A, Bräuninger H, Aleshcheva G, Edler C, Meissner K, et al. Association of cardiac infection with SARS-CoV-2 in confirmed COVID-19 autopsy cases. JAMA Cardiol. 2020; https://doi.org/10.1001/jamacardio.2020.3551.
42. Channappanavar R, Perlman S. Pathogenic human coronavirus infections: causes and consequences of cytokine storm and immunopathology. Semin Immunopathol. 2017;39:529–39. https://doi.org/10.1007/s00281-017-0629-x.
43. Qin C, Zhou L, Hu Z, Zhang S, Yang S, Tao Y, et al. Dysregulation of immune response in patients with COVID-19 in Wuhan, China. Clin Infect Dis. 2020; https://doi.org/10.1093/cid/ciaa248.
44. Schoenhagen P, Tuzcu EM, Ellis SG. Plaque vulnerability, plaque rupture, and acute coronary syndromes: (multi)-focal manifestation of a systemic disease process. Circulation. 2002;106:760–2. https://doi.org/10.1161/01.cir.0000025708.36290.05.
45. Dominguez-Erquicia P, Dobarro D, Raposeiras-Roubín S, Bastos-Fernandez G, Iñiguez-Romo A. Multivessel coronary thrombosis in a patient with COVID-19 pneumonia. Eur Heart J. 2020;41:2132. https://doi.org/10.1093/eurheartj/ehaa393.
46. Wang Y, Zhang D, Du G, Du R, Zhao J, Jin Y, et al. Remdesivir in adults with severe COVID-19: a randomised, double-blind, placebo-controlled, multicentre trial. Lancet. 2020;395:1569–78. https://doi.org/10.1016/S0140-6736(20)31022-9.
47. Pappa S, Ntella V, Giannakas T, Giannakoulis VG, Papoutsi E, Katsaounou P. Prevalence of depression, anxiety, and insomnia among healthcare workers during the COVID-19 pandemic: a systematic review and meta-analysis. Brain Behav Immun. 2020; https://doi.org/10.1016/j.bbi.2020.05.026.
48. Godinić D, Obrenovic B, Khudaykulov A. Effects of economic uncertainty on mental health in the COVID-19 pandemic context: social identity disturbance, job uncertainty and psychological well-being model. Int J Innov Econ Dev. 2020;6:61–74. https://doi.org/10.18775/ijied.1849-7551-7020.2015.61.2005.
49. Ackerman KD, Martino M, Heyman R, Moyna NM, Rabin BS. Immunologic response to acute psychological stress in MS patients and controls. J Neuroimmunol. 1996;68:85–94. https://doi.org/10.1016/0165-5728(96)00077-x.
50. Vedhara K, McDermott MP, Evans TG, Treanor JJ, Plummer S, Tallon D, et al. Chronic stress in nonelderly caregivers: psychological, endocrine and immune implications. J Psychosom Res. 2002;53:1153–61. https://doi.org/10.1016/s0022-3999(02)00343-4.
51. Pedersen A, Zachariae R, Bovbjerg DH. Influence of psychological stress on upper respiratory infection—a meta-analysis of prospective studies. Psychosom Med. 2010;72:823–32. https://doi.org/10.1097/PSY.0b013e3181f1d003.
52. Lambert EA, Lambert GW. Stress and its role in sympathetic nervous system activation in hypertension and the metabolic syndrome. Curr Hypertens Rep. 2011;13:244–8. https://doi.org/10.1007/s11906-011-0186-y.
53. van Westerloo DJ, Choi G, Löwenberg EC, Truijen J, de Vos AF, Endert E, et al. Acute stress elicited by bungee jumping suppresses human innate immunity. Mol Med. 2011;17:180–8. https://doi.org/10.2119/molmed.2010.00204.
54. Locke S, Hurst M, Heisel J, Kraus L, Williams M. The influence of stress and other psychosocial factors on human immunity [abstract]. Psychosomatic Society 36th Annual Meeting, Dallas, TX. 1979, Mar 23.
55. Vedhara K, Cox NK, Wilcock GK, Perks P, Hunt M, Anderson S, et al. Chronic stress in elderly carers of dementia patients and antibody response to influenza vaccination. Lancet. 1999;353:627–31. https://doi.org/10.1016/S0140-6736(98)06098-X.
56. Joseph JJ, Golden SH. Cortisol dysregulation: the bidirectional link between stress, depression, and type 2 diabetes mellitus. Ann N Y Acad Sci. 2017;1391:20–34. https://doi.org/10.1111/nyas.13217.
57. Miller GE, Cohen S, Ritchey AK. Chronic psychological stress and the regulation of pro-inflammatory cytokines: a glucocorticoid-resistance model. Health Psychol. 2002;21:531–41. https://doi.org/10.1037//0278-6133.21.6.531.
58. Miller GE, Chen E, Fok AK, Walker H, Lim A, Nicholls EF, et al. Low early-life social class leaves a biological residue manifested by decreased glucocorticoid and increased proinflammatory signaling. Proc Natl Acad Sci U S A. 2009;106:14716–21. https://doi.org/10.1073/pnas.0902971106.
59. Furman D, Campisi J, Verdin E, Carrera-Bastos P, Targ S, Franceschi C, et al. Chronic inflammation in the etiology of disease across the life span. Nat Med. 2019;25:1822–32. https://doi.org/10.1038/s41591-019-0675-0.
60. Rao RM, Nagendra HR, Raghuram N, Vinay C, Chandrashekara S, Gopinath KS, et al. Influence of yoga on mood states, distress, quality of life and immune outcomes in early stage breast cancer patients undergoing surgery. Int J Yoga. 2008;1:11–20. https://doi.org/10.4103/0973-6131.36789.
61. Agnihotri S, Kant S, Kumar S, Mishra RK, Mishra SK. Impact of yoga on biochemical profile of asthmatics: a randomized controlled study. Int J Yoga. 2014;7:17–21. https://doi.org/10.4103/0973-6131.123473.
62. Koh KB, Lee Y. Reduced anxiety level by therapeutic interventions and cell-mediated immunity in panic disorder patients. Psychother Psychosom. 2004;73:286–92. https://doi.org/10.1159/000078845.

63. Nagata T, Yamada H, Iketani T, Kiriike N. Relationship between plasma concentrations of cytokines, ratio of CD4 and CD8, lymphocyte proliferative responses, and depressive and anxiety state in bulimia nervosa. J Psychosom Res. 2006;60:99–103. https://doi.org/10.1016/j.jpsychores.2005.06.058.
64. Michopoulos V, Powers A, Gillespie CF, Ressler KJ, Jovanovic T. Inflammation in fear- and anxiety-based disorders: PTSD, GAD, and beyond. Neuropsychopharmacology. 2017;42:254–70. https://doi.org/10.1038/npp.2016.146.
65. Gerra G, Monti D, Panerai AE, Sacerdote P, Anderlini R, Avanzini P, et al. Long-term immune-endocrine effects of bereavement: relationships with anxiety levels and mood. Psychiatry Res. 2003;121:145–58. https://doi.org/10.1016/s0165-1781(03)00255-5.
66. Atanackovic D, Kröger H, Serke S, Deter HC. Immune parameters in patients with anxiety or depression during psychotherapy. J Affect Disord. 2004;81:201–9. https://doi.org/10.1016/S0165-0327(03)00165-4.
67. Irwin MR, Levin MJ, Carrillo C, Olmstead R, Lucko A, Lang N, et al. Major depressive disorder and immunity to varicella-zoster virus in the elderly. Brain Behav Immun. 2011;25:759–66. https://doi.org/10.1016/j.bbi.2011.02.001.
68. Olff M. Stress, depression and immunity: the role of defense and coping styles. Psychiatry Res. 1999;85:7–15. https://doi.org/10.1016/s0165-1781(98)00139-5.
69. Rothermundt M, Arolt V, Fenker J, Gutbrodt H, Peters M, Kirchner H. Different immune patterns in melancholic and non-melancholic major depression. Eur Arch Psychiatry Clin Neurosci. 2001;251:90–7. https://doi.org/10.1007/s004060170058.
70. Targum SD, Sullivan AC, Byrnes SM. Neuroendocrine interrelationships in major depressive disorder. Am J Psychiatry. 1982;139:282–6. https://doi.org/10.1176/ajp.139.3.282.
71. Naoroibam R, Metri KG, Bhargav H, Nagaratna R, Nagendra HR. Effect of integrated yoga (IY) on psychological states and CD4 counts of HIV-1 infected patients: a randomized controlled pilot study. Int J Yoga. 2016;9:57–61. https://doi.org/10.4103/0973-6131.171723.
72. Gopal A, Mondal S, Gandhi A, Arora S, Bhattacharjee J. Effect of integrated yoga practices on immune responses in examination stress—a preliminary study. Int J Yoga. 2011;4:26–32. https://doi.org/10.4103/0973-6131.78178.
73. Hari Chandra BP, Ramesh MN, Nagendra HR. Effect of yoga on immune parameters, cognitive functions, and quality of life among HIV-positive children/adolescents: a pilot study. Int J Yoga. 2019;12:132–8. https://doi.org/10.4103/ijoy.IJOY_51_18.
74. Chen PJ, Yang L, Chou CC, Li CC, Chang YC, Liaw JJ. Effects of prenatal yoga on women's stress and immune function across pregnancy: a randomized controlled trial. Complement Ther Med. 2017;31:109–17. https://doi.org/10.1016/j.ctim.2017.03.003.
75. Kiloor A, Kumari S, Metri K. Impact of yoga on psychopathologies and QoLin persons with HIV: a randomized controlled study. J Bodyw Mov Ther. 2019;23:P278–83. https://doi.org/10.1016/j.jbmt.2018.10.005.
76. Yadav RK, Magan D, Mehta N, Sharma R, Mahapatra SC. Efficacy of a short-term yoga-based lifestyle intervention in reducing stress and inflammation: preliminary results. J Altern Complement Med. 2012;18:662–7. https://doi.org/10.1089/acm.2011.0265.
77. Kiecolt-Glaser JK, Bennett JM, Andridge R, Peng J, Shapiro CL, Malarkey WB, et al. Yoga's impact on inflammation, mood, and fatigue in breast cancer survivors: a randomized controlled trial. J Clin Oncol. 2014;32:1040–9. https://doi.org/10.1200/JCO.2013.51.8860.
78. Chen N, Xia X, Qin L, Luo L, Han S, Wang G, et al. Effects of 8-week Hatha yoga training on metabolic and inflammatory markers in healthy, female Chinese subjects: a randomized clinical trial. Biomed Res Int. 2016;2016:5387258. https://doi.org/10.1155/2016/5387258.
79. Rajbhoj PH, Shete SU, Verma A, Bhogal RS. Effect of yoga module on pro-inflammatory and anti-inflammatory cytokines in industrial workers of lonavla: a randomized controlled trial. J Clin Diagn Res. 2015;9:CC01–5. https://doi.org/10.7860/JCDR/2015/11426.5551.
80. Zhang C, Wu Z, Li JW, Zhao H, Wang GQ. Cytokine release syndrome in severe COVID-19: interleukin-6 receptor antagonist tocilizumab may be the key to reduce mortality. Int J Antimicrob Agents. 2020;55:105954. https://doi.org/10.1016/j.ijantimicag.2020.105954.
81. Nagarathna R, Nagendra H, Majumdar V. A perspective on yoga as a preventive strategy for coronavirus disease 2019. Int J Yoga. 2020;13:89–98. https://doi.org/10.4103/ijoy.IJOY_22_20.
82. Luo P, Liu Y, Qiu L, Liu X, Liu D, Li J. Tocilizumab treatment in COVID-19: a single center experience. J Med Virol. 2020;92:814–8. https://doi.org/10.1002/jmv.25801.
83. Pullen PR, Thompson WR, Benardot D, Brandon LJ, Mehta PK, Rifai L, et al. Benefits of yoga for African American heart failure patients. Med Sci Sports Exerc. 2010;42:651–7. https://doi.org/10.1249/MSS.0b013e3181bf24c4.
84. Bower JE, Greendale G, Crosswell AD, Garet D, Sternlieb B, Ganz PA, et al. Yoga reduces inflammatory signaling in fatigued breast cancer survivors: a randomized controlled trial. Psychoneuroendocrinology. 2014;43:20–9. https://doi.org/10.1016/j.psyneuen.2014.01.019.
85. Vijayaraghava A, Doreswamy V, Narasipur OS, Kunnavil R, Srinivasamurthy N. Effect of yoga practice on levels of inflammatory markers after moderate and strenuous exercise. J Clin Diagn

Res. 2015;9:CC08–12. https://doi.org/10.7860/JCDR/2015/12851.6021.
86. Bradley PA, Bourne FJ, Brown PJ. The respiratory tract immune system in the pig. I. Distribution of immunoglobulin-containing cells in the respiratory tract mucosa. Vet Pathol. 1976;13:81–9. https://doi.org/10.1177/030098587601300201.
87. West J, Otte C, Geher K, Johnson J, Mohr DC. Effects of Hatha yoga and African dance on perceived stress, affect, and salivary cortisol. Ann Behav Med. 2004;28:114–8. https://doi.org/10.1207/s15324796abm2802_6.
88. Janakiramaiah N, Gangadhar BN, Naga Venkatesha Murthy PJ, Harish MG, Subbakrishna DK, Vedamurthachar A. Antidepressant efficacy of Sudarshan Kriya Yoga (SKY) in melancholia: a randomized comparison with electroconvulsive therapy (ECT) and imipramine. J Affect Disord. 2000;57:255–9. https://doi.org/10.1016/s0165-0327(99)00079-8.
89. Naveen GH, Varambally S, Thirthalli J, Rao M, Christopher R, Gangadhar BN. Serum cortisol and BDNF in patients with major depression—effect of yoga. Int Rev Psychiatry. 2016;28:273–8. https://doi.org/10.1080/09540261.2016.1175419.
90. Streeter CC, Gerbarg PL, Saper RB, Ciraulo DA, Brown RP. Effects of yoga on the autonomic nervous system, gamma-aminobutyric-acid, and allostasis in epilepsy, depression, and post-traumatic stress disorder. Med Hypotheses. 2012;78:571–9. https://doi.org/10.1016/j.mehy.2012.01.021.
91. Sarubin N, Nothdurfter C, Schüle C, Lieb M, Uhr M, Born C, et al. The influence of Hatha yoga as an add-on treatment in major depression on hypothalamic-pituitary-adrenal-axis activity: a randomized trial. J Psychiatr Res. 2014;53:76–83. https://doi.org/10.1016/j.jpsychires.2014.02.022.
92. Vempati RP, Telles S. Yoga-based guided relaxation reduces sympathetic activity judged from baseline levels. Psychol Rep. 2002;90:487–94. https://doi.org/10.2466/pr0.2002.90.2.487.
93. Sharma P, Poojary G, Dwivedi SN, Deepak KK. Effect of yoga-based intervention in patients with inflammatory bowel disease. Int J Yoga Therap. 2015;25:101–12. https://doi.org/10.17761/1531-2054-25.1.101.
94. Luu K, Hall PA. Hatha yoga and executive function: a systematic review. J Altern Complement Med. 2016;22:125–33. https://doi.org/10.1089/acm.2014.0091.
95. Musher DM, Abers MS, Corrales-Medina VF. Acute infection and myocardial infarction. N Engl J Med. 2019;380:171–6. https://doi.org/10.1056/NEJMra1808137.
96. Veerabhadrappa SG, Baljoshi VS, Khanapure S, Herur A, Patil S, Ankad RB, et al. Effect of yogic bellows on cardiovascular autonomic reactivity. J Cardiovasc Dis Res. 2011;2:223–7. https://doi.org/10.4103/0975-3583.89806.
97. Santaella DF, Lorenzi-Filho G, Rodrigues MR, Tinucci T, Malinauskas AP, Mion-Júnior D, et al. Yoga relaxation (savasana) decreases cardiac sympathovagal balance in hypertensive patients. MedicalExpress. 2014;1:233–8.
98. Krishna BH, Pal P, Pal GK, Balachander J, Jayasettiaseelon E, Sreekanth Y, et al. Effect of yoga therapy on heart rate, blood pressure and cardiac autonomic function in heart failure. J Clin Diagn Res. 2014;8:14–6. https://doi.org/10.7860/JCDR/2014/7844.3983.
99. Bowman AJ, Clayton RH, Murray A, Reed JW, Subhan MM, Ford GA. Effects of aerobic exercise training and yoga on the baroreflex in healthy elderly persons. Eur J Clin Invest. 1997;27:443–9. https://doi.org/10.1046/j.1365-2362.1997.1340681.x.
100. Pullen PR, Nagamia SH, Mehta PK, Thompson WR, Benardot D, Hammoud R, et al. Effects of yoga on inflammation and exercise capacity in patients with chronic heart failure. J Card Fail. 2008;14:407–13. https://doi.org/10.1016/j.cardfail.2007.12.007.
101. Rajak C, Verma R, Singh P, Singh A, Shiralkar M. Effect of yoga on serum adrenaline, serum cortisol levels and cardiovascular parameters in hyper-reactors to cold pressor test in young healthy volunteers. Eur J of Pharm Med Res. 2016;3:496–502.
102. Arora S, Bhattacharjee J. Modulation of immune responses in stress by yoga. Int J Yoga. 2008;1:45–55. https://doi.org/10.4103/0973-6131.43541.

Part V

Appendix

Dinacharya the Daily Routine and Ritucharya the Seasonal Routine for Yogic Lifestyle

30

Dilip Sarkar

A *dinacharya*, or daily routine, is one of the best practices that one can do to prevent and manage cardiovascular disease (*swastha Raksha*-maintenance of health and *rogir chikitsa*-treatment of patient). *Din* means "day" and *charya* means "routine," making a literal translation from Sanskrit of "daily routine." It means merging the daily cycle with the natural cycle of the solar system. The *yogic rishi* (a person who practices self-realization as a *yogi* or *yogini*) considers daily routine to be a stronger healing force than any other curative medicine. *Dinacharya* activates relaxation response and parasympathetic tone to counteract the sympathetic overdrive of stress the cause of cardiovascular disease.

It is best to adopt these daily practices into one's life slowly, so they are manageable, which encourages sustainability. Try beginning with one or two simple practices and adapting them daily, over the course of 3 weeks or so, since it takes 21 days to create a new habit through neuroplasticity. Then add a few more items to routine and so on. Before a person knows it, they will have a regular *dinacharya*. These daily practices are designed to bring the body to optimal health through proper digestion, elimination, and sleep which are the signs of health in yoga. As one adds these practices, pay attention to how the body and mind feel and observe what is happening. Many people feel immediate results with cardiovascular health.

30.1 Yogic and Ayurvedic Clock

The outcome of yoga practice is self-realization and the health benefits are byproduct. During the yoga practice, it became infused with *mudras* (hand gesture), *bandhas* (spiritual locks), *kriyas* (cleansing the body-mind), acupressure, and *Ayurvedic* philosophy to become yoga therapy (*yoga chikitsa*). It is helpful to understand the philosophy of *Ayurvedic* Medicine (Indian healing tradition) which has the same *vedic* root as yoga. The *dinacharya* is based on *Ayurvedic* philosophy. *Ayurveda* is a balance between microcosm (*pinda*) and macrocosm (*brahmanda*). The universe or macrocosm has five elements, space, air, fire, water and earth, and all these elements are also present in our body or microcosm. The attributes of these elements create a psycho-physiological energy body type called

D. Sarkar (✉)
American Association of Integrative Medicine (AAIM), American College of Surgeons (ACS), Virginia, MD, USA

American Heart Association, Virginia Beach, VA, USA

International Association of Yoga Therapists (IAYT), Little Rock, AR, USA

Life in Yoga Institute, Silver Spring, MD, USA

Center for Integrative Medicine and Yoga, Taksha Institute, Hampton, VA, USA

I. Basu-Ray, D. Mehta (eds.), *The Principles and Practice of Yoga in Cardiovascular Medicine*,
https://doi.org/10.1007/978-981-16-6913-2_30

doshas. Predominance of attributes of air in the body is called *vata* with a mobile catabolic energy, predominance of fire attributes is called *pitta* a fiery metabolic energy and a person with water attributes is called *kapha* a grounding anabolic energy. The concept of *doshas* breaks up the day into energy blocks associated with *vata*, *pitta*, and *kapha* and their energy of digestive fire (*jathar agni*). These three types of energies are derived after proper digestion of food. The end product of metabolism is glucose, which combines with oxygen and through aerobic glycolysis produces carbon dioxide, water, and energy as ATP (adenosine triphosphate). This energy performs all the functions of the body as catabolic, metabolic, and anabolic and the person tuned to these energies remains healthy. The breakdown of these energy cycles (*Ayurvedic* clock) is as follows:

30.1.1 First Cycle

- 6:00 a.m. to 10:00 a.m.—*Kapha* time, low digestive fire (*jathar agni*)
- 10:00 a.m. to 2:00 p.m.—*Pitta* time, strong digestive fire
- 2:00 p.m. to 6:00 p.m.—*Vata* time, variable digestive fire

30.1.2 Second Cycle

- 6:00 p.m. to 10:00 p.m.—*Kapha* time, low digestive fire
- 10:00 p.m. to 2:00 a.m.—*Pitta* time, strong digestive fire
- 2:00 a.m. to 6:00 a.m.—*Vata* time, variable digestive fire

The *Ayurvedic* daily routine centers on maximizing these daily energy cycles.

30.2 Morning

As mentioned before the person with cardiovascular disease should practice these daily routines slowly and in stages. A healthy person will try to get up 2 h before sunrise (between 4 and 6), which is called *Brahma Muhurta*, or the time of *Brahma*, the Supreme Being. This is the time when there is the most *sattva*, or purifying energy, in the air and environment. It is the freshest and purest time of the day. Practice waking up at this time of the day and the person will be rewarded with a much healthier and satisfying life.

30.2.1 Proper Hydration

Drinking a healthy amount of water is vital to our health. One of the easiest daily practices to add is proper hydration. Proper hydration is antithrombotic and anti-inflammatory; inflammation is the root cause of all cardiovascular diseases. Our bodies are composed mostly of water. We need water to break down food, clear our systems, and facilitate optimal function of vital organs. When one is dehydrated, the body cannot function optimally. Bodily functions slow or shut down, brain function is interrupted, and we become drowsy, lethargic, and disoriented. As we age, our perception of thirst, the indicator that more water is needed, becomes less sensitive and we may forget to consume enough water. To maintain proper hydration throughout the day, drink a glass of tepid water 1 h after every meal, drinking additional water as thirst dictates. A simple formula to determine the amount of water that should be consumed daily is half an ounce of water per pound of body weight. For example, a person weighing 150 pounds should drink 75 ounces of water per day. The total quantity of water also includes other fluid intakes.

One reason we are groggy when we wake up in the morning is dehydration from loss of body fluid while we were sleeping called insensible perspiration. Drinking a glass of water after waking up replenishes the body with water lost overnight and helps relieve grogginess, maintain fluid balance, stimulate the brain, and trigger elimination. Drink a comfortable amount of water at room temperature after waking up (*ushapan*). One should drink up to 12 ounces of water, but it might be wise to start with a half glass of water and work up to that amount. The water is ideally imbibed from a copper vessel, which encourages

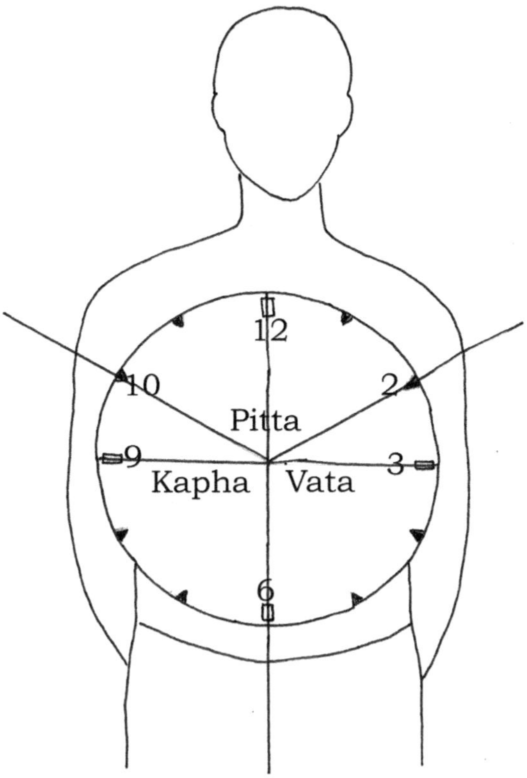

Fig. 30.1 *Ayurvedic* clock

elimination. Drinking water before bed prepares the body for the overnight release of water, creating a reservoir. If one has trouble drinking so much water at first, start with a smaller amount and build up to the full amount over time. *Ayurvedic* theory recommends water at room temperature because it is believed that cold water interferes with the *jathar agni*, or digestive fire, in the stomach (Fig. 30.1).

30.2.2 Elimination

Drinking a glass or two of lukewarm water at room temperature immediately after getting up from bed and sitting in squatting position (*malasana*) helps with elimination by triggering the gastro-colic reflex (stretching of stomach which causes contraction of colon). As soon as possible, one should empty colon and bladder. The gut is connected to the mind (thus the term "gut feeling"), bringing awareness to the colon for early morning elimination. Proper elimination is a sign of health that ensures body's proper functioning. If one waits until later in the morning or during the day, they are slowly poisoning themself due to the accumulation of toxins and wastes and creating an opportunity for cardiovascular disease to arise.

30.2.3 Cleansing of the Senses

Cleansing the senses allows one to experience the sights, sounds, tastes, smells, and touch of daily living to the fullest potential. As part of a daily *dinacharya*, one should wash the eyes and face and clear the mouth and nasal passages of toxins. The following is a road map for these activities.

30.2.4 Eyes and Face

Wash the eyes and face with water.

30.2.5 Mouth

Brush the teeth and scrape the tongue with a tongue scraper to remove the coating on the tongue. This purifies the mouth and allows the taste buds to function optimally. *Ayurveda* considers the coating of the tongue as an indicator of *ama*, or toxins in the colon from undigested food, and the functional status of the gut. *Ayurveda* prescribes the cleansing of the tongue by scraping it with a tongue scraper every morning. Scraping the tongue in the morning clears it of these toxins, helping decrease the likelihood of cardiovascular disease (Fig. 30.2).

Taste is also an important concept in *Ayurveda*. In fact, *Ayurvedic* philosophy associates the beginning of digestive function with the tastes of foods. The body recognizes initiation of the digestive process by tasting the six tastes in food. When excess residue is cleared from the taste buds, the tongue is better able to recognize these tastes, which assists in proper digestion and helps the body feel satisfied with smaller portions of food. By increasing the efficiency of digestion and contributing to the experience of the six tastes, the body feels satisfied with less food,

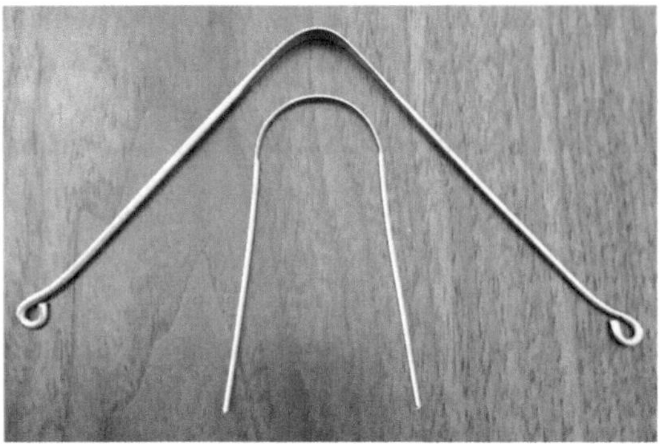

Fig. 30.2 Tongue scraper

translating into fewer calories consumed. In this manner, the body is better prepared to discover and maintain its correct function and weight.

Clearing away the *ama* that accumulates on the tongue by scraping it makes for nicer-smelling breath; just like with brushing teeth, it decreases the chances of bacteria causing gum infection, presumed cause of coronary artery disease the inflammation. It is as important as flossing. The color of the tongue scraping will give hints about what foods one may need to change in diet and what one needs to change in daily routine to balance the psycho-physiological body types (*doshas*) and prevent cardiovascular problems: whitish tongue coating (*kapha*), yellowish (*pitta*), or brownish (*vata*). The tongue scrapers are U-shaped and are generally made from metal or plastic and tend to last a long time.

30.2.6 Nasal Passages

It is important to clear away mucus, bacteria, and allergens gathered in the nasal passages to help reduce the likelihood of upper-respiratory infection another cause of cardiovascular disease. In the practice of *Ayurveda*, this cleansing process, which is gaining popularity in Western medicine due to its effectiveness, is called *jal neti*, which means "water cleansing of the nose." Better known in the West as nasal irrigation, this process uses a saline solution to thin and move mucus out of the nasal passages, increasing the cleansing efficiency of cilia, and is ideally followed by a short *kapalbhati pranayama* practice. Cleansing the nasal passages also improves the sense of smell and taste. A small plastic or ceramic pot resembling a small teapot with a thin, tapered spout called a *neti* pot is used for this practice and may be purchased at most drugstores. Irrigating the nasal passages clears them without dryness or rebound congestion, which occurs with the use of decongestants (Fig. 30.3).

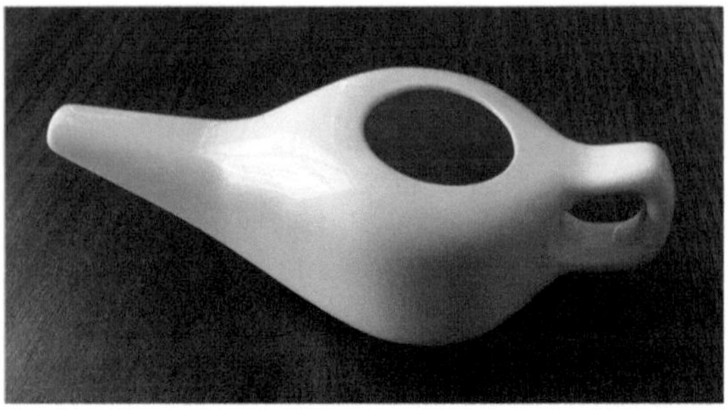

Fig. 30.3 *Neti* pot

Initially, when practicing *jal neti*, there will be a lot of irritation, a strange sensation inside the nose and mouth, flushing of the face, perhaps even a cough, and watering of the eyes, but stay with it as a daily practice. The body will become accustomed to the sensation and irritation will cease. Over time, the sensation will diminish. After a few times, especially when the relaxation response and parasympathetic activation starts, it becomes easier and will actually feel good. The body-mind will adapt slowly, and no mental or physical irritation will cause any detriment to the body-mind. The blood pressure or heart rate will not go up when facing an irritating boss or a teenager's attitude and is useful as prevention and management of cardiovascular disease (Fig. 30.4).

30.3 Yoga and Exercise

Exercise is important for keeping the mind and body in their best possible health. There are three prongs to optimal physical health: cardiovascular, strength, and flexibility. One must have an exercise routine that includes activities that accomplish all three of these elements like swim-

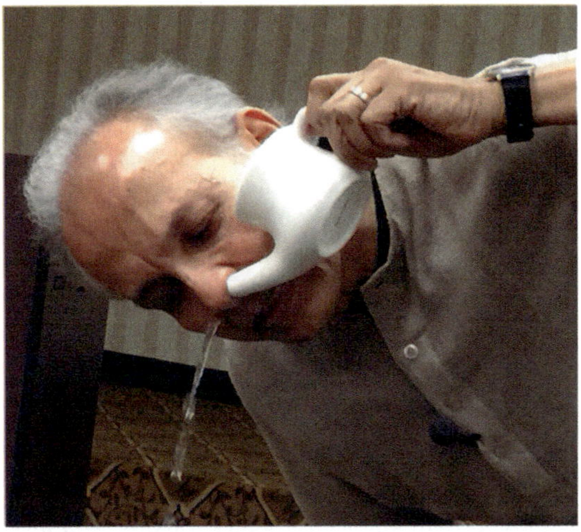

Fig. 30.4 *Jal neti*

ming, walking, or running for cardiovascular health, weight training to maintain muscle strength and encourage bone density, and yoga for relaxation and flexibility.

30.3.1 Yoga

Yoga is a practice with effortless breathing and awareness to achieve relaxation. The morning is the best time to stretch the body, and a slow yoga practice is the best exercise for encouraging suppleness in the joints and muscles. The comparatively long hold time of a yoga pose allows muscles time to truly relax after initial contraction into a stretch, while tandem breathing provides those engaged muscles with ample oxygenation, encouraging optimal relaxation and a higher level of function. The breathing associated with yoga asana practice creates a mind-body connection that is also unique to yoga, triggering a relaxation response that reduces stress. Yoga theory prescribes that the mind and the body are one connected unit. As the body does, so does the mind, and vice versa. So, if one is expanding, nurturing, stretching, strengthening, balancing, and relaxing with the body, one is also doing all of those things with the mind.

The breathing practice called *pranayama* helps to improve lung function. In yoga philosophy, lung and heart are the same organ and improving lung function improves heart function. Lungs are like a balloon with 6-l capacity, the vital capacity of four and half liter and one and half liter residual volume. We breathe only half a liter per breath as tidal volume. So, the lung has 80% reserve, able to do exhalation longer than inhalation effortlessly clears the body of toxins and brings fresh oxygen which is good for the heart. Exhalation is parasympathetic and inhalation is sympathetic. Able to practice longer exhalation increases parasympathetic tone. *Pranayama* also balances the three bodies (*sarira*) and the five sheaths (*koshas*) around us, activates the seven *chakras* of the subtle body, and still the mind for meditation. Meditation quiets the mind, increasing mental, emotional, and spiritual health while physically calming the body through the trigger of the parasympathetic response, the therapy for cardiovascular diseases. For optimal cardiac health, daily one hour practice of yoga is recommended, 25 min of *asana*, 25 min of *pranayama*, and 10 min of meditation.

30.3.2 Exercise

Vyayama is the Sanskrit word for physical exercise. One should augment daily yoga *asana–pranayama*–meditation practice with conventional exercise. This can be walking, swimming, jogging, or other light exercises. This early morning exercise removes stagnation in the body and mind, strengthens the digestive fire, reduces fat, and gives an overall feeling of lightness and joy as it fills body with good, fresh, and pure *prana*. The exercise should be moderate rather than strenuous. In fact, exercising at one-half of capacity with effortless breathing is recommended. Strength training and cardiovascular aerobic exercise are best performed in the afternoon every other day.

30.4 Cleansing the Body

30.4.1 Massage

Ayurveda recommends a daily oil massage called *abhyanga*. Typically, a self-massage is one of the main ways that *Ayurveda* keeps us strong and prevents us from aging. It is a short massage performed with oil to match *dosha* (psychophysiological body type): sesame oil for *vata*, liquid coconut oil for *pitta*, and mustard oil for *kapha* mixed with lukewarm water. A gentle 5-min massage of the scalp, forehead, temples, hands, and feet before showering or bathing is sufficient. At the end of the massage, put a drop of oil in each ear canal, in each nostril, and in the umbilicus.

30.4.2 Bath/Shower

After yoga, exercise, and *abhyanga*, one should bathe or shower to remove any excess oil and dirt from the skin. Warm water should be used for the body, while tepid water for the head and neck is highly recommended. Hot water on the head increases *pitta* and also affects vision, which is a function of *pitta*. Put on clean clothing after the bath or shower.

30.4.3 Ears

If you do not do *abhyanga* before bathing, make sure to put a drop of oil in each ear after bathing (*karna darpan*). This prevents hearing loss and keeps the ears free of wax.

30.4.4 Prayer and Meditation

Prayer and meditation are best practiced after cleansing the body and before breakfast. Praying and worshipping God by offering flowers and food is done to purify one's mind and surrender ego and the results of all actions to God. Meditate for a few minutes to an hour to put your attention toward awareness. This is the most important aspect of *dinacharya*. Simply being quiet and sitting in peace improves cardiovascular function.

30.4.5 Breakfast

This should be warm, nourishing, and wholesome. A light breakfast is best since this is *kapha* time and digestive fire is low. A late breakfast around nine or ten, close to *pitta* time, maybe more substantial since there is more digestive fire available at that time of day. A typical breakfast for cardiovascular health would consist of complex carbohydrates like oatmeal mixed with yogurt, brown sugar or jaggery, raisins, walnuts, and dates. Sip warm water or light tea with breakfast and drink a glass of water at room temperature one hour after breakfast.

30.4.6 Work/Study

Do what one does for occupation from now until noon.

30.5 Afternoon

30.5.1 Midday Meal

In *Ayurveda*, lunch is the main meal of the day because *pitta* time, which occurs between 10 and 2, is the best time to digest food. As yogis say, it is a time of high levels of *agni* (*tikshna agni*). Lunch is ideally consumed 3–4 hours after breakfast for optimal digestion because it is believed that eating food before the previous meal is digested produces *ama*, the toxin which is the main cause of endothelial dysfunction and formation of plaque in the arteries. The foods eaten at lunch should be *dosha*-specific, or *tridoshic*, and consist of complex carbohydrates, lean protein, and unsaturated fat. All six tastes (astringent, bitter, pungent, salty, sour, and sweet) and seven colors (colors of the rainbow) of fruits and vegetables should be included. Try to eat lighter foods before heavy foods. Refined carbohydrates like white sugar, white flour, and white rice should be omitted (three white poisons: white salt, sugar, and flour). Eating refined carbohydrates causes a sugar spike and the release of insulin. Insulin lowers blood sugar, while remaining or extra insulin converts carbohydrates to omental fat, which is fat stored inside the abdomen, causing truncal or abdominal obesity. The omental fat secretes proinflammatory molecules causing inflammation which manifests as metabolic syndrome (truncal obesity, diabetes, hypertension, atherosclerotic heart disease, dyslipidemia).

Fruit juice interferes with the absorption of trace elements and metabolism of drugs and elements, so it is ideal to eat fruits separate from other foods. If fresh fruit is included in the main meal, eat the fruit first. After the meal, it is good to take a little walk, a couple hundred steps only, to help the food digest. Drink water one hour after the meal so that water intake avoids the dilution of digestive enzymes.

30.5.2 Work/Study

Do what one does for occupation from now until supper.

30.5.3 Siesta

A short midday nap increases *kapha*, which is helpful for people younger than 15 years of age because they need *kapha* to grow. Midday naps are also good for people over 50 years of age because they need *kapha* to balance the *vata* time of life. Short naps are also beneficial for cardiovascular health. Anything more than a short nap should be avoided because sleeping in the day is prohibited in *Ayurveda*, due to the fear of accumulation of vitiated *kapha*.

30.5.4 Exercise and Snacking

The afternoon is an excellent time for more strenuous exercise like strength training and cardiovascular aerobic exercise. It is also a good time for a snack with fresh, seasonal, local, organic and multicolored fruit, waiting at least 30 min before eating anything else.

30.6 Evening

Sundown is a special time of balance between day and night. At this time, it is easier for the mind to stop long enough so that one can see themself introspectively. This is the time for evening prayers and meditations in many cultures around the world. It is nice to take some time to meditate or read something inspirational as the sun is setting.

30.6.1 Dinner

The evening meal should be taken around 6 or 7 or within 2 hours of sunset and 2 or 3 hours before bedtime, which gives the body ample time for food to leave the stomach. It should be lighter, about half the size of lunch. Sleeping just after dinner with a heavy stomach may inhibit sound sleep, insomnia and sleep apnea are the root cause of metabolic syndrome. Food is also not digested properly during sleep. If possible, take a 10- or 15-min walk following dinner to aid digestion. As the saying goes: after lunch, rest a while, after dinner, walk a mile. From dinner to bedtime, just take it easy. Spend time with family, interact with friends, read, and generally relax.

30.6.2 Bedtime

Sometimes it might be good to practice *jal neti* before going to bed, to help relieve nasal congestion and to sleep better with sleep apnea. Massaging the inside of both nostrils with the little finger dipped in *ghee* (clarified butter) keeps the nostril open from dried-up mucus, prevents mouth breathing, and corrects snoring or sleep apnea. Drinking a glass of water at room temperature or warm milk with honey, nutmeg, and turmeric before going to bed helps induce sleep and assists the body with the overnight cleansing process. Ideally, bedtime is between 9 and 10 o'clock.

During *pitta* time (10:00 p.m. to 2:00 a.m.), the body is like a self-cleaning oven. It is assimilating nutrients and eliminates toxins, so overnight fasting is necessary for the body to do its proper cleansing. The human body has profound internal manufacturing power to convert food into all the tissues of the body. Cells from every type of body tissue are constantly replaced by apoptosis (programmed cell death). This internal power can be tapped into with *dinacharya* for proper healing of the body when it is not working properly.

One should try to keep a routine as close to the recommended *dinacharya* as possible. The body might resist the change for the first few days, but persistence will be rewarded with the prevention and management of cardiovascular diseases.

30.7 Ritucharya

Ritucharya (*ritu*–season, *charya*–routine) is an *Ayurvedic* philosophy meaning the seasonal routine also affects our cardiac health as the body is a miniature reflection of nature. With the change in season, the change is very evident in the environment, like flowering in spring, leaf shedding in autumn, hibernation of many animals in winter. As human being is also part of the same ecology, the body is greatly influenced by the external environment. Cardiac health is also achieved when the body (microcosm or *pinda*) remains in balance with the universe (macrocosm or *brahmando*). In contrast to the four seasons of the west, *Ayurveda* divides a year into six seasons (*ritus*) and each *ritu* is 2 months long. The six seasons also have same attributes of psychophysiological energy body types called *doshas*. Summer and rainy seasons are *pitta dosha*, a fire attribute with hot metabolic energy, autumn and fall are *vata dosha*, air attribute with mobile catabolic energy, winter and spring are *kapha dosha*, water attribute with grounding anabolic energy. *Ayurveda*, which is primarily a preventive medicine, suggests changing diet and lifestyle patterns to suit the distinct attributes of the seasons based on the digestive fire (*jathar agni*) of the body. During summer and rainy seasons, when it is hot outside, the digestive fire is low, a person will eat light, cooling food. In fall and winter, when the weather is cold, the digestive fire is strong and keeps the body warm. Heavy, warm foods may be consumed. In autumn and spring, digestive fire is at medium strength, therefore the diet also is moderate in heaviness. Cardiovascular diseases are primarily due to imbalance of *pitta and vata doshas*. A person with cardiovascular disease will balance *pitta* and *vata dosha* tied to the seasons primarily with diet and lifestyle.

30.8 Yoga Protocol for Cardiac Health

For prevention and management of cardiovascular disease 1 hour of yoga practice daily is recommended, 25 min of *asanas*, 25 min of *pranayama*, and 10 min of meditation. *Asanas* from the list below and change daily with fixed *pranayama* and meditation practice from the list.

***Asanas* 25 min daily for cardiac health, various relaxing *asanas* (*sthiram sukhom asanam*, stillness happy poses) alternating with standing, seated, supine, and prone *asanas*.**

Beginning of Daily Practice: Activating Relaxation Response

- *Sukhasana* (easy pose), *Sidhasana* (perfect pose), *Ardha Padmasana* (half lotus pose), or *Padmasana* (lotus pose)
- *Jnana* or *Dhyana Mudra* (meditation gesture)
- Relaxation of the eyes (palming of the hands and cupping of the eyes)
- *Adhi Mudra* or *Bala Mushti Mudra* (yogic fist or infant's fist *mudra*)
- *Manibandha Naman* (wrist bending with breathing)
- *Paschim Namaskarasana* (reverse prayer pose)
- *Skanda Chalanasana* (moving shoulder)
- *Brahma Mudra* (neck rotations)

- *Yoga Mudra* (lotus pose with forward bend)
- *Dandasana* (staff pose)
- *Pada Mushtikasana* (make fist with toes)
- *Pada Chalanasana* (feet rotation)
- *Kulha Chalanasana* or *Shroni Chakra* (hip rotation)
- *Baddhakonasana* (feet together, knees on side) with *Titliasana* (butterfly pose)
- *Malasana* (sit in a squat, sit/rise test)

Standing Poses

- *Tadasana* (mountain pose)
- *Utthita Tadasana* (upward mountain pose)
- *Triyaka Tadasana* (oblique mountain pose)
- *Kati Chakrasana* (waist-rotating pose)
- *Chandra Namaskar* (moon salutation)
- Modified *Tadasana* (stand on one foot with the eyes closed)
- *Dhandayaman Paschim Baddha Hastasana* (back bound hand)
- *Vrksasana* (tree pose, standing on one foot)
- *Natarajasana* (dancer pose)
- *Virabhadrasana* I, II, and III (Warrior pose I, II, and III)
- *Trikonasana* (triangle pose)

Seated Poses

- *Paschimuthtanasana* (seated forward bend pose)
- *Vajrasana* (thunderbolt pose)
- *Mandukasana* (frog pose)
- *Shashankasana* (moon pose)
- *Vakrasana* (spinal twisted pose)
- *Ardha Matsyendrasana* (half spinal twist pose)
- *Gomukhasana* (cow face pose)

Supine Poses

- *Jasthiasana* (stick pose)
- *Pavan Muktasana* (wind-releasing pose)
- *Markatasana* (spinal twist pose)
- *Setu Bandhasana* (bridge pose)
- *Utthita Padasana* (feet-raising pose)
- *Naukasana* (boat pose)
- *Padvrittasana* (feet-rotating pose)
- *Dwichakrikasana* (cycling pose)

Prone Poses

- *Makarasana* (crocodile pose)
- *Bhujangasana* (cobra pose)
- *Shalabhasana* (locust pose)
- *Dhanurasana* (bow pose)

Inversions/Finishing Asanas

- *Yoga Mudra* (lotus pose with forward bend)
- *Savasana* (corpse pose)
- *Sarvangasana* (shoulder stand)
- *Yoga Nidra*

Advanced Asanas

- *Halasana* (plough pose)
- *Sirsasana* (headstand)
- *Simhasana* (lion pose)
- *Hasyasana* (laughing)

Pranayama for 25 min Daily for Cardiac Health

- *Bhastrika* (bellows)
- *Kapalbhati* (forehead shining)
- *Anulom-Vilom* (alternate-nostril breathing)
- *Chandra Bhedana* Pranayama (pranayama to generate cold)
- *Bhramari* (bumble bee)
- *Ujjayi* (victorious breath)
- *Udgeeth* or *Om*
- *Sheetali*, *Sheetkari*, and *Shadanta* (cooling)
- *Murcha* (fainting) Pranayama
- *Karna* (ear) *Rogantak* (treat) Pranayama

Meditation for 10 min Daily for Cardiac Health

- Silent meditation
- Breath-centered meditation
- *Chakra*-awakening meditation

Bandhas, Mudras, and Kriyas for Cardiac Health
Bandhas

- *Mula bandha* (root lock)
- *Uddiyana bandha* (abdominal lock)
- *Jalandhar bandha* (chin lock)
- *Maha bandha* (great lock)

Mudras

- *Jnana/Dhyana/Chin Mudra* (Meditation Gesture)
- *Shakti Mudra* (*Mudra* of Strength)
- *Apana Mudra* (*Mudra* of Digestion)
- *Apana Vayu Mudra* (*Mudra* of the Heart)
- *Vyana Mudra* (*Mudra* of Circulation)
- *Udan Mudra* (*Mudra* of Upward Movement)

Kriyas

- *Tratak*
- *Neti*
- *Kapalbhati*

Cardiac health is achieved by increasing parasympathetic tone through activation of the branches of the Vagus nerve with various yoga practices

- Activate auricular branch of vagus nerve by massaging tragus, auricle, and external auditory canal of ear
- Palming and cupping for the eyes
- Release of Nitric Oxide (NO) a potent vasodilator and endothelial relaxation by producing cyclic GMP and Acetylcholine mediator of parasympathetic tone—Breathing through the nose, *Bhramri Pranayama* (bumble bee breathing) and *Udgeet pranayama* (om chanting), the mucous membrane of sinuses secretes NO
- Activate pharyngeal branch of vagus nerve by Valsalva maneuver, forced exhalation with closed nose and mouth and bear down by constricting pharyngeal and laryngeal sphincter same as *Karna Rogantak Pranayama*
- Activate cricothyroid muscle supplied by the superior laryngeal nerve and intrinsic muscles of the larynx supplied by inferior laryngeal branch of recurrent laryngeal nerve branch of vagus nerve with *Ujjayi pranayama* (victorious breathing)
- Activate Carotid Sinus, site of baroreceptor to reduce heart rate and blood pressure by chin lock (*Jalandhar Bandha*) and neck massage
- Hering-Breuer reflex, prevent over inflation of lung by activating pulmonary stretch receptor supplied by vagus nerve to start exhalation by breath holding in inhalation (*Abhyantara Kumbhaka*)

  Combining *Jalandhar Bandha* and *Abhyantara Kumbhaka* is called *Murcha pranayama* (unconscious)
- Three-part breath, *Dirgha* (long) *Swash* (breath)
- Activate anterior and posterior vagus nerve at the gastroesophageal junction by slow *Kapalbhati Pranayama*
- *Chandra Bhedi pranayama*, breathing through the left nostril is parasympathetic
- Abdominal lock (*Uddiyana Bandha*), root lock (*Mula Bandh*), and great lock (*Maha Bandh*) activates vagus nerve
- *Jal-Neti, Vaman Dhauti*

Further Reading

1. Ornish D. Dr. Dean Ornish's program for reversing heart disease. New York: Ballantine Books.
2. Ramdev S. Yoga for heart disease. Haridwar: Patanjali Yogpeeth.
3. Manchanda SC, Narang R, Reddy KS, Sachdeva U, Prabhakaran D, Dharmanand S, Rajani M, Bijiani R. Retardation of coronary atherosclerosis with yoga lifestyle intervention. J Assoc Physicians India. 2000;48(7):687–94.
4. Rao MV, Harti S, Ghildiyal S, Rai S. AYUSHSHARYA 2018—A National Conference on Dinacharya and Ritucharya for public health promotion. J Ayurveda Integr Med. 2019;10(3):230–1.
5. Thakkar J, Chaudhari S, Sarkar PK. Ritucharya: answer to the lifestyle disorders. Ayu. 2011;32(4):466–71.
6. Bhavanani AB, Madanmohan SZ. Immediate effect of chandra nadi pranayama (left unilateral forced nostril

breathing) on cardiovascular parameters in hypertensive patients. Int J Yoga. 2011;21:4–7.
7. Gould KL, Ornish D, Scherwitz L, Brown S, Edens RP, Hess MJ, Mullani N, Bolomey L, Dobbs F, Armstrong WT, et al. Changes in myocardial perfusion abnormalities by positron emission tomography after long-term, intense risk factor modification. J Am Med Assoc. 1995;274:894–901.
8. Benson H. The relaxation response. New York: Harper Collins Publishers.
9. Sarkar D. Yoga as a therapeutic tool. J Sci Healing Outcome. 2015;7(27):5–9.
10. Swami Vivekananda Yoga Anusandhana Samsthana (S-VYASA), Bengaluru, India: Yoga Therapy for Common Ailments.
11. McCall T. Yoga as medicine. New York: Bantam Dell Publishers.
12. Joseph CN, Porta C, Casucci G, Casiraghi N, Maffeis M, Rossi M, Bernardi L. Slow breathing improves arterial baroreflex sensitivity and decreases blood pressure in essential hypertension. Hypertension. 2005;46:714–8.
13. Sharma H, Chandola HM, Singh G, Basisht G. Utilization of Ayurveda in health care: an approach for prevention, health promotion and treatment of disease. Part 1—Ayurveda, the science of life. J Altern Complement Med. 2007;13(9):1011–20. https://doi.org/10.1089/acm.2007.7017-A.
14. Sarlar D. Yoga therapy, Ayurveda, and Western medicine: a healthy convergence. Nataraj Books; 2018. http://www.natarajbooks.com/
15. Levine GN, Lange RA, Bairey-Merz CN, Davidson RJ, Jamerson K, Mehta PK, Michos ED, Norris K, Ray IB, Saban KL, Shah T, Stein R, Smith SC, The American Heart Association Council on Clinical Cardiology, Council on Cardiovascular and Stroke Nursing, and Council on Hypertension. Meditation and cardiovascular risk reduction: a scientific statement from the American Heart Association. J Am Heart Assoc. 2017; https://doi.org/10.1161/JAHA.117.002218.
16. Manchanda SC, et al. Yoga—a promising technique to control cardiovascular disease. Indian Heart J. 2014;66(5):487–9.
17. Manchanda SC, et al. Yoga and meditation in cardiovascular disease. Clin Res Cardiol. 2014;103(9):675–80.
18. Manchanda SC, et al. Reversal of early atherosclerosis in metabolic syndrome by yoga—a randomized controlled trial. J Yoga Phys Ther. 2013;3(1):132.

Yogic Diet and its Anti-inflammatory Effect in Relation to CVD

31

Kanwal Preet Kochhar, Sunil, Tamoghna Ghosh, and Jyoti Arora

31.1 Introduction

In response to illness, injury, lipid peroxidation, and infection, our body generates an immune response, a part of which occurs as inflammation in the vasculature [1]. In contrast to a belief that atherosclerosis represents a consequence of lipid accumulation as a degenerative and aging process, various studies have proven the critical role of inflammation in CVD and that of inflammatory cascade in atherosclerotic process [2]. Chronic inflammation is characterized by invasion of inflammatory macrophages in tissues that induces the expression of various growth factors as well as inflammatory cytokines which, in turn, are also related to the pathophysiology of various lifestyle-related diseases including diabetes, cardiovascular disease (CVD), obesity, chronic obstructive pulmonary disease (COPD), and diabetes [1, 2].

CVD is one of the leading causes of death all across the globe. Types of cardiovascular disease include peripheral arterial disease, coronary heart disease, deep vein thrombosis, cerebrovascular disease, pulmonary embolism, rheumatic heart disease, and congenital heart disease [3]. A quarter of all mortality in India is attributable to CVD. A study by "The Global Burden of Disease" has estimated that the age-standardized CVD death rate in India is 272 per 100,000 population which is higher than the global average of 235 per 100,000 population. Predominant causes of CVD deaths are stroke and Ischemic heart disease which are responsible for more than 80% of cardiovascular disease deaths [4, 5].

31.2 Role of Traditional Diet and Lifestyle Practices

Dietary factors have played an important part in both preventive and therapeutic medicine over the ages. Currently, the global interest has been increased to identify culinary herbs and spices that are pharmacologically effective against various degenerative and chronic metabolic illnesses including diabetic, gastrointestinal, cancerous, cardiovascular, dermatological, pulmonary, and autoimmune diseases along with having very less or no side effects for use in preventive medicine [6–8]. Culinary herbs and spices are an important part of human nutrition in all the cultures of the world. There has been extensive research within the last few decades concerning the herbs and spices in potential health benefits, especially in conferring protection against CVD [9, 10].

In the Indian traditional system of medicine, various spices and herbs have been described to

K. P. Kochhar (✉) · Sunil · T. Ghosh
Cognitive Neurophysiology and Nutrition Lab, Department of Physiology, AIIMS, New Delhi, India

J. Arora
All India Institute of Ayurveda, Ministry of Ayush, New Delhi, India

I. Basu-Ray, D. Mehta (eds.), *The Principles and Practice of Yoga in Cardiovascular Medicine*,
https://doi.org/10.1007/978-981-16-6913-2_31

possess medicinal properties, such as being hypoglycemic, hypolipidemic, antithrombotic, antioxidant, anti-inflammatory, anti-atherosclerotic, antibacterial, and antiarthritic [11]. Spices are dried parts of plants such as bud, root, seed, leaf, berry, bark, and stigma of flowers usually originating in the tropics generally used for culinary purpose.

A wide variety of phenolic compounds and salicylates present in spices that are extensively used as food adjuncts have been scientifically proven to possess potent antimutagenic, anti-inflammatory, oxidant, and cancer preventive activities [10]. The action of spices on reproductive functions as well as their potential role on regulations of fertility and/or conception also is an area holding great future promise.

Modern nutrition has undergone an epidemiologic shift and a significant transition in dietary practices and preferences including increased use of beverages, sugar, fast foods, processed food, beverages, and animal source foods which have impacted health adversely. This is where back to basics and increasing use of traditional Indian foods like coarse cereals, indigenous herbs, and plant-based natural food ingredients as well as spices, curd, and fermented food products can help. Knowledge of plant-derived spices and their myriad health benefits are extremely essential; especially for food security in low resource settings as a shift to traditional medicines, slow foods, and indigenous cooking styles will reduce the cost of healthcare and will have a better impact on the environment and epigenetics (Table 31.1, Fig. 31.1).

Table 31.1 Dietary spices, their constituents and usefulness (adapted from Kochhar [10], Gupta [7], Kunnumakkara et al. [12])

Spice	Major constituents	Traditional uses	Potential biological activity
Cinnamon (*Cinnamomum zeylanicum*) 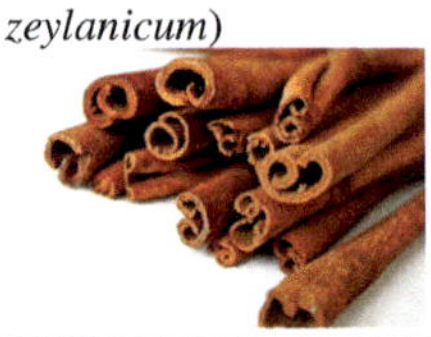	Cinnamaldehyde, eugenol, linalool, cinnamyl acetate, cineole, coumarin, humulene, β-caryophyllene, ethyl cinnamate, τ-cadinol	Its stem bark has been traditionally used in pain, obesity, dental and asthma, oral problems, bad breath, and tuberculosis	– Anti-inflammatory and antioxidant effects – Antibacterial and antifungal activity – Blood glucose control
Turmeric (*Curcuma longa*) 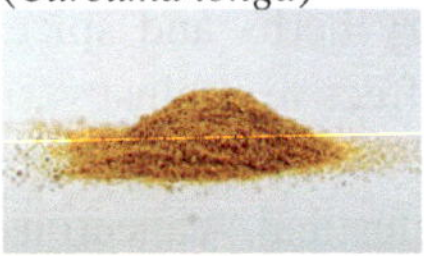	Curcumin (diferuloylmethane), demethoxycurcumin, bisdemethoxycurcumin	The rhizomes of turmeric have been traditionally used in cough, skin diseases, worm infestation, blood impurities, asthma, obesity, diabetes, and deficient lactation	– Antihistamine – Antifungal – Hypocholesterolemic – Antibacterial – Antihepatotoxic – Antiarthritic and anti-inflammatory
Saffron (*Crocus sativus*) 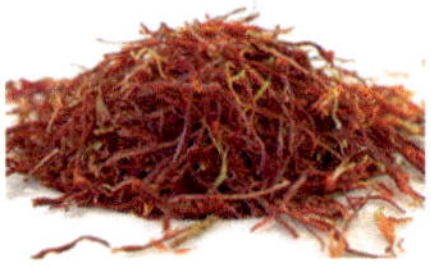	Safranal, crocin, crocetin, and picrocrocin	Its flowers have been traditionally used for vertigo, bleeding disorder, inflammation, headache, skin, and eye diseases	– Anti-convulsant – Anti-dermatogenic – Anti-inflammatory – anti-tumor and anti-nociceptive
Ginger (*Zingiber officinale*) 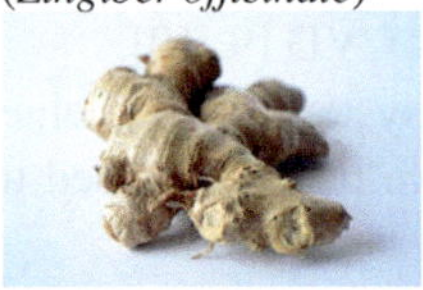	Gingerol, gingerdione, paradol, shogoal, 6-gingerdiol, bisabolene, zingiberene, cineole, citral (geranial and neral), α-farnesene, β-phellandrene, zingerone	Its rhizomes have been traditionally used in anorexia, asthma, colic pain, piles, cough, pyrexia, and rheumatic disease	– Anti-inflammatory – Carminative – Antipyretic – Analgesic – Antitussive and hypotensive

Table 31.1 (continued)

Spice	Major constituents	Traditional uses	Potential biological activity
Garlic/onion (*Allium sativum*)/ (*Allium cepa*) 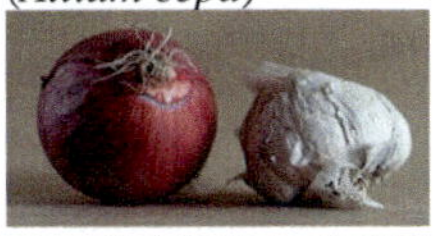	Diallyl sulfides, ajoene, diallyl disulfides, diallyl trisulfide, cycloalliin, allicin, alliin, methiin, S-allyl cysteine, isoalliin, S-allyl mercaptocysteine	Its bulbs are traditionally used in colic pain, rheumatic disease, obesity, worm infestation, anorexia, flatulence, and liver disorders	– Antifertility – Antihyperglycemic – Antihyperlipidemic – Antioxidant – Antiproliferative
Clove (*Syzygium aromatic*) 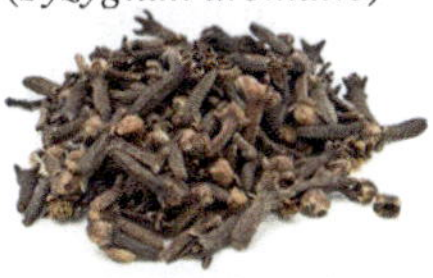	Eugenol, α-humulene, β-caryophyllene, eugenyl acetate	Its flower buds have been traditionally used in dental and oral diseases, cough, throat infections, colic pain, asthma, and hiccoughs	– Stimulant – Carminative – Local anesthetic – Analgesic – Anticarcinogenic – Anticonvulsant and antimicrobial
Black pepper (*Piper nigrum*) 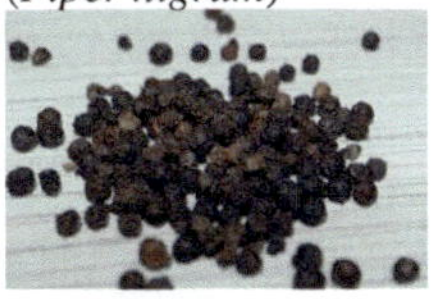	Piperine, β-caryophyllene, myrcene, limonene, δ-3-carene, α-phellandrene, β-pinene, α-pinene, terpinolene	Its fruits have been traditionally used in worm infestation, anorexia, pyrexia, cough, asthma, liver disease, and obesity	– Analgesic – Antimicrobial – Antioxidative – Stimulant and carminative
Coriander (*Coriandrum sativum*) 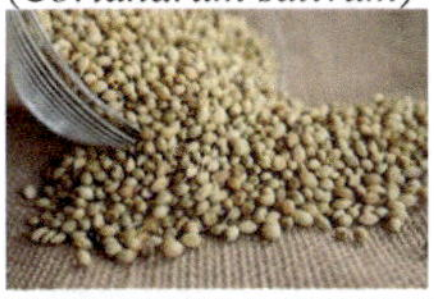	Petroselinic acid, oleic acid, linoleic acid, myristic acid, palmitic acid, vaccenic acid, and stearic acid	Traditionally used in pyrexia, colic pain, burning sensation, flatulence, anorexia, indigestion, thirst, headache, and oral diseases	– Antifertility – Antihyperglycemic – Antihyperlipidemic – Antioxidant – Antiproliferative
Mustard (*Brassica campestris*) 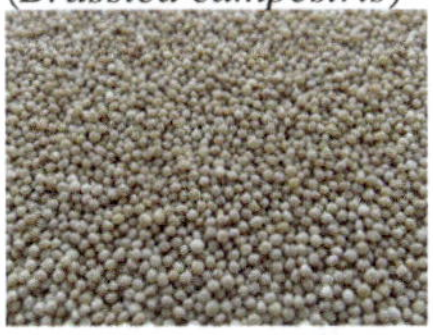	Fixed oils, myrosin, sinalbin, sinigrin, and lecithin	Its seeds have been traditionally used in anorexia, skin disease, obesity, dental disorders, worm infestation, and dry skin	– Chemo preventive – Antioxidant – Antineoplastic

31.3 Beneficial Effects on Atherosclerosis and Lipid Metabolism

Atherosclerosis is a progressive and chronic disease of arteries that derives from epigenetic disorders, lipid deregulation, inflammatory responses, and oxidative stress (OS), and is characterized by the accumulation of lipids and fibrous elements in arteries [8, 13]. It is related to other forms of CVDs, such as hypertension, coronary artery disease, peripheral arterial disease, and ischemic stroke, accounting for the majority of CVDs mortality. Atherosclerosis develops due to hyperlipidemia which induces the increase and deposition of oxidized low-density lipoproteins in the subendothelial area [13].

Staple Indian dietary spices, e.g., Turmeric, Garlic, Cinnamon, and Chili pepper have been reported to reduce the incidence of atherosclerosis through their various constituting active compounds as described below [14–16].

Treatment with cinnamaldehyde, one of the active ingredients of *Cinnamomum cassia* (*cin-*

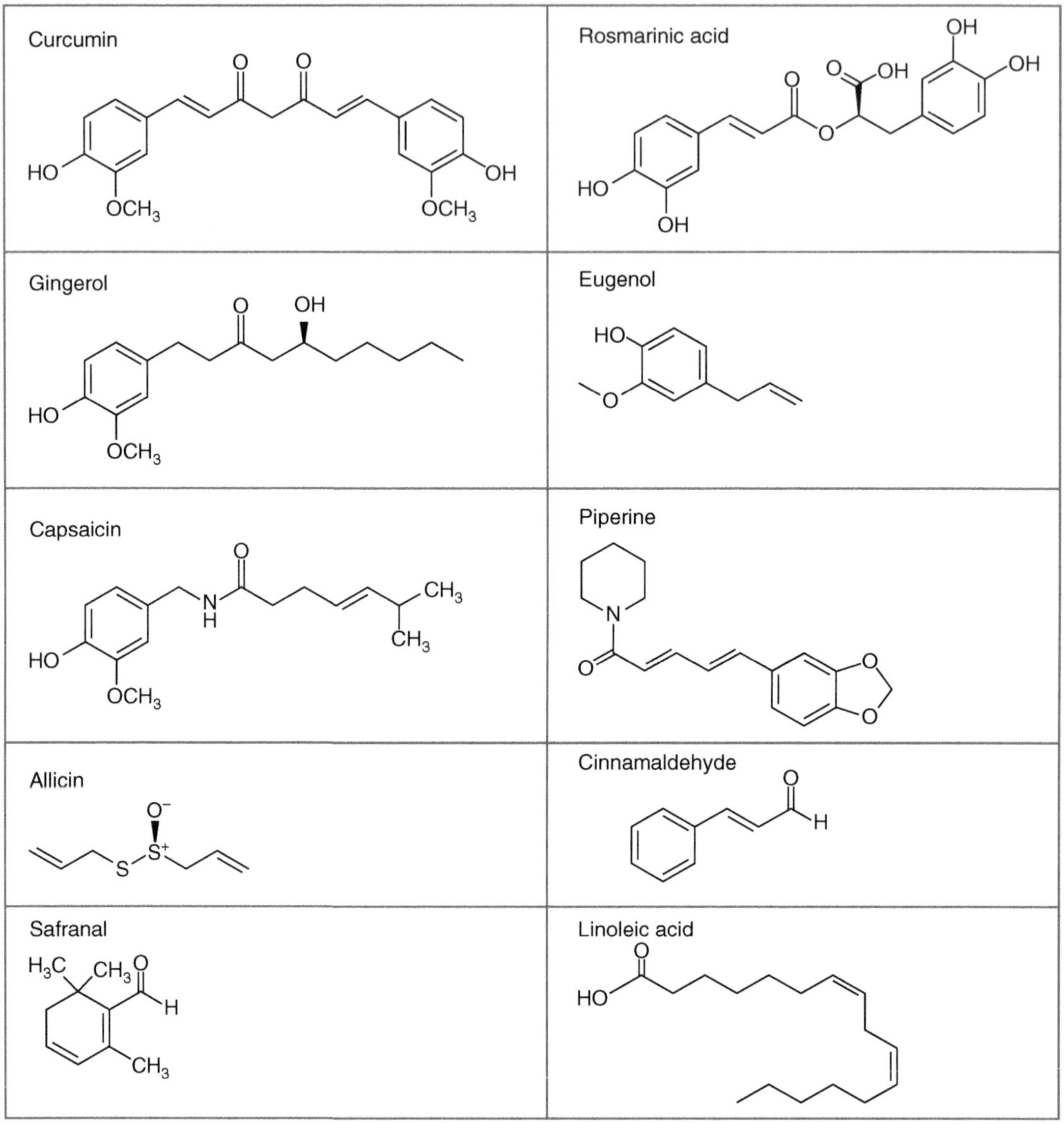

Fig. 31.1 Chemical structural similarities in spices (Adapted from Kochhar [10])

namon), has been shown to significantly decrease inflammatory cytokine (NO, TNF-α, MCP-1, and IL-6) overproduction along with reduction of atherosclerotic plaque area in ApoE−/− mice [14]. Anti-atherosclerotic effect of cinnamaldehyde via the IκB/NF-κB signaling pathway has also been proposed [14]. Various species of cinnamon possess anti-inflammatory properties via different molecular mechanisms including inhibition of NF-κB pathway and by suppression of the expression of inducible nitric oxide (NO) production, cyclooxygenase-2 (COX-2), and nitric oxide synthesis (iNOS), production [17].

Curcumin exhibits hypolipidemic effects, which together with its anti-inflammatory and antioxidant activity, leads to reduced incidence of atherosclerosis [18, 19]. The remarkable antioxidant capacity of curcumin reduces lipid peroxidation and the generation of oxLDL, and consequently, reduces the inflammatory response, ultimately the progression of atherosclerosis [20]. Curcumin treatment (0.3 mg/d/

mouse) significantly attenuated the incidence along with progression of atherosclerosis while another study reported significant changes in gene expression that were associated with leukocyte adhesion and trans-endothelial migration in aortic tissues [21]. These effects of curcumin seemed to be mediated by increased expression of inhibitor of NF-κB (IκB) protein and a decrease in NF-κB binding and transcriptional activity after stimulation with tumor necrosis factor-α (TNF-α). Moreover, it was evidenced that curcumin downregulated the activation of toll-like receptor 4 (TLR4 which in turn, reduced the NF-κB activation and the production of pro-inflammatory mediators, which protected against atherogenesis [22]. In a rat model of coronary atherosclerosis heart disease, curcumin (100 mg/kg/day, for 4 weeks) significantly improved the permeability of coronary artery through inhibition of CD40L, C-reactive protein (CRP), TNF-α, and matrix metalloproteinase 9 (MMP-9) expression [23, 24].

A study by Bharti et al., on the active ingredient of the world's most expensive spice, Saffron, demonstrated how safranal offers protection in a rat model of myocardial ischemia-reperfusion injury by enhancing phosphorylation of eNOS/glycogen synthase kinase-3β (GSK-3β)/protein kinase B (Akt) pathway, attenuation of NF-κB/IKK-β activity, normalization of the antioxidant reserve and upregulation of the anti-apoptotic route by enhancing Bcl2 expression [25].

Finally, the active ingredient in *Chilli pepper*, i.e., capsaicin, significantly decreased CRP levels in adults with low HDL-C, which suggested that capsaicin performed anti-inflammatory effect in humans [26]. Capsaicin modulates the functions of ECs, macrophages, and VSMCs. Kim et al. suggested that capsaicin inhibits NF-κB signalling in lipopolysaccharide (LPS)-stimulated peritoneal macrophages. Additionally, capsaicin upregulates NO/Ca2+/Akt/PI3K/eNOS signalling thereby inhibiting the expression of inflammatory cytokines and adhesion molecules in endothelial cells. Dihydrocapsaicin, a chili pepper extract, has also been proven to reduce the arterial plaque formation through the LXRα/PPARγ pathway in ApoE−/− mice [16].

Various ingredients of the Indian diet such as clove, coriander, mustard seed, garlic, and ginger, have also been reported to possess anti-atherosclerotic effects [6, 8, 27].

31.4 Benefits on Hypertension and Actions on Vascular Smooth Muscles

Hypertension or high blood pressure is defined as having a systolic blood pressure (SBP) of ≥140 mmHg and a diastolic blood pressure (DBP) of ≥90 mmHg [28]. Every 20/10 (SBP/DBP) mmHg increase indicates a higher risk stage of hypertension; stage 1 (140–159/90–99 mmHg), stage 2 (≥160/≥100 mmHg; with the latter stage requiring immediate medical attention [28, 29]. Over the last decade, the use of herbal medicine as a treatment modality for hypertension has significantly increased.

In a study by Vazquez-Prieto et al., the addition of a daily dose of aqueous garlic extracts caused a reduction of VCAM-1 in fructose-fed rats [30]. The constituents of Garlic dampen Ang II-induced vasoconstrictor responses, antagonize endothelin-1-induced vasoconstriction, inhibit VSMCs proliferation in smooth muscles isolated from SHR and downregulate the activation of NF-κB [31–33]. Allicin modulates these effects after the reaction of Alliin with the enzyme Alliinase.

Coriander acts as an anti-inflammatory agent by reducing the activities of iNOS and NF-κB [29, 34].

Saffron and its constituents also possess an inherent ability to inhibit TNF-α expression, inflammatory pathways, and NF-κB [25, 35].

In the powder form, cardamom decreases SBP, DBP as well as mean arterial blood pressure (MAP), in pre-hypertensive subjects where SBP and DBP were dramatically decreased by 19 and 12 mmHg, respectively. The reason for this hypotensive action can be attributed due to its ability to enhance total antioxidant status [36, 37].

Curcuma longa has also been reported to lower blood pressure, thus reducing the risk of hypertension by lowering the expression of COX-

2, which further leads to decreased levels of inflammatory cytokines, MMP-2, MMP-9. The reduction in the levels of cytokines leads to vasodilatation and consequently decreased blood pressure.

31.5 Beneficial Effects on Myocardial Infarction (MI) Through Action on Cardiac Muscle and Vasculature

Myocardial infarction (MI) is an acute condition of necrosis of the myocardium that occurs as a result of imbalance between myocardial demand and coronary blood supply. Myocardial infarction occurs due to coronary artery obstruction, thrombotic occlusion, and coronary vasospasm associated with myocardial ischemia [38, 39]. It is well established that high oxidative stress and inflammation play a key role in the pathogenesis of myocardial infarction [40]. Acute myocardial infarction is associated with sudden chest pain radiating to the left arm and shoulder, shortness of breath, palpitation, sweating, vomiting, and nausea [41, 42].

Gingerol, a phytoconstituent in *Ginger*, shows cardioprotection via stimulating blood flow through relaxing blood vessels [6]. Gingerol inhibits thromboxane formation as well as gingerols and shogaols attribute the potent antiplatelet aggregation through the blockade of COX and Lipo-oxygenase (LOX) pathway [43, 44]. Ginger exhibits potent anti-inflammatory activity by inhibiting endogenous prostaglandins through COX inhibition and by reducing the inflammatory mediated pathway [42].

Black Pepper contains Piperine which acts to protect against oxidative damage by inhibiting free radicals and ROS maintains and enhances the levels and efficacy of important antioxidant compounds. Black pepper is a source of effective antioxidants and contains several powerful. Piperine also attributes potent anti-inflammatory action to inhibit the production of proinflammatory mediators: PGE_2, IL-6, and IL-1β [42].

Cinnamon, a traditional medicine, helps in the improvement of blood circulation responsible for prevention of myocardial infarction. Methoxy cinnamaldehyde (MCA) reduced the expression of High mobility group box 1 (HMGB1), an activator of the inflammatory cascade when released into the extracellular space and VCAM-1 in I/R myocardium along with increase of Haem-oxygenase-1 (HO-1) induction. MCA also significantly inhibited NF-κB luciferase activity in TNF-activated endothelial cells [42].

Curcumin possesses anti-inflammatory effects due to which it prevents atrial arrhythmias which are mostly mediated through inhibition of COX-2, iNOS, and LOX. Curcumin shows potent anti-inflammatory activity through downregulation of NF-κB, consequently decreasing in the expression of IL-6, IL-1, and TNF-α. Curcumin also inhibits the independent Mitogen-Activated Protein Kinase (MAPK) pathways, which plays a crucial role in the activation of inflammatory stimuli [42, 45].

31.6 Beneficial Effects on Microangiopathy and Cardiac Myopathy in Diabetes Mellitus

Diabetic cardiomyopathy is characterized by cardiac structural and functional damage, including myocardial fibrosis, myocyte hypertrophy, and consequent heart failure.

Inflammatory mediators are strongly recognized as diabetes risk factors; elevated inflammatory cytokines may contribute to insulin resistance [46, 47]. In a study, ginger could reduce inflammation through suppression of inflammatory cytokines, enzyme prostaglandin synthase, and nitric oxide. Thomson et al. confirmed the inhibitory action of ginger on prostaglandin by daily administration of ginger to rats; as in their research they reported that ginger significantly reduced serum prostaglandin-E2. In an in vitro study, cardamom has exerted significantly anti-inflammatory properties through reducing NO production [48]. Ahmad et al. showed cardamom to significantly suppress COX-2 expression and inhibit tumor necrosis factor α (TNF-α) production [49]. Saffron has potentially bioactive components such as anthocyanin, flavonoids, alkaloids, saponins, and tannins, which may have contributed to the anti-inflammatory effects seen in mice [50].

In an animal study, cinnamon treatment inhibited the postprandial overproduction of apoB48-containing lipoproteins and inflammation in hamsters and rats [50]. Another study demonstrated that cinnamon may significantly decrease mRNA expression of inflammatory factors, including IL-6, IL-1, and TNF-α.

Soetikno et al. showed that curcumin ameliorated diabetic cardiomyopathy by regulating ERK1/2 pathway, p38, and protein kinase C (PKC) with reduced inflammation and oxidative stress. Consistently, another study found that curcumin supplementation reversed diabetes-induced endothelial dysfunction via inhibiting PKC pathway and superoxide production, curcumin supplementation reversed diabetes-induced endothelial dysfunction [19, 51] (Table 31.2).

31.7 Conclusion and Future Prospects

Herbal medicine is one of the most important aspects of complementary medicines. There are many studies that have asserted the role of several herbs in inflammation remission. We introduce some herbs with their anti-inflammatory effects that have been evaluated in experimental and clinical studies.

Inflammation process has various mechanisms and consequently numerous treatment methods. Plenty of cytokines participate in enzyme activation (such as phospholipase), mediator release, fluid extravasation and vasodilation, cell migration, and finally tissue damage, which generally have been named inflammation. Biochemical outcomes of the experimental studies clearly show the potential role of herbs in activation or inhibition of proinflammatory cytokines. It should be noted that the word "natural anti-inflammatory" refers to natural compounds, exercise, lifestyle, sleeping, and eating habits. There are numerous studies on natural compounds and herbal medicines issues but those outcomes are varied and inconsistent; sometimes, the method of evoking extract has a direct impact on the chemical constituents and it must be considered because the pharmacological effect of each phytomedicine herb is the net result of a diverse combination of primary and secondary metabolites along with their synergistic effects as well as dose dependence, tachyphylaxis, habituation, and physiological individuality.

Thus, complementary and adjunct use of food-based products with modern medicine may

Table 31.2 Mechanisms of anti-inflammatory effects of dietary spices

	Inhibition of								
Herb	TNF-α	COX-2	iNOS	NF-kB	PGE2	NO	LOX	Complement	IFN-γ
Curcuma longa	✓	✓	✓				✓		
Zingiber officinale	✓	✓				✓	✓		
Oenothera biennis	✓	✓				✓			✓
Borago officinalis	✓				✓				
Boswellia serrata	✓				✓	✓	✓	✓	✓
Urtica dioica		✓		✓					
Rosa canina		✓			✓	✓	✓		
Salvia officinalis					✓		✓		
Azadirachta indica		✓					✓		
Commiphora wightii				✓					

Note: Other mechanisms may also exist

provide lasting personalized effective and efficacious integral health benefits.

Acknowledgments The authors express their sincere gratitude to the Departments of Physiology, All India Institute of Medical Sciences, New Delhi, India for their assistance and motivation. The authors are thankful to Dr. Raj Kumar Yadav, Ms. Shweta Sharma, Mr. Sunil, Mr. Aman Tilak, Ms. Riya Madan, and Mr. Kushankur Pandit for their help in drafting the manuscript.

Competing Interests The authors declare that they have no competing interests.

Funding This was an investigator-initiated non-funded study.

References

1. Willerson JT, Ridker PM. Inflammation as a cardiovascular risk factor. Circulation. 2004; https://doi.org/10.1161/01.cir.0000129535.04194.38.
2. Katsiari CG, Bogdanos DP, Sakkas LI. Inflammation and cardiovascular disease. World J Transl Med. 2019;8:1–8.
3. Cardiovascular diseases. https://www.who.int/health-topics/cardiovascular-diseases/#tab=tab_1. Accessed 13 Mar 2020.
4. Prabhakaran D, Jeemon P, Roy A. Cardiovascular diseases in India: current epidemiology and future directions. Circulation. 2016;133:1605–20.
5. Whiteford H, Ferrari A, Degenhardt L. Global burden of disease studies: implications for mental and substance use disorders. Health Aff. 2016;35:1114–20.
6. Vasanthi HR, Parameswari RP. Indian spices for healthy heart - an overview. Curr Cardiol Rev. 2010;6:274–9.
7. Gupta M. Pharmacological properties and traditional therapeutic uses of important Indian spices: a review. Int J Food Prop. 2010;13:1092–116.
8. Tsui PF, Lin CS, Ho LJ, Lai JH. Spices and atherosclerosis. Nutrients. 2018; https://doi.org/10.3390/nu10111724.
9. Kochhar KP. Dietary spices in health and diseases (II). Indian J Physiol Pharmacol. 2008;52(4):327–54.
10. Kochhar KP (1996) An experimental study on some physiological effects of dietary spices. AIIMS.
11. Kochhar KP. Dietary spices in health and diseases: I. Indian J Physiol Pharmacol. 52:106–22.
12. Kunnumakkara AB, Sailo BL, Banik K, Harsha C, Prasad S, Gupta SC, Bharti AC, Aggarwal BB. Chronic diseases, inflammation, and spices: how are they linked? J Transl Med. 2018;16:14.
13. Lusis AJ. Atherosclerosis. Nature. 2000;407:233–41.
14. Li W, Zhi W, Zhao J, Li W, Zang L, Liu F, Niu X. Cinnamaldehyde attenuates atherosclerosis: via targeting the IκB/NF-κB signaling pathway in high fat diet-induced ApoE−/− mice. Food Funct. 2019;10:4001–9.
15. Stabler SN, Tejani AM, Huynh F, Fowkes C. Garlic for the prevention of cardiovascular morbidity and mortality in hypertensive patients. Cochrane Database Syst Rev. 2012; https://doi.org/10.1002/14651858.cd007653.pub2.
16. Kim CS, Kawada T, Kim BS, Han IS, Choe SY, Kurata T, Yu R. Capsaicin exhibits anti-inflammatory property by inhibiting IkB-a degradation in LPS-stimulated peritoneal macrophages. Cell Signal. 2003;15:299–306.
17. Rao PV, Gan SH. Cinnamon: a multifaceted medicinal plant. Evid Based Complement Alternat Med. 2014; https://doi.org/10.1155/2014/642942.
18. Shimizu K, Funamoto M, Sunagawa Y, Shimizu S, Katanasaka Y, Miyazaki Y, Wada H, Hasegawa K, Morimoto T. Anti-inflammatory action of curcumin and its use in the treatment of lifestyle-related diseases. Eur Cardiol Rev. 2019;14:117–22.
19. Li H, Sureda A, Devkota HP, Pittalà V, Barreca D, Silva AS, Tewari D, Xu S, Nabavi SM. Curcumin, the golden spice in treating cardiovascular diseases. Biotechnol Adv. 2020;38:107343.
20. Sahebkar A. Dual effect of curcumin in preventing atherosclerosis: the potential role of pro-oxidant-antioxidant mechanisms. Nat Prod Res. 2015;29:491–2.
21. Coban D, Milenkovic D, Chanet A, Khallou-Laschet J, Sabbe L, Palagani A, Vanden Berghe W, Mazur A, Morand C. Dietary curcumin inhibits atherosclerosis by affecting the expression of genes involved in leukocyte adhesion and transendothelial migration. Mol Nutr Food Res. 2012;56:1270–81.
22. Wang L, Li N, Lin D, Zang Y. Curcumin protects against hepatic ischemia/reperfusion induced injury through inhibiting TLR4/NF-κB pathway. Oncotarget. 2017;8:65414–20.
23. Kang H, Park SH, Yun JM, Nam TG, Kim YE, Kim DO, Kim YJ. Effect of cinnamon water extract on monocyte-to-macrophage differentiation and scavenger receptor activity. BMC Complement Altern Med. 2014; https://doi.org/10.1186/1472-6882-14-90.
24. Li X, Lu Y, Sun Y, Zhang Q. Effect of curcumin on permeability of coronary artery and expression of related proteins in rat coronary atherosclerosis heart disease model. Int J Clin Exp Pathol. 2015;8:7247–53.
25. Bharti S, Golechha M, Kumari S, Siddiqui KM, Arya DS. Akt/GSK-3β/eNOS phosphorylation arbitrates safranal-induced myocardial protection against ischemia-reperfusion injury in rats. Eur J Nutr. 2012;51:719–27.
26. Qin Y, Ran L, Wang J, Yu L, Lang HD, Wang XL, Mi MT, Zhu JD. Capsaicin supplementation improved risk factors of coronary heart disease in individuals

with low HDL-C levels. Nutrients. 2017; https://doi.org/10.3390/nu9091037.
27. Sobenin IA, Andrianova IV, Lakunin KY, Karagodin VP, Bobryshev YV, Orekhov AN. Anti-atherosclerotic effects of garlic preparation in freeze injury model of atherosclerosis in cholesterol-fed rabbits. Phytomedicine. 2016;23:1235–9.
28. Duggan KA. Management of hypertension. Med Today. 2010;11:16–23.
29. Al Disi SS, Anwar MA, Eid AH. Anti-hypertensive herbs and their mechanisms of action: part I. Front Pharmacol. 2016;6:323.
30. Vazquez-Prieto MA, González RE, Renna NF, Galmarini CR, Miatello RM. Aqueous garlic extracts prevent oxidative stress and vascular remodeling in an experimental model of metabolic syndrome. J Agric Food Chem. 2010;58:6630–5.
31. Banerjee SK, Maulik M, Mancahanda SC, Dinda AK, Gupta SK, Maulik SK. Dose-dependent induction of endogenous antioxidants in rat heart by chronic administration of garlic. Life Sci. 2002;70:1509–18.
32. Castro C, Lorenzo AG, González A, Cruzado M. Garlic components inhibit angiotensin II-induced cell-cycle progression and migration: involvement of cell-cycle inhibitor p27Kip1 and mitogen-activated protein kinase. Mol Nutr Food Res. 2010;54:781–7.
33. Pan LL, Liu XH, Gong QH, Yang HB, Zhu YZ. Role of cystathionine γ-Lyase/hydrogen sulfide pathway in cardiovascular disease: a novel therapeutic strategy? Antioxid Redox Signal. 2012;17:106–18.
34. Jungbauer A, Medjakovic S. Anti-inflammatory properties of culinary herbs and spices that ameliorate the effects of metabolic syndrome. Maturitas. 2012;71:227–39.
35. Nam KN, Park Y-M, Jung H-J, et al. Anti-inflammatory effects of crocin and crocetin in rat brain microglial cells. Eur J Pharmacol. 2010;648:110–6.
36. Verma SK, Jain V, Katewa SS. Blood pressure lowering, fibrinolysis enhancing and antioxidant activities of cardamom (Elettaria cardamomum). Indian J Biochem Biophys. 2009;46:503–6.
37. Anwar MA, Al Disi SS, Eid AH. Anti-hypertensive herbs and their mechanisms of action: part II. Front Pharmacol. 2016; https://doi.org/10.3389/fphar.2016.00050.
38. Horimoto M, Takenaka T, Igarashi K, Fujiwara M, Batra S. Coronary spasm as a cause of coronary tllrombosis and myocardial infarction. Jpn Heart J. 1993;34:627–31.
39. Martin JF, Kristensen SD, Mathur A, Grove EL, Choudry FA. The causal role of megakaryocyte-platelet hyperactivity in acute coronary syndromes. Nat Rev Cardiol. 2012;9:658–70.
40. Ueda SI, Yamagishi SI, Matsui T, Jinnouchi Y, Imaizumi T. Administration of pigment epithelium-derived factor inhibits left ventricular remodeling and improves cardiac function in rats with acute myocardial infarction. Am J Pathol. 2011;178:591–8.
41. Upaganlawar A, Gandhi H, Balaraman R. Isoproterenol induced myocardial infarction: protective role of natural products. J Pharmacol Toxicol. 2011;6:1–17.
42. Banewal L, Khanna D, Mehan S. Spices, fruits, nuts and vitamins: preventive interventions for myocardial infarction. Pharmacologia. 2013;4:553–70.
43. Guh J-H, Ko F-N, Jong T-T, Teng C-M. Antiplatelet effect of gingerol isolated from Zingiber officinale. J Pharm Pharmacol. 1995;47:329–32.
44. Bordia A, Verma SK, Srivastava KC. Effect of ginger (Zingiber officinale Rosc.) and fenugreek (Trigonella foenumgraecum L.) on blood lipids, blood sugar and platelet aggregation in patients with coronary artery disease. Prostaglandins Leukot Essent Fatty Acids. 1997;56:379–84.
45. Soni KB, Kuttan R. Effect of oral curcumin administration on serum peroxides and cholesterol levels in human volunteers. Indian J Physiol Pharmacol. 1992;36:273–5.
46. Azimi P, Ghiasvand R, Feizi A, Hariri M, Abbasi B. Effects of cinnamon, cardamom, saffron, and ginger consumption on markers of glycemic control, lipid profile, oxidative stress, and inflammation in type 2 diabetes patients. Rev Diabet Stud. 2014;11:258–66.
47. Qin B, Panickar KS, Anderson RA. Cinnamon: potential role in the prevention of insulin resistance, metabolic syndrome, and type 2 diabetes. J Diabetes Sci Technol. 2010;4:685–93.
48. Majdalawieh AF, Carr RI. In vitro investigation of the potential immunomodulatory and anti-cancer activities of black pepper (Piper nigrum) and cardamom (Elettaria cardamomum). J Med Food. 2010;13:371–81.
49. Ahmad S, Israf DA, Lajis NH, et al. Cardamonin, inhibits pro-inflammatory mediators in activated RAW 264.7 cells and whole blood. Eur J Pharmacol. 2006;538:188–94.
50. Hosseinzadeh H, Younesi HM. Antinociceptive and anti-inflammatory effects of Crocus sativus L. stigma and petal extracts in mice. BMC Pharmacol. 2002;2:7.
51. Rahimi HR, Mohammadpour AH, Dastani M, Jaafari MR, Abnous K, Ghayour Mobarhan M, Kazemi Oskuee R. The effect of nano-curcumin on HbA1c, fasting blood glucose, and lipid profile in diabetic subjects: a randomized clinical trial. Avicenna J Phytomed. 2016;6:567–77.

Principles of Diet for a Yogic Lifestyle

32

Gauri Junnarkar

The practice of yoga is ancient and developed in India more than 5000 years ago. It focuses on the union of mind and body. Ayurveda the sister science of Yoga and developed in India and is also more than 5000 years old. Ayurveda comes from two Sanskrit words "Ayur" meaning life and "Veda" meaning "Knowledge or Science" and hence it is known as the knowledge or science of life. While Yoga focuses on the mind and Ayurveda focuses on the physiological aspects. Yoga and Ayurveda both emphasize the principle of balance which is apparent in their diet and lifestyle recommendations. Diet and Lifestyle play an integral part in reducing risk factors as well as disease prevention when it comes to cardiovascular disease and Diabetes. Both Yoga and Ayurveda as a combined holistic and complementary approach could play a role in disease prevention and risk reduction in cardiovascular disease and Diabetes through diet, lifestyle, and use of spices.

Yoga and Ayurveda texts provide a wealth of knowledge on Dietetics. According to the references found in Gherand Samhita and Hathpradipika, a yoga practitioner needs to consume foods such as rice, barley, ghee, milk, honey, wheat, green gram, horse gram, black gram, leafy greens, and dry ginger which are considered nourishing and less stimulating. The emphasis is on a bland diet or "Satvik Ahara." The Satvik diet is considered balanced, less stimulatory to senses and is believed to increase calmness and energy and mental clarity. The Satvik diet focuses on including fresh foods, fruits, vegetables, honey, milk, nuts, tubers, and curd. The food needs to be easy to digest, soft, unctuous, and consumed in small and moderate amounts. A Yogi is asked to avoid foods that are salty, pungent, sour, mustard and sesame oils, curds, garlic, eggs, and meat that are considered stimulating to the senses and irritate the nervous system [1, 2]. Three types of diets have been described in Yoga and Ayurveda based on their qualities, which are Sattvic Diet, Rajasic Diet, and Tamasic Diet [2].

The Rajasic Diet is believed to trigger the senses. It may create feelings such as agitation, rage and is usually recommended for people meant to lead and warriors. The foods included in this diet are pungent, hot, high in salt and sugar, bitter to taste, dry, and include a lot of fried foods [2]. The Tamasic Diet is heavy. It can make a person lazy, could be sleep inducing and create weightiness. The people doing Yoga state that this diet could slow down spiritual growth, increase angriness, and make a person less sharp. The food included in this diet are onions, deep fried, stale, foods high in salt and sugar, meats, and alcohol. The overconsumption of foods in this diet category may decrease good health and could decrease expectancy of life [2].

G. Junnarkar (✉)
Ayurnutrition, Dallas, TX, USA
e-mail: gauri@ayurnutrition.com

I. Basu-Ray, D. Mehta (eds.), *The Principles and Practice of Yoga in Cardiovascular Medicine*,
https://doi.org/10.1007/978-981-16-6913-2_32

Ayurveda focuses on the mind–body relation and the importance of balance between the various physiological components to ensure health. Ayurveda is one of the oldest sciences to talk about personalized wellness in form of *Prakriti*. According to Ayurveda, every person is born with a Prakriti (constitution) which is dominated by the presence of doshas in various ranges. The three doshas or body physiologies described in Ayurveda are Vata, Pitta, and Kapha. According to Ayurveda, every person is born with a Prakriti (constitution) which is dominated by the presence of doshas in various ranges. The doshas that are most prominent define a person's prakriti. Ayurveda texts such as "Charak Samhita" go in great depth about the typical characteristics of each dosha Prakriti. Ayurveda emphasis that a person's *ahara* (food), *Dincharya* (daily routine), and in fact *rutucharya* (seasonal routine) should be in harmony with a person's Prakriti. Way before the world discovered vitamins, minerals, and their physiological role in the body, the concept of balanced diet was written in Ayurveda. The emphasis is to eat foods belonging to all the six tastes such as sweet, salty, sour, pungent, bitter, and astringent at every meal. This is to ensure that a balanced diet is being consumed. The goal of Ayurveda is "*Swasthasya Swathya rakshanam, aturasya vicar prashmanam cha*." It means protecting the health of a healthy individual and eliminating the imbalances [3–7].

The dietary intake of a person can be an important predictor of one's health. There is a lot of evidence that a diet with higher intake of foods such as whole grain cereals, fruits, vegetables, and lean proteins can reduce the risk of chronic disease states such as cardiovascular disease, cancer, and diabetes. In a study conducted by Agte and Chiplonkar, they categorized foods according to their properties or gunas, i.e., Satvik foods, Rajasic food, and Tamasic foods. They found that the Satvik foods had the highest amount of micronutrient content, followed by Rajasic and Tamasic foods. Also, the fat content was lower in Satvik foods and highest in Tamasic foods. Based on the findings of the study the authors state that Satvik food could have a better choice with regard to increased health benefits. The authors have provided a sample diet plan in their study to increase intake of Satvik foods and decrease the intake of Tamasic and Rajasic foods. It is important to note that the study showed that Satvik foods included more functional foods like red amaranth, tomato, soy milk, and herbal teas [8].

Cross-sectional studies have shown that people who practice yoga had better diet intake than people who were sedentary. The studies show that yoga practitioners had lower intakes of fats and lower BMI. Interventions including better dietary habits, physical activity, and stress management showed a greater improvement in overall health [9, 10]. A study by Ross et al. shows that practice of yoga at home may increase the intake of fresh fruits and vegetables and could be a predictor of a healthy lifestyle [11]. The study on Yoga and Bioenergetics showed that Mexican Hatha Yoga practitioners made changes towards healthy diet choices and started slowly increasing functional foods such as flavonoids, lignans, and fiber foods [2].

The chapter presented by the author talks about how effective dyslipidemia management with non-drug therapy and effective diet and lifestyle intervention can prevent the risk of cardiovascular disease in the person. The chapter talks about how ancient lifestyles could benefit people in having good health [12]. Studies have shown that Yoga can help with better stress management and positive outcomes for reducing risk for cardiovascular disease. Studies show that people who follow a vegan diet or a vegetarian diet could have stable emotions which may include a feeling of wellbeing and less depression and anxiety [13]. The study on yoga-based lifestyle intervention showed that the yoga intervention consisting of asanas, pranayama, stress management, and nutrition showed significant improvement in anxiety in a patient with history of hypertension and coronary artery disease [14]. Another study on yoga-based lifestyle intervention and risk factors for Diabetes and Cardiovascular disease showed that parameters such as fasting blood glucose, total cholesterol levels, LDL, and triglycerides were lower, and HDL was higher on the last day of the course as compared to the first day. Significant results were noted in patients who had hyperglycemia and hypercholesterolemia [15].

Another study was done on cardiovascular risk profile in middle-aged men and women by using yoga practices showed a decrease in blood pressure, blood glucose, cholesterol, and triglycerides and showed increased feeling of wellbeing. This study showed that yoga could help in modifying the risk of cardiovascular disease [15, 16]. The article on the therapeutic role of Yoga in type 2 diabetes states that including yoga and pranayama were found to be helpful in improving food habits. This could be correlated with eating more fruits and vegetables and being mindful. The article also states that eating mindfully could help in diabetes outcomes by improving dietary intake, inducing moderate weight loss and better blood glucose control. Yoga may help with stress management and activation of Parasympathetic system which could further enhance glucose tolerance, lipid metabolism, and make a person more sensitive to insulin. The article further states that yoga practices combined with relaxation techniques were shown to improve glycemic control, manage comorbidities resulting in better clinical results [17].

Another study on Ayurveda and Yoga in Type 2 Diabetes showed favorable results in treatment goals for Type 2 Diabetes with the use of Ayurveda and Yoga intervention [18]. Ayurvedic herbs such as ginger, cinnamon, fenugreek, and turmeric have been studied for their role in the management of type 2 Diabetes. A study on intake of dietary ginger in type 2 Diabetes showed improvement in HbA1c from baseline to follow-up [19]. The article on the review of medicinal plants and their role in type 2 diabetes describes the benefits of Ayurvedic herbs such as cinnamon, fenugreek, and turmeric. The article states that the antidiabetic activity of cinnamon could be due to decrease in insulin resistance, enhancing glycogen formation in the liver thereby showing the blood glucose-lowering effect. Fenugreek's antidiabetic effect could be contributed to the presence of phytochemicals such as diosgenin, galactomannan, and more. Fenugreek has also shown to increase sensitivity to insulin. Curcumin is the phytochemical in turmeric. The glucose-lowering activity of Curcumin can be correlated to improved beta-cell function and controlling insulin resistance [20].

Yoga and Ayurvedic diet principles focus on including more plant-based foods, food high in fiber, and least processed foods. Satvik diet emphasizes the consumption of foods that are less stimulatory. Ayurveda talks about creating a balance with including foods from all the six tastes, foods more suitable according to the prakriti of a person and including spices such as ginger, turmeric, cinnamon, and fenugreek for better digestion. Yoga and Ayurveda with their emphasis on Diet and lifestyle management can play a key role in reducing risk factors for both cardiovascular disease and diabetes. Integrating both these practices could increase the overall wellbeing and reduce disease risk and could be a good resource in disease prevention.

References

1. Desai BP. Place of nutrition in yoga. Anc Sci Life. 1990 Jan;9(3):147–53.
2. Ramos-Jiménez A, Wall-Medrano A, Corona-Hernández RI, Hernández-Torres RP. Yoga, bioenergetics and eating behaviors: a conceptual review. Int J Yoga. 2015;8(2):89–95. https://doi.org/10.4103/0973-6131.158469.
3. Junnarkar G. (15 Mar 2016) Why Ayurveda makes sense? AyurNutrition. https://ayurnutrition.com/2016/03/15/ayurveda-makes-sense/
4. Sastri K, Chaturvedi G. Charak Samhita. 22nd ed. Varanasi: Chaukahmba Bharati Academy; 1996.
5. Govindaraj P, Nizamuddin S, Sharath A, Jyothi V, Rotti H, Raval R, Nayak J, Bhat BK, Prasanna BV, Shintre P, Sule M, Joshi KS, Dedge AP, Bharadwaj R, Gangadharan GG, Nair S, Gopinath PM, Patwardhan B, Kondaiah P, Satyamoorthy K, Valiathan MV, Thangaraj K. Genome-wide analysis correlates Ayurveda Prakriti. Sci Rep. 2015;5:15786. https://doi.org/10.1038/srep15786.
6. Shastri KA. Susruta Samhita. 11th ed. Varanasi: Chaukhamba Sanskrit Sansthan; 1997.
7. Gupta KA, Upadhyaya Y. Ashtangahridayam. 12th ed. Varanasi: Chaukhamba Sanskrit Sansthan; 1997.
8. Agte V, Chiplonkar S. Linkages of concepts of good nutrition in yoga and modern science. Curr Sci. 2007;2007:956–61.
9. Palasuwan A, Margaritis I, Soogarun S, Rousseau AS. Dietary intakes and antioxidant status in mindbody exercising pre- and postmenopausal women. J Nutr Health Aging. 2011;15:577–84.

10. Toobert DJ, Glasgow RE, Strycker LA, Barrera M Jr, Ritzwoller DP, Weidner G. Long-term effects of the Mediterranean lifestyle program: a randomized clinical trial for postmenopausal women with type 2 diabetes. Int J Behav Nutr Phys Act. 2007;4:1.
11. Ross A, Friedmann E, Bevans M, Thomas S. Frequency of yoga practice predicts health: results of a national survey of yoga practitioners. Evid Based Complement Alternat Med. 2012;2012:983258.
12. Sharma R, Moffatt R. Diet and nutrition therapy in dyslipidemia management. In: Dyslipidemia: causes, diagnosis and treatment. Nova Publisher; 2012. p. 1–40.
13. Michalak J, Zhang XC, Jacobi F. Vegetarian diet and mental disorders: results from a representative community survey. Int J Behav Nutr Phys Act. 2012;9:67. https://doi.org/10.1186/1479-5868-9-67.
14. Gupta N, Khera S, Vempati RP, Sharma R, Bijlani RL. Effect of yoga based lifestyle intervention on state and trait anxiety. Indian J Physiol Pharmacol. 2006;50(1):41–7.
15. Bijlani RL, Vempati RP, Yadav RK, Ray RB, Gupta V, Sharma R, Mehta N, Mahapatra SC. A brief but comprehensive lifestyle education program based on yoga reduces risk factors for cardiovascular disease and diabetes mellitus. J Altern Complement Med. 2005;11(2):267–74. https://doi.org/10.1089/acm.2005.11.267.
16. Damodaran A, Malathi A, Patil N, Shah N, Suryavansihi MS. Therapeutic potential of yoga practices in modifying cardiovascular risk profile in middle aged men and women. J Assoc Physicians India. 2002;50(5):633–40.
17. Raveendran AV, Deshpandae A, Joshi SR. Therapeutic role of yoga in type 2 diabetes. Endocrinol Metab (Seoul). 2018;33(3):307–17. https://doi.org/10.3803/EnM.2018.33.3.307.
18. Sharma R, Shahi VK, Khanduri S, Goyal A, Chaudhary S, Rana RK, Singhal R, Srikanth N, Dhiman KS. Effect of Ayurveda intervention, lifestyle modification and *Yoga* in prediabetic and type 2 diabetes under the national programme for prevention and control of cancer, diabetes, cardiovascular diseases and stroke (NPCDCS)-AYUSH integration project. Ayu. 2019;40(1):8–15. https://doi.org/10.4103/ayu.AYU_105_19.
19. Huang FY, Deng T, Meng LX, Ma XL. Dietary ginger as a traditional therapy for blood sugar control in patients with type 2 diabetes mellitus: a systematic review and meta-analysis. Medicine (Baltimore). 2019;98(13):e15054. https://doi.org/10.1097/MD.0000000000015054.
20. Unuofin JO, Lebelo SL. Antioxidant effects and mechanisms of medicinal plants and their bioactive compounds for the prevention and treatment of type 2 diabetes: an updated review. Oxidative Med Cell Longev. 2020;2020:1356893. https://doi.org/10.1155/2020/1356893.

GPSR Compliance

The European Union's (EU) General Product Safety Regulation (GPSR) is a set of rules that requires consumer products to be safe and our obligations to ensure this.

If you have any concerns about our products, you can contact us on ProductSafety@springernature.com

In case Publisher is established outside the EU, the EU authorized representative is:

Springer Nature Customer Service Center GmbH
Europaplatz 3
69115 Heidelberg, Germany

Batch number: 10731383

Printed by Printforce, the Netherlands